Bionanocomposites for Biomedical Applications

This book examines bionanocomposites in the biomedical field from a fundamental level to in-depth applications using an interdisciplinary approach that combines polymer technology, nanotechnology, biomedical science, and pharmaceutical research. Advancements of bionanocomposites in biomedical applications, such as wound dressings, tissue engineering, drug delivery, bioimaging, biosensing, 3D-printing, medical implants, and many more, are comprehensively summarized and supported by a number of case studies.

Features:

- Discusses properties, classifications, and synthesis of bionanocomposites in addition to applications.
- Each chapter focuses on the application of bionanocomposites.
- Reviews cytotoxicity and biocompatibility of bionanocomposites.
- Explores safety aspects of bionanocomposites.
- Covers wound healing, nerve regeneration, biosensors, skin regeneration, drug delivery, and so forth.

This book is aimed at graduate students and researchers in chemical, polymer, tissue, and biomedical engineering.

Bionanocomposites for Biomedical Applications

Fundamental Concepts, Impacts, and Clinical Applications

Edited by

Shakeel Ahmed

CRC Press
Taylor & Francis Group
Boca Raton London New York

CRC Press is an imprint of the
Taylor & Francis Group, an **informa** business

First edition published 2026
by CRC Press
2385 NW Executive Center Drive, Suite 320, Boca Raton FL 33431

and by CRC Press
4 Park Square, Milton Park, Abingdon, Oxon, OX14 4RN

CRC Press is an imprint of Taylor & Francis Group, LLC

ISBN: 978-1-032-55557-7 (hbk)
ISBN: 978-1-041-09577-4 (pbk)
ISBN: 978-1-003-65081-2 (ebk)

DOI: 10.1201/9781003650812

Typeset in Times
by SPi Technologies India Pvt Ltd (Straive)

Contents

Preface

Within the field of biomedical engineering, the primary focus is on developing new materials and technologies in order to push the boundaries of healthcare forward. The convergence of nanotechnology and composite materials has expanded the range of potential applications, providing solutions that were previously considered to be limited to the realm of speculative fiction. *Bionanocomposites for Biomedical Applications* examines the applications of bionanocomposites that have the potential to greatly impact different aspects of medicine.

This book is an extensive manual that consolidates the combined knowledge of researchers, engineers, and practitioners who are leading the way in this rapidly growing sector. This statement highlights the importance of working together and using a variety of disciplines to address the intricate problems in the field of biomedical engineering.

The chapters in this book encompass a wide array of subjects, ranging from the basic concepts of bionanocomposites to their customized design for specific biological purposes such as bone tissue engineering, wound healing, drug delivery, biomarkers, and gene delivery. Readers will explore the applications of bionanocomposites acquiring a deep understanding of the complexities of materials science and engineering. The multifunctionality of bionanocomposites is one of its most fascinating features. These materials provide flexible platforms that can be customized to tackle various healthcare concerns, ranging from targeted drug delivery systems to wound healing scaffolds. This book highlights the potential of bionanocomposites in diagnostics, and treatments emphasizing their ability to bring about significant transformations.

I, as editor, am pleased to bring this collection of research and technical progress to the scientific community, students, and practitioners. This book aims to be a valuable resource, encouraging further exploration and invention in the captivating field of bionanocomposites for biomedical applications.

About the Editor

Shakeel Ahmed (PhD), is Assistant Professor of Chemistry at the Higher Education Department, Government of Jammu and Kashmir, India and Assistant Professor at Postgraduate Department of Chemistry, Government Postgraduate College Rajouri, Jammu and Kashmir, India. He obtained a first degree in general science from Government Postgraduate College Rajouri (University of Jammu) followed by a master's degree and a doctoral degree in chemistry from Jamia Millia Islamia, a central university, in New Delhi, India. He gained post-doctoral experience in biocomposite materials at the Indian Institute of Technology, Delhi. He has published several research publications in the area of green nanomaterials and biopolymers for various applications including biomedical, packaging, and water treatment. He is an active reviewer and member of the editorial board of many reputed journals. He has published more than 40 books in the area of nanomaterials and green materials with publishers of international repute. He is a fellow of The Linnean Society of London and the International Society for Development and Sustainability (ISDS), Japan and the recipient of many awards from different agencies.

Contributors

Aminu Abdullahi
Department of Biotechnology
Modibbo Adama University
Nigeria

RajaSekhar Reddy Alavala
Shobhaben Pratapbhai Patel School of Pharmacy and Technology Management
SVKM's NMIMS
Mumbai, India

Sarfaraz Ahmad
Howard University
USA

Emad Abdulrahman Alsaedi
College of Medicine
Al Rayyan Colleges
Al-Madinah, Saudi Arabia

Farrukh Jawad Alvi
University Institute of Public Health
The University of Lahore
Pakistan

Zainab Anis
School of Food and Agriculture Sciences
University of Management and Technology
Lahore, Pakistan

Iqra Arooj
Department of Microbiology and Molecular Genetics
The Women University
Multan, Pakistan

Atif Amin Baig
School of Pain and Regenerative Medicine
The University of Lahore
Pakistan

Roja Rani Budha
H.K. College of Pharmacy
Mumbai, India

Jeba Sweetly Dharmadhas
Department of Biochemistry and Biotechnology
Avinashilingam Institute for Home Science and Higher Education for Women
Coimbatore, India

Ujwala Desai
Modern College of Pharmacy
Pune, India

Şeyma Duman
Department of Metallurgical and Materials Engineering
Bursa Technical University
Bursa, Türkiye

Basma Ellahi
Department of Social Work and Inter-Professional Education
Faculty of Health, Medicine and Society
University of Chester
UK

Sehrish Fiaz
Department of Microbiology and Molecular Genetics
The Women University
Multan, Pakistan

S. N. Koteswara Rao Gudhanti
Shobhaben Pratapbhai Patel School of Pharmacy and Technology Management
SVKM's NMIMS
Mumbai, India

Pushpalatha Ganesh
Department of Biotechnology
M.S. Swaminathan School of Agriculture
Centurion University of Technology and Management
Odisha, India

Maryum Hamayoun
School of Biochemistry and Biotechnology
University of Punjab
Lahore, Pakistan

Nimra Idrees
School of Pain and Regenerative Medicine
The University of Lahore
Pakistan

Saadia Ijaz
Department of Microbiology and Molecular Genetics
The Women University
Multan, Pakistan

Nida Islam
School of Food and Agriculture Sciences
University of Management and Technology
Lahore, Pakistan

Sangita Kale
Modern College of Pharmacy
Pune, India

Diya Karbhari
Shobhaben Pratapbhai Patel School of Pharmacy and Technology Management
SVKM's NMIMS
Mumbai, India

Selva Kumar T.
Centre for Interfaces and Nanomaterials
Department of Biotechnology
Vel Tech Rangarajan Dr. Sagunthala R&D Institute of Science and Technology
Chennai, India

Sree Harsha Nagaraja
Department of Pharmaceutical Sciences
College of Clinical Pharmacy
King Faisal University
Al-Ahsa, Saudi Arabia

Meysam Naseri
Department of Mining Engineering
Amirkabir University of Technology
Tehran, Iran

Rahele Khosravi Nessiani
Department of Chemical Engineering
Sahand University of Technology
Tabriz, Iran

Momina Maitla
Center of Agriculture Biochemistry and Biotechnology
University of Agriculture
Faisalabad, Pakistan

Tanzeela Mariam
Institute of Molecular Biology and Biotechnology
The University of Lahore
Pakistan

Farwa Munir
Faculty of Medicine
University of Sultan Zainal Abidin
Malaysia

Büşra Mutlu
Department of Metallurgical and Materials Engineering
Bursa Technical University
Bursa, Türkiye

Issac Abraham Sybiya Vasantha Packiavathy
Department of Biotechnology
Karunya Institute of Technology and Sciences
Coimbatore, India

Rajiv Periakaruppan
Department of Biotechnology
PSG College of Arts and Science
Coimbatore, India

B. Rabi Prasad
Department of Biotechnology
School of Engineering and Technology
GIET University
Gunupur, India

Ghanistha Prusty
Department of Biotechnology
School of Engineering and Technology
GIET University
Gunupur, India

Gomathi Renga Raj
Department of Biochemistry
Holy Cross College
Trichy, India

Saeid Sabzehali
Department of Materials Science and Engineering
Isfahan University of Technology
Isfahan, Iran

Hamna Shahid
Department of Microbiology and Molecular Genetics
The Women University
Multan, Pakistan

Muhammad Shahzaib
Surraya Azeem Teaching Hospital
Lahore, Pakistan

Karimunnisa Shaikh
Modern College of Pharmacy
Pune, India

Saniya Sameer Shaikh
Poona College of Pharmacy
Pune, India

Muniza Shehzad
Institute of Molecular Biology and Biotechnology
The University of Lahore
Pakistan

Polaki Suman
Department of Biotechnology
M.S. Swaminathan School of Agriculture
Centurion University of Technology and Management
Odisha, India

Pınar Terzioğlu
Department of Polymer Materials Engineering
Bursa Technical University
Bursa, Türkiye

Khushwant S. Yadav
Shobhaben Pratapbhai Patel School of Pharmacy and Technology Management
SVKM's NMIMS
Mumbai, India

Serap Yalcin
Department of Medical Pharmacology
Kırsehir Ahi Evran University
Kırsehir, Turkey

Mehmethan Yıldırım
Department of Molecular Biology and Genetics
Kırsehir Ahi Evran University
Kırsehir, Turkey

Fatima Tul Zahra
University Institute of Medical Laboratory Technology
The University of Lahore
Pakistan

1 Bionanocomposites for Biomedical Applications: Fabrication and Properties

Rahele Khosravi Nessiani, Saeid Sabzehali and Meysam Naseri

1.1 INTRODUCTION

Green composites or biohybrids are the same old phrases used to explain bionanocomposites. Together, these hybrid substances convey the information of biology, nanotechnology, and materials technology. They are regarded as environmentally friendly substitutes for petroleum-primarily based merchandise, presenting a bunch of benefits together with a large surface area, cost-effectiveness, and advanced mechanical, chemical, and organic properties. Biodegradable substances, which include herbal or biopolymers, are referred to as green composites [1, 2]. The components of bionanocomposites, which consist of inorganic substances, herbal nanomaterials, and the biopolymers themselves, decide their composition (Figure 1.1). This is due to the fact that in the presence of nature, they decompose without problems when left unprotected. Bionanocomposites have the ability to make use of tissue engineering, wound restoration, cancer prognosis, medicinal drug delivery systems, and more. One wonderful use of bionanocomposite materials has been within the controlled release of pharmaceuticals [3, 4].

The first time that nanoparticles (NPs) in nanocarriers were used to improve therapeutic performance in pharmaceuticals was in 1965. This method has shown certain benefits, including increased drug solubility, controlled drug release into the body, focused medication delivery, and continuous drug absorption into the circulation. Liposomes, polymeric NPs, dendrimers, and inorganic NPs are examples of NP drug transport architectures that are increasingly being employed to increase the efficacy of various antibiotics and medications [5, 6]. Nanotechnologies have rapidly expanded in the biomedical field, with potential applications in improving long-term bioavailability, tissue distribution or concentration (biodistribution), pharmacological profile (pharmacokinetics/pharmacodynamics), and period of motion (sustained launch). Thus, reading, creating, developing, and describing materials that absorb dimensions among multiple atoms up to 100 nm are all included in nanotechnology. Nanomaterials have unique physical habitats due to their small size and high floor area-to-volume ratio. This appears to be a major accomplishment in the field of science [7, 8].

Scientists are working hard to combine inorganic fillers, which are smaller than nanoscale, to be able to deal with the limitations of biopolymers. A variety of biopolymers have been explored as capacity substitutes for artificial substances, further to alginate, starch, cellulose, collagen, and chitosan, among other substances. Because those biopolymers are biocompatible and biodegradable, they are ideal for utilization in biomedical packages. The main reasons chitosan is remarkable are its special qualities, which include its exceptional biocompatibility and biodegradability, which are mostly caused by the presence of top amines along its structure. Because of these materials' ability to be used as remedies, there has been significant interest in their utilization in recent years [9, 10].

Natural polymers, such as cellulose and chitosan, are identified for their availability and first-rate features such as non-toxicity, biocompatibility, and degradability. In the human body, those biopolymers break down and are comfortably absorbed as harmless amino sugars. Chitosan and its

DOI: 10.1201/9781003650812-1

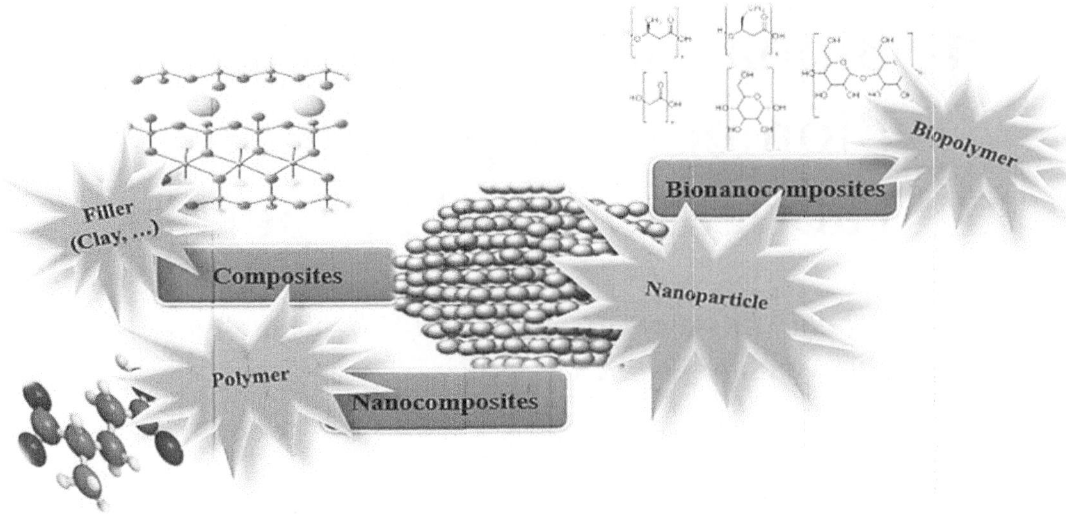

FIGURE 1.1 Bionanocomposites.

derivatives are drastically used in remedies to make contact lenses, mobile encapsulation, wound dressings, and drug delivery structures, among other things [11, 12]. By modifying its physical and chemical characteristics, nanotechnology has significantly advanced the biotechnology and pharmaceutical sectors [7]. Wound dressings, antimicrobial agents, remedy transport structures, and medical equipment are a few examples of bionanocomposites [11]. Because of their antibacterial properties, chitosan-primarily based nanocomposites have become appealing materials for use in biomedical packages with tissue engineering, wound recovery, and drug transport [13]. Biodegradable polymers, such as PGLAs, PGA, and PLA, were utilized in surgical fixation tools, as well as pins, clips, bone plates, and sutures, in the 1960s. There are already more than 40 one-of-a-kind forms of biodegradable polymers, additionally known as copolymers or biocomposites, which offer superb substitutes for steel implants. These bionanocomposite materials deal with the limitations of metallic implants, eliminating the need for surgical implant elimination. The improvement of bionanocomposites has made them useful as tissue engineering scaffolds and tissue culturing, fulfilling the desires of each smooth and difficult tissue. Scientists are working hard to supply and modify primarily bio-based substances with a variety of programs in many domains [14, 15].

1.2 FABRICATION METHODS

Depending on the intended ultimate shape—bulk, thin films, or fibers—a variety of methods are available for creating bionanocomposites. In the production of thin movies, it has been shown that assembly techniques may produce nanomaterials with high dispersion and nanofiller content. The widely used layer-through-layer assembly technique entails precisely controlling the thickness of discrete, strongly interacting additive layers as they are deposited alternately [16]. Spin coating is another well-liked method that uses high rotation speed evaporation of the solvent to create ultrathin films from the nanocompound's solution or dispersion. A number of variables, including solvent properties, rotational velocity, viscosity, and attentiveness, determine the thickness of the film [17].

The Langmuire-Blodgett movie or Langmuire Schaefer movie can be used to construct one or more monolayers of a naturally occurring amphiphilic molecule, producing a very exact film thickness. This involves submerging successive monolayers in a liquid solution containing the natural component to adsorb them onto a robust substrate [18]. These methods have been successfully used to produce layers of cellulose nanocrystals. In addition to thin films, electrospinning can be used to easily obtain micro- and nanofibers. With this method, a solution of viscous polymers is exposed to a high voltage, which causes a liquid jet to form. The jet is constantly expanded due to solvent evaporation, as well as the electrostatic charges produced on its floor as it hardens [18].

The method offers enormous adaptability given that it may be used with a broad range of polymers and provides varying degrees of control over the final morphology, diameter length, and surface roughness. This control is carried out by the deliberate selection of solution resistances, polymer concentration, conductivity, and viscosity, as well as the precise modification of processing factors such as voltage, glide fee, and the separation between the collector and the solution. Furthermore, temperature and humidity are two other important environmental elements [19].

Several nanocrystals and composite systems with unique polymer matrices can be employed to generate hydrogels, provided that robust molecular interactions such as ionic and hydrogen bonding are able to form. Utilizing polysaccharides like chitin and nanocellulose, novel hydrogels with superior water absorption, elastic modulus, and structural balance have been created [20].

A variety of methods, including solvent casting, melt processing, and in situ polymerization, may be utilized to create bionanocomposites that comprise NPs such as HAp detritus, silver, and clay. Solvent casting can occur under various circumstances. In one scenario, pre-made NPs are dispersed in a polymer solution, and the process is monitored through solvent evaporation. In another scenario, NPs are created within the polymer solution. For example, silver NPs ($AgNO_3$) can be reduced among polymers in an ethanolic solution, where the polymer acts as a stabilizing agent and the solvent serves as a reductant [21].

In the second scenario, heating occurs either in batch mode or under continuous shear, such as in an extruder, for the polymer matrix and particles. The process typically starts with mixing NPs with powdered polymer at high speed. Another approach called in situ polymerization involves initially dispersing inorganic particles with a nanometer size in a monomer, which is then polymerized using a bulk or solution procedure with the addition of a small catalyst. By using a low-viscosity monomer to achieve a homogeneous distribution of the NPs, this technique results in a more uniform dispersion of the particles within the final nanocomposites [22].

Efforts to develop new thermoformable bionanocomposites have included attempts to decrease the softening factor of natural polymers like cellulose. One particular instance is the development of nanocomposites that can be thermoformed or injection molded. In these instances, cellulose nanocrystals were coated with dense polymer brushes (such as PCL) to enhance the material's ability to take shape under heat [23].

An excellent method for improving the dispersion of clay NPs in polylactide (PLA) matrices is ultrasonic micromolding production. This process utilizes ultrasonic waves to enhance the mixing, considering how the NPs are dispersed throughout the PLA matrix, aiming to improve the material's overall performance and characteristics as a nanocomposite [24].

1.3 PROPERTIES

1.3.1 Mechanical

The inclusion of natural resins in polymer matrices leads to a shift in Young's modulus and an increase in the tensile strength of nanocomposites. For example, Adarmanabadi et al. demonstrated a noteworthy alteration in the nanocomposites' mechanical characteristics by incorporating nanoclay (NC), nanographene oxide (NGO), and carbon nanotubes (CNT) with varying percentages of weight in the epoxy matrix. Additionally, mixing NC and NGO can enhance the mechanical properties of graphene nanocomposites. The study suggests incorporating NC into the epoxy/NG composite can potentially double the crack strength and increase the pressure and tensile energy at the point of failure. But there was no appreciable change in Young's modulus [25].

Eghbalian et al. performed studies on polymer nanocomposites reinforced using molecular dynamics (MD) simulations with silicon carbide nanotubes (SiCNTs H and F-fSiCNT) functionalized with hydrogen (H) and fluorine (F). The findings indicated that as the degree of subordination increases, there is a decrease in most pressure, maximum stress, elastic modulus, and stress strength. In comparison to pure polymers and polymers containing functionalized silicon carbide nanotubes (fSiCNT), polymer nanocomposites, including SiCNT, exhibit superior tensile electricity. Furthermore, adding fSiCNT to the polymer matrix (fSiCNT/polymer) significantly complements the very last power of pure polymer against nanocomposites. Polymer nanocomposites reinforced with fSiCNTs and armchair SiCNTs exhibit better strain tolerance and decrease Young's modulus inside the longitudinal course than the same systems containing zigzag nanotubes. At each subordination percentage, zigzag F-fSiCNT/polymer may additionally have a better Young's modulus than zigzag polymer/H-fSiCNT. Armchair fSiCNTs introduced into a polyethylene (PE) matrix (F-fSiCNTs/PE) exhibit greater stiffness in comparison to H-fSiCNTs/PE. Additionally, armchair fSiCNT polymer nanocomposites store more pressure energy than their zigzag opposite numbers [26].

Processing conditions can significantly affect the exfoliation degree, thereby impacting the reinforcing effectiveness of nanocomposites. Factors such as processing temperature, blending strategy, and shear intensity can influence filler dispersion and, consequently, the final nanocomposite materials' mechanical characteristics [27].

A substantial increase in the polymer matrix's molecular weight improves the nanocomposites' modulus and yield strength. This is because of the increased shear stress caused by higher molecular weights, leading to the exfoliation of big clay fragments into platelets. The increased degree of exfoliation, facilitated by stronger interfacial bonding, allows for an efficient stress transmission from the polymer matrices to nanofiller [28].

Layered silicates and compatibilizers play a vital part in raising the nanocomposites' tensile strength and Young's modulus. Tanpichai et al. studied the operational mechanism of ENR nanofiber nanocomposites strengthened with CNFs from the water plant Eichhornia crassipes. The results showed that strong bonding from interactions between the stiff CNFs and the functional groups of ENR led to significant improvements in mechanical properties, which successfully transmitted stress from the ENR matrix to the CNFs. Tensile strength and Young's modulus of ENR nanocomposites containing 2 phr of CNFs improved by 80% and 39%, respectively, in comparison to pure ENR, without any reduction in tensile strength at failure. Additionally, the addition of CNFs increased the nanocomposites' resistance to oil [28].

Zhang et al. explored nanocomposite performance by incorporating poly(methyl methacrylate) (PMMA) and poly(butyl acrylate) (PBA) with CNCs. The findings revealed that the modification of CNCs led to improvements. The hydrophobic ground modification combined with the crystalline structure and morphology of CNCs, as well as the thermal stability of modified CNCs (MCNCs), contributed to these enhancements. 7 wt%M CNCs/PBA-co-PMMA nanocomposites exhibited over a 25-fold growth in Young's modulus and approximately a 3-fold growth in tensile electricity as compared to herbal PBA-co-PMMA copolymer. Furthermore, the MCNCs/PBA-co-PMMA nanocomposites displayed a microphase-separated morphology, with soft PBA domain names and tough PMMA and CNC domains. The considerable boom in the garage, the normal shape of MCNCs/PBA-co-PMMA nanocomposites, and their moduli (glass transition temperature) further clarified the connection between most of the mechanical houses and the morphology of the remoted microphase [29].

In polymer structures, the enhancements in the loading, dispersion, and adhesion between HNTs and polymer matrices determine the modulus and tensile energy. Increasing the amount of HNTs generally results in reinforcement and higher tensile energy in nanocomposites. However, difficulties in dispersing HNTs inside polymer matrices may hinder these improvements, especially in nonpolar polymers. Rubavich et al. examined how MWCNTs and HNTs affected the EVA copolymer's mechanical, electrical, thermal, and physical characteristics. The EVA copolymer matrix's crystallization behavior was not appreciably changed by the addition of nanotubes. The tensile strength of nanocomposites based on EVA improved using the content of CNTs, reaching 40% at an 8 wt% loading. HNTs notably improved the tension upon failure. Cyclic mechanical tensile tests showed that composites reinforced with these fillers exhibited reinforcing behavior. The combined effect of both types of NPs became noticeable at elongations of 100% and 200%. Additionally, it was observed that there was an enhancement in conductivity as the amount of MWCNTs increased in the nanocomposites of EVA/CNTs [30].

Improved dispersion by surface preparation, such as polymer grafting or silane, can improve hydrogen bonding and interfacial bonding between HNTs and nonpolar polymers. Studies have shown that using modified HNTs increased the starch/HNT nanocomposites' modulus by 26% compared to unmodified HNTs. Additionally, treating HNTs, when compared to clean PLA, the tensile modulus and energy of PLA/HNT nanocomposites were improved by 25% and 29%, respectively, using quaternary ammonium salt [31].

Additionally, the bonding of polymer matrices across interfacial halloysite nanotubes (HNTs) may be greatly increased by the inclusion of a compatibilizer, improving the characteristics of the nanocomposites. The study conducted by Song et al. focused on the alteration of urea formaldehyde (UF) resin with multiwalled halloysite nanotubes (HNTs). The results showed a notable improvement in the nanocomposite's thermal stability, with a significant reduction in formaldehyde emission from UF wood glue by 62%. Additionally, the water resistance of UF wood glue experienced a significant increase of 84%. Notably, the nanocomposites were able to incorporate HNTs up to a weight percent of 60% [32].

The even distribution of CNT in polymer/CNT nanocomposites improves Young's modulus and tensile strength with the aid of increasing the CNT loading. Sando et al. have looked at the impact of mechanical recovery on the acetylene vinyl acetate (EVA)/CNT nanocomposites' thermal, rheological, mechanical, and electric properties and discovered that mechanical restoration did not cause enormous changes within the thermal and float conduct of EVA/CNT nanocomposites. After 3 recuperation cycles, the EVA/CNT nanocomposites retained approximately 75% of the initial elastic modulus and between 80% and 90% of the distinct tensile power, with the CNT loading directly influencing those values. Furthermore, compared to the unique nanocomposites, the electrical conductivity of the recovered nanocomposites has decreased by around a factor of 10, transitioning from insulating to semiconducting residences (10^{-9} S/m–10^{-2} S/m). Moreover, the conductivity of the EVA/CNT nanocomposite is proportional to CNT loading. These findings propose that by controlling the casting temperature and CNT loading, a mechanically stable electric house can be finished in recovered EVA nanocomposites [32].

The reinforcement configuration and compositions of nanocomposites are influenced by using diverse styles of CNTs and their manufacturing techniques. Currently, because of their superior polymer bonding, single-walled carbon nanotubes (SWCNTs) are preferred over multi-walled carbon nanotubes (MWCNTs). Furthermore, research has been done on the impact of different MWCNT diameters on the mechanical houses of PCL/MWCNT nanocomposites. The effects imply that thick MWCNTs with an outer diameter of 25 nm and 7% oxygen content material show better overall performance in comparison to skinny MWCNTs with an outer diameter of 10 nm and comparable oxygen content. The modulus of PCL/thick MWCNT nanocomposites elevated from 290 GPa (neat polymer) to 715 GPa, while PCL/skinny MWCNT nanocomposites confirmed an increase up to 610 GPa. These findings underscore the significance of considering the diameter and properties of CNTs within the design of nanocomposites [31].

Additionally, the inclusion of functionalized SWCNTs notably influences improvement by raising the interfacial shear energy, nanocomposites' modulus, and tensile strength. Demski et al. carried out a study to investigate the carbon fiber reinforced polymer properties for mechanical and electrical systems (CFRP) SWCNTs combined with ELIUM® thermoplastic acrylic resin. The incorporation of SWCNTs into the structure of CFRP brought about upgrades in impact resistance, interlayer shear energy, and Young's modulus. Furthermore, as compared to the reference laminate, dynamic mechanical analysis (DMA) revealed that the glass transition temperature of the SWCNT/CFRP nanocomposites remained mostly consistent [33].

The primary mechanical characteristics of CNTs-based nanocomposites are strongly encouraged by using the selected fabrication approach. Yun et al. primarily focused on ethylene-co-acid-co-sodium acid copolymer-based ionomer and cyanuric acid. Research was done on the effects of constituents on the antistatic, mechanical, thermal, and rheological properties of extruded MWCNT/polyoxymethylene (POM) nanocomposites. The study verified that although there was a slight decrease in mechanical properties, the POM/CNT nanocomposites' advanced dispersion of CNTs was attributed to the ionomer (coating on CNTs) and/or cyanuric acid (causing π-π interaction between CNTs and cyanuric acid). As a result, this caused more suitable electrical properties, which include electrical conductivity (inclusive of floor resistance) and unmarried scattering electrical conductivity. They took a look and concluded that the most fulfilling mixture for achieving the very best electrical properties consisted of 3.0 weight% ionomer/3.5% weight% POM/0.5 weight% cyanuric acid [34].

In the world of cellulose-based total nanocomposites, various factors affect their overall mechanical performance, together with characteristics of polymers and nanofibers made of cellulose. Xia et al. conducted a look at a nanocomposite film designed to be long-lasting, flame-retardant, and biodegradable. This film was made of inorganic hydroxyapatite nanowires (HNWs) and TEMPO-oxidized cellulose nanofibers (TOCNFs). They had a study and discovered that each TOCNF and HNW possessed a revamp of the one-dimensional microstructure to form a unique microstructure of natural inorganic communities. This network mounted robust interactions characterized by bodily entanglement and numerous chemical bonds, contributing to the outstanding mechanical houses discovered inside the film on nanocomposite materials. The nanocomposite film specifically showed a Young's modulus of 9.18 GPa and a tensile energy of 223.68 MPa, surpassing the mechanical resistances of the maximum previously mentioned cellulose-based total nanocomposites. Additionally, the movie established fantastic properties with thermal stability and flame resistance, credited to the mineral structure created with the aid of the inclusion of HNWs. Remarkably, even with a 30% HNW content, the nanocomposite film maintained high optical transmittance. Furthermore, the film exhibited rapid degradation in soil, making it promising for environmentally pleasant packages [35].

Additionally, the incorporation of nanocellulose filler is important in figuring out the modulus and tensile electricity of the very last nanocomposites. However, it's critical to be aware that increasing the nanocellulose content does not always cause stepped-forward houses. In positive cases, the compatibility among polymer matrices and fillers could have a substantial impact on precise properties. Sharif et al. carried out an observation to discover that they have an impact on graphene oxide encapsulated with biodegradable chitosan (CGO) at the characteristics and form of epoxy composites. The composites were organized by the use of solution mixing with various filler hundreds. The study found that the composition of CGO and the arrangement of fillers inside the epoxy matrix were motivated by its content material, as discovered through microstructural evaluation. Mechanical and thermal checks have been conducted, displaying that the chitosan-GO ratio and the CGO loading stage have proven crucial in raising the power of the epoxy/CGO composites. According to tensile testing, CGO-containing nanocomposites had an impressive 65% higher elastic modulus. This is thought to be the result of better load transmission caused by the interfacial interactions between the CGO and matrix. Additionally, it was shown by dynamic mechanical thermal analysis (DMTA) that the addition of CGO to the epoxy matrix increased the composite's glass transition temperature (Tg) by up to 30°C [36].

The intrinsic brittleness or poor sturdiness of nanocomposite systems, which results from the failure-induced debonding of the polymer matrices and clay, is one of their main drawbacks. Anstey et al. conducted a study to enhance PLA composites' mechanical performance by incorporating thermoplastic polyester elastomer (TPEE) nanofibrils. These nanofibrils had a high aspect ratio, allowing them to form physical penetration networks in the material, despite being present in low weight proportions (2.8% by weight). The formation of these networks caused the material's mechanical properties to drastically change. The material's behavior changed from brittle to ductile due to the network creation, leading to a notable increase in toughness while experiencing a very little reduction in Young's modulus. This discovery underscores the significant potential of TPEE nanofibrils in improving PLA composites' mechanical performance [37].

The production method used for nanocomposites can significantly impact the elongation at failure of the material. In the case of ethylene-vinyl acetate copolymer (EVA-12) nanocomposites, the addition of organoclays produced a noticeable increase in the lengthening at the break. Behian et al. conducted a study on the synthesis of hectorite nanocomposites, MWCNTs, and ethylene-co-vinyl acetate (EVA) using the solution interpolation technique. The incorporation of 4 wt% filler content led to remarkable improvements in various tensile properties. Specifically, the tensile strength increased from 1.78 MPa to 6.11 MPa (243%), the elongation at break increased from 366% to 750% (105%), and the toughness improved from 3.36 MPa to 17.67 MPa (426%). Interestingly, Young's modulus remained relatively unchanged, with a slight increase from 1.12 MPa to at least 1.31 MPa. To further enhance the understanding of the nanocomposites, the researchers employed differential scanning calorimetry, revealing significant increases in crystallinity, crystallization temperature (Tc), and crystallite melting temperature (Tm) compared to neat EVA. The observed changes in Tc (~87 to ~98°C) and Tm (~118 to ~151°C), amounting to over 10°C and 30°C, respectively, validate the enhanced nanocomposites' thermal stability. Furthermore, the inclusion of a hybrid filler content of 5 wt% resulted in a maximum improvement of 25% in the dielectric constant and a 50% improvement in AC conductivity. These findings demonstrate the enhanced electrical properties of the nanocomposites [38].

1.3.2 Dynamic Mechanical

Semitela et al. carried out a study on the bionanocomposites of graphene oxide (GO) functionalized with polyethyleneimine (GOPEI) and montmorillonite (MS). The investigation worried about the use of mechanodynamic stimulation, especially a 2-hour sinusoidal compression biking interval at a stress range and 0.5 Hz in frequency of 0–10%, for a period of 14 days. Osteoblasts (MC3T3-E1) were applied within the examination to assess the bioactivity of the GOPEI@MS bionanocomposites. The consequences revealed a large bioactivity, with cell proliferation occurring under dynamic settings ten times faster than under static ones. Furthermore, dynamic experiments demonstrated that GOPEI@MS bionanocomposites are capable of functioning as mechanical stimuli-responsive scaffolds, efficaciously meeting the physiological needs of the extracellular matrix. The presence of the bionanocomposites strongly stimulated the mineralization of the bone matrix by way of the bone cells (ECM), in addition to validating their potential as an appropriate surrounding for controlling the mechanisms regulating mobile proliferation induced by using mechanical stimulation. These findings spotlight the promising possibilities of the cellular-GOPEI@MS system in regulating cellular proliferation via mechanical stimulation and provide a foundation for ability in vivo experiments [39].

Sharma et al. carried out a study on the nanocomposite of polylactic acid (PLA), polyethylene glycol (PEG), and halloysite nanotubes (HNT). The research used dynamic thermomechanical evaluation (DMTA) to assess the PLA/PEG/HNT films' mechanical properties inside the rubbery area. The results showed that the PLA/PEG/HNT films' storage modulus had significantly increased, indicating advanced mechanical performance. The advent of PEG as a plasticizer inside the films resulted in a decrease in the glass transition temperature, making them more flexible. Moreover, the incorporation of HNT caused a development in the crystallinity of the nanocomposite in contrast to clean PLA. When compared to movies containing PLA alone, PLA/PEG, and PLA/HNT, the PLA/PEG/HNT movies' thermal stability is shown to be superior. This implies that PEG and HNT are present and contribute to better thermal resistance and durability of the nanocomposite structure. The degree of crystallinity determined through X-ray diffraction analysis confirmed appropriate agreement with the outcomes obtained from differential scanning calorimetry (DSC), in addition to confirming the impact of PEG and HNT on the crystalline nanocomposite's characteristics. Overall, the look demonstrates the potential of the PLA/PEG/HNT nanocomposite in improving mechanical houses, crystallinity, and thermal stability, thereby paving the way for its utility in numerous fields [40].

1.3.3 Thermal Stability

In polymer/clay nanocomposites, the polymer matrices' inclusion of layered silicates has been shown to enhance thermal stability. These silicates act as insulators and impediments to mass transit, effectively hindering the release of unstable byproducts during degradation. For example, chitosan/montmorillonite (MMT) nanocomposites exhibit significant improvements in thermal stability. Studies have revealed that the decomposition temperature, corresponding to a 50% weight reduction, is up to 94.3°C higher in nitrogen flow and 85.5°C higher in airflow compared to natural chitosan alone. This demonstrates the substantial enhancement achieved by incorporating MMT into the chitosan matrix. [41].

Papadopoulou et al. carried out research on the bionanocomposites of poly(butylene succinate) (PBSu), including 1%, 2.5%, and 5% of biochar (MSP700) by weight. All of the materials showed excellent thermal stability, with degradation starting at about 300°C, according to the TGA thermograms. Nonetheless, the results indicated that the PBSu biochar nanocomposites' little loss in thermal stability could have been caused by the biochar's catalytic action. The thermal degradation process of PBSu nanocomposites packed with biochar was investigated using Py-GC/MS analysis. After a thermal breakdown at 450°C, the decomposition components were detected by this technique, which also showed that the degradation route mostly includes the breaking of beta hydrogen bonds, similar to Neat PBSu. Subtle differences in the peak intensities of certain thermal degradation products were noticed at a greater biochar concentration (5 wt%), though, indicating the possibility of α-hydrogen bond scission [42].

Ahuja et al. conducted a study on the thermal balance and degradation kinetics of cellulose nanofibers (CNFs) derived from wheat straw that were added to glycerol plasticized starch (GPS) nanocomposites for reinforcement. The findings tested that the m-CNF/GPS bionanocomposite films exhibited advanced morphology in contrast to other movies, with superior floor bonding. Additionally, the inclusion of m-CNFs resulted in an impressive 81% reduction in water vapor transmission charge (WVP) relative to pristine GPS movies. Moreover, the thermal stability skilled a sizeable growth, with the addition of CNFs contributing to an extensive upward push of up to 52% in activation energy. The observation successfully hooked up a correlation between morphology and thermal stability [43].

1.3.4 Biodegradation

Biodegradation, the technique of chemically breaking down materials in the presence of bacteria or under organic conditions, may be notably extra beneficial in bionanocomposite systems. Gohargani et al. performed a study on a composite fabric made from TiO_2 NPs in combination with Shirazi thyme vital oil (ZEO) and whey protein isolate (WPI)/chitosan. The study discovered that because the content material of NPs accelerated, the composite samples confirmed a higher degree of crystallinity. However, the presence of ZEO had minimum impact on the purposeful houses and crystallinity of the composite samples. In phrases of visible characteristics, the addition and growth of TiO_2 and TiO_2-ZEO drastically extended the lightness and transparency of the samples. The inclusion of TiO_2 brought about full-size upgrades in the composite samples' mechanical and water vapor characteristics; however, adding ZEO significantly reduced those attributes independent of the TiO_2 content. Furthermore, when it came to *Staphylococcus aureus*, *Escherichia coli*, and *Listeria monocytogenes*, composite films containing 2% TiO_2 in addition to ZEO showed stronger antibacterial qualities than films having 1% NPs combined with ZEO. Overall, the findings imply that while TiO_2 augments the antibacterial properties of the composite layers, ZEO's synergistic impact contributes to their ability to fight germs. Thus, these biodegradable composite samples might be employed as colorful food packaging materials [44].

Singh et al. performed an examination aimed at growing and figuring out active nanocomposite biofilms with the use of cornstarch with a lime oil nanoemulsion (LNE-2%) and montmorillonite filler (MMT-1.5% and 2.5%). The analysis revealed that adding 1.5% MMT significantly improved the movie's tensile houses (by 50.85%). However, an increase in MMT to 2.5% resulted in a loss in tensile energy (using 31.25%), making the films seem opaque and brittle. Additionally, by decreasing water solubility (by 4.65), absorption (by 27.26%), and water vapor transmission rate (WVTR) (by 26.49%), as well as by extending their degradation rate to fourteen days in comparison to the managed pattern, the addition of MMT improved the film's water resistance. Voids formed in the film microstructure as a result of combining LNE with starch/MMT. As a result, the advancements in barrier and mechanical resistances shown in the starch/MMT film lost some of their prominence. However, the addition of LNE resulted in increased water absorption (by 3.37%), decreased film solubility (by 5.22%), and increased tensile electricity (by 37%). WVTR was not significantly impacted, though. Furthermore, the combination of MMT and LNE had a synergistic effect, reducing soil degradation and increasing antioxidant activity (by ~279.31%) and antibacterial actions taken to combat *Escherichia coli* (ZOI-8.19 mm) and *Staphylococcus aureus* (ZOI-11.71 mm). X-ray diffraction and FT-IR spectroscopy related the observed alterations to the intercalation and exfoliation between maize starch and MMT in the presence of LNE. Even as a totally biodegradable end product, the findings indicate that the maize starch movie reinforced with MMT and LNE successfully increased the movie's physicochemical, structural, barrier, and functional characteristics [45].

Rahim et al. conducted an observation on Fe_3O_4@tannic acid-Cu. The significant hydroxyl and phenolic hydroxyl organizations of this bionanocomposite are one of the main elements that determine its novelty, which successfully beautifies its catalytic pastime and cooperative interplay for the selective oxidation of alcohols. Another crucial element of this bionanocomposite is that it's synthesized from biomaterials, making the technique of oxidizing alcohol to aldehydes and ketones safe for the environment and simple to use. Furthermore, the unique structure of the bionanocomposite makes it an effective bionanocatalyst. As a result, the bionanocomposite that was created was employed as a relatively green heterogeneous catalyst for the alcohols' selective oxidation. The procedure has a number of benefits, including high to extremely high efficiency, fast response times, simple nanocatalyst separation, straightforward operation, and non-toxicity. Furthermore, the computed turnover frequency (TOF) and turnover range (TON) values supported the bionanocomposite's excellent overall performance in the production of aldehydes and ketones. Moreover, the bionanocomposite's unique form is responsible for the massively energetic floor proximity of Fe_3O_4@tannic acid-Cu, which enhances its catalytic hobby [46].

1.3.5 Physical Properties

Wu et al. carried out a study on environmentally pleasant bionanocomposite movies by means of introducing phlorotannins from sargassum (PS) that were incorporated into composites of konjac glucomannan (KGM) and cellulose cotton nanocrystals (CNC). The results of Fourier transform infrared spectroscopy, X-ray diffraction, and scanning electron microscopy revealed excellent compatibility between PS and the KGM/CNC composite matrix, leading to the development of compact and homogeneous layers. The use of PS significantly enhanced the thermal balance of the KGM/CNC bionanocomposite movies, as shown by thermal analysis and differential scanning calorimetry. Additionally, the appropriate amount of PS applied improved the mechanical strength and water vapor barrier properties of the bionanocomposite film. Notably, the KGM/CNC/PS bionanocomposite film's tensile electricity increased by 33.9% with a PS content material of 9%, while the water vapor transmission decreased by 41.67% when compared to KGM/CNC films [47].

Bratovcic et al. carried out a comprehensive study on bionanocomposite films and safe-to-eat coatings incorporating steel NPs into biopolymers. The consequences tested that using these fruits and vegetables with bionanocomposite films and edible coatings can have a number of benefits, such as fewer color changes, a lower respiration rate, and weight loss, which will prolong their usable lives and postpone ripening. Moreover, those movies and coatings exhibited environmental compatibility. Extensive studies have been carried out on diverse physicochemical residences, which include moisture barrier effectiveness, oxygen scavenging abilities, and antimicrobial properties. The research additionally included physicochemical properties consisting of floor traits, shape, touch attitude, thickness, transparency, color traits, and thermal stability. Furthermore, the findings showcased that these progressive nanocomposite films suitable for eating coatings can decorate texture, enhance product look, and prolong shelf lifestyles via forming semipermeable obstacles that include carbon dioxide and oxygen, as well as gases and moisture [48].

Shahvlizadeh et al. performed a study wherein gelatin and crucible were applied to increase antimicrobial nanocomposites containing distinct concentrations (1%, 3%, and 5%) of zinc oxide NPs (ZnO-NPs). The results found a large enhancement within the melting factor temperature (Tm), with values growing from about 90°C to around 101°C–93°C following the addition of 1–5% ZnO-NPs, as indicated by means of DSC analysis. Furthermore, the incorporation of 1%, 3%, and 5% ZnO-NPs led to extraordinary development inside the closing tensile energy (UTS) to values of 31.21 MPa, 34.57 MPa, and 35.06 MPa, respectively. Similarly, Young's modulus confirmed tremendous improvements to 287.44 MPa, 335.47 MPa, and 367.04 MPa for the corresponding ZnO-NP concentrations. Notably, the films' water vapor permeability (WVP) reduced in a dose-dependent way with the presence of ZnO-NPs, indicating progressed water resistance residences. FE-SEM analysis of the floor and move-phase of the nanocomposites validated a compact and homogeneous structure despite the very best attention of 5% ZnO-NPs [49].

In their study, Wu et al. examined the consequences of adding zein NPs (ZNPs) at different concentrations directly into a konjac glucomannan (KGM) and chitosan (CS) composite matrix to produce organic nanocomposite biofilms. Along with testing the resulting bionanocomposite movies' mechanical, morphological, thermal, and moisture barrier properties, the scientists also examined the film-forming solutions' (FFSs) rheological behavior. The findings demonstrated that the inclusion of ZNPs caused a sizable enhancement in the properties of the composite movies. These upgrades encompassed moisture resistance, mechanical power, and thermal balance. It is really worth noting, though, that an immoderate overload of ZNPs ought to decrease those upgrades. Therefore, the strategic reinforcement of ZNPs within the composite film matrices represents an ability to strive for growing biodegradable movie additives that showcase remarkable overall performance for meal packaging applications [50].

1.3.6 Biological Properties

The use of natural polymer matrices in food packaging materials and medical equipment has grown in popularity as concern about plastic pollution has grown. In response, there have been significant advancements in the development of two-part or three-part structures that blend natural elements in an effort to produce products of a caliber similar to those made entirely of synthetic materials. Novel bionanocomposites made of starch, chitosan, and graphene oxide (GO) are presented by Kristajan et al. in their work, and they show improved biological activity. Cell-based analyses revealed that the composites did not exhibit any toxic effects on HaCat keratinocytes and HepG2 hepatocytes. Additionally, the nanocomposites showed a strong bacteriostatic effect against various pathogenic bacterial species. In conclusion, the starch/chitosan/GO nanocomposites possess a range of beneficial physicochemical and biological characteristics, establishing them as a potential substitute for materials that are entirely manufactured [51].

Erol et al. performed a study wherein they correctly synthesized a like-minded combination of chitosan (CS) using poly 2-(4-fluorophenyl)-2-oxoethyl-2-methylprop-2-enoate (PFPAMA), an artificial polymer largely based on methacrylate. The researchers finished an antibiogram check on the usage of the disk diffusion approach, revealing that the nanocomposites show strong resistance toward the pathogens *Escherichia coli* and *Staphylococcus aureus*. Furthermore, the nanocomposites verified antioxidant and oxidant houses that were comparable to those of the reference material used. These findings suggest that CS-primarily based nanocomposites possess favorable biological properties, making them viable biomaterials [52].

The field of bone regeneration has garnered significant interest lately with the goal of replacing and fixing the human body's broken and damaged bones. In this context, Swaminathan et al. have successfully developed highly porous bionanocomposite scaffolds using a combination of polyetheretherketone (PEEK), hydroxyapatite (HA), carbon fiber (CF), and CNTs. The study findings indicate that the enhanced nanocomposites demonstrate remarkable biocompatibility, as they were found to be non-hazardous and showed improved viability of cells. Furthermore, the scaffolds allowed for the development of bone marrow cells, exhibiting enhanced cell attachment when carbon elements were incorporated into the PEEK/HA biocomposites compared to PEEK/HA composites alone. During cellular viability assessments, the bionanocomposites containing 0.5 wt% CNTs showed significantly improved cell attachment at the discs, surpassing the performance of PEEK/HA biocomposites. Similar results were observed in bone marrow cell culture experiments involving osteoblasts and osteoclasts. 0.5 wt% CF exhibited higher cell attachment for osteoblasts, while 1 wt% CNTs displayed greater cell attachment for osteoclasts. It has been determined that incorporating carbon-based NPs into PEEK/HA is a successful method for improving its mechanical, biological, and cell attachment qualities. The PEEK/HA/CNTs and CF bionanocomposites that were created showed remarkable biocompatibility, as they showed improved cell adhesion, vitality, and proliferation. As a result, these materials have a lot of potential for use in biological contexts, such as bone scaffolding [53].

In their studies, Maqsood Lu et al. centered on bone regrowth and investigated the capacity of a biological nanocomposite tissue bolstered with bioactive NPs for addressing femur defects in remedy. The observed findings discovered that the MTT test revealed that scaffolds made with various doses of the scaffold extract were not cytotoxic. These results suggest that the scaffold under investigation has potential for use in bone tissue engineering projects. Its adequate porosity and structural resemblance to human bone contribute to its usefulness in this field. By leveraging the blessings of bioactive NPs, this nanocomposite-primarily based scaffold demonstrates viability as a solution for femur disorder remedies [54].

1.4 NATURAL POLYMERS AS NANOCOMPOSITES FOR BIOMEDICAL APPLICATIONS

1.4.1 Cellulose

The consensus is that the most common renewable polymer on Earth is cellulose. This amazing structural component clumps into cellulose fibers and spontaneously produces microfibrils. Many living things, including bacteria, fungi, amoebae, and marine life, as well as higher and lower plants, create it through biosynthesis. The primary component of cellulose is a linear homopolysaccharide made up of β-D-glucopyranose units joined by β-1-4 linkages. Figure 1.2 shows the underlying

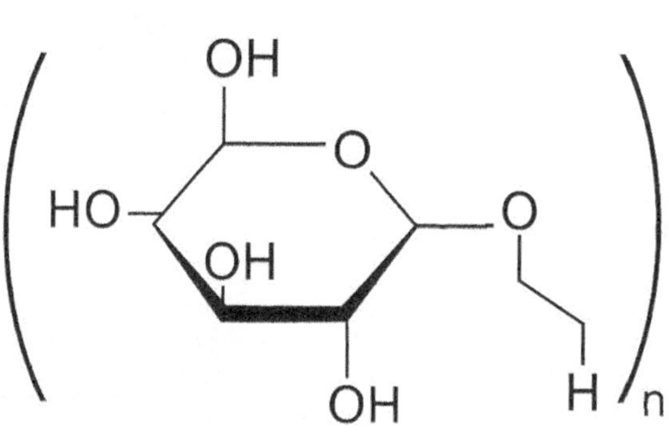

FIGURE 1.2 Cellulose's chemical structure.

chemical structure of cellulose. Each monomer has three hydroxyl groups, which are crucial for hydrogen bonding and significantly influence the crystalline structure and physical properties of cellulose [55].

In cotton, the degree of polymerization (DP) of native cellulose is around 15,000 glucopyranose units, whereas it is typically 10,000 in wood. It's important to keep in mind that the length of the polymer chains may vary depending on the source of the cellulose, including the plant section from which it originates. The cellulose microfibril is the main structural component of cellulose and is created during biosynthesis. As shown in Figure 1.3, a fibril is really formed by poly-β-(1→4)-D-glucosyl residue chains. This fibril can be thought of as a lengthy, thread-like bundle of molecules held together laterally by hydrogen bonds [56].

Individual cellulose microfibrils usually range in diameter from 2 to 20 nm. Each microfibril includes cellulose crystals related alongside twists and kinks along the microfibril axis via amorphous, disordered areas. Studies utilizing X-ray diffraction and infrared spectroscopy have found that cellulose enterprise in flowers predominantly comprises crystallites interspersed with amorphous regions of low order [58]. Cellulose I is the term for cellulose in its native crystalline form, while regenerated cellulose derived from answers, specifically alkali solutions, is known as cellulose II. These polymorphs represent the primary styles of cellulose. Based on contemporary know-how of cellulose crystallography and biosynthesis, cellulose structure is normally composed of parallel chains. Conversely, cellulose II's crystalline structure is referred to as anti-parallel. It is significant to remember that cellulose I is not the most thermodynamically solid form of cellulose. This type of cellulose II is the most energetically favorable because it has an extra hydrogen bond that is consistent with the glucose residue [56].

Since Mercer discovered the cellulose I to cellulose II conversion in 1850, when local cellulose was treated with a strong alkali, it has been a pastime and the topic of several studies. The mechanism behind this transformation has been the problem of severe debate that continues to this day.

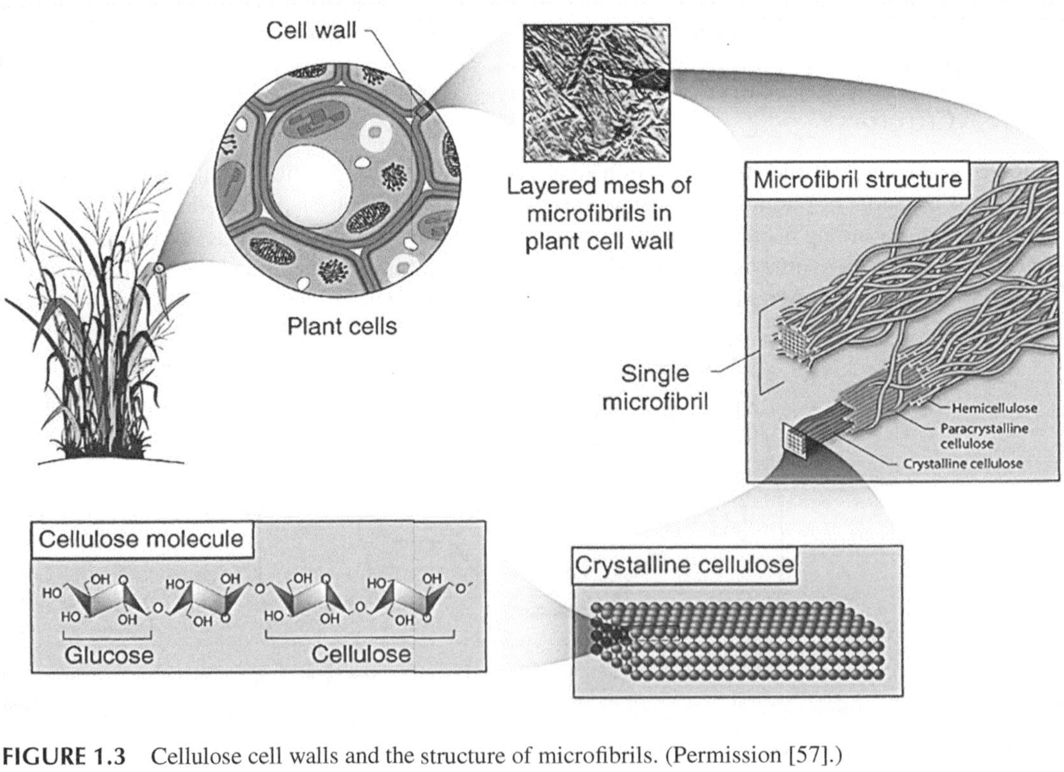

FIGURE 1.3 Cellulose cell walls and the structure of microfibrils. (Permission [57].)

Attala and VanderHart were the first to use move polarization/magic perspective spinning (CP-MAS) nuclear magnetic resonance (NMR) studies to illustrate the lifetimes of two superb crystalline bureaucracies in natural cellulose, namely Iα and Iβ. The ratio of those allomorphs can affect numerous bodily properties of cellulose fibers. Notably, it's been determined that both bureaucracy, Iα and Iβ, can coexist within the same cellulose pattern in addition to alongside a single microfibril. While cellulose Iα is taken into consideration as a metastable shape, annealing treatment can convert it into the Iβ form. Even though the two lattices' polysaccharide chains' conformations are identical, Iα and Iβ, there are differences in their hydrogen-bonding styles [59].

The material hired as local cellulose, namely as cellulose nanofiller, cellulose I is made from lignocellulosic fibers using conventional bleaching techniques. Known for its superior mechanical qualities, cellulose I is characterized by its high modulus and crystallinity. Furthermore, nanoscale fillers have exhibited remarkable potential as reinforcing factors for approximately 15 years. Essentially, there are fundamental classes of nanosized cellulosic debris: cellulose nanocrystals and microfibrillated cellulose (MFC) [60].

1.4.1.1 Nanocomposites Based on Cellulose

A rapidly developing field of study is the reinforcing of nanocomposites with cellulose NPs, such as whiskers and MFC. In addition to the raw fabric's affordability, cellulosic particles offer several nicely installed blessings in nanocomposites, which include low density, renewable nature, availability of a various variety of fillers worldwide, low strength intake, high unique houses, minimal abrasiveness in the course of processing, biodegradability, and a quite reactive floor that permits for grafting particular organizations [61]. However, there are some drawbacks to take into account for cellulose NPs in reinforcement programs: excessive moisture absorption, bad wetting ability, incompatibility with maximum polymeric matrices, and processing temperature limits. Notably, the degradation of lignocellulosic materials starts at around 220°C, which restricts the types of matrix materials that may be combined with natural filler [62].

Because of its polar floor features, cellulose whiskers have an inherent difficulty distributing internal nonpolar media in polymer nanocomposites. This is one drawback of using them. Put more simply, cellulose nanocrystals have often only been used in polar or aqueous conditions when included as reinforcing materials. The following are the main methods for creating polysaccharide nanocomposite films: 1) Solvent casting for evaporating water or natural solvents, and 2) extrusion using freeze-dried cellulose NPs [63].

According to the polymer utilized in the matrix, the first technique—which is the one most usually used—can be classified into three systems: polymer emulsions, non-hydrosoluble polymers, and water-soluble polymers [64]. Two strategies may be taken into consideration for non-hydrosoluble polymers to gain from cellulose nanocrystal dispersions in a suitable natural media that are not flocculated: i) Applying surfactants to the floor of cellulose nanocrystals that have polar heads and long hydrophobic tails, or ii) Grafting hydrophobic chains onto the surface of the cellulose nanocrystals [65].

These methods allow the creation of polymer nanocomposites by combining a polymer solution with NP suspensions in a natural medium. A melting compounding process called extrusion may be utilized to make nanocomposites reinforced with cellulose NPs. This strategy is especially novel, and only a small amount of thorough study has been done in this field. Consequently, it is becoming more and more feasible to expand laboratory research to a commercial scale [66].

However, there is a big challenge when using cellulose NPs in a dry environment. When these polysaccharide NPs dry, strong hydrogen bonds form quickly, which leads to the formation of aggregates and reduces the use of nanoscale reinforcement. It has been shown that nanocomposites containing a mixture of cellulose whiskers and artificial latex, formed by casting and evaporating, have better mechanical properties than nanocomposites containing the same mixture, freeze-dried and hot-pressed. The formation of an inflexible community linking the whiskers is responsible for the considerable reinforcing impact observed in cast and evaporated materials. This community is most likely enabled by the presence of hydrogen bonds. The theory is that community creation is more noticeable when videos evaporate because they process more quickly [67].

1.4.1.1.1 Cellulose Sources

According to where it comes from, cellulose may be divided into five categories: the different types of cellulose include wood-based (WC), plant-based (PC), microorganism-based (BC), algae-based (WC), and tunicate-based (Figure 1.4). Due to their accessibility and cost, WC and PC have been the most well-known forms of cellulose throughout their extensive history, compared to BC, tunicate-based cellulose, and algae-based cellulose. [68].

1.4.1.1.1.1 Plant Cellulose and Wood A variety of materials may be used to extract cellulose, including hardwoods like oak and beech, and softwoods like pine, cedar, and spruce. Furthermore, cellulose extraction from numerous plant materials has been studied, such as potato peel waste, cotton, flax, pineapple leaves, maize, hemp, jute, bagasse, ramie, and biomass from oil palms (Figure 1.4) [69].

Plant fibers consist of biodegradable polymers of carbohydrates, such as cellulose, hemicellulose, and lignin, and resemble wood in both composition and structure. In both wood and plants, cellulose molecules have a multifaceted, intricate form (Figure 1.5), and they are linked to other biopolymers such as lignin and hemicellulose (Figure 1.6). Despite having the same composition as cellulose obtained from different sources, cellulose derived from wood and plants has a unique microstructural commercial operation [70]. A matrix of hemicellulose and lignin holds the cellulose chains in the cases of WC and PC together in the form of layers called nanofibrils (Figure 1.6). Nevertheless, cotton fiber lacks significant levels of lignin and hemicellulose while being entirely plant-based. Similar to wood, where it ranges from 40% to 50%, flowers often have cellulose contents between 30% and 75%. In addition to differing in their chemical makeup, softwoods and hardwoods also differ in their structural structure and in the quantity of lignin, hemicellulose, and cellulose that they contain [71].

1.4.1.1.1.2 Bacterial Cellulose Bacteria create cellulose, which is sometimes referred to as "microbial cellulose," "bacterial nanocellulose," "biocellulose," or, more precisely, "bacterial cellulose" (BC). BC is created in a nearly pure form (approximately 90%) by employing the terminal

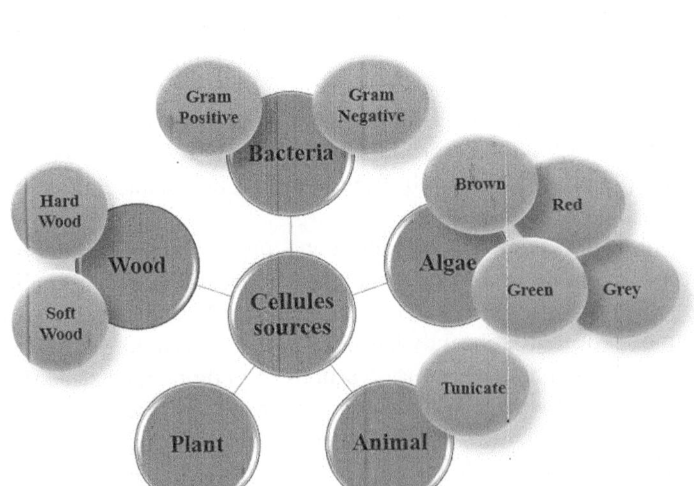

FIGURE 1.4 Cellulose is categorized based on its source, which includes wood, plants, algae, animals, and microbes.

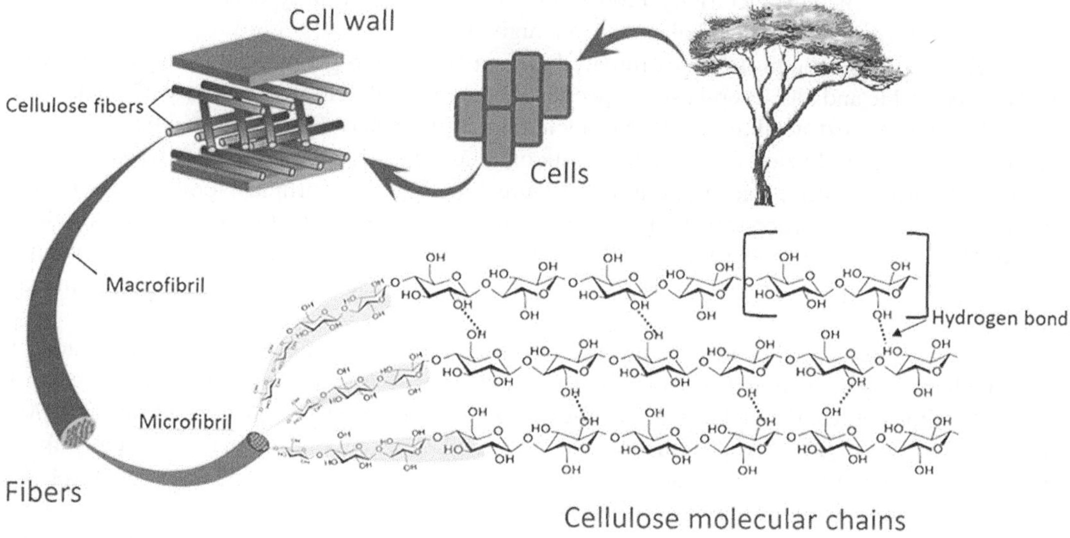

FIGURE 1.5 Diagram shows the structure of wood from the cellulose molecule to the tree. (Permission [72].)

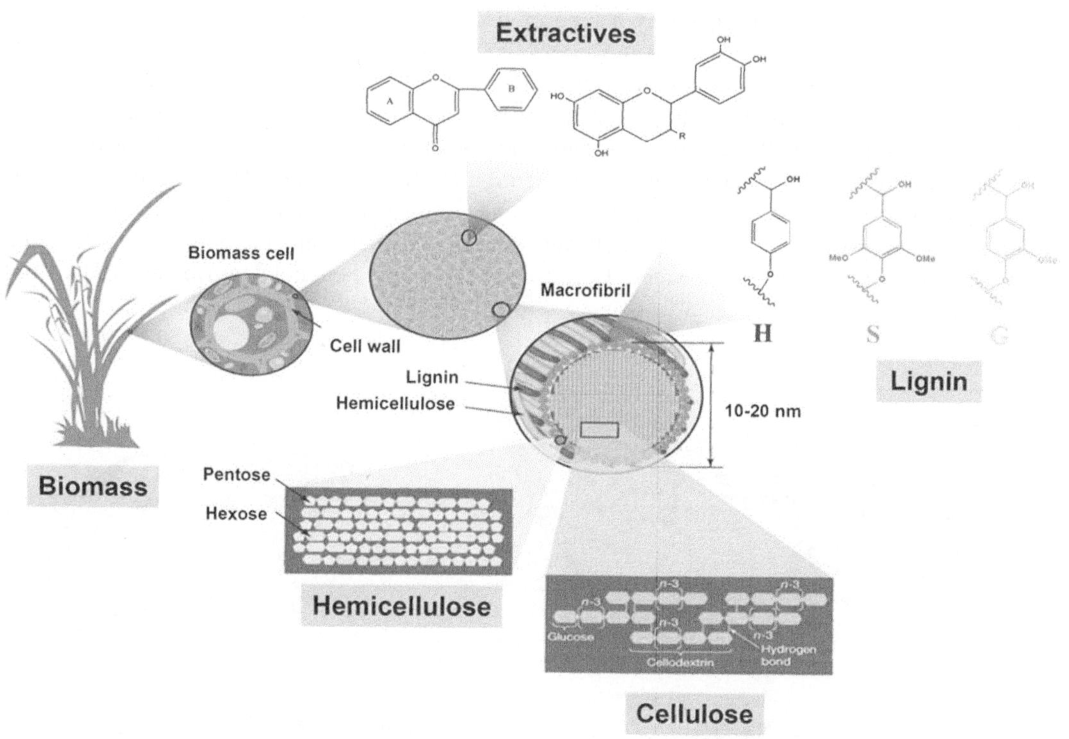

FIGURE 1.6 Microstructure of a cellulosic fiber. (Permission [73].)

complex, which is incapable of binding to lignin, hemicellulose, or other polymers (Figure 1.7). Consequently, the separation and purification of BC are quite simple and do not require big chemicals or other forms of treatment, in contrast to WC and PC. Since its discovery, BC has drawn attention for a variety of reasons, including its high purity, ultrafine fiber shapes, unusually crystalline structure, high mechanical electricity, biodegradability, biocompatibility, excessive water-maintaining capacity, favorable chemical balance, and a high DP [74].

Crucially, BC is thought to be extremely biocompatible, non-genotoxic, and cytotoxic, which makes it desirable and has several uses, especially in the medical field. The majority of the time, BCs are produced by extracellular bacteria, including Agrobacterium, Komagataeibacter xylinus, Achromobacter, Aerobacter, Azotobacter, Pseudomonas, and Rhizobium, in addition to one genus of superior Gram-positive bacteria, Sarcina (Figure 1.4). The three primary food sources for these bacteria are nitrogen, carbon (mostly D-glucose), and air. The most widely used microbe species for BC synthesis is Komagataeibacter xylinus (previously known as Acetobacter xylinum), which can produce notably high quantities of BC from a range of carbon and nitrogen resources in liquid life [74].

Common carbon supplies include rotting fruit, pineapple peel juice, agroindustrial wastes, and, as a medium, sugar. Although large-scale BC production is frequently costly, depending on the original carbon source, the yield of BC synthesis can reach up to 40%. High crystallinity (80–90%), an excessive DP (7,000–16,000 glucose residues), and an excessive mechanical force linked to unique CNFs (metallic or Kevlar) are some of BC's key properties. BC has a versatile morphology that can be processed into fleeces, films, spheres, and hollow particles, giving it the ability to be used in the creation of biomedical materials. Despite having the same chemical building blocks, WC, PC, and BC differ in their structural organization, which causes differences in their mechanical characteristics [75].

In addition, BC degrades at a somewhat faster pace than WC and PC. In artificial and non-synthetic settings, BC is produced by a type of bacteria that produces acetic acid. A haphazard nanofibrillar population of crystalline and disordered cellulose strand areas generates a pellicle that BC develops throughout biosynthesis (Figure 1.7). Furthermore, BC may form solid hydrogels and has an exceptional capacity to retain water (up to 99% in certain cases). A large surface area is provided by well-separated BC nanofibers, creating an incredibly porous structure. BC is made up of randomly arranged ribbon-shaped fibrils that are around 100 nm in size. These fibrils are made up of typical nanofibrils that are 7–8 nm in length and grouped in bundles [76]. This precise nanomorphology has good conformability, high wet strength, elasticity, and a large surface area that can store a substantial quantity of water. Because of its many beneficial attributes, BC is being

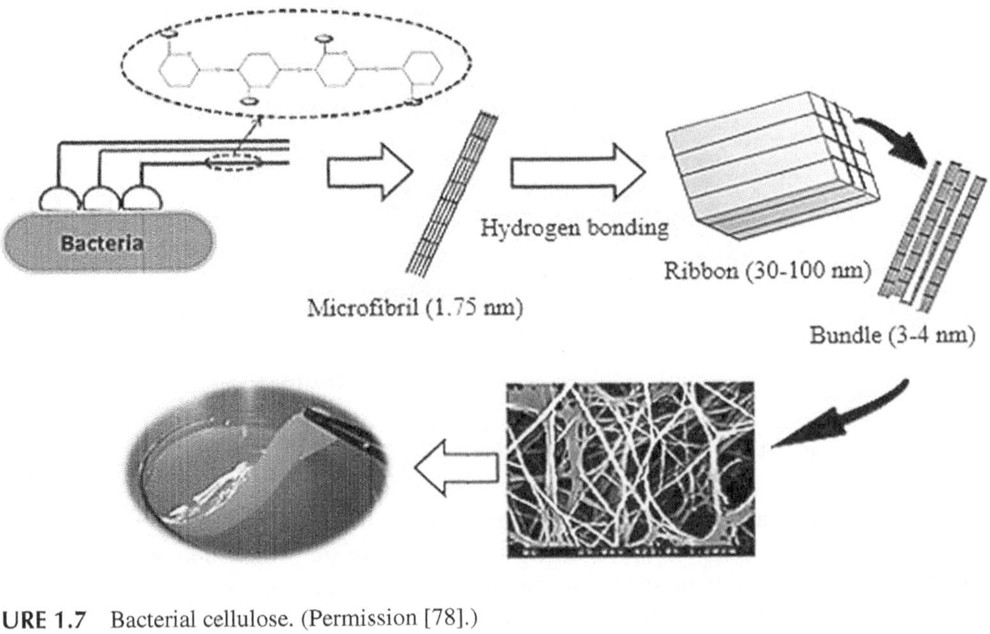

FIGURE 1.7 Bacterial cellulose. (Permission [78].)

considered as a material for biomedical applications, particularly in the areas of tissue engineering and medicine. These applications include implant and scaffold construction, emulsion and hydrogel stabilization, drug delivery systems, clever treatments for wound healing or artificial skin, and the immobilization of enzymes and biomolecules to enhance activity and balance in vivo [77].

1.4.1.1.1.3 Algal Cellulose Since cellulose makes up a large portion of the cellular partitions of algae, several algae species that are good sources of cellulose include brown species (Posidonia oceanica), green species (Cladophora), and red species (Gelidium elegans) (Figure 1.4). Carbohydrates make up the majority of the material of red algae, such as Gelidium elegans, along with cellulose that is highly concentrated in power and mucilaginous materials like agar [79]. Algae may be grown on a large scale, which benefits the environment. Moreover, they are able to use nutrients from waste streams (such as flue fuel and wastewater) to provide an alternative and sustainable supply of cellulose. Cellulose from Valonia or Cladophora is well known for having an exceptionally high crystallinity (over 95%). However, algal cellulose is not pure and is typically combined with protein, lignin, and hemicellulose [80].

The cellulose derived from green algae presents notable benefits in comparison to WC, PC, and BC because of its elevated crystallinity level (over 70%), reduced capacity to adsorb moisture, high mesoporous porosity, and correspondingly elevated specific surface area. Because algal nanocellulose is non-poisonous and easily manipulated chemically, it has great promise for use in biomedical programs and tissue engineering [81].

1.4.1.1.1.4 Animal Cellulose Tunicates are the most easily recognized animal source of cellulose; they are invertebrate organisms that live in large quantities in the ocean (Figure 1.4). The tunicate epidermal cells' plasma membrane contains a variety of enzyme complexes that are responsible for producing cellulose. Cellulose that is predominantly derived from tunicates is obtained from the outer layer of the plant known as "tunic," from which pure cellulose, known as "tunicin," may be isolated (Figure 1.8) [82]. Tunic cellulose, also known as tunicin, is the refined cellulose that has been isolated from the tunic. Over 2300 species of tunicates belong to the class known as Ascidiacea, or sea squirts; this has been the main subject of this field's research. Hundreds of cellulose nanofibrils (CNFs) are crammed inside the tunic. The shape and size of a nanofibril bundle differ among species. Nanofibril bundles are deposited in a multilayered manner parallel to the surface of the epidermis. Tunic CNFs have dimensions of 10 to 30 nm in width, 60 to 70 tiers in element ratio, and lengths ranging from 100 nm to several micrometers (often 2 μm) [82].

Typically, 27% of the components in a dry tunic contain nitrogen, while 60% of the material is cellulose. Nevertheless, after treatment and extraction, tunicate cellulose is extremely crystalline (approximately 95%) and is composed of almost pure cellulose within the morphological form of high-issue ratio fibrils. Tunicate cellulose has a highly unique surface area of 170–150 m^2/g.

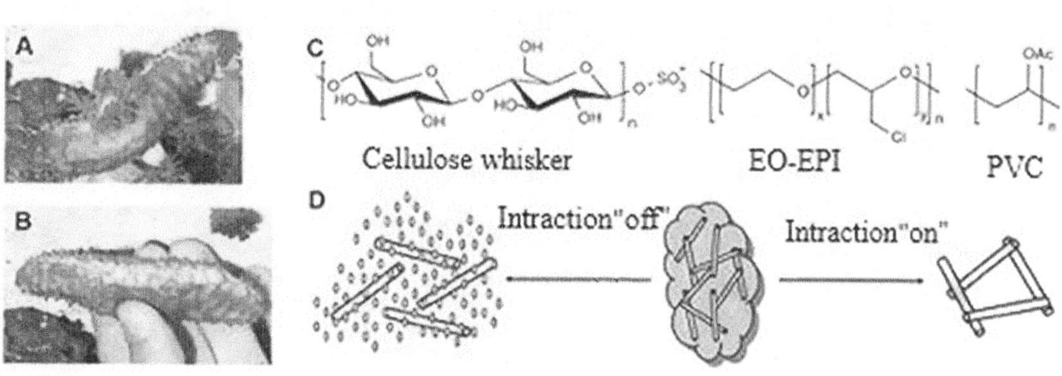

FIGURE 1.8 Tunicate cellulose. (Permission [84].)

Considering it has the hydroxyl groups, its surface is also reactive. It has been determined that the tunic cellulose polymerization degree falls between 700 and 3500 [83].

1.4.1.2 Types of Nanocellulose

Herbal cellulose, which is found in a variety of plants, animals, and microorganisms, is the source of nanocellulose. According to Figure 1.9, it may be categorized into four types: fibers, filaments, crystals, and micro/nanofibrils. These types are seen in the accompanying electron microscope image [85].

1.4.1.2.1 Cellulose Fibers

Cellulose is produced within the shape of microfibrils throughout the process of wood biosynthesis or flowers, and they subsequently combine to create cellulose fibers (Figure 1.9). Three geometries may be distinguished from cellulosic fibers: pulp fibers, which are extremely short fibers measuring 1–10 mm; staple fibers, which are rapid fibers measuring around 60 mm; and strand fibers, which are lengthy fibers measuring 20–100 cm [85]. A single, undamaged cell makes up a staple fiber, whereas a few cells make up a strand fiber. Staple fibers range in size from 25 to 45 mm, such as cotton fibers. Conversely, the short, few-millimeter-long threads that stay connected to the cotton seed are called cotton linters. Water retting is a technique used to concurrently extract staple and strand fibers from cultivated or wild plants. Conversely, the pulp fibers are often extracted by a pulping process from wood character cells and, on rare occasions, from plant sources including bananas, cotton linters, sisal, and fique. Pulping produces individual plant cells that may only be a few millimeters long by removing lignin from between cells with a huge volume of solution. [86].

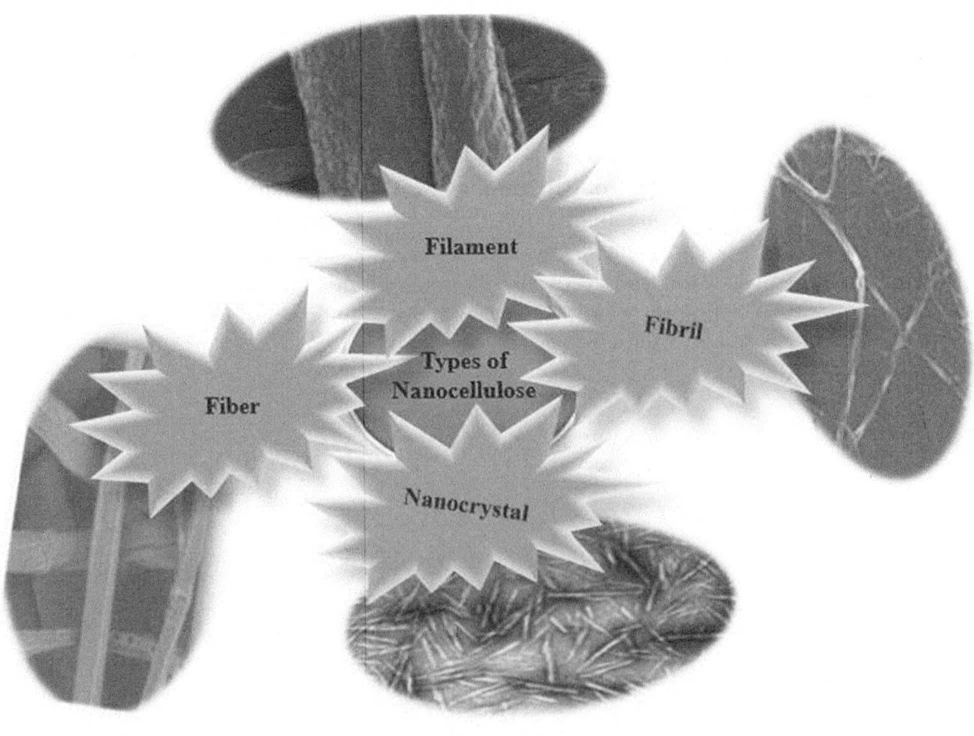

FIGURE 1.9 Types of nanocellulose.

1.4.1.2.2 Cellulose Filaments

The formation of filaments may be achieved by CNFs in a number of ways, such as wet extrusion, flow focusing, or spinning. Allomorph, crystallinity, and distinct physicochemical homes are displayed by these cellulose filaments; yet, they all share remarkable mechanical electricity, ductility, and high element ratios (Figure 1.9). These filaments are functional and show promise as biomedical application building blocks [87].

Additionally, there exists an awesome sort of cellulose filament that is received otherwise from the aforementioned techniques. This opportunity technique entails peeling cellulose fibers from wood or vegetation, the usage of merely mechanical methods, without the need for chemical substances, enzymes, or the era of effluent. The unique traits of those robotically peeled filaments cause them to be particularly attractive for biomedical packages [87].

1.4.1.2.3 Cellulose Crystals

It is possible to remove the highly crystalline sections of cellulose microfibrils by using the right mix of enzymatic, chemical, and/or mechanical treatments. This results in the creation of cellulose nanocrystals (CNCs; with a diameter in nanoscale) or microcrystalline cellulose (MCC; with a diameter on micron scale). The rigid rod-like detritus known as MCC and CNCs contains segments of cellulose chains that are almost perfectly crystalline [88]. MCC was initially marketed under the name Avicel®. The pharmaceutical industry was first exposed to Avicel® PH in 1964 by the Food Machinery Corporation as a direct tableting component. The Avicel® PH MCC period falls within the micrometer range. Presently, MCC is produced globally through around 10 sources. The most often used source of medicinal MCC is wood cellulose [89].

Through the hydrolysis of hydrochloric acid, alpha cellulose is partially depolymerized and refined into MCC. Because of its propensity for hydrolysis, MCC, a shorter and more crystalline fragment, is produced when the disordered areas of cellulose are partially depolymerized by acid hydrolysis. Because of its innate delivery protection, physiological inertness, manageability, and biodegradability, MCC is very compatible with active pharmaceutical ingredients (APIs). The round or rod-like particles in commercial MCC range in size from 10 to 200 μm [90]. The components of pharmaceutical MCC include cotton, hardwood, and softwood. MCC is an ideal choice for use as a filler in biocomposites because of its many advantages, including biodegradability, thermal balancing, pleasant mechanical characteristics, excessive elastic modulus, excessive component ratio, and occasional density. Furthermore, MCC's enormous floor area and high internal porosity offer the right cohesion for wetted bulk [91].

The cellulose microfibrils' removed crystalline portions are known as CNC debris. Native cellulose is hydrolyzed with sulfuric acid to produce purified CNCs. Forceful hydrolysis of sulfuric acid combined with ultrasonication of bulk cellulose causes a notable amount of crystalline CNC debris to break down, which may subsequently be recovered. Notable characteristics of CNCs include their high capacity to generate stable suspensions in a range of low-polarity solvents when a surfactant is introduced, thin ratio, huge exact surface area, high precise electricity and modulus, abundance, and reactive surfaces [92]. The form, length, and width of nanocrystals, for example, are dependent on the cellulose's availability and the extraction method, regulated acid hydrolysis temperature and duration, high-pressure homogenization conditions, and further adjustments such as neutralization and dialysis. Special sources can be organized into CNCs, including WC, PC, BC, algae, and tunicate cellulose [93].

Breaking down MCC debris can help isolate CNC debris. Following the sulfuric acid treatment of MCC particles, a robust CNC dispersion in water or other natural solvents is formed. Because the acid hydrolysis is diffusion-managed, CNCs often have a notably broad period distribution. Typically, the width is a few nanometers, the period is a few hundred nanometers, and the element ratio is between 10 and 67 for cotton, tunicin, and Capim dourado (golden grass) [94]. CNCs made from WC and PC typically have a period of 100–500 nm and a width of 3–30 nm, whereas cellulose generated from tunicates and microorganisms typically has a period of 100 nm to several microns and a width of 5–50 nm. In CNCs, the cellulose polymerization ranges from 500 to 15000. It has been proposed that CNC has a tensile strength of 7500–7700 MPa and an elastic modulus of 60–220 GPa [95]. Some nanocrystals possess extremely high specific energy, elastic moduli, excessive surface vicinity, and exact liquid crystalline characteristics in contrast to bulk cellulose, which contains larger, well-sized, disordered fractions. A lot of interest has been shown in CNC as an NP reinforcement due to its attractive properties, which include low density, excellent homogeneity and durability, and biodegradability. The far-reaching reinforcing influence on the whole matrix structure is facilitated by the nanocrystalline cellulose's short dimensions, high strength, and elastic modulus. Bionanocomposites, which are composed of nanocrystalline cellulose, are a versatile and flexible material that may be applied to several biological applications. These uses include wound dressings, medication administration, therapeutic implants, and scaffolds for tissue engineering and vascular grafts [96].

1.4.1.2.4 Cellulose Fibrils

The initial terminology for cellulose microfibrils was microfibrillated cellulose (MFC). These microfibrils are created by utilizing technologies like homogenization to robotically break down cellulose fibers, usually derived from wood, into micro- and nanofibrils. CNFs, which have a width of around 100 nm, are typically derived at low concentrations from wood or plant pulp aqueous solutions. However, CNFs may still contain substantial quantities of hemicellulose and lignin long after they disintegrate (Figure 1.9) [97].

A variety of methods, including enzymatic treatments and mechanical disintegration via homogenization and micro-fluidization, have been employed to get individual fibrils. In addition to carboxymethylation and TEMPO-catalyzed oxidation, chemical treatments have also been used to give the fibrils new functions and effectively disintegrate CNF. Commonly, the breadth of CNFs varies between 2 and 100 nm, contingent upon the source of cellulose, the traumatic inflammatory process, and the therapy. CNFs often have a period greater than 1 μm. Frequently, a series of crystalline and disordered domain names make up CNFs. In terms of mechanical characteristics, CNFs normally show an elastic modulus between 14 and 36 GPa and a final tensile electricity of around 1 GPa under ambient conditions. However, very high thresholds have been indicated [28].

1.4.1.3 Characteristics of Nanocomposites Based on Cellulose

1.4.1.3.1 Mechanical

The use of cellulose-based materials and their composites with inorganic materials and polymers is being used to build high-performance mechanical and functional materials. The strong intrinsic stiffness and strength of cellulose I crystals, when appropriately fabricated, result in materials with exceptional mechanical properties that are perfect for biomedical applications needing high mechanical performance. For example, intermolecular interactions like hydrogen bonding between cellulose chains give CNFs their amazing intrinsic mechanical characteristics (high specific modulus and strength) and exceptional crystallinity [98].

Along the cellulose chain axis, the elastic modulus of crystalline cellulose I has been shown to range from 124 to 155 GPa. The moduli of the rigid crystalline CNCs are similar to those of steel and Kevlar. Moreover, never-dried BC has amazing mechanical properties akin to soft tissue, and dried BC has been found to have a high elastic modulus of 60–115 GPa. Research on the mechanical properties of BC and how it interacts with smooth muscle cells shows that the geometry of individual nanofibrils, the network topologies of BC, and the stress-strain response are similar to those of a collagen network. Numerous studies have been conducted to improve collagen-based constructs because of their enormous potential for use in biological applications [99].

This offers chances for creative biomimetic scaffold design in which BC takes the role of the extracellular matrix's collagen network. Details on the mechanical properties of different types of cellulose from different sources are provided in Table 1.1. The data in Table 1.1 and the preceding

TABLE 1.1
Mechanical Characteristics of Various Cellulose

Type Cellulose	Method	Material	Young's Modulus (MPa)	Tensile Strength σ_{max}, (MPa)	Elongation at Break (ε_{max}) (%)	Reference
Bacterial cellulose (BC)	Dehydrated	Office paper (80 g/m^2)	302 ± 20.9	12.5 ± 0.9	6.0 ± 0.4	[101]
Bacterial cellulose (BC)	Dehydrated	Crude dry BC	180.3 ± 10.6	11.6 ± 0.8	8.2 ± 0.6	[101]
Bacterial cellulose (BC)	Dehydrated	Decellularized dry BC	428.0 ± 24.1	26.0 ± 1.6	7.5 ± 0.4	[101]
Bacterial cellulose (BC)	Dehydrated	Decellularized dry BC with calcium phosphate	491.8 ± 23.8	31.3 ± 2.2	6.1 ± 0.3	[101]
Bacterial cellulose (BC)	Dehydrated	Decellularized dry BC with colloid silver	432.8 ± 26.2	24.1 ± 2.8	8.0 ± 0.4	[101]
Bacterial cellulose (BC)	Wet (fresh and rehydrated)	Crude fresh BC	3.1 ± 0.5	1.2 ± 0.2	46.2 ± 3.5	[101]
Bacterial cellulose (BC)	Wet (fresh and rehydrated)	Decellularized wet BC	1.5 ± 0.3	0.28 ± 0.02	49.0 ± 3.6	[101]
Bacterial cellulose (BC)	Wet (fresh and rehydrated)	Crude rehydrated BC	127.2 ± 13.9	25.1 ± 1.8	21.1 ± 0.9	[101]
Bacterial cellulose (BC)	Wet (fresh and rehydrated)	Decellularized rehydrated BC	250.4 ± 20.1	31.4 ± 2.3	18.5 ± 0.8	[101]
Wood cellulose	Dehydrated	Senbo provided the hardwood pulpboard	—	77.22	14%	[102]
Wood cellulose	Esterified	—	—	45.4	318.4%	[103]
Cellulose	—	Ethyl cellulose (EC)	6.94	—	—	[104]
Cellulose	—	Cellulose nanofiber (CNF)	0.24	—	—	[104]
Plant cellulose	Prepared by AM	Wheat straw	0.32 ± 0.07–1.41 ± 0.07	29.1 ± 6.6–46.1 ± 15.0	—	[105]
Plant cellulose	Prepared by EM	Wheat straw	0.56 ± 0.10–1.21 ± 0.12	38.0 ± 1.8–65.1 ± 2.2	—	[105]
Plant cellulose	Distilled water	Raw bagasse (CNF and AgNPs were incorporated in PVA matrix)	—	0.004	—	[106]
Wood cellulose	Chemical precipitation	Cellulose (bleached softwood kraft pulp)—ZnO	—	202.0	—	[107]

discussion demonstrate how remarkable and promising cellulosic reinforcements' elastic modulus and tensile strength are for biomedical applications like tissue engineering, wound healing, and drug delivery—applications where robust and stable structures are essential [100].

1.4.1.3.2 Solubility

One major disadvantage of cellulose for biological applications is that it is insoluble in water and other common solvents due to the strong hydrogen bonds that hold its molecules together. Because of these connections, cellulose becomes intractable because it forms strong bundles with plenty of hydroxyl groups in combination with electrostatics and hydrophobic interactions. Although the precise function of hydrogen bonds in stabilization remains unclear, new research indicates that hydrophobic and electrostatic interactions are also important [108].

Complex solvents that dissolve cellulose with the least amount of energy are necessary to remedy this. It has been discovered that ionic liquids dissolve cellulose effectively and are well known for their low toxicity, thermal stability, recyclability, and environmental friendliness. These ionic liquids are 1-butyl-3-methylimidazolium formate (BMIMFmO), 1-butyl-3-methylimidazolium chloride (BmimCl), LiOH/urea, NaOH-urea, and N, N-dimethylacetamide/lithium chloride (DMAc/LiCl). Furthermore, 1-Ethyl3-methylimidazolium diethyl phosphate ([EMIM] DEP) is a helpful cellulose solvent due to its low viscosity, melting point, and stability in a cellulose solution over time [109].

Although these solvents have potential, their use is restricted by issues, including high energy consumption, expense, and solvent recovery problems. Because of its great recyclability and non-toxicity, N-methylmorpholine-N-oxide monohydrate ($NMMO \cdot H_2O$) has also been used as a solvent for the dissolving of cellulose. Innovative cellulose solvents with advantageous characteristics for biomedical usage are still of interest, given the diverse needs for various applications. Apart from the previously stated obstacles, the requirement for specific attributes, including non-toxicity, biocompatibility, and effortless extraction from the end result, has propelled the advancement of inventive cellulose solvents for biomedical applications [110]. Scholars are investigating new solvent solutions that satisfy these particular conditions and dissolve cellulose efficiently. In order to create and evaluate novel solvents that can get around the drawbacks of the available alternatives, this endeavor combines computational and experimental methods. By overcoming these challenges, the intention is to advance the use of cellulose in a range of biomedical applications, such as drug delivery systems and tissue engineering [111].

Gunathilake et al. investigated the application of biocompatible polymers in simulated drug delivery to enhance the release of nonionic/poorly soluble medicines. The results showed that when the concentration of CMC in the film grew, so did the film's ionic conductivity. The tensile characteristics of the film were successfully recovered with the addition of a tiny quantity of ZnO NPs (2%). The composite films showed a nearly linear drug release profile when exposed to an electric field. The picture had very little passive drug release when there was no electric field. The findings of this work made it easier to create an electrically sensitive nanocomposite platform for the delivery of nonionic, poorly water-soluble medications [112].

1.4.1.3.3 Hygroscopic

Although cellulose has remarkable mechanical qualities when dry, many applications are limited by its poor wet strength. This problem arises from the innate hygroscopic characteristic of cellulose, which causes water molecules to be drawn to and retained inside its structure through hydrogen bond formation. Water seeps mostly into the disordered domains; the proportion of these domains to the fiber saturation point is usually around 30%. Because cellulose swells in the water, aqueous processing of cellulose and cellulose-based hybrid and composite products can be beneficial [113].

Nevertheless, the hydrophilic surface of cellulose or embedded hydrophilic polymers allows liquid water or moist air to stick to it, which can cause products made from these materials to expand considerably. Materials based on nanocellulose have a higher surface area than fiber-based materials, which allows them to absorb more water and swell more. Moreover, water absorption is influenced by the osmotic swelling pressure generated by charged groups in chemically modified cellulose-based materials. These hygroscopic properties of cellulose are crucial in determining if a certain set of biological functions is suitable for it [114].

1.4.1.3.4 Toxicity

When it comes to biological applications, toxicity is a worry. Although cellulosic particles are obtained from non-toxic or low-toxic sources, their size, surface modification, hydrophilization, hydrophobization, and aggregation may all have an impact on their cytotoxicity and biocompatibility. It has been established that the nanoscale dimension of particles may have a role in producing toxicity in materials containing these particles. There are conflicting results on in vitro studies on the immunotoxicity, genotoxicity, and cytotoxicity of cellulose NPs. Furthermore, as a typical biological reaction to a foreign substance, inflammation frequently develops upon exposure to cellulose NPs, albeit it may eventually go away. Although attempts have been made to link cell toxicity in acute testing to the size and stiffness of cellulose NPs, no conclusive evidence of this relationship has been found. Thus, further investigation is required to fully understand the long-term effects of cellulose nanomaterials in vivo, as these effects can be different from the results of acute and in vitro studies [115, 116].

1.4.1.4 Applications in Biomedicine

A careful evaluation of a material's biocompatibility and cellular interactions is necessary for biomedical applications, particularly when the substance will be in close proximity to live tissue. Cytotoxic or other negative effects shouldn't occur. Among its many special qualities are its biodegradability, biocompatibility, abundance, sustainable resource availability, cheap production cost in comparison to synthetic biopolymers, non-toxicity, and superior mechanical capabilities. Because of these characteristics, cellulose can be a viable option for bioresorbable polymers, which are becoming more and more significant in biomedical applications. This is because cellulose can fully resorb in time periods that are predetermined, ranging from a few months to many years [117–119] (Figure 1.10).

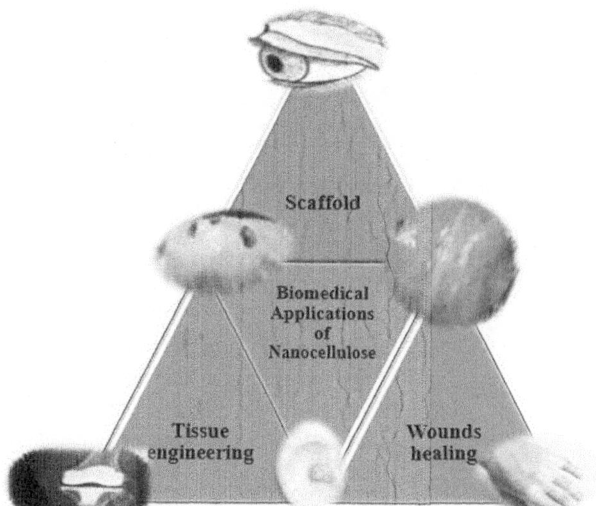

FIGURE 1.10 Biomedical applications of nanocellulose.

1.4.1.4.1 Tissue Engineering

The multidisciplinary area of tissue engineering uses concepts from the biology and engineering disciplines to create biological replacements that enhance, preserve, and repair damaged tissue functions. Biomaterials are typically used in this discipline to create medical intervention constructions. These structures interact with a variety of living biological entities, including the biomolecules, physiological fluids, cells, tissues, and organs of the human body (Table 1.2). It must have the optimal physical properties of regenerating tissue material, such as compressive strength for the production of bone tissue or tensile strength for the development of artificial blood vessels and soft tissue repairs. Chemical considerations are crucial, and the choice of material must take the intended usage into account. Examples of these include the surface chemistry of the materials. For instance, nanocellulosic materials may have their porosity, thickness, and interconnectivity changed without compromising their mechanical properties [117, 118, 120].

Tissue engineering commonly uses biomaterials to create physiologically appropriate scaffolds that aid in the attachment, growth, and differentiation of live cells. This facilitates tissue regeneration in in vivo and laboratory settings. Mammalian cells have trouble adhering to the hydrophilic cellulosic surfaces used in artificial tissue scaffolds; however, this can be improved by adding matrix ligands. For example, cellulose membranes can have ionic charges added to them to promote cellular adhesion and help absorb collagen [121]. Positively charged BC has demonstrated significant promise in dental and oral applications by improving cell adhesion without the need for proteins. The human body's functioning tissues and organs have been developed, repaired, and rejuvenated through the use of affordable biopolymeric materials. It has been proposed to utilize cellulose composites in place of [122].

With a β-glucose bond, hydroxyethyl cellulose is a nonionic polymer that dissolves in water and may be used in tissue engineering. Especially at high doses, it promotes cell proliferation and

TABLE 1.2
Biomedical Applications of Nanocellulose

Source	Type Cellulose	Application	Reference
Softwood cellulose	Nanocrystal	Bone tissue	[125]
Carboxymethyl cellulose (CMC)	—	Bone tissue	[126]
Rice husks biomass	Nanocrystals	Bone tissue	[127]
Bacterial cellulose	—	Bone tissue	[128]
Hydroxyethyl cellulose/CNC	Nanocrystal	Bone tissue	[129]
Microcrystalline cellulose powder (MCC)	Nanocrystals	Scaffold for cartilage tissue regeneration	[130]
Oxidized cellulose nanofibers suspension	Nanofibers	Scaffolds for tissue regeneration	[131]
Cellulose	Nanofiber	Scaffold	[132]
Bacterial cellulose	—	Scaffold	[133]
Cellulose acetate(CA)	Nanofiber	Bone tissue	[134]
Acetylated cellulose	Nanofiber	Scaffold for soft tissue	[135]
Cellulose acetate (CA)	Nanofiber	Bone tissue	[136]
Wood cellulose	Nanocrystals	Skin tissue	[137]
Cellulose	Nanocrystals	Scaffold for bone tissue	[138]
Ficus thonningii (FT)	Nanocrystals	Robust biomimetic scaffolds for bone tissue	[139]
Wheat straw	Nanofibers	Bone tissue	[140]
Bacterial cellulose	—	Scaffolds for bone repair	[141]

increases the viability of cells. Biomedical materials and equipment must have mechanical qualities that are appropriate for their intended use. For instance, the material's elastic modulus must roughly match that of the medium or tissue it reinforces or replaces. Nanocrystalline cellulose possesses exceptional mechanical properties and is biocompatible, which makes it a promising material for enhancing cell adhesion and proliferation [123]. Its high aspect ratio construction components are mechanically entangled and hydrogen bonded together to produce a natural fiber network. One way to strengthen this network even further is to cross-link individual nanofibers. Regarding biomaterials made of nanocellulose, including hydrogels, electrospun nanofibers, composites, and membranes, a variety of biological species are cultivated. A common option for cell culture is bacterial nanocellulose, which is renowned for its excellent porosity, biodegradability, and low toxicity. In order to allow wounded tissue to be restored to function and be replaced by healthy tissue, it is imperative that the pace of scaffold degradation under particular conditions matches the rate of tissue creation [124].

1.4.1.4.2 Wound Dressing

In order to minimize dehydration, lower the risk of bacterial infection, and restore barrier functioning, the process of wound healing involves a vast array of biological processes. Skin grafting and burn wounds require the development of new materials for wound dressings. The use of cellulose-based polymers in wound dressings has several potential uses [142]. When it comes to wound dressing materials, they ought to encourage porosity and dryness, which deters bacterial adhesion, as well as high water absorption capacity or water retention. In this case, the cellulosic material has to be formed into a sheet and applied to wounds as a dressing (Table 1.3). Making bandages with drugs embedded in them made of cellulose is a very good idea. Because nanocellulose may be applied directly to the site, it has significant potential for use in wound-healing applications [143]. By absorbing and holding onto water, it can lessen inflammatory responses and promote fibroblast proliferation in the wound-healing cascade. Nanofibrillar cellulose is an ideal matrix for wound healing because of its high porosity, high water-holding capacity, and high surface area-to-volume ratio. Moreover, its design allows for the replication of extracellular matrix, tissues, and organs. Nanofibrillar cellulose hydrogel is a novel material for controlling excessive wound contraction both in vivo and in vitro [144].

The most promising materials for wound dressings are Because of their high water bonding affinity, swelling capacity, biodegradability, biocompatibility with mucosal membranes and skin, and lack of

TABLE 1.3
Biomedical Applications of Nanocellulose

Source	Type Cellulose	Application	Reference
Bacterial cellulose	—	Wound dressing	[149]
Cellulose nanofibrils	Nanofibers	Topical wound delivery	[150]
Cellulose nanofibrils	Nanofibers	Wound therapy	[151]
Cellulose acetate	Nanofibers	Wound dressing	[152]
Wood cellulose	Nanofibers	Wound dressing	[153]
Bacterial cellulose	—	Antibacterial wound dressing	[154]
Plantago ovata (PO) seed husk	Hemicellulose (Arabinoxylan (AX))	Antibacterial wound-dressing	[155]
Cellulose nanofibrous gel	Nanofiber	Hemorrhage control material	[156]
Rosemary dried	Nanofibrils	Wound dressing	[157]
Oxidated sodium carboxymethyl cellulose	—	Hemostasis and infected wound treatment	[158]

toxicity, nanofibrillar cellulosics—such as CMC and CA—have gained attention in the scientific community. Because oxidized CNF has well-dispersed cellulose fibrils and a substantial water absorption capacity, it is also a good choice for wound healing. In order to reduce the resulting pain load in patients, several adjustments must be made while using CMC in wound healing [145]. There have been reports of synechia, postoperative hemorrhage, and modest degrees of localized discomfort associated with dissolvable CMC foam dressing. The minimal amounts of postoperative bleeding and synechia development that have been noted allow it to be utilized as a wound dressing following sinus surgery. BC-based nanocomposites are made by mixing magnetic NPs with cellulose culture medium for efficient chronic wound healing. It has been proposed that plant-based CNC-containing bionanocomposites, which accelerate tissue regeneration, might function as useful templates for wound healing [146]. In biocomposites, CA is also a good option for the scaffold used in wound healing once electrospun nanofibers are developed. Because of its hydrophilicity and bioactivity, CA can interact with fibroblasts intracellularly, which encourages cell division. BC's advantageous qualities, including biocompatibility, non-toxicity, and mechanical stability, make it an attractive option for wound-healing applications. Furthermore, BC keeps the wound wet, hastening the healing process. Although BCs provide an acceptable environment on-site when used as wound dressings, their capacity to promote healing may be hampered by the pH levels. To create biomaterials based on BC that have improved qualities and are appropriate for wound dressing, several materials have been combined. Without causing any negative side effects, for use in therapeutic applications, BC-montmorillonite-reinforced composites have been developed as materials for wound healing and regeneration [143, 147].

BC-chitosan membranes have demonstrated a high degree of wound dressing compatibility and antibacterial activity. Membranes derived from BC have surpassed TegadermTM, a commercial wound dressing product, in terms of epithelialization and skin regeneration. In addition, the BC membrane accelerates wound healing in a burn model system by regulating angiogenesis and connective tissue formation. Hydrogel microparticles based on BC have been employed as a dressing material for burn wounds that are somewhat thick, both in vitro and in vivo. Because of its strong ability to absorb water, antimicrobial properties, and evenly distributed cellulose fibers, oxidized BC is an additional cellulose substance that is valuable for the healing of wounds [148].

1.4.1.4.3 Drug Delivery

The exact amount of medication released at predetermined times to certain organs is known as a drug delivery system. These systems distribute drugs to certain organs, tissues, or cells by processes that may be tuned to respond to environmental signals such as light, temperature, pH, chemical reactions, and electric and magnetic fields. Cellulose has long been used in the pharmaceutical industry to coat tablets after being mixed with various excipients for oral administration. Research is currently ongoing to determine how cellulose and its derivatives could be used in complex drug-loaded systems; extended drug release as novel carriers or tablet dissolving rates as excipients are given special attention. As a means of delivering medication, cellulosic materials have to possess controlled diffusive properties and dissolvability (Table 1.4). For example, cellulose and its derivatives have proven certain drug delivery patterns, such as immediate, controlled, or delayed release in oral dosage forms. Furthermore, because cellulosic materials are naturally resistant to the stomach's acidic environment, they can be used as enteric coatings on tablets or capsules [159, 160].

Compound drugs are used ad hoc when a certain dosage or form is desired but not available commercially, or when adherence to a specific regimen is necessary. In compounded pharmaceuticals, powdered cellulose and MCC function as thickening, stabilizing, and capsule diluents. MCC responds to the strain rate and exhibits viscoelastic characteristics. Elastic effects are especially important in high-speed tableting since there is less time for plastic deformation. As a result, the reliance of MCC on the strain rate needs to be considered in the formulation design and dose [160].

Because of their elasticity, low toxicity, low density, reactive surface, and flexibility, CNFs hold great promise for use in biomedicine as carriers for regulated drug administration. They are cheap,

TABLE 1.4
Biomedical Applications of Nanocellulose

Source	Application	Reference
Carboxymethyl cellulose	Oral anticancer drug	[164]
Bacterial cellulose	Carrier materials for controlled protein drug	[165]
Polyethylene oxide-cellulose	Drug delivery vehicle	[166]
Cellulose	pH-controlled delivery of curcumin	[167]
Rice straw waste(nanowhisker)	Colorectal cancer treatment	[168]
Hydroxypropyl cellulose	Drug delivery	[169]
Carboxymethyl cellulose	pH-sensitive nanocarrier for curcumin drug	[170]
WTP	Drug delivery	[171]
Eucalyptus globulus cellulose nanofibrils (CNF)	Vancomycin drug release	[172]
Mucoadhesive cellulose nanocrystal	Delivery of hydrophobic compounds	[173]
Carboxymethyl cellulose	Improved 5-FU delivery	[174]
Cellulose nanocrystals (CNCs)	Hard capsule for drug delivery	[175]

renewable, and useful for grafting certain groupings. It is believed that the rheological, barrier, and physicochemical characteristics of CNFs enable them to stabilize the interfaces between oil and water as well as air and water. Moreover, the higher surface area per mass unit of CNFs aids in the stabilization of NPs and raises the possibility of a beneficial chemical interaction with poorly soluble pharmaceuticals. CNFs have been used as film formers with immediate release properties for medicines that are poorly soluble, as matrix formers for long-term sustained drug release, and as stabilizers for crystalline drug NPs. After drug adsorption, CNFs can be freeze-dried to turn into an aerogel. Plant-based CNFs have been successfully used as an injectable drug-releasing hydrogel in mice, demonstrating potential as a matrix for targeted local distribution or controlled release of medicinal substances in humans [161, 162].

One of the most popular hydrophilic biodegradable polymers, hydroxypropyl methylcellulose, is approved by the US Food and Drug Administration (FDA) for use in controlled-release formulations. Injectable chitosan/glycerophosphate thermosensitive solutions containing hydroxypropyl methylcellulose microparticles loaded with vancomycin are developed for the local treatment of osteomyelitis. Because of its porous and spongy structure, hydroxypropyl methylcellulose hydrogel has a long-term release profile in vitro, making it an extremely promising substance for sustained antibiotic treatment [163].

1.4.2 Chitosan

Chitosan, whose chemical formula is $(C_6H_{11}O_4N)_n$, is chitin in a deacetylated state. Poly β (1-4-→) structural units make up its constitution. -2-amino-2-deoxy-D-glucopyranose and various degrees of deacetylation (DD) can be found. It shares a structure with cellulose, but chitosan has an amine functional group (2NH) at carbon number 2 in lieu of cellulose's hydroxy group (OH) (Figure 1.11) [176].

1.4.2.1 Characteristics of Nanocomposites Based on Chitosan

1.4.2.1.1 Physical–Chemical Properties

Many unique characteristics of chitosan encompass mucosal adhesion, movie formation, chelation, viscosity, solubility in exclusive substrates, polyelectrolyte conduct, and salt polyoxygenation. The annealing situations can be changed to change the viscosity of chitosan. Because it affects both its

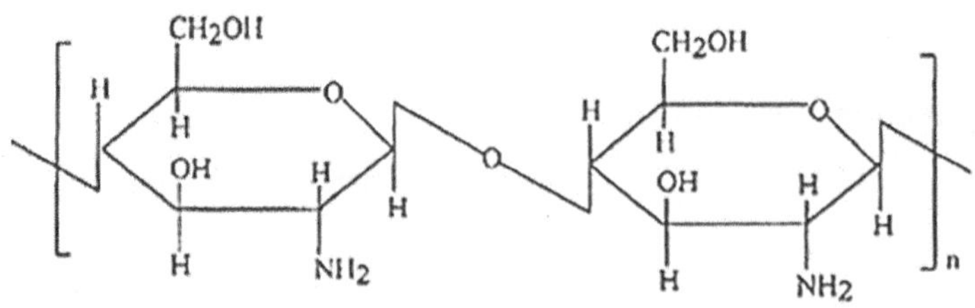

FIGURE 1.11 Structure of chitosan. (Permission [177].)

chemical and bodily traits, chitosan's structure is crucial. Because of its low crystalline region attention and excessive diploma of deacetylation, it's far from an applicable choice for a wide variety of actual-global packages, which include biotechnology and pharmaceuticals [178].

A wide variety of variables, consisting of the degree of deacetylation (DD), crystallinity, molecular weight, and breakdown techniques, have an effect on the chemical and bodily traits of chitosan. The percent of acetyl groups in chitin which can be converted to amine agencies in chitosan is called the deacetylation degree. It has been mentioned that the order and distribution of metal corporations, as well as DD, have an inverse dating with the fee of chitosan breakdown. Significantly slower degradation charges are produced by way of better DD, while faster degradation rates are produced via lower DD. Both high molecular weight and coffee molecular weight industrial chitosan are available [179]. The system of dissolving chitosan in diluted SD entails leaving the amino practical organization in its molecular chain with the protons of hydrogen present within the aqueous solution, turning it right into a polyelectrolyte with a fantastic charge. Chitosan molecules are eliminated by the solvent's cations, which causes them to dissolve in water. Furthermore, the molecular weight and DD of chitosan have an impact on its solvent. Higher DD often results in less complex disintegration and a higher degree of protonation of useful amino structures within the molecular chain. Larger molecular weight chitosan forms greater intramolecular bonds and intermolecular bonds in its chains, making them more intertwined and tough to dissolve [180].

1.4.2.1.2 Characteristics of Chitosan Nanostructures

Chitosan nanostructures are non-toxic, biodegradable, hydrophilic, and quite powerful in getting rid of dye waste. In the separation procedure, nano-sized adsorbents feature better than micro-sized adsorbents [181].

1.4.2.1.3 Solubility

Deacetylating chitin results in the conversion of certain N-acetylglucosamine moieties into glucosamine units, which is how chitosan is made. The high concentration of protonated -NH2 groups in the chitosan structure allows it to dissolve in acidic aqueous conditions, with a pKa of around 6.5. A few factors that influence chitosan solubility are temperature, pH, polymer crystallinity, degree of acetylation, and polymer molecular weight. When chitin is deacetylated homogeneously (by alkali treatment at 0°C), it can produce polymers that are soluble in aqueous acetic acid solutions, even at low DD values of 28%. This is not achievable with heterogeneous deacetylation (by alkali treatment at high temperatures) [182–184]. Furthermore, the samples exhibit water solubility at a DD of 49%. This effect is hypothesized to be caused by homogeneous deacetylation, which increases the quantity of glucosamine units and alters the polymer's crystalline structure. Depending on the polymer DD, these modifications can range from a reduction in crystal size and perfection to the emergence of a new crystal structure that resembles β-chitin [185].

1.4.2.1.4 Biological Characteristics

Because of its unique characteristics, chitosan can be utilized in a variety of methods. Its non-poisonous, biodegradable, functional, biocompatible, exceptionally antibacterial, and antiseptic features are responsible for its explosive upward thrust inside the scientific enterprise. Because of these characteristics, chitosan is the best packaging cloth for retaining the safety and quality of food. Its negative water solubility, however, limits its use (Table 1.5) [186].

1.4.2.2 Applications in Biomedicine

1.4.2.2.1 Drug Delivery

Chitosan is a great medication carrier since it is non-toxic, readily forms a film, is biocompatible, and can be absorbed by the body. Chitosan's complete absorption by the tissue as a result of its breakdown by lysozyme in the human body after drug release is the main advantage of employing it as a drug carrier. This advantage has led to it being the primary area of study in this subject. Generally speaking, chitosan can be used to dissolve, coat, or combine medications to provide sustained-release films, gels, pills, microspheres, microcoatings, etc. (Figure 1.12) (Table 1.6) [198, 199].

1.4.2.2.2 Wound Dressing

Preventing wound infection throughout the healing process is essential, as it is a multifaceted and ever-changing process. The 6 stages of wound healing include hemostasis, inflammation, cell migration, vascularization, collagen deposition, and re-epithelialization. Skin tissue requires the N-subunit (NAG) in chitosan to be repeated in order for wounds to heal. Because of its high surface positive charge, chitosan encourages cell proliferation, which causes blood clotting and thrombosis. Additionally, unbound amine functional groups on the chitosan film's surface have the ability to combine with the acidic groups in blood cells to create a complex. Because of this property, chitosan is a substance that may be used to treat wounds and hasten their healing (Table 1.7) [234, 235].

TABLE 1.5
Biological Chitosan

Microorganism(s)	Findings	Reference
P. aeruginosa *E. coli* *S. aureus* *Salmonella typhi* *Klebsiella pneumoniae*	Significant antibacterial activity	[187]
E. coli *S. aureus*	Shows significant antibacterial effects	[188]
S. epidermidis	Inhibits bacterial biofilm and exhibits synergism with antibiotics	[189]
S. aureus	Shows antibacterial activity	[190]
E. coli	Inhibits bacterial growth	[191]
E. faecalis	Enhances the antibacterial properties	[192]
C. albicans *E. coli* *S. aureus*	Shows significant antimicrobial activity	[193]
E. coli *S. aureus*	Provides bactericidal activity directly to the wound site	[194]
Candida glabrata	Acts synergistically with clotrimazole against non-albicans Candida strains	[195]
Methicillin-resistant S. aureus	Antibacterial activity against resistant strains	[196]
Candida species	Anti-Candida activity	[197]

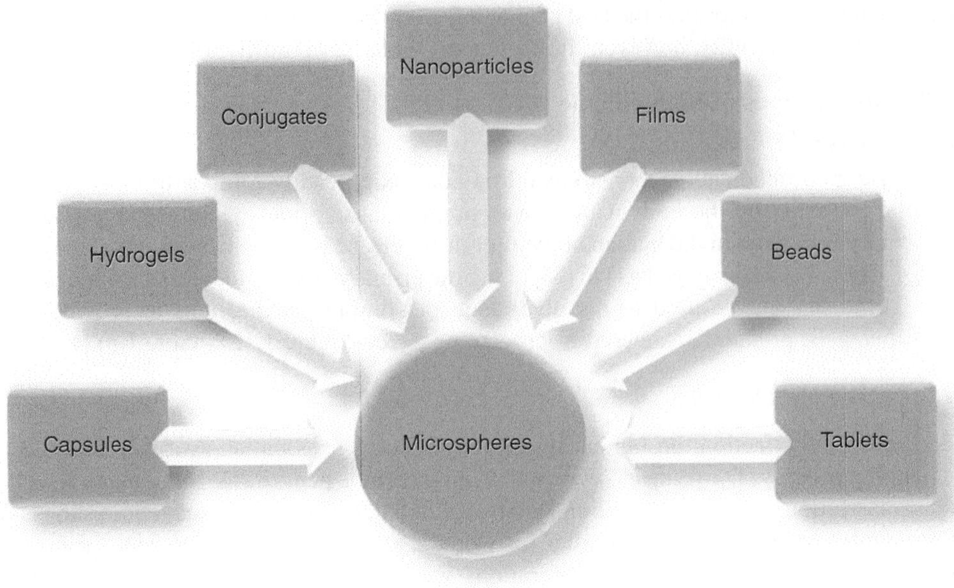

FIGURE 1.12 Chitosan-based medication delivery methods.

1.4.3 Chitin

French professor Henri Braconnot made the initial discovery of chitin, a naturally occurring polymer, in mushrooms in 1811. With an annual output of 1010 to 1011 tons, after cellulose, it is the second most common biopolymer. Chitin resembles cellulose in many aspects and is thought of as a derivative of cellulose with acetamido residues instead of the C_2 hydroxyl groups. Natural crystalline microfibrils, which are structural components found in a large range of animals, are known to include chitin. The commercial value of chitin has recently increased due to the beneficial properties of its soluble derivatives, which are helpful for a variety of industrial applications in biotechnology, agriculture, food processing, cosmetics, veterinary care, medicine, dentistry, environmental protection, and paper or textile production [246, 247].

Chitin is a widely dispersed polymer that is found in many one-of-a-kind types of animals, along with the cuticles of bugs, the endoskeleton of cephalopods discovered in mollusks, and the cell partitions of fungi and algae. It is a broadly diagnosed element determined in mushrooms and plays a sizeable position inside the exoskeletons of bugs and different arthropods. Crustaceans (shrimp, crabs, prawns, lobsters, and krill) provide over 75% of their whole weight as waste that is often applied to isolate chitin. In actuality, there may be an annual surplus of over 10,000 lots of shellfish waste that may be used as a suitable uncooked cloth to supply chitin [247, 248]. Amino sugars, or N-acetylglucosamine and glucosamine, are monomeric additives discovered in chitin. It is made of linear, unbranched chains of polysaccharide residues that are β-(1 → 4) related to 2-acetamido-2-deoxy-D-glucose (N-Acetyl-D-glucosamine). Because chitin incorporates extremely little glucosamine, it's miles much less soluble in water and solvents [249].

Chitin's linear structure, stability, and stiffness are attributed to the β-1,4-linkage that exists between monomeric gadgets. The several hydroxyl and amino corporations within the polymer have the tendency to create hydrogen bonds in each interior and between molecules, which results in the improvement of linear aggregates with a massive degree of crystallinity [250]. Chitin's molecular weight (Mw) can reach up to 10 Da. Figure 1.13 indicates the structure of chitin. Three distinct polymeric forms of chitin—α, β, and γ—each with precise bodily characteristics, may be discovered

TABLE 1.6
Chitosan-Based Medication Delivery Methods

Nanocomposite Type	Drug Used	Drug Type	Reference
Thiolated chitosan nanoparticles	Insulin	Oral	[200]
Snail mucin/CS NPs	Insulin	Oral	[201]
CS/Dz13Scr NPs	insulin	Oral	[202]
CS NPs	Polydatin	Oral	[203]
FD/CS NPs	Methotrexate (MTX)	Oral	[204]
Cys/PLA/CS NPs	Paclitaxel (PTX)	Oral	[205]
TPGS/HPMC/CS NPs	Paclitaxel (PTX)	Oral	[206]
CS/WP-NPs	Polysaccharides from Ophiopogon japonicus (OJPs)	Oral	[207]
ALG/CS NPs anchored with lipopolysaccharide (LPS) as an adjuvant	HBsAg antigen	Oral	[208]
Soy lecithin/CS hybrid NPs	Raloxifene hydrochloride (RLX)	Oral	[209]
GCS NPs	Dexamethasone (DEX)	Ocular	[210]
CS/LIP	Triamcinolone acetonide (TA)	Ocular	[211]
CS or CS maleimide NPs	Japanese encephalitis-chimeric virus vaccineNasal vaccine	Nasal	[212]
PLGA NPs and PLGA/CS NPs	Ropinirole hydrochloride	Nose	[213]
N,O-CMC NPs	Dopamine (DOPA) or Tyrosine (Tyr)	Nose	[214]
CS NPs	Therapy for Huntington's disease	Nose	[215]
CS NPs	Zolmitriptan (ZOL)	Nose	[216]
CS NPs	Rotigotine (R)	Nose	[217]
CS NPs	Nicotine hydrogen tartrate (NHT)	Pulmonary	[218]
CS/PLGA NPs followed by coating with chitosan	Catechin hydrate (CTH)	Pulmonary	[219]
CS/SLNs	Rifampicin (RIF)	Pulmonary	[220]
Mn-TMC NPs	Etofylline (ETO)	Pulmonary	[221]
HA/CS NPs	Ferulic acid (FA)	Pulmonary	[222]
CS NPs	Oxiplatin	Buccal	102
CS/PEO NFs	Sublingval delivery	Buccal	[223]
Core-sheath NFs: shell layer: CS Core: PVA containing drug	Etracycline hydrochloride (TH)	Periodontal	[224]
CS/IO NPs	Chlorhexidine (CHX)	Periodontal	[225]
CS NPs	Nicotinamide	Dermal	[226]
CS NFs	Colchicine	Transdermal	[227]
PCL/CS NFs	Curcumin (CUR)	Wound	[228]
Hydrogel membranes based on HA/PU/PVA loaded with cefepime-CS NPs	Cefepime	Wound	[229]
CS and spicules NPs	Calophycin A (Cal A)	Vaginal	[230]
CS and ALG-coated CS NPs	Hepatitis A vaccine (HAV)	Vaccine	[231]
TMC/DS or ALG NPs	hSET1 antisense—silencing oligonucleotide	Gene	[232]
CS NPs	Doxorubicin (DOX) and Bcl-2 siRNA co-delivery of therapeutics and si-RNA	Gene	[233]

TABLE 1.7
Chitosan-Based Wound Dressing

System Wound Dressings	Application	Reference
Chitosan/polyvinyl alcohol with tea tree	Anti-infection wound dressing	[236]
Chitosan, gelatin, and polyhydroxybutyrate	The regeneration of rat excisional wounds	[237]
N,N,N-trimethyl chitosan capped bimetallic nanoparticles	MDR microbial-infected wounds	[238]
Vanillin-infused chitosan-PVA hydrogel reinforced by nanocellulose and CuO-Ag nanoparticles	Antibacterial wound dressing	[239]
Polycaprolactone membrane and chitosan-carrageenan hydrogel incorporating storax balsam	Wound healing	[240]
Chitosan-based emulgel and xerogel film with Thymus pubescens	Wound dressing	[241]
Chitosan-based POSS-PEG hybrid hydrogel	Promote diabetic wound healing	[242]
Chitosan hydrogel	Antibacterial properties for skin wound dressing	[243]
Carboxymethyl chitosan	Wound antibacterial and hemostasis	[244]
Chitosan/calcium phosphate	Hemostatic wound dressing	[245]

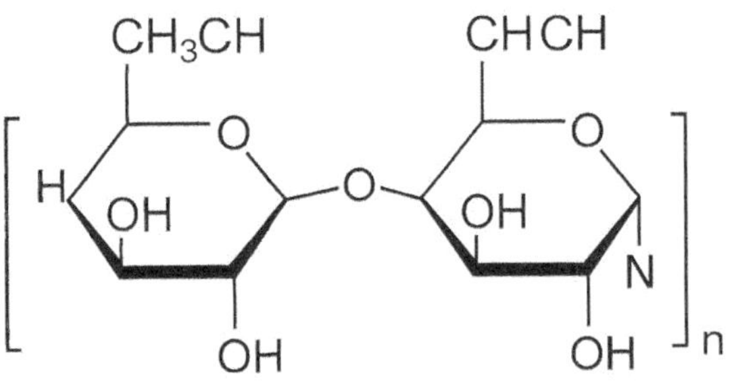

FIGURE 1.13 Different polymeric configurations of chitin.

in nature [251]. Figure 1.14 illustrates how the polymeric chain is organized otherwise in this bureaucracy. α-chitin reveals anti-parallel chain arrangements, β-chitin shows parallel chain arrangements, and γ-chitin shows a random chain arrangement. Together, those polymeric chains create a polymeric structure along with parallel chains and one anti-parallel chain [252].

Crustaceans like shrimp and crabs are the principal supply of α-chitin, whereas loligo is the supply of γ-chitin and squids of β-chitin. Chitin's molecular mass and degree of deacetylation (DDA) are its distinguishing characteristics. These might trade relying on the chitin's origin, method, and separation method [253]. The degree of deacetylation is the molar percentage of deacetylated monomer devices in the chitin polymer chain. The difference between chitosan and chitin is made feasible by using the DDA content material. It is called chitin if the DDA is much less than 50% and chitosan if the DDA is more than 50%. The maximum extensive detail influencing chitin's solubility, flexibility, polymer conformation, and viscosity is DDA [254].

Traditionally, three primary chemical steps—deproteinization, demineralization, and bleaching—are used to dispose of chitin from the exoskeletons of crustaceans. While demineralization is typically finished at temperatures between 90°C and 100°C with the use of acidic solutions like HCl, HNO_3, H_2SO_4, CH_3COOH, and HCOOH, deproteinization includes treating the shells in alkaline solutions like NaOH and KOH. Lastly, colorless chitin is finished by means of bleaching. As an

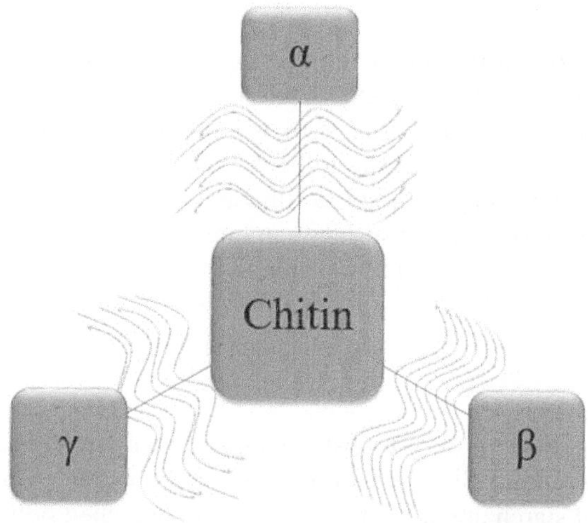

FIGURE 1.14 Chemical structure of chitin. (Permission [177].)

opportunity, biological strategies for extracting chitin may be used, in which microbial extracellular proteases instead of alkaline answers are used to induce deproteinization [255].

Crustacean shell demineralization is accomplished by employing natural probiotic organisms in conjunction with enzymatic and microbiological techniques. For the extraction of chitin, the microbiological approach works better than the chemical approach. In the biological process, demineralization and deproteinization occur together. When lactic acid bacteria break down the shell waste of shrimp (Penaeus monodon) to recover chitin, they utilize carbohydrates as a natural energy source [256].

1.4.3.1 Applications in Biomedicine

1.4.3.1.1 Tissue Engineering

Chitin can be used to create scaffolds for tissue engineering of bone and cartilage. Similar methods might be used to use chitin scaffolds to regenerate other tissues or organs. Moreover, the adaptability of chitin in 3D scaffolds and as an injectable hydrogel customized with particular biomolecules presents a multitude of opportunities for various tissue engineering applications (Table 1.8) [257].

TABLE 1.8
Chitin for Tissue Engineering Applications

System	Application	Reference
Apatite/chitin/pectin	Scaffolds in orthopedics	[257]
Chitosan/chitin	Cartilage tissue engineering	[258]
Chitinous	3D Scaffold	[259]
Chitin whisker/poly(l-lactide)	Bone tissue	[260]
Chitin-glucan polysaccharide	Fungal-scaffolds	[261]
Chitin/glucan-and cellulose	3D Scaffolds for skin	[262]
Chitin	Dental pulp regeneration	[263]
Chitin	Dental pulp stem cells	[264]
Chitin	Scaffold combined with autologous repairs sciatic nerve defects	[265]
Carboxymethyl chitin	Osteoinduction effect on the human periodontal ligament stem cells	[266]

1.4.3.1.2 Wound Healing

Preventing wound infection during the healing process is crucial, given its complex and dynamic nature. Inflammation, cell migration, vascularization, temporary bed preparation, collagen deposition, and re-epithelialization are the 6 stages of wound healing. The repetition of the N-subunit (NAG) in chitin is essential for skin tissue to heal wounds. Chitin's high positive surface charge promotes cell proliferation, leading to blood clotting and thrombosis. Moreover, the unbound amine functional groups on the chitosan film's surface can interact with acidic groups in blood cells, forming a complex. This property makes chitin a suitable material for wound dressings and expediting wound healing (Table 1.9) [267].

1.4.4 Starch

Depending on the source, plant tissues store starch as insoluble semicrystalline granules with unique sizes, shapes, and architectures. Starch is a polymeric carbohydrate. The two homopolymers (glucans) that make up local starch are amylopectin, a highly branched polymer, and amylose, a linear polymer, together with minor additions like lipids and proteins (Figure 1.15). The distribution of amylose and amylopectin, whose ratios vary depending on the starch supply due to differences in cultivation conditions and geographic starting point, impacts the granule form of starch [275].

With a molecular weight of 10^5–10^6 and a DP that can exceed 600, amylose is a linear polymer. It is mostly composed of α-D (1, 4) repeating units. The structure's many hydroxyl groups demonstrate the polymer's hydrophilic qualities, giving the substance a significant affinity for moisture. The highly branched polymer amylopectin, on the other hand, is made up of short α-1, 4 chains connected by α-1, 6 bonds holding between 10 and 60 glucose units, and side chains holding between 15 and 45 glucose units. Amylopectin has a molecular weight between 10^7 and 10^9 [276].

Starch exhibits three distinct types of crystallinity. The C type, which is frequently seen in beans and other root starches, combines the polymorphic A and B type crystallinity patterns. The B type is derived from tubers like potatoes, cassava, and sago, whereas the A type is mostly found in cereal starches like maize, wheat, and rice. The concentration of amylose/amylopectin and the size of its granules dictate the properties of starch, including its ability to absorb water, gelatinize and paste, undergo retrogradation, and be vulnerable to enzyme attacks. The functional properties of starches

TABLE 1.9
Chitin for Wound Healing

System	Application	Reference
Gold@Halloysite nanotubes-chitin	Antibacterial and hemostatic	[267]
Imidazolium salt chitin	Antimicrobial activity for infected wound healing	[268]
β-Chitin nanofibers	Construct-oriented cryogel for wound healing	[269]
Chitin/PEGDE-tannic acid	Antibacterial, antioxidant, hemostatic	[270]
Hydroxypropyl chitin	Antibacterial, non-invasive visualization, and wound healing	[271]
Silver NPs-incorporated quaternized chitin	Antibacterial for infected wound healing	[23]
AgNP@ zeolite/chitin/bamboo	Antibacterial hemostatic for wound healing without heat injury	[272]
Corn stalk-modified chitin	Hemostasis and promoting wound healing	[68]
β-Chitin nanofiber	Promote wound healing in rats	[273]
Chitin derivatives, egg white protein, and montmorillonite	Antibacterial and hemostatic effects for promoting wound healing	[274]

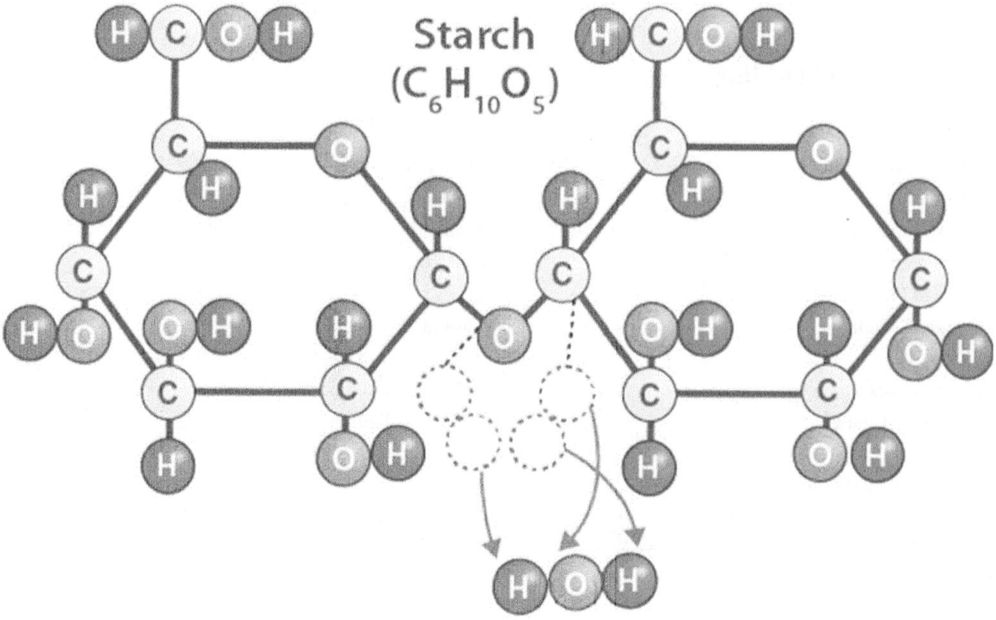

FIGURE 1.15 Chemical structure of starch.

are also influenced by factors such as chemical modification, system composition, pH, and medium ionic strength [277].

1.4.4.1 Applications in Biomedicine

1.4.4.1.1 Drug Delivery

Natural polysaccharides, such as starch, cellulose, and their derivatives, have been thoroughly studied and assessed by researchers for many years, both in vitro and in vivo, and their results have demonstrated that they are safe and well-tolerated drug carriers. The significant potential of these polymers for the development of innovative and secure therapeutic formulations is demonstrated by recent advancements in the manufacturing of starch-loaded medicine microparticles (Table 1.10) [278].

1.4.5 Polylactide

Aliphatic polyesters like PLA are made from renewable resources, including potatoes, maize, and sugar (Figure 1.16). Temperature of production, molecular weight, and isomer composition are some of the variables that affect its qualities. Poly(D-lactic acid) (PDLA), poly(L-lactic acid) (PLLA), and the racemic mix D,L-PLA (PDLLA) are the three primary forms of PLA. Each has a unique microstructure. Whereas PDLA is always amorphous, semicrystalline PLLA and PDLLA have somewhat differing glass transition temperatures. The ratio of D to L enantiomers determines the degree of crystallization and polymer reactivity. These PLA variations' particular uses are determined by their distinct architectures. For example, because of its monophasic structure, PDLLA is chosen in drug delivery systems, while PLLA is recommended in applications that need strong mechanical qualities. However, pure PLA materials have drawbacks such as poor osteoinduction, brittleness, and unpredictable rates of breakdown [287, 288].

PLA-based nanocomposites, which are made up of PLA-based copolymers at the nanoscale, as well as nanocomposites with PLA or PLA copolymers as the matrix and nanofillers as annexing agents, have shown a lot of promise in the biomedical field. Because of the small-scale and surface

TABLE 1.10
Chitin for Wound Healing

System	Drug	Reference
2-Hydroxyethyl starch	Ketoprofen, ofloxacin	[279]
Freeze-dried potato starch	Resveratrol	[280]
Crosslinked retrograded starch	Ketoprofen	[275]
Cassava starch	S. guianensis essential oil	[281]
Debranched lentil starch	Rutin	[282]
Retrograded starch	5-Fluorouracil	[278]
Starch	Camelia sinensis extract	[283]
Corn and tapioca starch	Bovine serum albumin	[284]
Carboxymethyl starch	Bovine serum albumin	[276]
Starch/zein	Fucoxanthin	[285]
Taro succinylated starch	Pomegranate seed oil	[286]
Maltodextrin, sweet potato starch	Lactiplantibacillus plantarum (probiotics)	[277]

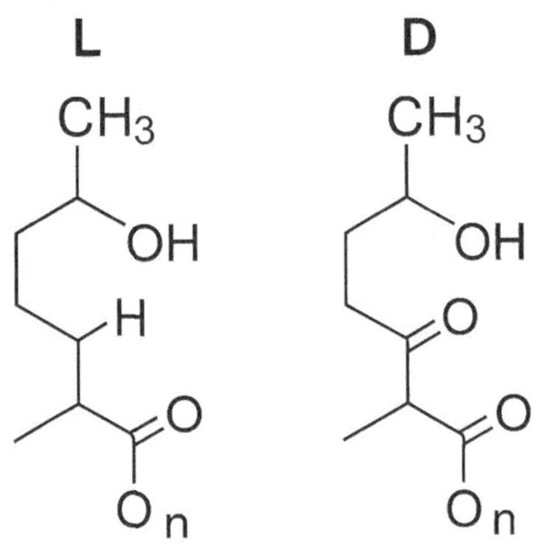

FIGURE 1.16 Chemical structure of polylactide. (Permission [290].)

effects of NPs, PLA-based nanocomposites are more common than pure PLA materials in tissue engineering, drug delivery systems, and synthetic bone replacements and repairs [289].

1.4.5.1 Applications in Biomedicine

1.4.5.1.1 Tissue Engineering

Because PLA materials are so biocompatible, they are frequently used as scaffolds (Table 1.11).

1.4.5.1.2 Drug Delivery

Four primary methods are employed to convert PLA into biodegradable NPs: solvent evaporation, solvent displacement, salting-out, and solvent diffusion. Because of this, these drug carriers have proven to be incredibly effective in encapsulating a variety of medications, such as hormones (progesterone), proteins (BSA), psychotic medications (savoxepine), and restenosis medications (tyrphostins), and drugs pertaining to restenosis. Additionally, these drug carriers enhance the

TABLE 1.11
Polylactide for Tissue Engineering Applications

System	Application	Reference
PLA/β-TCP nanofiber	GelMA scaffold for tissue engineering	[291]
Core-shell PLA/Kef hybrid	Scaffolds for skin tissue engineering	[292]
PLA-bioglass	3D Scaffold	[293]
Zeolite-nHA blended PCL/PLA nanofibers	Dental tissue engineering	[294]
PLA/n-HA	3D scaffolds for bone tissue engineering	[295]
Polyaniline, polydopamine, and polylactide	Scaffolds	[296]
Emulsion electrospun PLA/calcium alginate nanofibers	Periodontal tissue engineering	[297]
PCL/PLA and PCL/PLLA	Tissue engineering	[298]
PLA/nano-HA	Bone tissue engineering application	[299]
PLA	Soft tissue engineering	[300]

TABLE 1.12
Polylactide for Drug Delivery

System	Drug	Reference
PLA/TiO_2	Norfloxacin	[302]
Polylactide dipyridamole	5-Fluorouracil and 4-piperidinopiperidine	[303]
PLA/HAP	Doxycycline	[304]
PLGA/PLA	Peptide and protein	[305]
Polylactide	mRNA delivery	[306]
PLGA/PLA	Protein/peptide delivery	[307]
Cashew gum-graft-polylactide	Amphotericin B delivery	[308]
PLA stereocomplexed with methyl-β-cyclodextrin	Atropine	[309]

drug-to-carrier ratio and mitigate hepatic and renal damage. Furthermore, the looser structure of PLA may result in enhanced drug release as it progressively deteriorates, offsetting the decreased drug delivery brought on by lower overall drug dosages and creating a sustained drug delivery system (Table 1.12) [301].

1.4.6 Collagen

The fundamental structural protein in an animal's frame is collagen, which makes up the majority of the extracellular matrix in connective tissues (Figure 1.17). In animals, it makes up 25–35% of the whole protein of our bodies; in human beings, there are 28 different kinds [310].

1.4.6.1 Applications in Biomedicine

1.4.6.1.1 Tissue Engineering

Electrospun (ES) scaffolds based on collagen have been used in several in vitro and in vivo tissue engineering applications, including replacing bone, muscle, neuronal, skin, and blood vascular tissues, as well as assisting in the healing process following damage. Every instance involves tailoring the scaffold's crosslinking, composition, and structure to the unique needs of the target tissue (Table 1.13) [311].

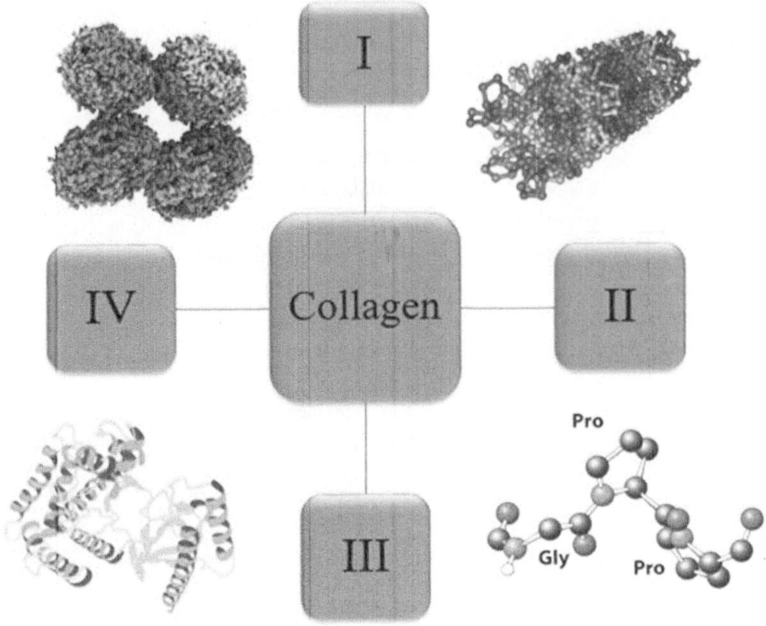

FIGURE 1.17 Different types of collagen.

TABLE 1.13
Collagen for Tissue Engineering Applications

System	Application	Reference
Collagen	Bone tissue engineering	[312]
Marine collagen	Scaffolds	[313]
Collagen type I	Scaffold for bone tissue engineering	[314]
Collagen by glycation	Tissue engineering	[315]
Collagen gelation	Tissue engineering	[316]
Chitosan-collagen-hydroxyapatite	Tissue engineering	[317]
Collagen/GelMA	Tissue engineering	[318]
Collagen and gelatin	Tissue engineering	[319]

1.4.6.1.2 Drug Delivery

Because it functions as a matrix, the characteristics of marine collagen can be used to transport drugs. These characteristics include biocompatibility, fluidity, and ease of manipulation (Table 1.14) [320].

1.4.6.1.3 Wound Dressing

The benefits of collagen dressings for wound healing are numerous. First off, because of their well-preserved main sequence and helix shape, they show less immunological rejection in people. Second, collagen interacts with platelets to restrict blood flow and promote the development of clots by starting a coagulation cascade and functioning as a mechanical hemostatic agent. Third, these dressings may absorb fluids several times their weight due to the unusual three-dimensional structure of collagen, which encourages gelation and creates a moist wound environment that facilitates dressing

TABLE 1.14
Collagen for Drug Delivery

System	Drug	Reference
Collagen	Allopurinol	[321]
Hydroxyapatite-collagen	BMP-2 and alendronate	[322]
Chitosan/collagen	5-Fluorouracil	[323]
Collagen	Gentamicin	[324]
Collagen	Doxorubicin	[325]
Silica/bioglass/collagen	Antibiotic	[326]
PVA/anionic collagen	Ciprofloxacin	[327]
Collagen	Metalloproteinase 14	[328]

TABLE 1.15
Collagen for Wound Dressing

System	Application	Reference
Collagen	Skin regeneration and wound dressing	[329]
Collagen and chitosan	Hemostatic and wound healing	[330]
Collagen	Accelerated wound healing	[331]
Collagen	Diabetes-related foot ulcers	[332]
Collagen	Promoting infected wound healing	[333]
Collagen	Wound dressings for burns	[143]
3D PCL/collagen	One-time treatment of diabetic foot ulcers	[334]
Collagen and ethanolic extract of hypericum perforatum	Wound dressing	[335]

changes. Moreover, collagen serves as a competitive substrate for collagenase, reducing the amount of tissue degradation brought on by enzymes [329]. Moreover, low-pH collagen dressings aid in lowering the pH around the wound, lowering the risk of bacterial infection and preventing protease action. Collagen breakdown products also aid in lowering type I collagenase activity. Collagen dressings' scaffold structure draws macrophages, fibroblasts, and epithelial cells, which promotes wound healing. Moreover, the collagen in the dressings promotes angiogenesis and collagen deposition, which quickens the healing process for wounds. A moist wound environment not only facilitates dressing changes but also enhances the patient's quality of life by promoting healing. Because collagen is beneficial for wound healing, it is employed in skin substitutes (Table 1.15) [330].

1.4.7 Hydroxyapatite

A naturally occurring kind of calcium apatite that is a member of the phosphate mineral institution is known as hydroxyapatite (HA). Because of its structural and chemical resemblance to bone phosphates, HA is one of the major calcium phosphates. Interestingly, at room temperature, HA is the most solid by-product of calcium phosphate salt within the pH variety of 4–14. Because of its unique features, HA is widely utilized in a huge variety of industries, together with biomedicine, water treatment, protein chromatography, prescription drugs, and fertilizer manufacturing [336].

Because HA is bioactive and biocompatible, it has found widespread application in the biomedical industry. It is frequently used in processes involving the regeneration of bone tissue. To increase the bioactivity of implant materials, HA is often coated on them. Furthermore, HA is a great option for drug delivery, especially when it comes to delivering proteins to certain locations or establishing

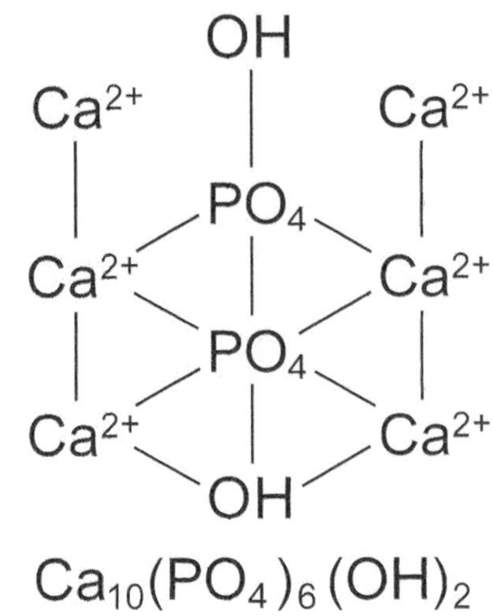

FIGURE 1.18 Hydroxyapatite structure.

a regulated and progressive release of medications. Osteoblastic cell development may be efficiently stimulated by this regulated release mechanism [337].

HA is a member of the apatite's own family, which is made of phosphates and calcium. Its unit cell formulation is $Ca_{10}(PO_4)_6(OH)_2$, at the same time as its widespread component is $Ca_5(PO_4)_3OH$. The arrangement of calcium and phosphates inside the HA unit mobile is as follows: at the M_1 position, 9 oxygen atoms of the phosphate businesses encircle 4 calcium atoms, and in the M_2 role, the remaining 6 calcium atoms are encircled with the aid of the closing 6 oxygen atoms of the phosphate agencies. All calcium atoms have crystallographic positions M_1 and M_2, respectively (Figure 1.18). Not to be counted in what it comes from, HA usually has trace ranges of contaminants such as hydroxyl ions (OH^-), fluoride ions (F^-), phosphite ions (PO_3^{3-}), and chloride ions (Cl^-) [338].

1.4.7.1 Applications in Biomedicine

1.4.7.1.1 Drug Delivery

Because of the remaining components that are still inside of them, many biological calcium apatites have asymmetric morphologies. On the other hand, hydroxyapatite (HA) is distinguished by its rough surface, which makes it very useful in biological applications. During the mineralization process, the surface roughness and the "P" and "C" sites of HA are essential for facilitating protein binding. The interaction between amino acids and HA highlights the importance of the rough surface and these particular locations (Table 1.16) [338].

TABLE 1.16
HA for Drug Delivery

System	Drug	Reference
Serum albumin–hydroxyapatite nanoflowers	Ciprofloxacin	[339]
Hydroxyapatite	Ciprofloxacin	[340]
Hydroxyapatite	Doxycycline	[341]
Hydroxyapatite/zein	Doxorubicin hydrochloride	[342]
Poly (ethylene glycol)-poly (ε-caprolactone)-hydroxyapatite	Doxorubicin	[343]
Chitosan hydroxyapatite	Protein	[344]
Polyvinyl alcohol/whey protein isolate/hydroxyapatite	Gentamicin	[345]

TABLE 1.17
HA for Tissue Engineering Applications

System	Application	Reference
Hydroxyapatite/polyurethane	Bone tissue engineering	[346]
Polycaprolactone-hydroxyapatite	Bone tissue engineering	[347]
Polycaprolactone-hydroxyapatite	Bone tissue engineering	[348]
Mg-Hydroxyapatite	Bone tissue engineering	[349]
Chitosan-collagen-hydroxyapatite	Tissue engineering	[317]
Hydroxyapatite/ethanolamine	Bone tissue engineering	[350]
GelMA-gelatin-hydroxyapatite	Bone tissue engineering	[351]
Polyvinyl alcohol/whey protein isolate/hydroxyapatite	Gentamicin	[345]

1.4.7.1.2 Tissue Engineering

Water, collagen, and calcium phosphate are the main constituents of natural bone, which functions as a ceramic composite. Apart from these components, natural bone also contains trace quantities of proteins, lipids, and polysaccharides. Bone structure is made stiff by calcium phosphate, which is found in the form of hydroxyapatite (HA) crystals. Trace Na^+, Mg^{2+}, and F^- ion impurities are among the components of HA, much like in bone. The length and breadth of HA crystals found in bones are usually measured in nanometers. Implanting HA boosts the osteoinductive characteristics of the device as well as the osteoconductive interactions it has with bone cells, especially osteoblastic cells. This similarity between HA and the inorganic cement found in natural bone emphasizes how well-suited they are for use in implant applications (Table 1.17) [338].

1.5 CHALLENGES AND LIMITATIONS

The integration of nanostructured materials into biocompatible matrices has opened doors for the creation of innovative bio-based nanocomposites that hold significant promise in various biomedical applications. Nevertheless, the transition of these groundbreaking materials from the research laboratory to clinical settings faces a multitude of challenges that necessitate comprehensive investigation and resolution. While specific challenges have been addressed in separate reviews, some overarching issues are outlined below:

1. Biocompatibility: The biocompatibility of bio-based nanocomposites remains a primary focal point, demanding extensive research to ensure seamless interactions with biological systems while averting adverse reactions or toxicity.
2. Uniform Dispersion: Attaining and sustaining the uniform dispersion of NPs within bionanocomposites is crucial for optimal performance and stable material properties. Advanced techniques are essential to overcome dispersion challenges effectively.
3. Degradation Control: Regulating the degradation rate of bio-based nanocomposites presents a significant obstacle in biomedical applications. Material degradation must align with the healing process timeline without compromising structural integrity.
4. Cost Considerations: The financial implications linked to the development and manufacturing of bionanocomposites for biomedical purposes represent a substantial barrier to widespread adoption. This underscores the importance of implementing cost-effective production methods and strategies.

1.6 CONCLUSION AND FUTURE DIRECTIONS

In the end, bionanocomposites show off giant promise for biomedical packages due to their unique combination of biocompatibility, mechanical properties, and drug shipping competencies. The fusion of NPs into biopolymer matrices complements functionalities that can revolutionize diverse sectors of biomedicine, from tissue engineering to drug delivery structures.

By leveraging the synergistic outcomes of biopolymers and NPs, bionanocomposites have the potential to address crucial challenges in cutting-edge healthcare, inclusive of enhancing implant overall performance, promoting tissue regeneration, and facilitating focused drug shipping with minimized facet consequences. The customizable nature of bionanocomposite properties similarly elevates their enchantment for personalized medication applications.

Looking forward, advancements in the realm of bionanocomposites for biomedical applications should concentrate on the following key areas:

- Enhanced Characterization: Develop sophisticated techniques for characterizing bionanocomposite properties at the nanoscale to better comprehend structure-property relationships and optimize performance.
- Biodegradability and Sustainability: Investigate the use of biodegradable and sustainable NP sources to produce environmentally friendly bionanocomposites with improved end-of-life considerations.
- Clinical Translation: Bridge the gap between laboratory investigation and clinical implementation by conducting thorough preclinical studies and refining production processes for scalability and regulatory approval.
- Multifunctionality: Create multifunctional bionanocomposites capable of providing mechanical support, controlled therapeutic release, imaging capabilities, and antibacterial properties simultaneously for comprehensive biomedical applications.
- Clinical Trials and Commercialization: Allocate resources to clinical trials to validate the safety and efficacy of bionanocomposites in human subjects and explore pathways for commercialization to introduce these innovative technologies to the market.

In essence, bionanocomposites represent a state-of-the-art approach with the potential to transform the landscape of biomedical applications. Sustained innovation and collaborative efforts across interdisciplinary domains will be instrumental in fully realizing the potential of bionanocomposites to enhance human health and well-being. Exciting prospects lie ahead for this dynamic field!

REFERENCES

[1] Al-Handarish, Y. et al., "A survey of tactile-sensing systems and their applications in biomedical engineering," *Adv. Mater. Sci. Eng.*, vol. 2020, 2020.

[2] Alcântara, A. C. S. & Darder, M., "Building up functional bionanocomposites from the assembly of clays and biopolymers," *Chem. Rec.*, vol. 18, no. 7–8, pp. 696–712, 2018.

[3] Filip, D. et al., "Hybrid green bionanocomposites based on chitosan/starch/gelatin and metallic nanoparticles for biological applications," *Int. J. Biol. Macromol.*, vol. 253, p. 127571, 2023.

[4] Bertolino, V., Cavallaro, G., Milioto, S., & Lazzara, G., "Polysaccharides/halloysite nanotubes for smart bionanocomposite materials," *Carbohydr. Polym.*, vol. 245, p. 116502, 2020.

[5] Yanar, F., Carugo, D., & Zhang, X., "Hybrid nanoplatforms comprising organic nanocompartments encapsulating inorganic nanoparticles for enhanced drug delivery and bioimaging applications," *Molecules*, vol. 28, no. 15, p. 5694, 2023.

[6] Shariati, L. et al., "Nanobased platform advances in cardiovascular diseases: Early diagnosis, imaging, treatment, and tissue engineering," *Environ. Res.*, vol. 238, p. 116933, 2023.

[7] Asl, F. D. et al., "Nano drug-delivery systems for management of AIDS: Liposomes, dendrimers, gold and silver nanoparticles," *Nanomedicine*, vol. 18, no. 3, pp. 279–302, 2023.

[8] Wang, D. et al., "Nanocarriers transport across the gastrointestinal barriers: The contribution to oral bioavailability via blood circulation and lymphatic pathway," *Adv. Drug Deliv. Rev.*, vol. 203, p. 115130, 2023.

[9] Perera, K. Y., Jaiswal, A. K., & Jaiswal, S., "Biopolymer-based sustainable food packaging materials: Challenges, solutions, and applications," *Foods*, vol. 12, no. 12, p. 2422, 2023.

[10] Mallakpour, S., Tukhani, M., & Hussain, C. M., "Sustainable plant and microbes-mediated preparation of Fe_3O_4 nanoparticles and industrial application of its chitosan, starch, cellulose, and dextrin-based nanocomposites as catalysts," *Int. J. Biol. Macromol.*, vol. 179, pp. 429–447, 2021.

[11] Bashir, S. M. et al., "Chitosan nanoparticles: A versatile platform for biomedical applications," *Materials (Basel)*, vol. 15, no. 19, p. 6521, 2022.

[12] Arif, Z. U. et al., "Additive manufacturing of sustainable biomaterials for biomedical applications," *Asian J. Pharm. Sci.*, p. 100812, 2023.

[13] Carvalho, J. R. G. et al., "Long-term evaluation of poly (lactic acid)(PLA) implants in a horse: An experimental pilot study," *Molecules*, vol. 26, no. 23, p. 7224, 2021.

[14] Kim, I., Viswanathan, K., Kasi, G., Sadeghi, K., Thanakkasaranee, S., & Seo, J., "Poly (lactic acid)/ZnO bionanocomposite films with positively charged ZnO as potential antimicrobial food packaging materials," *Polymers (Basel)*, vol. 11, no. 9, p. 1427, 2019.

[15] Braccini, S., Pecorini, G., Chiellini, F., Bakos, D., Miertus, S., & Frecer, V., "Adhesion of fibroblast cells on thin films representing surfaces of polymeric scaffolds of human urethra rationalized by molecular models of integrin binding: Cell adhesion on polymeric scaffolds for regenerative medicine," *J. Biotechnol.*, vol. 324, pp. 233–238, 2020.

[16] Boucher, M. C., Isaac, C. E., Sun, P., Borbat, P. P., & Marohn, J. A., "A non-perturbative, low-noise surface coating for sensitive force-gradient detection of electron spin resonance in thin films," *ACS Nano*, vol. 17, no. 2, pp. 1153–1165, 2023.

[17] Yano, H. et al., "Construction of multilayer films and superlattice-and mosaic-like heterostructures of 2D metal oxide nanosheets via a facile spin-coating process," *ACS Appl. Mater. Interfaces*, vol. 13, no. 36, pp. 43258–43265, 2021.

[18] Yuan, Q., Gu, S., Chi, Y., Zhao, L., & Wang, D., "Langmuir–Blodgett deposition of cellulose nanocrystal surfactants into ordered monolayers," *Langmuir*, vol. 38, no. 28, pp. 8495–8501, 2022.

[19] Carvalho da Silva, L., Castelo, R. M., Cheng, H. N., Biswas, A., Furtado, R. F., & Alves, C. R., "Methods of microencapsulation of vegetable oil: Principles, stability and applications-a minireview," *Food Technol. Biotechnol.*, vol. 60, no. 3, pp. 308–320, 2022.

[20] He, Y. et al., "Investigation of the effect and mechanism of nanocellulose on soy protein isolate-konjac glucomannan composite hydrogel system," *Int. J. Biol. Macromol.*, vol. 254, p. 127943, 2024.

[21] Berrabah, I. et al., "A bionanocomposite of poly (3-hydroxybutyrate-co-3-hydroxyhexanoate)/ZnO-nanoparticles intended for food packaging," *Int. J. Biol. Macromol.*, vol. 238, p. 124162, 2023.

[22] Xu, A. et al., "Nanocomposite polymer colloids prepared via emulsion polymerization and stabilized using polydopamine-coated silica particles," *Langmuir*, vol. 38, no. 18, pp. 5454–5463, 2022.

[23] Zhang, H., Yu, S., Wu, S., Xu, M., Gao, T., Wu, Q., … & Liu, Y. "Rational design of silver NPs-incorporated quaternized chitin nanomicelle with combinational antibacterial capability for infected wound healing," *Int. J. Biol. Macromol.*, vol. 224, pp. 1206–1216, 2023.

[24] Mahmoudi, A., Kesharwani, P., Majeed, M., Teng, Y., & Sahebkar, A., "Recent advances in nanogold as a promising nanocarrier for curcumin delivery," *Colloids Surf. B Biointerfaces*, vol. 215, p. 112481, 2022.

[25] Adarmanabadi, S. R., Jafari, M., Farrash, S. M. H., & Heidari, M., "Effect of nano clay, nano-graphene oxide and carbon nanotubes on the mechanical and tribological properties of crosslinked epoxy nanocomposite," *PLoS One*, vol. 16, no. 11, p. e0259401, 2021.

[26] Eghbalian, M., Ansari, R., & Haghighi, S., "On the mechanical properties and fracture analysis of polymer nanocomposites reinforced by functionalized silicon carbide nanotubes: A molecular dynamics investigation," *J. Mol. Graph. Model.*, vol. 111, p. 108086, 2022.

[27] Zotti, A. et al., "Effect of the mixing technique of graphene nanoplatelets and graphene nanofibers on fracture toughness of epoxy based nanocomposites and composites," *Polymers (Basel)*, vol. 14, no. 23, p. 5105, 2022.

[28] Tanpichai, S., Thongdeelerd, C., Chantaramanee, T., & Boonmahitthisud, A., "Property enhancement of epoxidized natural rubber nanocomposites with water hyacinth-extracted cellulose nanofibers," *Int. J. Biol. Macromol.*, vol. 234, p. 123741, 2023.

[29] Zhang, J. et al., "Cellulose nanocrystal driven microphase separated nanocomposites: Enhanced mechanical performance and nanostructured morphology," *Int. J. Biol. Macromol.*, vol. 130, pp. 685–694, 2019.
[30] Zubkiewicz, A., Szymczyk, A., Franciszczak, P., Kochmanska, A., Janowska, I., & Paszkiewicz, S., "Comparing multi-walled carbon nanotubes and halloysite nanotubes as reinforcements in EVA nanocomposites," *Materials (Basel)*, vol. 13, no. 17, p. 3809, 2020.
[31] Patel, V. et al., "Multi-walled carbon-nanotube-reinforced PMMA nanocomposites: An experimental study of their friction and wear properties," *Polymers (Basel)*, vol. 15, no. 13, p. 2785, 2023.
[32] Sandu, I.-L., Stan, F., & Fetecau, C., "Mechanical recycling of ethylene-vinyl acetate/carbon nanotube nanocomposites: Processing, thermal, rheological, mechanical and electrical behavior," *Polymers (Basel)*, vol. 15, no. 3, p. 583, 2023.
[33] Demski, S., Dydek, K., Bartnicka, K., Majchrowicz, K., Kozera, R., & Boczkowska, A., "Introduction of SWCNTs as a method of improvement of electrical and mechanical properties of CFRPs based on thermoplastic acrylic resin," *Polymers (Basel)*, vol. 15, no. 3, p. 506, 2023.
[34] Yun, S.-S., Shin, D., & Jang, K.-S., "Influence of ionomer and cyanuric acid on antistatic, mechanical, thermal, and rheological properties of extruded carbon nanotube (CNT)/polyoxymethylene (POM) nanocomposites," *Polymers (Basel)*, vol. 14, no. 9, p. 1849, 2022.
[35] Xia, L. et al., "Robust, biodegradable and flame-retardant nanocomposite films based on TEMPO-oxidized cellulose nanofibers and hydroxyapatite nanowires," *Carbohydr. Polym.*, vol. 324, p. 121495, 2024.
[36] Sharif, M. & Tavakoli, S., "Biodegradable chitosan-graphene oxide as an affective green filler for improving of properties in epoxy nanocomposites," *Int. J. Biol. Macromol.*, vol. 233, p. 123550, 2023.
[37] Anstey, A., Tuccitto, A. V., Lee, P. C., & Park, C. B., "Generation of tough, stiff polylactide nanocomposites through the in situ nanofibrillation of thermoplastic elastomer," *ACS Appl. Mater. Interfaces*, vol. 14, no. 12, pp. 14422–14434, 2022.
[38] Bhuyan, B., Srivastava, S. K., & Mittal, V., "Ethylene-co-vinyl acetate/MWCNTs/hectorite elastomeric nanocomposites: Characterization and electrical properties," *J. Nanosci. Nanotechnol.*, vol. 18, no. 6, pp. 4057–4064, 2018.
[39] Semitela, Â. et al., "Biomimetic graphene/spongin scaffolds for improved osteoblasts bioactivity via dynamic mechanical stimulation," *Macromol. Biosci.*, vol. 22, no. 1, p. 2100311, 2022.
[40] Sharma, S., Singh, A. A., Majumdar, A., & Butola, B. S., "Tailoring the mechanical and thermal properties of polylactic acid-based bionanocomposite films using halloysite nanotubes and polyethylene glycol by solvent casting process," *J. Mater. Sci.*, vol. 54, pp. 8971–8983, 2019.
[41] Divakaran, N., Kale, M. B., Dhamodharan, D., Mubarak, S., Wu, L., & Wang, J., "Effect of POSS-modified montmorillonite on thermal, mechanical, and electrical properties of unsaturated polyester nanocomposites," *Polymers (Basel)*, vol. 12, no. 9, p. 2031, 2020.
[42] Papadopoulou, K. et al., "The effect of biochar addition on thermal stability and decomposition mechanism of poly (butylene succinate) bionanocomposites," *Molecules*, vol. 28, no. 14, p. 5330, 2023.
[43] Ahuja, D., Kumar, L., & Kaushik, A., "Thermal stability of starch bionanocomposites films: Exploring the role of esterified cellulose nanofibers isolated from crop residue," *Carbohydr. Polym.*, vol. 255, p. 117466, 2021.
[44] Gohargani, M., Lashkari, H., & Shirazinejad, A., "Study on biodegradable chitosan-whey protein-based film containing bionanocomposite TiO_2 and Zataria multiflora essential oil," *J. Food Qual.*, vol. 2020, pp. 1–11, 2020.
[45] Singh, P., Kaur, G., Singh, A., & Kaur, P., "Starch based bio-nanocomposite films reinforced with montmorillonite and lemongrass oil nanoemulsion: Development, characterization and biodegradability," *J. Food Meas. Charact.*, vol. 17, no. 1, pp. 527–545, 2023.
[46] Rahimi, J., Bahrami, N., Niksefat, M., Kamalzare, M., & Maleki, A., "A novel biodegradable magnetic bionanocomposite based on tannic acid as a biological molecule for selective oxidation of alcohols," *Solid State Sci.*, vol. 105, p. 106284, 2020.
[47] Wu, Z. et al., "Investigation of the structural and physical properties, antioxidant and antimicrobial activity of konjac glucomannan/cellulose nanocrystal bionanocomposite films incorporated with phlorotannin from Sargassum," *Int. J. Biol. Macromol.*, vol. 192, pp. 323–330, 2021.
[48] Bratovcic, A., "Physical–chemical, mechanical and antimicrobial properties of bio-nanocomposite films and edible coatings," *Int. J. Res. Appl. Sci. Biotechnol.*, vol. 8, no. 5, pp. 151–161, 2021.
[49] Shahvalizadeh, R. et al., "Antimicrobial bio-nanocomposite films based on gelatin, tragacanth, and zinc oxide nanoparticles–Microstructural, mechanical, thermo-physical, and barrier properties," *Food Chem.*, vol. 354, p. 129492, 2021.

[50] Wu, H., Wu, H., Qing, Y., Wu, C., & Pang, J., "KGM/chitosan bio-nanocomposite films reinforced with ZNPs: Colloidal, physical, mechanical and structural attributes," *Food Packag. Shelf Life*, vol. 33, p. 100870, 2022.
[51] Krystyjan, M. et al., "Physicochemical, bacteriostatic, and biological properties of starch/chitosan polymer composites modified by graphene oxide, designed as new bionanomaterials," *Polymers (Basel)*, vol. 13, no. 14, p. 2327, 2021.
[52] Erol, I., Hazman, Ö., Aksu, M., & Uygur, I., "Novel bionanocomposites of chitosan-based blend containing LaB_6: Thermal, dielectric, and biological properties," *Polym. Adv. Technol.*, vol. 34, pp. 2721–2738, 2023.
[53] Swaminathan, P. D., Uddin, M. N., Wooley, P., & Asmatulu, R., "Fabrication and biological analysis of highly porous PEEK bionanocomposites incorporated with carbon and hydroxyapatite nanoparticles for biological applications," *Molecules*, vol. 25, no. 16, p. 3572, 2020.
[54] Maghsoudlou, M. A., Nassireslami, E., Saber-Samandari, S., & Khandan, A., "Bone regeneration using bio-nanocomposite tissue reinforced with bioactive nanoparticles for femoral defect applications in medicine," *Avicenna J. Med. Biotechnol.*, vol. 12, no. 2, p. 68, 2020.
[55] Babi, M., Williams, A., Reid, M., Grandfield, K., Bassim, N. D., & Moran-Mirabal, J. M., "Unraveling the supramolecular structure and nanoscale dislocations of bacterial cellulose ribbons using correlative super-resolution light and electron microscopy," *Biomacromolecules*, vol. 24, no. 1, pp. 258–268, 2022.
[56] Kong, L., Alqus, R., Yong, C. W., Todorov, I., Eichhorn, S. J., & Bryce, R. A., "Cellulose Iβ microfibril interaction with pristine graphene in water: Effects of amphiphilicity by molecular simulation," *J. Mol. Graph. Model.*, vol. 118, p. 108336, 2023.
[57] Siqueira, G., Bras, J., & Dufresne, A., "Cellulosic bionanocomposites: A review of preparation, properties and applications," *Polymers (Basel)*, vol. 2, no. 4, pp. 728–765, 2010.
[58] Song, B., Zhao, S., Shen, W., Collings, C., & Ding, S.-Y., "Direct measurement of plant cellulose microfibril and bundles in native cell walls," *Front. Plant Sci.*, vol. 11, p. 479, 2020.
[59] Holding, A. J. et al., "Thermo-reversible cellulose micro phase-separation in mixtures of methyltributylphosphonium acetate and γ-valerolactone or DMSO," *ChemPhysChem*, vol. 23, no. 7, p. e202100635, 2022.
[60] Zambrano-Mite, L. F. et al., "Optimization of microfibrillated cellulose isolation from cocoa pod husk via mild oxalic acid hydrolysis: A response surface methodology approach," *Heliyon*, vol. 9, no. 6, 2023.
[61] Bangar, S. P., Whiteside, W. S., Kajla, P., and Tavassoli, M., "Value addition of rice straw cellulose fibers as a reinforcer in packaging applications," *Int. J. Biol. Macromol.*, vol. 243, p. 125320, 2023.
[62] Chandan, V., Mishra, R. K., Kolář, V., Jirků, P., Müller, M., & Jamshaid, H., "Numerical and experimental analysis of mechanical properties in hybrid epoxy–basalt composites partially reinforced with cellulosic fillers," *Materials (Basel)*, vol. 16, no. 14, p. 4898, 2023.
[63] Redondo, A. et al., "Comparing percolation and alignment of cellulose nanocrystals for the reinforcement of polyurethane nanocomposites," *ACS Appl. Mater. Interfaces*, vol. 14, no. 5, pp. 7270–7282, 2022.
[64] Schver, G. C. R. M. & Lee, P. I., "Combined effects of supersaturation rates and doses on the kinetic-solubility profiles of amorphous solid dispersions based on water-insoluble poly (2-hydroxyethyl methacrylate) hydrogels," *Mol. Pharm.*, vol. 15, no. 5, pp. 2017–2026, 2018.
[65] Lin, F., Pignon, F., Putaux, J.-L., & Jean, B., "Temperature-triggered formation of a cellulose II nanocrystal network through regioselective derivatization," *Nanoscale*, vol. 13, no. 13, pp. 6447–6460, 2021.
[66] Völtz, L. R., Geng, S., Teleman, A., & Oksman, K., "Influence of dispersion and orientation on polyamide-6 cellulose nanocomposites manufactured through liquid-assisted extrusion," *Nanomaterials*, vol. 12, no. 5, p. 818, 2022.
[67] Zhu, G. & Dufresne, A., "Synergistic reinforcing and cross-linking effect of thiol-ene-modified cellulose nanofibrils on natural rubber," *Carbohydr. Polym.*, vol. 278, p. 118954, 2022.
[68] Liu, Y., Ma, X., Jiang, Q., & Yang, G., "Corn stalk modified chitin composite sponge for effective hemostasis and promoting wound healing," *Int. J. Biol. Macromol.*, vol. 242, p. 124882, 2023.
[69] Romruen, O., Karbowiak, T., Tongdeesoontorn, W., Shiekh, K. A., & Rawdkuen, S., "Extraction and characterization of cellulose from agricultural by-products of Chiang Rai Province, Thailand," *Polymers (Basel)*, vol. 14, no. 9, p. 1830, 2022.
[70] Senapitakkul, V. et al., "Pretreatment of cellulose from sugarcane bagasse with xylanase for improving dyeability with natural dyes," *Acs Omega*, vol. 5, no. 43, pp. 28168–28177, 2020.
[71] Chen, B. & Yang, Y., "Co-pyrolysis of algae with other carbon-based materials: A review on synergistic products and molecular reaction pathway," *J. Therm. Anal. Calorim.*, vol. 148, no. 6, pp. 2233–2249, 2023.

[72] Owonubi, S. J., Agwuncha, S. C., Malima, N. M., Shombe, G. B., Makhatha, E. M., & Revaprasadu, N., "Non-woody biomass as sources of nanocellulose particles: A review of extraction procedures," *Front. Energy Res.*, vol. 9, p. 608825, 2021.

[73] Huang, C., Xu, C., Meng, X., Wang, L., & Zhou, X., "Isolation, modification, and characterization of the constituents (cellulose, hemicellulose, lignin, et al.) in biomass and their bio-based applications," *Front. Bioeng. Biotechnol.*, vol. 10, p. 866531, 2022.

[74] Avcioglu, N. H., "Bacterial cellulose: Recent progress in production and industrial applications," *World J. Microbiol. Biotechnol.*, vol. 38, no. 5, p. 86, 2022.

[75] Mardawati, E. et al., "Pineapple core from the canning industrial waste for bacterial cellulose production by Komagataeibacter xylinus," *Heliyon*, vol. 9, no. 11, 2023.

[76] Narayanan, K. B., Bhaskar, R., Sudhakar, K., Nam, D. H., & Han, S. S., "Polydopamine-functionalized bacterial cellulose as hydrogel scaffolds for skin tissue engineering," *Gels*, vol. 9, no. 8, p. 656, 2023.

[77] de Amorim, J. D. P. et al., "Bacterial cellulose as a versatile biomaterial for wound dressing application," *Molecules*, vol. 27, no. 17, p. 5580, 2022.

[78] Eslahi, N., Mahmoodi, A., Mahmoudi, N., Zandi, N., & Simchi, A., "Processing and properties of nanofibrous bacterial cellulose-containing polymer composites: A review of recent advances for biomedical applications," *Polym. Rev.*, vol. 60, no. 1, pp. 144–170, 2020.

[79] Tarchoun, A. F., Trache, D., & Klapötke, T. M., "Microcrystalline cellulose from Posidonia oceanica brown algae: Extraction and characterization," *Int. J. Biol. Macromol.*, vol. 138, pp. 837–845, 2019.

[80] Husni, A. & Budhiyanti, S. A., "Effect of isolation method on characterization of microcrystalline cellulose from brown seaweed sargassum vulgare," *Indones. J. Pharm./Majalah Farm. Indones.*, vol. 33, no. 1, 2022.

[81] Khanra, A. et al., "Green bioprocessing and applications of microalgae-derived biopolymers as a renewable feedstock: Circular bioeconomy approach," *Environ. Technol. Innov.*, p. 102872, 2022.

[82] Song, G. et al., "Structure and composition of the tunic in the sea pineapple Halocynthia roretzi: A complex cellulosic composite biomaterial," *Acta Biomater.*, vol. 111, pp. 290–301, 2020.

[83] Jiang, C., Wu, M., Zhang, F., Liu, C., Sun, M., & Li, B., "All-tunicate cellulose film with good light management properties for high-efficiency organic solar cells," *Nanomaterials*, vol. 13, no. 7, p. 1221, 2023.

[84] Cao, L., Huang, J., Fan, J., Gong, Z., Xu, C., & Chen, Y., "Nanocellulose-a sustainable and efficient nanofiller for rubber nanocomposites: From reinforcement to smart soft materials," *Polym. Rev.*, vol. 62, no. 3, pp. 549–584, 2022.

[85] Mahur, B. K., Ahuja, A., Singh, S., Maji, P. K., & Rastogi, V. K., "Different nanocellulose morphologies (cellulose nanofibers, nanocrystals and nanospheres) extracted from Sunn hemp (Crotalaria Juncea)," *Int. J. Biol. Macromol.*, vol. 253, p. 126657, 2023.

[86] Jamshaid, H. et al., "Natural cellulosic fiber reinforced concrete: Influence of fiber type and loading percentage on mechanical and water absorption performance," *Materials (Basel)*, vol. 15, no. 3, p. 874, 2022.

[87] Rashwan, O. et al., "Extrusion and characterization of recycled polyethylene terephthalate (rPET) filaments compounded with chain extender and impact modifiers for material-extrusion additive manufacturing," *Sci. Rep.*, vol. 13, no. 1, p. 16041, 2023.

[88] Ma, L., Xu, Y., Chen, J., Dong, C., & Pang, Z., "Preparation of cellulose nanocrystals by synergistic action of ionic liquid and recyclable solid acid under mild conditions," *Molecules*, vol. 28, no. 7, p. 3070, 2023.

[89] Zhao, H., Zhao, L., Lin, X., & Shen, L., "An update on microcrystalline cellulose in direct compression: Functionality, critical material attributes, and co-processed excipients," *Carbohydr. Polym.*, vol. 278, p. 118968, 2022.

[90] Zhao, J. et al., "Room temperature preparation of cellulose nanocrystals with high yield via a new $ZnCl_2$ solvent system," *Carbohydr. Polym.*, vol. 278, p. 118946, 2022.

[91] Sinsukudomchai, P., Aht-Ong, D., Honda, K., & Napathorn, S. C., "Green composites made of polyhydroxybutyrate and long-chain fatty acid esterified microcrystalline cellulose from pineapple leaf," *PLoS One*, vol. 18, no. 3, p. e0282311, 2023.

[92] Lu, S. et al., "Facile extraction and characterization of cellulose nanocrystals from agricultural waste sugarcane straw," *J. Sci. Food Agric.*, vol. 102, no. 1, pp. 312–321, 2022.

[93] Chen, Z., Xu, H.-N., & Ouyang, X.-K., "The simultaneous production of two distinct types of cellulose nanocrystals," *Langmuir*, vol. 38, no. 19, pp. 5996–6003, 2022.

[94] Qian, H., "Major factors influencing the size distribution analysis of cellulose nanocrystals imaged in transmission electron microscopy," *Polymers (Basel)*, vol. 13, no. 19, p. 3318, 2021.
[95] Diem, L. N. et al., "Sugarcane Bagasse-Derived Cellulose Nanocrystal/Polyvinyl Alcohol/Gum Tragacanth Composite Film Incorporated with Betel Leaf Extract as a Versatile Biomaterial for Wound Dressing," *Int. J. Biomater.*, vol. 2023, 2023.
[96] Luo, Y., Ye, Z., Liao, S., Wang, F., & Shao, J., "Mechanically tunable spongy graphene/cellulose nanocrystals hybrid aerogel by atmospheric drying and its adsorption applications," *Materials (Basel)*, vol. 14, no. 20, p. 5961, 2021.
[97] Zhou, J., Fang, Z., Chen, K., Cui, J., Yang, D., & Qiu, X., "Improving the degree of polymerization of cellulose nanofibers by largely preserving native structure of wood fibers," *Carbohydr. Polym.*, vol. 296, p. 119919, 2022.
[98] Lou, S., Huang, Y., & Wu, M., "Regulation of hydrogen bonding network between cellulose nanofibers by rare earth ion Y3+," *Carbohydr. Polym.*, vol. 302, p. 120421, 2023.
[99] Sriplai, N., Mongkolthanaruk, W., Eichhorn, S. J., & Pinitsoontorn, S., "Magnetically responsive and flexible bacterial cellulose membranes," *Carbohydr. Polym.*, vol. 192, pp. 251–262, 2018.
[100] Horue, M., Silva, J. M., Berti, I. R., Brandão, L. R., Barud, H. da S., & Castro, G. R., "Bacterial cellulose-based materials as dressings for wound healing," *Pharmaceutics*, vol. 15, no. 2, p. 424, 2023.
[101] Pogorelova, N., Rogachev, E., Digel, I., Chernigova, S., and Nardin, D., "Bacterial cellulose nanocomposites: Morphology and mechanical properties," *Materials (Basel)*, vol. 13, no. 12, p. 2849, 2020.
[102] Zhu, Y., Wang, T., Dai, Y., Wang, Y., Ding, Y., & Zhang, L., "Surface engineering of regenerated cellulose nanocomposite films with high strength, ultraviolet resistance, and a hydrophobic surface," *Polymers (Basel)*, vol. 15, no. 6, p. 1427, 2023.
[103] Meng, L. et al., "Improved mechanical and antibacterial properties of polyvinyl alcohol composite films using quaternized cellulose nanocrystals as nanofillers," *Compos. Sci. Technol.*, vol. 232, p. 109885, 2023.
[104] Yu, T.-Y. et al., "Effect of cellulose compositions and fabrication methods on mechanical properties of polyurethane-cellulose composites," *Carbohydr. Polym.*, vol. 291, p. 119549, 2022.
[105] Bian, H., Yang, Y., Tu, P., & Chen, J. Y., "Value-added utilization of wheat straw: From cellulose and cellulose nanofiber to all-cellulose nanocomposite film," *Membranes (Basel)*, vol. 12, no. 5, p. 475, 2022.
[106] Madivoli, E. S., Kareru, P. G., Gichuki, J., & Elbagoury, M. M., "Cellulose nanofibrils and silver nanoparticles enhances the mechanical and antimicrobial properties of polyvinyl alcohol nanocomposite film," *Sci. Rep.*, vol. 12, no. 1, p. 19005, 2022.
[107] Li, X. et al., "Facile in situ fabrication of ZnO-embedded cellulose nanocomposite films with antibacterial properties and enhanced mechanical strength via hydrogen bonding interactions," *Int. J. Biol. Macromol.*, vol. 183, pp. 760–771, 2021.
[108] Wu, W. et al., "The effect of the degree of substitution on the solubility of cellulose acetoacetates in water: A molecular dynamics simulation and density functional theory study," *Carbohydr. Res.*, vol. 496, p. 108134, 2020.
[109] Wei, J., Wang, B., Yuan, H., Kang, Z., Gao, H., & Nie, Y., "Effects of glucose and coagulant on the structure and properties of regenerated cellulose fibers," *Biomacromolecules*, vol. 24, no. 4, pp. 1810–1818, 2023.
[110] Bagherjeri, M. A., Monhemi, H., Haque, A. N. M. A., & Naebe, M., "Molecular mechanism of cellulose dissolution in N-methyl morpholine-N-oxide: A molecular dynamics simulation study," *Carbohydr. Polym.*, vol. 323, p. 121433, 2024.
[111] Li, Y. et al., "UV and IR dual light triggered cellulose-based invisible actuators with high sensitivity," *Int. J. Biol. Macromol.*, vol. 238, p. 124031, 2023.
[112] Gunathilake, T. M. S. U., Ching, Y. C., Chuah, C. H., Hai, N. D., & Nai-Shang, L., "Electro-stimulated release of poorly water-soluble drug from poly (lactic acid)/carboxymethyl cellulose/ZnO nanocomposite film," *Pharm. Res.*, vol. 37, pp. 1–20, 2020.
[113] Sirviö, J. A., Haataja, R., Kantola, A. M., Suopajärvi, T., & Liimatainen, H., "Insights into the role of molar ratio and added water in the properties of choline chloride and urea-based eutectic mixtures and their cellulose swelling capacity," *Phys. Chem. Chem. Phys.*, vol. 24, no. 46, pp. 28609–28620, 2022.
[114] Jing, S., Wu, L., Siciliano, A. P., Chen, C., Li, T., & Hu, L., "The critical roles of water in the processing, structure, and properties of nanocellulose," *ACS Nano*, vol. 17, no. 22, pp. 22196–22226, 2023.
[115] Hamouda, R. A., Abd El Maksoud, A. I., Wageed, M., Alotaibi, A. S., Elebeedy, D., Khalil, H., … & Abdella, A., "Characterization and anticancer activity of biosynthesized Au/cellulose nanocomposite from Chlorella vulgaris," *Polymers (Basel)*, vol. 13, no. 19, p. 3340, 2021.

[116] Doustdar, F., Olad, A., & Ghorbani, M., "Development of a novel reinforced scaffold based on chitosan/cellulose nanocrystals/halloysite nanotubes for curcumin delivery," *Carbohydr. Polym.*, vol. 282, p. 119127, 2022.

[117] Liu, W., Du, H., Zheng, T., & Si, C., "Biomedical applications of bacterial cellulose based composite hydrogels," *Curr. Med. Chem.*, vol. 28, no. 40, pp. 8319–8332, 2021.

[118] Hosny, K. M., Alkhalidi, H. M., Alharbi, W. S., Md, S., Sindi, A. M., Ali, S. A., ... & Kurakula, M., "Recent trends in assessment of cellulose derivatives in designing novel and nanoparticulate-based drug delivery systems for improvement of oral health," *Polymers (Basel)*, vol. 14, no. 1, p. 92, 2021.

[119] Khosravi Nessiani, N., Karmegam, M., Jayakumar, R., "Antibacterial and antifungal properties of green herbal compounds for textile applications," in *Encyclopedia of Green Materials*, 2022, pp. 1–9.

[120] Ghafari, R., Jonoobi, M., Naijian, F., Ashori, A., Mekonnen, T. H., & Taheri, A. R., "Fabrication and characterization of bilayer scaffolds - nanocellulosic cryogels - for skin tissue engineering by co-culturing of fibroblasts and keratinocytes," *Int. J. Biol. Macromol.*, vol. 223, pp. 100–107, 2022.

[121] Raut, M. P., Asare, E., Syed Mohamed, S. M. D., Amadi, E. N., & Roy, I., "Bacterial cellulose-based blends and composites: Versatile biomaterials for tissue engineering applications," *Int. J. Mol. Sci.*, vol. 24, no. 2, p. 986, 2023.

[122] Cakmak, A. M., Unal, S., Sahin, A., Oktar, F. N., Sengor, M., Ekren, N., ... & Kalaskar, D. M., "3D printed polycaprolactone/gelatin/bacterial cellulose/hydroxyapatite composite scaffold for bone tissue engineering," *Polymers (Basel)*, vol. 12, no. 9, p. 1962, 2020.

[123] Opricǎ, G. M., Panaitescu, D. M., Usurelu, C. D., Vlǎsceanu, G. M., Stanescu, P. O., Lixandru, B. E., ... & Frone, A. N., "Nanocellulose sponges containing antibacterial basil extract," *Int. J. Mol. Sci.*, vol. 24, no. 14, p. 11871, 2023.

[124] Bai, F., Dong, T., Chen, W., Wang, J., & Li, X., "Nanocellulose hybrid lignin complex reinforces cellulose to form a strong, water-stable lignin-cellulose composite usable as a plastic replacement," *Nanomaterials*, vol. 11, no. 12, p. 3426, 2021.

[125] Hong, J. K., Cooke, S. L., Whittington, A. R., & Roman, M., "Bioactive cellulose nanocrystal-poly (ε-caprolactone) nanocomposites for bone tissue engineering applications," *Front. Bioeng. Biotechnol.*, vol. 9, p. 605924, 2021.

[126] Aminatun, A., Hikmawati, D., Widiyanti, P., Amrillah, T., Nia, W. A., Firdania, I. T., & Abdullah, C. A. C., "Study of mechanical and thermal properties in nano-hydroxyapatite/chitosan/carboxymethyl cellulose nanocomposite-based scaffold for bone tissue engineering: The roles of carboxymethyl cellulose," *Appl. Sci.*, vol. 10, no. 19, p. 6970, 2020.

[127] Patel, D. K., Dutta, S. D., Hexiu, J., Ganguly, K., & Lim, K. T., "Bioactive electrospun nanocomposite scaffolds of poly (lactic acid)/cellulose nanocrystals for bone tissue engineering," *Int. J. Biol. Macromol.*, vol. 162, pp. 1429–1441, 2020.

[128] Khan, M. U. A., Haider, S., Haider, A., Abd Razak, S. I., Kadir, M. R. A., Shah, S. A., ... & Al-Zahrani, A. A., "Development of porous, antibacterial and biocompatible GO/n-HAp/bacterial cellulose/β-glucan biocomposite scaffold for bone tissue engineering," *Arab. J. Chem.*, vol. 14, no. 2, p. 102924, 2021.

[129] Nizan, N. S. N. H. & Zulkifli, F. H., "Reinforcement of hydroxyethyl cellulose/poly (vinyl alcohol) with cellulose nanocrystal as a bone tissue engineering scaffold," *J. Polym. Res.*, vol. 27, pp. 1–9, 2020.

[130] Ghorbani, M., Roshangar, L., & Rad, J. S., "Development of reinforced chitosan/pectin scaffold by using the cellulose nanocrystals as nanofillers: An injectable hydrogel for tissue engineering," *Eur. Polym. J.*, vol. 130, p. 109697, 2020.

[131] Mirtaghavi, A., Baldwin, A., Tanideh, N., Zarei, M., Muthuraj, R., Cao, Y., ... & Luo, J., "Crosslinked porous three-dimensional cellulose nanofibers-gelatine biocomposite scaffolds for tissue regeneration," *Int. J. Biol. Macromol.*, vol. 164, pp. 1949–1959, 2020.

[132] Lohrasbi, S., Mirzaei, E., Karimizade, A., Takallu, S., & Rezaei, A., "Collagen/cellulose nanofiber hydrogel scaffold: Physical, mechanical and cell biocompatibility properties," *Cellulose*, vol. 27, pp. 927–940, 2020.

[133] Sharma, C., Bhardwaj, N. K., & Pathak, P., "Ternary nano-biocomposite films using synergistic combination of bacterial cellulose with chitosan and gelatin for tissue engineering applications," *J. Biomater. Sci. Polym. Ed.*, vol. 32, no. 2, pp. 166–188, 2021.

[134] Maharjan, B., Park, J., Kaliannagounder, V. K., Awasthi, G. P., Joshi, M. K., Park, C. H., & Kim, C. S., "Regenerated cellulose nanofiber reinforced chitosan hydrogel scaffolds for bone tissue engineering," *Carbohydr. Polym.*, vol. 251, p. 117023, 2021.

[135] Goudarzi, Z. M., Behzad, T., Ghasemi-Mobarakeh, L., & Kharaziha, M., "An investigation into influence of acetylated cellulose nanofibers on properties of PCL/Gelatin electrospun nanofibrous scaffold for soft tissue engineering," *Polymer (Guildf)*, vol. 213, p. 123313, 2021.

[136] Mousa, H. M., Hussein, K. H., Sayed, M. M., Abd El-Rahman, M. K., & Woo, H. M., "Development and characterization of cellulose/iron acetate nanofibers for bone tissue engineering applications," *Polymers (Basel)*, vol. 13, no. 8, p. 1339, 2021.

[137] Khadivar, P., Khajeniazi, S., & Karimi, A., "Preparation of a carboxymethylated diethyl aminoethyl cellulose-collagen nanocomposite scaffold as a candidate for skin tissue engineering," *J. Mater. Res. Technol.*, vol. 19, pp. 3966–3979, 2022.

[138] Ali, A., Bano, S., Poojary, S., Chaudhary, A., Kumar, D., & Negi, Y. S., "Effect of cellulose nanocrystals on chitosan/PVA/nano β-TCP composite scaffold for bone tissue engineering application," *J. Biomater. Sci. Polym. Ed.*, vol. 33, no. 1, pp. 1–19, 2022.

[139] N'Gatta, K. M., Belaid, H., El Hayek, J., Assanvo, E. F., Kajdan, M., Masquelez, N., … & Salameh, C., "3D printing of cellulose nanocrystals based composites to build robust biomimetic scaffolds for bone tissue engineering," *Sci. Rep.*, vol. 12, no. 1, p. 21244, 2022.

[140] Mohammadalipour, M., Karbasi, S., Behzad, T., Mohammadalipour, Z., & Zamani, M., "Effect of cellulose nanofibers on polyhydroxybutyrate electrospun scaffold for bone tissue engineering applications," *Int. J. Biol. Macromol.*, vol. 220, pp. 1402–1414, 2022.

[141] Cao, S., Li, Q., Zhang, S., Liu, K., Yang, Y., & Chen, J., "Oxidized bacterial cellulose reinforced nanocomposite scaffolds for bone repair," *Colloids Surf. B Biointerfaces*, vol. 211, p. 112316, 2022.

[142] Eskilson, O., Zattarin, E., Berglund, L., Oksman, K., Hanna, K., Rakar, J., … & Aili, D., "Nanocellulose composite wound dressings for real-time pH wound monitoring," *Mater. Today Bio*, vol. 19, p. 100574, 2023.

[143] Pasaribu, K. M., Ilyas, S., Tamrin, T., Radecka, I., Swingler, S., Gupta, A., … & Gea, S., "Bioactive bacterial cellulose wound dressings for burns with collagen in-situ and chitosan ex-situ impregnation," *Int. J. Biol. Macromol.*, vol. 230, p. 123118, 2023.

[144] Zahel, P., Beekmann, U., Eberlein, T., Schmitz, M., Werz, O., & Kralisch, D., "Bacterial cellulose-adaptation of a nature-identical material to the needs of advanced chronic wound care," *Pharmaceuticals*, vol. 15, no. 6, p. 683, 2022.

[145] Isopencu, G., Deleanu, I., Busuioc, C., Oprea, O., Surdu, V. A., Bacalum, M., … & Stoica-Guzun, A., "Bacterial cellulose-carboxymethylcellulose composite loaded with turmeric extract for antimicrobial wound dressing applications," *Int. J. Mol. Sci.*, vol. 24, no. 2, p. 1719, 2023.

[146] Ding, M., Wang, X., Man, J., Li, J., Qiu, Y., Zhang, Y., … & Li, J., "Antibacterial and hemostatic polyvinyl alcohol/microcrystalline cellulose reinforced sodium alginate breathable dressing containing Euphorbia humifusa extract based on microfluidic spinning technology," *Int. J. Biol. Macromol.*, vol. 239, p. 124167, 2023.

[147] Wan, J., Liang, Y., Wei, X., Liang, H., & Chen, X. L., "Chitosan-based double network hydrogel loading herbal small molecule for accelerating wound healing," *Int. J. Biol. Macromol.*, vol. 246, p. 125610, 2023.

[148] Ahovan, Z. A., Khosravimelal, S., Eftekhari, B. S., Mehrabi, S., Hashemi, A., Eftekhari, S., … & Gholipourmalekabadi, M., "Thermo-responsive chitosan hydrogel for healing of full-thickness wounds infected with XDR bacteria isolated from burn patients: In vitro and in vivo animal model," *Int. J. Biol. Macromol.*, vol. 164, pp. 4475–4486, 2020.

[149] Fu, R., Ren, Y., Fang, K., Sun, Y., Zhang, Z., & Luo, A., "Preparation, characterization and biocompatibility of chitosan/TEMPO-oxidized bacterial cellulose composite film for potential wound dressing applications," *Fibers Polym.*, vol. 22, no. 7, pp. 1790–1799, 2021.

[150] Balla, E. D., Bikiaris, N. D., Nanaki, S. G., Papoulia, C., Chrissafis, K., Klonos, P. A., … & Papageorgiou, G. Z., "Chloramphenicol loaded sponges based on PVA/nanocellulose nanocomposites for topical wound delivery," *J. Compos. Sci.*, vol. 5, no. 8, p. 208, 2021.

[151] Gou, L., Xiang, M., & Ni, X., "Development of wound therapy in nursing care of infants by using injectable gelatin-cellulose composite hydrogel incorporated with silver nanoparticles," *Mater. Lett.*, vol. 277, p. 128340, 2020.

[152] Li, A., Han, Z., Li, Z., Li, J., Li, X., & Zhang, Z., "A PTHrP-2 loaded adhesive cellulose acetate nanofiber mat as wound dressing accelerates wound healing," *Mater. Des.*, vol. 212, p. 110241, 2021.

[153] Claro, F. C., Jordão, C., de Viveiros, B. M., Isaka, L. J. E., Villanova Junior, J. A., & Magalhães, W. L. E., "Low cost membrane of wood nanocellulose obtained by mechanical defibrillation for potential applications as wound dressing," *Cellulose*, vol. 27, pp. 10765–10779, 2020.

[154] Shahriari-Khalaji, M., Hong, S., Hu, G., Ji, Y., & Hong, F. F., "Bacterial nanocellulose-enhanced alginate double-network hydrogels cross-linked with six metal cations for antibacterial wound dressing," *Polymers (Basel)*, vol. 12, no. 11, p. 2683, 2020.

[155] Ahmad, N., Tayyeb, D., Ali, I. K., Alruwaili, N., Ahmad, W., ur Rehman, A., … & Iqbal, M. S., "Development and characterization of hemicellulose-based films for antibacterial wound-dressing application," *Polymers (Basel)*, vol. 12, no. 3, p. 548, 2020.

[156] Tavakoli, S., Kharaziha, M., Nemati, S., & Kalateh, A., "Nanocomposite hydrogel based on carrageenan-coated starch/cellulose nanofibers as a hemorrhage control material," *Carbohydr. Polym.*, vol. 251, p. 117013, 2021.

[157] Rooholghodos, S. H., Pourmadadi, M., Yazdian, F., & Rashedi, H., "Optimization of electrospun CQDs-Fe_3O_4-RE loaded PVA-cellulose nanofibrils via central composite design for wound dressing applications: Kinetics and in vitro release study," *Int. J. Biol. Macromol.*, vol. 237, p. 124067, 2023.

[158] Wang, Y., Xiao, D., Yu, H., Zhong, Y., Zhang, L., Sui, X., … & Mao, Z., "Composite hydrogel based oxidated sodium carboxymethyl cellulose and gelatin loaded carboxymethylated cotton fabric for hemostasis and infected wound treatment," *Int. J. Biol. Macromol.*, vol. 224, pp. 1382–1394, 2023.

[159] Sheikhy, S., Safekordi, A. A., Ghorbani, M., Adibkia, K., & Hamishehkar, H., "Synthesis of novel superdisintegrants for pharmaceutical tableting based on functionalized nanocellulose hydrogels," *Int. J. Biol. Macromol.*, vol. 167, pp. 667–675, 2021.

[160] Krivokapić, J., Ivanović, J., Djuriš, J., Medarević, D., Potpara, Z., Maksimović, Z., & Ibrić, S., "Tableting properties of microcrystalline cellulose obtained from wheat straw measured with a single punch bench top tablet press." *Saudi Pharm. J.*, vol. 28, no. 6, pp. 710–718, 2020.

[161] Löbmann, K. & Svagan, A. J., "Cellulose nanofibers as excipient for the delivery of poorly soluble drugs," *Int. J. Pharm.*, vol. 533, no. 1, pp. 285–297, 2017.

[162] Paukkonen, H., Kunnari, M., Laurén, P., Hakkarainen, T., Auvinen, V. V., Oksanen, T., … & Laaksonen, T., "Nanofibrillar cellulose hydrogels and reconstructed hydrogels as matrices for controlled drug release," *Int. J. Pharm.*, vol. 532, no. 1, pp. 269–280, 2017.

[163] Wang, T., Chen, L., Shen, T., & Wu, D., "Preparation and properties of a novel thermo-sensitive hydrogel based on chitosan/hydroxypropyl methylcellulose/glycerol," *Int. J. Biol. Macromol.*, vol. 93, pp. 775–782, 2016.

[164] Rakhshaei, R., Namazi, H., Hamishehkar, H., & Rahimi, M., "Graphene quantum dot cross-linked carboxymethyl cellulose nanocomposite hydrogel for pH-sensitive oral anticancer drug delivery with potential bioimaging properties," *Int. J. Biol. Macromol.*, vol. 150, pp. 1121–1129, 2020.

[165] Ji, L., Zhang, F., Zhu, L., & Jiang, J., "An in-situ fabrication of bamboo bacterial cellulose/sodium alginate nanocomposite hydrogels as carrier materials for controlled protein drug delivery," *Int. J. Biol. Macromol.*, vol. 170, pp. 459–468, 2021.

[166] Prusty, K. & Swain, S. K., "Polypropylene oxide/polyethylene oxide-cellulose hybrid nanocomposite hydrogels as drug delivery vehicle," *J. Appl. Polym. Sci.*, vol. 138, no. 9, p. 49921, 2021.

[167] Anirudhan, T. S., Manjusha, V., & Sekhar, V. C., "A new biodegradable nano cellulose-based drug delivery system for pH-controlled delivery of curcumin," *Int. J. Biol. Macromol.*, vol. 183, pp. 2044–2054, 2021.

[168] Yusefi, M., Shameli, K., Lee-Kiun, M. S., Teow, S. Y., Moeini, H., Ali, R. R., … & Abdullah, N. H., "Chitosan coated magnetic cellulose nanowhisker as a drug delivery system for potential colorectal cancer treatment," *Int. J. Biol. Macromol.* vol. 233, p. 123388, 2023.

[169] Chen, Y., Cheng, H., Wang, W., Jin, Z., Liu, Q., Yang, H., … & Gupta, V. K., "Preparation of carbon dots-hematite quantum dots-loaded hydroxypropyl cellulose-chitosan nanocomposites for drug delivery, sunlight catalytic and antimicrobial application," *J. Photochem. Photobiol. B Biol.*, vol. 219, p. 112201, 2021.

[170] Parvaneh, S., Pourmadadi, M., Abdouss, M., Pourmousavi, S. A., Yazdian, F., Rahdar, A., & Díez-Pascual, A. M., "Carboxymethyl cellulose/starch/reduced graphene oxide composite as a pH-sensitive nanocarrier for curcumin drug delivery," *Int. J. Biol. Macromol.*, vol. 241, p. 124566, 2023.

[171] Ghayour, N. et al., "Nanoencapsulation of quercetin and curcumin in casein-based delivery systems," *Food Hydrocoll.*, vol. 87, pp. 394–403, 2019.

[172] Cabrera-Barjas, G., Becheran, L., Valdés, O., Giordano, A., Segura-del Río, R., Bravo-Arrepol, G., … & Delattre, C., "Effect of cellulose nanofibrils on vancomycin drug release from chitosan nanocomposite films," *Eur. Polym. J.*, vol. 197, no. 112371, 2023.

[173] Kim, D. S., Haji, F., Jun, J., Baek, J., Han, L., Wu, P., … & Tam, K. C., "Mucoadhesive cellulose Nanocrystal-chitosan nanocomposite for the delivery of hydrophobic compounds," *JCIS Open*, vol. 11, p. 100092, 2023.

[174] Ghasemizadeh, H., Pourmadadi, M., Yazdian, F., Rashedi, H., Navaei-Nigjeh, M., Rahdar, A., & Díez-Pascual, A. M., "Novel carboxymethyl cellulose-halloysite-polyethylene glycol nanocomposite for improved 5-FU delivery," *Int. J. Biol. Macromol.*, vol. 232, p. 123437, 2023.

[175] Mariia, K., Arif, M., Ding, Y., Chi, Z., & Liu, C., "Preparation of novel hard capsule using water-soluble polysaccharides and cellulose nanocrystals for drug delivery," *J. Pharm. Innov.*, vol. 18, no. 2, pp. 675–686, 2023.

[176] Sivanesan, I., Muthu, M., Gopal, J., Hasan, N., Kashif Ali, S., Shin, J., & Oh, J. W., "Nanochitosan: Commemorating the metamorphosis of an exoskeletal waste to a versatile nutraceutical," *Nanomaterials*, vol. 11, no. 3, p. 821, 2021.

[177] Gupta, K. C. & Ravi Kumar, M. N., "An overview on chitin and chitosan applications with an emphasis on controlled drug release formulations," *J. Macromol. Sci. Part C Polym. Rev.*, vol. 40, no. 4, pp. 273–308, 2000.

[178] Burgos-Díaz, C., Opazo-Navarrete, M., Palacios, J. L., Barahona, T., Mosi-Roa, Y., Anguita-Barrales, F., & Bustamante, M., "Synthesis of new chitosan from an endemic Chilean crayfish exoskeleton (Parastacus Pugnax): Physicochemical and biological properties," *Polymers (Basel)*, vol. 13, no. 14, p. 2304, 2021.

[179] Asrahwi, M. A., Rosman, N. A., Shahri, N. N. M., Santos, J. H., Kusrini, E., Thongratkaew, S., … & Usman, A., "Solid-state mechanochemical synthesis of chitosan from mud crab (Scylla serrata) chitin," *Carbohydr. Res.*, vol. 534, p. 108971, 2023.

[180] Yu, M., Zhang, K., Guo, X., & Qian, L., "Effects of the degree of deacetylation on the single-molecule mechanics of chitosans," *J. Phys. Chem. B*, vol. 127, no. 19, pp. 4261–4267, 2023.

[181] Fu, B., Mei, S., Su, X., Chen, H., Zhu, J., Zheng, Z., … & Yang, D. P., "Integrating waste fish scale-derived gelatin and chitosan into edible nanocomposite film for perishable fruits," *Int. J. Biol. Macromol.*, vol. 191, pp. 1164–1174, 2021.

[182] Li, F., You, X., Li, Q., Qin, D., Wang, M., Yuan, S., … & Bi, S., "Homogeneous deacetylation and degradation of chitin in NaOH/urea dissolution system," *Int. J. Biol. Macromol.*, vol. 189, pp. 391–397, 2021.

[183] Araújo, D., Alves, V. D., Marques, A. C., Fortunato, E., Reis, M. A., & Freitas, F., "Low temperature dissolution of yeast chitin-glucan complex and characterization of the regenerated polymer," *Bioengineering*, vol. 7, no. 1, p. 28, 2020.

[184] Huang, J., Zhong, Y., Zhang, X., Xu, H., Zhu, C., & Cai, J., "Continuous pilot-scale wet-spinning of biocompatible chitin/chitosan multifilaments from an aqueous KOH/urea solution," *Macromol. Rapid Commun.*, vol. 42, no. 16, p. 210052, 2021.

[185] Saravanan, V., Davoodbasha, M., Rajesh, A., Nooruddin, T., Lee, S. Y., & Kim, J. W., "Extraction and characterization of Chitosan from Shell of Borassus flabellifer and their antibacterial and antioxidant applications," *Int. J. Biol. Macromol.*, vol. 253, p.126592, 2023.

[186] Al-Absi, M. Y., Caprifico, A. E., & Calabrese, G., "Chitosan and its structural modifications for siRNA delivery," *Adv. Pharm. Bull.*, vol. 13, no. 2, p. 275, 2023.

[187] Asghar, M. A., Yousuf, R. I., Shoaib, M. H., Asghar, M. A., Ansar, S., Zehravi, M., & Abdul Rehman, A., "Synergistic nanocomposites of different antibiotics coupled with green synthesized chitosan-based silver nanoparticles: Characterization, antibacterial, in vivo toxicological and biodistribution studies," *Int. J. Nanomed.*, vol. 15, pp. 7841–7859, 2020.

[188] Brasil, M., Filgueiras, A., Campos, M., Neves, M., Eugênio, M., Sena, L., Sant'Anna, C., da Silva, V., Diniz, C., & Sant'Ana, A., "Synergism in the antibacterial action of ternary mixtures involving silver nanoparticles, chitosan and antibiotics," *J. Braz. Chem. Soc.*, vol. 29, pp. 2026–2033, 2018.

[189] Ong, T. H., Chitra, E., Ramamurthy, S., Ling, C. C. S., Ambu, S. P., & Davamani, F., "Cationic chitosan-propolis nanoparticles alter the zeta potential of S. epidermidis, inhibit biofilm by modulating gene expression and exibit synergism with antibiotics," *PLoS One*, vol. 14, p. e0213079, 2019.

[190] Golmohamadi, M., Ghorbani, H. R., & Otadi, M., "Synthesis of chitosan nanoparticles loaded with antibiotics as drug carriers and the study of antibacterial activity," *J. Nanoanalysis*, vol. 6, no. 1, pp. 72–79, 2019.

[191] Sharma, P. K., Halder, M., Srivastava, U., & Singh, Y., "Antibacterial PEG-chitosan hydrogels for controlled antibiotic/protein delivery," *ACS Appl. Bio Mater.*, vol. 2, no. 12, pp. 5313–5322, 2019.

[192] Aksel, H., Mahjour, F., Bosaid, F., Calamak, S., & Azim, A., "Antimicrobial activity and biocompatibility of antibiotic-loaded chitosan hydrogels as a potential scaffold in regenerative endodontic treatment," *J. Endod.*, vol. 46, no. 12, pp. 1867–1875, 2020.

[193] Nimal, T. R., Mohandas, A., Riju, R. M., Arun, S. M., Raja, B., & Rangasamy, J., "Ciprofloxacin- and fluconazole-containing fibrin-nanoparticle-incorporated chitosan bandages for the treatment of polymicrobial wound infections," *ACS Appl. Bio Mater.*, vol. 2, no. 1, pp. 243–254, 2018.

[194] Goller, S. & Turner, N., "The antimicrobial effectiveness and cytotoxicity of the antibiotic-loaded chitosan: ECM scaffolds," *Appl. Sci.*, vol. 10, no. 10, p. 3446, 2020.

[195] Grimling, B., Karolewicz, B., Nawrot, U., Wlodarczyk, K., & Gorniak, A., "Physicochemical and antifungal properties of clotrimazole in combination with high-molecular weight chitosan as a multifunctional excipient," *Mar. Drugs*, vol. 18, no. 2, p. 591, 2020.

[196] Shahiwala, A. F., Khan, G. A., & Bostanooei, N. M., "Efficacy of levofloxacin, chitosan and EDTA combination against methicillin resistant Staphylococcus aureus skin infections: In vitro and in vivo evaluations," *Int. J. Clin Medation*, vol. 2, p. 119, 2017.

[197] Perinelli, D. R., Campana, R., Skouras, A., Bonacucina, G., Cespi, M., Mastrotto, F., Baffone, W., & Casettari, L., "Chitosan loaded into a hydrogel delivery system as a strategy to treat vaginal co-infection," *Pharmaceutics*, vol. 10, p. 23, 2018.

[198] Sun, H., Choi, D., Heo, J., Jung, S. Y., & Hong, J., "Studies on the drug loading and release profiles of degradable chitosan-based multilayer films for anticancer treatment," *Cancers (Basel)*, vol. 12, no. 3, p. 593, 2020.

[199] Li, X., Zeng, D., Ke, P., Wang, G., & Zhang, D., "Synthesis and characterization of magnetic chitosan microspheres for drug delivery," *RSC Adv.*, vol. 10, no. 12, pp. 7163–7169, 2020.

[200] Sudhakar, S., Chandran, S. V., Selvamurugan, N., & Nazeer, R. A., "Biodistribution and pharmacokinetics of thiolated chitosan nanoparticles for oral delivery of insulin in vivo biological macromolecules," *Int. J. Biol. Macromol.*, vol. 150, pp. 281–288, 2020.

[201] Mumuni, M. A., Kenechukwu, F. C., Ofokansi, K. C., Attama, A. A., & Díaz Díaz, D., "Insulin-loaded mucoadhesive nanoparticles based on mucin-chitosan complexes for oral delivery and diabetes treatment," *Carbohydr. Polym*, vol. 229, p. 115506, 2020.

[202] Wong, C. Y., Al-Salami, H., & Dass, C., "Formulation and characterisation of insulin-loaded chitosan nanoparticles capable of inducing glucose uptake in skeletal muscle cells in vitro," *J. Drug Deliv. Sci. Technol.*, vol. 57, p. 101738, 2020.

[203] Abdel-Moneim, A., El-Shahawy, A., Yousef, A. I., Abd El-Twab, S. M., Elden, Z. E., & Taha, M., "Novel polydatin-loaded chitosan nanoparticles for safe and efficient type 2 diabetes therapy: In silico, in vitro and in vivo approaches," *Int. J. Biol. Macromol.*, vol. 154, pp. 1496–1504, 2020.

[204] Coutinho, A. J., Costa Lima, S. A., Afonso, C. M. M., & Reis, S., "Mucoadhesive and pH responsive fucoidan-chitosan nanoparticles for the oral delivery of methotrexate," *Int. J. Biol. Macromol.*, vol. 158, pp. 180–188, 2020.

[205] Du, X., Yin, S., Xu, L., Ma, J., Yu, H., Wang, G., & Li, J., "Polylysine and cysteine functionalized chitosan nanoparticle as an efficient platform for oral delivery of paclitaxel," *Carbohydr. Polym.*, vol. 229, p. 115484, 2020.

[206] Tran, P. H. L., Wang, T., Yang, C., Tran, T. T. D., & Duan, W., "Development of conjugate-by-conjugate structured nanoparticles for oral delivery of docetaxel," *Mater. Sci. Eng. C*, vol. 107, p. 110346, 2020.

[207] Lin, C., Kuo, T. C., Lin, J. C., Ho, Y. C., & Mi, F., "Delivery of polysaccharides from Ophiopogon japonicus (OJPs) using OJPs/chitosan/whey protein co-assembled nanoparticles to treat defective intestinal epithelial tight junction barrier," *Int. J. Biol. Macromol.*, vol. 160, pp. 558–570, 2020.

[208] Saraf, S., Jain, S., Sahoo, R. N., & Mallick, S., "Lipopolysaccharide derived alginate coated Hepatitis B antigen loaded chitosan nanoparticles for oral mucosal immunization," *Int. J. Biol. Macromol.*, vol. 154, pp. 466–476, 2020.

[209] Murthy, A., Ravi, P. R., Kathuria, H., & Vats, R., "Self-Assembled lecithin-chitosan nanoparticles improve the oral bioavailability and alter the pharmacokinetics of raloxifene," *Int. J. Pharm.*, vol. 588, p. 119731, 2020.

[210] Yu, A., Shi, H., Liu, H., Bao, Z., Dai, M., Lin, D., Lin, D., Xu, X., Li, X., & Wang, Y., "Mucoadhesive dexamethasone-glycol chitosan nanoparticles for ophthalmic drug delivery," *Int. J. Pharm.*, vol. 575, p. 118943, 2020.

[211] Khalil, M., Hashmi, U., Riaz, R., & Abbas, S., "Chitosan coated liposomes (CCL) containing triamcinolone acetonide for sustained delivery: A potential topical treatment for posterior segment diseases," *Int. J. Biol. Macromol.*, vol. 143, pp. 483–491, 2020.
[212] Dumkliang, E., Pamornpathomkul, B., Patrojanasophon, P., Ngawhirunpat, T., Rojanarata, T., Yoksan, S., & Opanasopit, P., "Feasibility of chitosan-based nanoparticles approach for intranasal immunisation of live attenuated Japanese encephalitis vaccine," *Int. J. Biol. Macromol.*, vol. 183, pp. 1096–1105, 2021.
[213] Chatzitaki, A. T., Karavasili, S. J. C., Andreadis, D., Fatouros, D. G., & Borges, O., "Chitosan-coated PLGA nanoparticles for the nasal delivery of ropinirole hydrochloride: In vitro and ex vivo evaluation of efficacy and safety," *Int. J. Pharm.*, vol. 589, p. 119776, 2020.
[214] Cassano, R., Trapani, A., Di Gioia, M. L., Mandracchia, D., Pellitteri, R., Tripodo, G., Trombino, S., & Di Gioia, S., "Synthesis and characterization of novel chitosan-dopamine or chitosantyrosine conjugates for potential nose-to-brain delivery," *Int. J. Pharm.*, vol. 589, p. 119829, 2020.
[215] Sava, V., Fihurka, O., Khvorova, A., & Sanchez-Ramos, J., "Enriched chitosan nanoparticles loaded with siRNA are effective in lowering Huntington's disease gene expression following intranasal administration," *Nanomed. Nanotechnol. Biol. Med.*, vol. 24, p. 102119, 2020.
[216] Khezri, F. A. N. Z., Lakshmi, C. S. R., Bukka, R., Nidhi, M., & Nargund, S., "Pharmacokinetic study and brain tissue analysis of Zolmitriptan loaded chitosan nanoparticles in rats by LC-MS method," *Int. J. Biol. Macromol.*, vol. 142, pp. 52–62, 2020.
[217] Bhattamisra, S. K., Shak, A. T., Xi, L. W., Safian, N. H., Choudhury, H., Lim, W. M., Shahzad, N., Alhakamy, N. A., Anwer, K., & Radhakrishnan, A. K., "Nose to brain delivery of rotigotine loaded chitosan nanoparticles in human SH-SY5Y neuroblastoma cells and animal model of Parkinson's disease," *Int. J. Pharm.*, vol. 579, p. 119148, 2020.
[218] Wang, H., Holgate, J., Bartlett, S., & Islam, N., "Assessment of nicotine release from nicotine-loaded chitosan nanoparticles dry powder inhaler formulations via locomotor activity of C57BL/6 mice," *Eur. J. Pharm. Biopharm.*, vol. 154, pp. 175–185, 2020.
[219] Ahmad, N., Ahmad, R., Alrasheed, R. A., Almatar, H. M. A., Al-Ramadan, A. S., Buheazah, T. M., Al-Homoud, H. S., Al-Nasif, H. A., & Alam, A., "A Chitosan-PLGA based catechin hydrate nanoparticles used in targeting of lungs and cancer treatment," *Saudi J. Biol. Sci.*, vol. 27, pp. 2344–2357, 2020.
[220] Vieira, A. C. C., Chaves, L. L., Pinheiro, M., Costa Lima, S., Rolim Neto, P. J., Ferreira, D., Sarmento, B., & Reis, S., "Lipid nanoparticles coated with chitosan using a one-step association method to target rifampicin to alveolar macrophages," *Carbohydr. Polym*, vol. 25, p. 116978, 2021.
[221] Pardeshi, C. V., Agnihotri, V. V., Patil, K. Y., Pardeshi, S. R., & Surana, S., "Mannose-Anchored N,N,N-trimethyl chitosan nanoparticles for pulmonary administration of etofylline," *Int. J. Biol. Macromol.*, vol. 165, pp. 445–459, 2020.
[222] Dhayanandamoorthy, Y., Antoniraj, M. G., Kandregula, C. A. B., & Kandasamy, R., "Aerosolized hyaluronic acid decorated, ferulic acid loaded chitosan nanoparticle: A promising asthma control strategy," *Int. J. Pharm.*, vol. 591, p. 119958, 2020.
[223] Stie, M. B., Gätke, J. R., Wan, F., Chronakis, J. S., Jacobsen, J., & Nielsen, H., "Swelling of mucoadhesive electrospun chitosan/polyethylene oxide nanofibers facilitates adhesion to the sublingual mucosa," *Carbohydr. Polym*, vol. 24, p. 116428, 2020.
[224] Dos Santos, D. M., Chagas, P. A. M., Leite, I. S., Inada, N. M., de Annunzio, S. R., Fontana, C. R., Campana-Filho, S. P., & Correa, D., "Core-sheath nanostructured chitosan-based nonwovens as a potential drug delivery system for periodontitis treatment," *Int. J. Biol. Macromol.*, vol. 142, pp. 521–534, 2020.
[225] Araujo, H. C., Gomes da Silva, A. C., Paião, L. I., Magario, M. K. W., Frasnelli, F. C. T., Oliveira, S. H. P., Pessan, J. P., & Monteiro, D., "Antimicrobial, antibiofilm and cytotoxic effects of a colloidal nanocarrier composed by chitosan-coated iron oxide nanoparticles loaded with chlorhexidine," *J. Dent.*, vol. 101, p. 103453, 2020.
[226] Abd-Allah, H., Abdel-Aziz, R. T. A., & Nasr, M., "Chitosan nanoparticles making their way to clinical practice: A feasibility study on their topical use for acne treatment," *Int. J. Biol. Macromol.*, vol. 156, pp. 262–272, 2020.
[227] Morad, H., Jahanshahi, M., Akbari, J., Saeedi, M., Gill, P., & Enayatifard, R., "Novel topical and transdermal delivery of colchicine with chitosan based biocomposite nanofiberous system; formulation, optimization, characterization, ex vivo skin deposition/permeation, and anti-melanoma evaluation," *Mater. Chem. Phys.*, vol. 263, p. 124381, 2021.

[228] Fahimirad, S., Abtahi, H., Satei, P., Ghaznavi-Rad, E., Moslehi, M., & Ganji, A., "Wound healing performance of PCL/Chitosan based electrospun nanofiber electrosprayed with curcumin loaded chitosan nanoparticles," *Carbohydr. Polym*, vol. 259, p. 117640, 2021.

[229] Shafique, M., Sohail, M., Minhas, M. U., Khaliq, T., Kousar, M., Khan, S., Hussain, Z., Mahmood, A., Abbasi, M., & Aziz, H. C., "Bio-functional hydrogel membranes loaded with chitosan nanoparticles for accelerated wound healing," *Int. J. Biol. Macromol.*, vol. 170, pp. 207–221, 2021.

[230] Arumugam, G. & Rajendran, R., "Callophycin A loaded chitosan and spicules based nanocomposites as an alternative strategy to overcome vaginal candidiasis," *Int. J. Biol. Macromol.*, vol. 161, pp. 656–665, 2020.

[231] Abdel Allah, N. H., Gaber, Y., Rashed, M. E., Azmy, A. F., Abou-Taleb, H. A., & Abdel Ghani, S., "Alginate-Coated chitosan nanoparticles act as effective adjuvant for hepatitis A vaccine in mice," *Int. J. Biol. Macromol.*, vol. 152, pp. 904–912, 2020.

[232] Baghaei, M., Tekie, F. S. M., Khoshayand, M. R., Varshochian, R., Hajiramezanali, M., Kachousangi, M. J., Dinarvand, R., & Atyabiet, F., "Optimization of chitosan-based polyelectrolyte nanoparticles for gene delivery, using design of experiment: In vitro and in vivo study," *Mater. Sci. Eng. C*, vol. 118, p. 111036, 2021.

[233] Yan, T., Zhu, S., Hui, W., He, J., Liu, Z., & Cheng, J., "Chitosan based pH-responsive polymeric prodrug vector for enhanced tumor targeted co-delivery of doxorubicin and siRNA," *Carbohydr. Polym*, vol. 250, p. 116781, 2020.

[234] Yang, Y., Dong, Z., Li, M., Liu, L., Luo, H., Wang, P., … & Lei, S., "Graphene oxide/copper nanoderivatives-modified chitosan/hyaluronic acid dressings for facilitating wound healing in infected full-thickness skin defects," *Int. J. Nanomedicine*, pp. 8231–8247, 2020.

[235] Huang, J., Lu, D., Wu, C., Pei, D., Guo, C., Guo, H., … & Gao, B., "Guanidinylated bioactive chitosan-based injectable hydrogels with pro-angiogenic and mechanical properties for accelerated wound closure," *Int. J. Biol. Macromol.*, vol. 258, p. 128943, 2024.

[236] Jiang, T., Wang, D., Zhang, X., Yang, Q., Huang, Q., Ju, X., … & Li, C., "Electrospinning of chitosan/polyvinyl alcohol Pickering emulsion with tea tree essential oil loaded for anti-infection wound dressings," *Mater. Chem. Phys.*, vol. 311, p. 128561, 2024.

[237] Barbosa, J. L., de Melo, M. I. A., da Silva Cunha, P., de Miranda, M. C., Barrioni, B. R., Moreira, C. D. F., … & de Goes, A. M., "Development of a membrane and a bilayer of chitosan, gelatin, and polyhydroxybutyrate to be used as wound dressing for the regeneration of rat excisional wounds," *J. Biomed. Mater. Res. Part A*, vol. 112, no. 1, pp. 82–98, 2024.

[238] Malik, A. K., Singh, C., Tiwari, P., Verma, D., Mehata, A. K., Setia, A., … & Muthu, M. S., "Nanofibers of N, N, N-trimethyl chitosan capped bimetallic nanoparticles: Preparation, characterization, wound dressing and in-vivo treatment of MDR microbial infection and tracking by optical and photoacoustic imaging," *Int. J. Biol. Macromol.*, vol. 263, p. 130154, 2024.

[239] Amir, F., Niazi, M. B. K., Malik, U. S., Jahan, Z., Andleeb, S., Ahmad, T., & Mustansar, Z., "A multifunctional vanillin-infused chitosan-PVA hydrogel reinforced by nanocellulose and CuO-Ag nanoparticles as antibacterial wound dressing," *Int. J. Biol. Macromol.*, vol. 258, 2024.

[240] Nakipoglu, A., Özkabadayı, Y., Karahan, S., & Tezcaner, A., "Bilayer wound dressing composed of asymmetric polycaprolactone membrane and chitosan-carrageenan hydrogel incorporating storax balsam," *Int. J. Biol. Macromol.*, vol. 254, p. 128020, 2024.

[241] Karami, F., Torabiardekani, N., Moradi, M., Zare, A., Mojahedtaghi, M., Khorram, M., … & Zareshahrabadi, Z., "Chitosan-based emulgel and xerogel film containing Thymus pubescens essential oil as a potential wound dressing," *Carbohydr. Polym.*, vol. 318, p. 121156, 2023.

[242] Li, C., Jiang, T., Zhou, C., Jiang, A., Lu, C., Yang, G., … & Chen, Z., "Injectable self-healing chitosan-based POSS-PEG hybrid hydrogel as wound dressing to promote diabetic wound healing," *Carbohydr. Polym.*, vol. 299, p. 120198, 2023.

[243] Liu, F., Wang, L., Zhai, X., Ji, S., Ye, J., Zhu, Z., … & Wei, W., "A multi-functional double cross-linked chitosan hydrogel with tunable mechanical and antibacterial properties for skin wound dressing," *Carbohydr. Polym.*, vol. 322, p. 121344, 2023.

[244] Chen, Z., Yao, J., Zhao, J., & Wang, S., "Injectable wound dressing based on carboxymethyl chitosan triple-network hydrogel for effective wound antibacterial and hemostasis," *Int. J. Biol. Macromol.*, vol. 225, pp. 1235–1245, 2023.

[245] Akram, A. M., Omar, R. A., & Ashfaq, M., "Chitosan/calcium phosphate-nanoflakes-based biomaterial: A potential hemostatic wound dressing material," *Polym. Bull.*, vol. 80, no. 5, pp. 5071–5086, 2023.

[246] Piekarska, K., Sikora, M., Owczarek, M., Jóźwik-Pruska, J., & Wiśniewska-Wrona, M., "Chitin and Chitosan as polymers of the future-obtaining, modification, life cycle assessment and main directions of application," *Polymers (Basel)*, vol. 15, no. 4, p. 793, 2023.

[247] Al Shaqsi, N. H. K., Al Hoqani, H. A. S., Hossain, M. A., & Al Sibani, M. A., "Optimization of the demineralization process for the extraction of chitin from Omani Portunidae segnis," *Biochem. Biophys. Rep.*, vol. 23, p. 100779, 2020.

[248] Jabeen, A. S., Younis, T., Sidra, S., Muneer, B., Nasreen, Z., Saleh, F., … & Abbas, A. S., "Extraction of chitin from edible crab shells of Callinectes sapidus and comparison with market purchased chitin," *Braz. J. Biol.*, vol. 83, 2021.

[249] Subramanian, K., Sadaiappan, B., Aruni, W., Kumarappan, A., Thirunavukarasu, R., Srinivasan, G. P., … & Subramanian, M., "Bioconversion of chitin and concomitant production of chitinase and N-acetylglucosamine by novel Achromobacter xylosoxidans isolated from shrimp waste disposal area," *Sci. Rep.*, vol. 10, no. 1, p. 11898, 2020.

[250] Madland, E., Forsberg, Z., Wang, Y., Lindorff-Larsen, K., Niebisch, A., Modregger, J., … & Courtade, G., "Structural and functional variation of chitin-binding domains of a lytic polysaccharide monooxygenase from Cellvibrio japonicus," *J. Biol. Chem.*, vol. 297, no. 4, 2021.

[251] Montroni, D., Sparla, F., Fermani, S., & Falini, G., "Influence of proteins on mechanical properties of a natural chitin-protein composite," *Acta Biomater.*, vol. 120, pp. 81–90, 2021.

[252] Al-Hmoud, L., Abu Fara, D., Rashid, I., Chowdhry, B. Z., & Badwan, A. A., "Influence of Chitin source and polymorphism on powder compression and compaction: Application in drug delivery," *Molecules*, vol. 25, no. 22, p. 5269, 2020.

[253] Kim, H., Kim, H., Ahn, Y., Hong, K. B., Kim, I. W., Choi, R. Y., … & Han, S. H., "The preparation and physiochemical characterization of tenebrio molitor chitin using alcalase," *Molecules*, vol. 28, no. 7, p. 3254, 2023.

[254] Turley, J. L., Moran, H. B., McEntee, C. P., O'Grady, K., Muñoz-Wolf, N., Jin, L., … & Lavelle, E. C., "Chitin-derived polymer deacetylation regulates mitochondrial reactive oxygen species dependent cGAS-STING and NLRP3 inflammasome activation," *Biomaterials*, vol. 275, p. 120961, 2021.

[255] Rahayu, A. P., Islami, A. F., Saputra, E., Sulmartiwi, L., Rahmah, A. U., & Kurnia, K. A., "The impact of the different types of acid solution on the extraction and adsorption performance of chitin from shrimp shell waste," *Int. J. Biol. Macromol.*, vol. 194, pp. 843–850, 2022.

[256] Gharibzadeh, M., Osfouri, S., Jamekhorshid, A., & Jafari, S. A., "Microbial chitin extraction and characterization from green tiger shrimp waste: A comparative study of culture mediums along with bioprocess optimization," *Int. J. Biol. Macromol.*, vol. 242, p. 125213, 2023.

[257] Cui, Y., Wu, Q., He, J., Li, M., Zhang, Z., & Qiu, Y., "Porous nano-minerals substituted apatite/chitin/pectin nanocomposites scaffolds for bone tissue engineering," *Arab. J. Chem.*, vol. 13, no. 10, pp. 7418–7429, 2020.

[258] Zubillaga, V., Alonso-Varona, A., Fernandes, S. C., Salaberria, A. M., & Palomares, T., "Adipose-derived mesenchymal stem cell chondrospheroids cultured in hypoxia and a 3D porous chitosan/chitin nanocrystal scaffold as a platform for cartilage tissue engineering," *Int. J. Mol. Sci.*, vol. 21, no. 3, p. 1004, 2020.

[259] Machałowski, T., Rusak, A., Wiatrak, B., Haczkiewicz-Leśniak, K., Popiel, A., Jaroszewicz, J., … & Jesionowski, T., "Naturally formed chitinous skeleton isolated from the marine demosponge Aplysina fistularis as a 3D scaffold for tissue engineering," *Materials (Basel)*, vol. 14, no. 11, 2021.

[260] Liu, K., Zhu, L., Tang, S., Wen, W., Lu, L., Liu, M., … & Luo, B., "Fabrication and evaluation of a chitin whisker/poly (L-lactide) composite scaffold by the direct trisolvent-ink writing method for bone tissue engineering," *Nanoscale*, vol. 12, no. 35, pp. 18225–18239, 2020.

[261] Narayanan, K. B., Zo, S. M., & Han, S. S., "Novel biomimetic chitin-glucan polysaccharide nano/microfibrous fungal-scaffolds for tissue engineering applications," *Int. J. Biol. Macromol.*, vol. 149, pp. 724–731, 2020.

[262] Narayanan, K. B., Bhaskar, R., Kim, H., & Han, S. S., "In vitro cytocompatibility assessment of novel 3D chitin/glucan-and cellulose-based decellularized scaffolds for skin tissue engineering," *Sustainability*, vol. 15, no. 21, p. 15618, 2023.

[263] Wang, S., Xing, X., Peng, W., Huang, C., Du, Y., Yang, H., & Zhou, J., "Fabrication of an exosome-loaded thermosensitive chitin-based hydrogel for dental pulp regeneration," *J. Mater. Chem. B*, vol. 11, no. 27, pp. 1580–1590, 2023.

[264] Zawadzka-Knefel, A., Rusak, A., Mrozowska, M., Machałowski, T., Zak, A., Haczkiewicz-Leśniak, K., … & Skośkiewicz-Malinowska, K., "Chitin scaffolds derived from the marine demosponge Aplysina fistularis stimulate the differentiation of dental pulp stem cells," *Front. Bioeng. Biotechnol.*, vol. 11, p. 1254506, 2023.

[265] Wang, B., Lu, C. F., Liu, Z. Y., Han, S., Wei, P., Zhang, D. Y., … & Jiang, B. G., "Chitin scaffold combined with autologous small nerve repairs sciatic nerve defects," *Neural Regen. Res.*, vol. 17, no. 5, p. 1106, 2022.

[266] Fan, C., Li, Z., Ji, Q., Sun, H., Liang, Y., & Yang, P., "Carboxymethyl chitin or chitosan for osteoinduction effect on the human periodontal ligament stem cells," *Dent. Mater. J.*, vol. 41, no. 3, pp. 392–401, 2022.

[267] Zhao, P., Feng, Y., Zhou, Y., Tan, C., & Liu, M., "Gold@ Halloysite nanotubes-chitin composite hydrogel with antibacterial and hemostatic activity for wound healing," *Bioact. Mater.*, vol. 20, pp. 355–367, 2023.

[268] Ma, Y., Xu, S., Yue, P., Cao, H., Zou, Y., Wang, L., … & Ye, Q., "Synthesis and evaluation of water-soluble imidazolium salt chitin with broad-spectrum antimicrobial activity and excellent biocompatibility for infected wound healing," *Carbohydr. Polym.*, vol. 306, p. 120575, 2023.

[269] Guo, X., Shi, X., Chen, L., Wang, L., Deng, H., & Du, Y., "Electro-assembly of β-chitin nanofibers to construct oriented cryogel for wound healing," *Chem. Eng. J.*, vol. 471, p. 144346, 2023.

[270] Cao, H., Xiang, D., Zhou, X., Yue, P., Zou, Y., Zhong, Z., … & Ye, Q., "High-strength, antibacterial, antioxidant, hemostatic, and biocompatible chitin/PEGDE-tannic acid hydrogels for wound healing," *Carbohydr. Polym.*, vol. 307, p. 120609, 2023.

[271] Huang, L., Cai, M., Qiao, Q., Li, T., Chen, J., & Jiang, X., "Water soluble AIEgen-based thermosensitive and antibacterial hydroxypropyl chitin hydrogels for non-invasive visualization and wound healing," *Carbohydr. Polym.*, vol. 319, p. 121186, 2023.

[272] Zheng, L., Li, X., Xu, C., Xu, Y., Zeng, Y., Tam, M., … & Wang, X., "High-efficiency antibacterial hemostatic AgNP@ zeolite/chitin/bamboo composite sponge for wound healing," *Adv. Healthc. Mater.*, vol. 12, p. 2300075, 2023.

[273] Liu, Y., Liu, Y., Wu, M., Zou, R., Mao, S., Cong, P., … & Bao, Y., "Adipose-derived mesenchymal stem cell-loaded β-chitin nanofiber hydrogel promote wound healing in rats," *J. Mater. Sci. Mater. Med.*, vol. 33, no. 2, p. 12, 2022.

[274] Yang, Y., Zhang, H., Zeng, F., Jia, Q., Zhang, L., Yu, A., & Duan, B., "A quaternized chitin derivatives, egg white protein and montmorillonite composite sponge with antibacterial and hemostatic effect for promoting wound healing," *Compos. Part B Eng.*, vol. 234, p. 109661, 2022.

[275] de Oliveira Cardoso, V. M., Evangelista, R. C., Gremião, M. P. D., & Cury, B. S., "Insights into the impact of cross-linking processes on physicochemical characteristics and mucoadhesive potential of gellan gum/retrograded starch microparticles as a platform for colonic drug release," *J. Drug Deliv. Sci. Technol.*, vol. 55, p. 101445, 2020.

[276] Quadrado, R. F., & Fajardo, A., "Microparticles based on carboxymethyl starch/chitosan polyelectrolyte complex as vehicles for drug delivery systems," *Arab. J. Chem.*, vol. 13, pp. 2183–2194, 2020.

[277] De Almeida Costa, N., Silveira, L. R., de Paula Amaral, E., Pereira, G. C., de Almeida Paula, D., Vieira, É. N. R., Martins, E. M. F., Stringheta, P. C., Júnior, B. R. D. C. L., & Ramos, A., "Use of maltodextrin, sweet potato flour, pectin and gelatin as wall material for microencapsulating Lactiplantibacillus plantarum by spray drying: Thermal resistance, in vitro release behavior, storage stability and physicochemical properties," *Food Res. Int.*, vol. 164, p. 112367, 2023.

[278] Dos Santos, A. M., Meneguin, A. B., Akhter, D. T., Fletcher, N., Houston, Z. H., Bell, C., Thurecht, K. J., & Gremião, M. P., "Understanding the role of colon-specific microparticles based on retrograded starch/pectin in the delivery of chitosan nanoparticles along the gastrointestinal tract," *Eur. J. Pharm. Biopharm*, vol. 158, pp. 371–378, 2021.

[279] Obireddy, S. R., & Lai, W., "Preparation and characterization of 2-hydroxyethyl starch microparticles for co-delivery of multiple bioactive agents," *Drug Deliv.*, vol. 28, pp. 1562–1568, 2021.

[280] Choi, I., Li, N., & Zhong, Q., "Enhancing bioaccessibility of resveratrol by loading in natural porous starch microparticles," *Int. J. Biol. Macromol*, vol. 194, pp. 982–992, 2022.

[281] Moura, W. S., Oliveira, E. E., Haddi, K., Correa, R. F., Piau, T. B., Moura, D. S., Santos, S. F., Grisolia, C. K., Ribeiro, B. M., & Aguiar, R. W., "Cassava starch-based essential oil microparticles preparations: Functionalities in mosquito control and selectivity against non-target organisms," *Ind. Crop. Prod*, vol. 162, p. 113289, 2021.

[282] Ren, N., Ma, Z., Li, X., & Hu, X., "Preparation of rutin-loaded microparticles by debranched lentil starch-based wall materials: Structure, morphology and in vitro release behavior," *Int. J. Biol. Macromol.*, vol. 173, pp. 293–306, 2021.

[283] Baltrusch, K. L., Torres, M. D., Domínguez, H., & Flórez-Fernández, N., "Spray-drying microencapsulation of tea extracts using green starch, alginate or carrageenan as carrier materials," *Int. J. Biol. Macromol*, vol. 203, pp. 417–429, 2022.

[284] Kusonwiriyawong, C., "Development of spray-dried corn and tapioca starch microparticles for protein delivery," *J. Curr. Sci. Technol*, vol. 11, pp. 375–391, 2021.

[285] Zhao, Y., Zhi, J., Huang, S., Zhang, X., Kim, Y. R., Xu, Y., Wang, D., & Luo, K., "Fabrication of starch/zein-based microcapsules for encapsulation and delivery of fucoxanthin," *Food Chem.*, vol. 392, p. 133282, 2022.

[286] Cortez-Trejo, M. C., Wall-Medrano, A., Gaytán-Martínez, M., & Mendoza, S., "Microencapsulation of pomegranate seed oil using a succinylated taro starch: Characterization and bioaccessibility study," *Food Biosci.*, vol. 41, p. 100929, 2021.

[287] Ren, Q., Wu, M., Weng, Z., Zhu, X., Li, W., Huang, P., ... & Ohshima, M., "Promoted formation of stereocomplex in enantiomeric poly (lactic acid) s induced by cellulose nanofibers," *Carbohydr. Polym.*, vol. 276, p. 118800, 2022.

[288] Chang, W. W., Niu, J., Peng, H., & Rong, W., "Preferential formation of stereocomplex crystals in poly (L-lactic acid)/poly (D-lactic acid) blends by a fullerene nucleator," *Int. J. Biol. Macromol.*, vol. 253, p. 127230, 2023.

[289] Bai, T., Zhu, B., Liu, H., Wang, Y., Song, G., Liu, C., & Shen, C., "Biodegradable poly (lactic acid) nanocomposites reinforced and toughened by carbon nanotubes/clay hybrids," *Int. J. Biol. Macromol.*, vol. 151, pp. 628–634, 2020.

[290] Ahmed, J., & Varshney, S. K., "Polylactides—chemistry, properties and green packaging technology: A review," *Int. J. Food Prop.*, vol. 14, no. 1, pp. 37–58, 2011.

[291] Joshi, M. K., Lee, S., Tiwari, A. P., Maharjan, B., Poudel, S. B., Park, C. H., & Kim, C. S., "Integrated design and fabrication strategies for biomechanically and biologically functional PLA/β-TCP nanofiber reinforced GelMA scaffold for tissue engineering applications," *Int. J. Biol. Macromol.*, vol. 164, pp. 976–985, 2020.

[292] Lopresti, F., Campora, S., Tirri, G., Capuana, E., Pavia, F. C., Brucato, V., ... & La Carrubba, V., "Core-shell PLA/Kef hybrid scaffolds for skin tissue engineering applications prepared by direct kefiran coating on PLA electrospun fibers optimized via air-plasma treatment," *Mater. Sci. Eng. C*, vol. 127, p. 112248, 2021.

[293] Alizadeh-Osgouei, M., Li, Y., Vahid, A., Ataee, A., & Wen, C., "High strength porous PLA gyroid scaffolds manufactured via fused deposition modeling for tissue-engineering applications," *Smart Mater. Med.*, vol. 2, pp. 15–25, 2021.

[294] Mohandesnezhad, S., Pilehvar-Soltanahmadi, Y., Alizadeh, E., Goodarzi, A., Davaran, S., Khatamian, M., ... & Akbarzadeh, A., "In vitro evaluation of Zeolite-nHA blended PCL/PLA nanofibers for dental tissue engineering," *Mater. Chem. Phys.*, vol. 252, p. 123152, 2020.

[295] Wang, W., Zhang, B., Li, M., Li, J., Zhang, C., Han, Y., ... & Zhang, X., "3D printing of PLA/n-HA composite scaffolds with customized mechanical properties and biological functions for bone tissue engineering," *Compos. Part B Eng.*, vol. 224, p. 109192, 2021.

[296] Massoumi, B., Abbasian, M., Jahanban-Esfahlan, R., Mohammad-Rezaei, R., Khalilzadeh, B., Samadian, H., ... & Jaymand, M., "A novel bio-inspired conductive, biocompatible, and adhesive terpolymer based on polyaniline, polydopamine, and polylactide as scaffolding biomaterial for tissue engineering application," *Int. J. Biol. Macromol.*, vol. 147, pp. 1174–1184, 2020.

[297] Ye, Z., Xu, W., Shen, R., & Yan, Y., "Emulsion electrospun PLA/calcium alginate nanofibers for periodontal tissue engineering," *J. Biomater. Appl.*, vol. 34, no. 6, pp. 763–777, 2020.

[298] Oztemur, J., Ozdemir, S., Tezcan-Unlu, H., Cecener, G., Sezgin, H., & Yalcin-Enis, I., "Investigation of biodegradability and cellular activity of PCL/PLA and PCL/PLLA electrospun webs for tissue engineering applications," *Biopolymers*, vol. 114, no. 11, p. e23564, 2023.

[299] Wang, W., Zhang, B., Zhao, L., Li, M., Han, Y., Wang, L., ... & Liu, L., "Fabrication and properties of PLA/nano-HA composite scaffolds with balanced mechanical properties and biological functions for bone tissue engineering application," *Nanotechnol. Rev.*, vol. 10, no. 1, pp. 1359–1373, 2021.

[300] Gangolphe, L., Leon-Valdivieso, C. Y., Nottelet, B., Déjean, S., Bethry, A., Pinese, C., ... & Garric, X., "Electrospun microstructured PLA-based scaffolds featuring relevant anisotropic, mechanical and degradation characteristics for soft tissue engineering," *Mater. Sci. Eng. C*, vol. 129, p. 112339, 2021.

[301] Mundel, R., Thakur, T., & Chatterjee, M., "Emerging uses of PLA–PEG copolymer in cancer drug delivery," *3 Biotech*, vol. 12, no. 2, p. 41, 2022.

[302] Salahuddin, N., Abdelwahab, M., Gaber, M., & Elneanaey, S., "Synthesis and design of norfloxacin drug delivery system based on PLA/TiO_2 nanocomposites: Antibacterial and antitumor activities," *Mater. Sci. Eng. C*, vol. 108, p. 110337, 2020.

[303] Moorkoth, D., Nampoothiri, K. M., Nagarajan, S., Ravindran Girija, A., Balasubramaniyan, S., & Kumar, D. S., "Star-shaped polylactide dipyridamole conjugated to 5-fluorouracil and 4-piperidinopiperidine nanocarriers for bioimaging and dual drug delivery in cancer cells," *ACS Appl. Polym.*, vol. 3, no. 2, pp. 737–756, 2021.

[304] Farkas, N. I., Marincaş, L., Barabás, R., Bizo, L., Ilea, A., Turdean, G. L., ... & Barbu-Tudoran, L., "Preparation and characterization of doxycycline-loaded electrospun PLA/HAP nanofibers as a drug delivery system," *Materials (Basel)*, vol. 15, no. 6, p. 2105, 2022.

[305] Zhang, C., Yang, L., Wan, F., Bera, H., Cun, D., Rantanen, J., & Yang, M., "Quality by design thinking in the development of long-acting injectable PLGA/PLA-based microspheres for peptide and protein drug delivery," *Int. J. Pharm.*, vol. 585, p. 119441, 2020.

[306] Lacroix, C., Humanes, A., Coiffier, C., Gigmes, D., Verrier, B., & Trimaille, T., "Polylactide-based reactive micelles as a robust platform for mRNA delivery," *Pharm. Res.*, vol. 37, pp. 1–12, 2020.

[307] Butreddy, A., Gaddam, R. P., Kommineni, N., Dudhipala, N., & Voshavar, C., "PLGA/PLA-based long-acting injectable depot microspheres in clinical use: Production and characterization overview for protein/peptide delivery," *Int. J. Mol. Sci.*, vol. 21, no. 16, p. 8884, 2021.

[308] Richter, A. R., Carneiro, M. J., de Sousa, N. A., Pinto, V. P., Freire, R. S., de Sousa, J. S., ... & de Paula, R. C., "Self-assembling cashew gum-graft-polylactide copolymer nanoparticles as a potential amphotericin B delivery matrix," *Int. J. Biol. Macromol.*, vol. 152, pp. 492–502, 2020.

[309] Kost, B., Brzeziński, M., Zimnicka, M., Socka, M., Wielgus, E., Słowianek, M., & Biela, T., "PLA Stereocomplexed microspheres modified with methyl-β-cyclodextrin as an atropine delivery system. Synthesis and characterizatio," *Mater. Today Commun.*, vol. 25, p. 101605, 2020.

[310] Zhao, C., Xiao, Y., Ling, S., Pei, Y., & Ren, J., "Synthesis and assembly of recombinant collagen," *Fibrous Proteins Des. Synth. Assem.*, pp. 83–96, 2021.

[311] Bertsch, C., Maréchal, H., Gribova, V., Lévy, B., Debry, C., Lavalle, P., & Fath, L., "Biomimetic bilayered scaffolds for tissue engineering: From current design strategies to medical applications," *Adv. Healthc. Mater.*, p. 2203115, 2023.

[312] Li, Y., Liu, Y., Li, R., Bai, H., Zhu, Z., Zhu, L., ... & Huang, L., "Collagen-based biomaterials for bone tissue engineering," *Mater. Des.*, vol. 210, p. 1100149, 2021.

[313] Liu, S., Lau, C. S., Liang, K., Wen, F., & Teoh, S. H., "Marine collagen scaffolds in tissue engineering," *Curr. Opin. Biotechnol.*, vol. 74, pp. 92–103, 2022.

[314] Rico-Llanos, G. A., Borrego-González, S., Moncayo-Donoso, M., Becerra, J., & Visser, R., "Collagen type I biomaterials as scaffolds for bone tissue engineering," *Polymers (Basel)*, vol. 13, no. 4, p. 599, 2021.

[315] Vaez, M., Asgari, M., Hirvonen, L., Bakir, G., Khattignavong, E., Ezzo, M., ... & Bozec, L., "Modulation of the biophysical and biochemical properties of collagen by glycation for tissue engineering applications," *Acta Biomater.*, vol. 155, pp. 182–198, 2023.

[316] Kim, J. & Bonassar, L. J., "Controlling collagen gelation pH to enhance biochemical, structural, and biomechanical properties of tissue-engineered menisci," *J. Biomed. Mater. Res. Part A*, vol. 111, no. 4, pp. 478–487, 2023.

[317] Becerra, J., Rodriguez, M., Leal, D., Noris-Suarez, K., & Gonzalez, G., "Chitosan-collagen-hydroxyapatite membranes for tissue engineering," *J. Mater. Sci. Mater. Med.*, vol. 33, no. 2, p. 18, 2022.

[318] Nagaraj, A., Etxeberria, A. E., Naffa, R., Zidan, G., & Seyfoddin, A., "3D-Printed hybrid collagen/GelMA hydrogels for tissue engineering applications," *Biology (Basel)*, vol. 11, no. 11, p. 1561, 2022.

[319] Alves, A. L., Costa-Gouveia, J., de Castro, J. V., Sotelo, C. G., Vázquez, J. A., Pérez-Martín, R. I., ... & Silva, T. H., "Study of the immunologic response of marine-derived collagen and gelatin extracts for tissue engineering applications," *Acta Biomater.*, vol. 141, pp. 123–131, 2022.

[320] Oslan, S. N. H., Li, C. X., Shapawi, R., Mokhtar, R. A. M., Noordin, W. N. M., & Huda, N., "Extraction and characterization of bioactive fish by-product collagen as promising for potential wound healing agent in pharmaceutical applications: Current trend and future perspectiv," *Int. J. Food Sci.*, vol. 2022, p. 9437878, 2022.

[321] Nguyen, C. T., Vu, M. Q., Phan, T. T., Vu, T. Q., Vo, Q. A., Bach, G. L., & Thai, H., "Novel pH-sensitive hydrogel beads based on carrageenan and fish scale collagen for allopurinol drug delivery," *J. Polym. Environ.*, vol. 28, pp. 1795–1810, 2020.

[322] Lee, D., Wufuer, M., Kim, I., Choi, T. H., Kim, B. J., Jung, H. G., ... & Yoon, D. S., "Sequential dual-drug delivery of BMP-2 and alendronate from hydroxyapatite-collagen scaffolds for enhanced bone regeneration," *Sci. Rep.*, vol. 11, no. 1, p. 746, 2021.

[323] Hongsa, N., Thinbanmai, T., Luesakul, U., Sansanaphongpricha, K., & Muangsin, N., "A novel modified chitosan/collagen coated-gold nanoparticles for 5-fluorouracil delivery: Synthesis, characterization, in vitro drug release studies, anti-inflammatory activity and in vitro cytotoxicity assay," *Carbohydr. Polym.*, vol. 277, p. 118858, 2022.

[324] Billings, C. & Anderson, D. E., "Comparison of three methods for assessment of drug elution: In vitro elution of gentamicin from a collagen-based scaffold," *Front. Drug Deliv.*, vol. 2, p. 958731, 2022.

[325] Druzhkova, I., Nikonova, E., Ignatova, N., Koryakina, I., Zyuzin, M., Mozherov, A., ... & Shirmanova, M., "Effect of collagen matrix on doxorubicin distribution and cancer cells' response to treatment in 3D tumor model," *Cancers (Basel)*, vol. 14, no. 22, p. 5487, 2022.

[326] Skwira, A., Szewczyk, A., Barros, J., Laranjeira, M., Monteiro, F. J., Sądej, R., & Prokopowicz, M., "Biocompatible antibiotic-loaded mesoporous silica/bioglass/collagen-based scaffolds as bone drug delivery systems," *Int. J. Pharm.*, vol. 645, p. 123408, 2023.

[327] Daza, J. H. U., Righetto, G. M., Chaud, M. V., da Conceição Amaro Martins, V., Lopes Baratella da Cunha Camargo, I., & Maria de Guzzi Plepis, A., "PVA/anionic collagen membranes as drug carriers of ciprofloxacin hydrochloride with sustained antibacterial activity and potential use in the treatment of ulcerative keratitis," *J. Biomater. Appl.*, vol. 35, no. 3, pp. 301–312, 2021.

[328] Wang, T. Y., Kendrick-Williams, L. L., Choy, M. Y., Gilmore, K. A., Bonnard, T., Pearce, H. A., ... & Harth, E., "Collagen-targeted theranostic nanosponges for delivery of the matrix metalloproteinase 14 inhibitor naphthofluorescein," *Chem. Mater.*, vol. 32, no. 9, pp. 3707–3714, 2020.

[329] Mbese, Z., Alven, S., & Aderibigbe, B. A., "Collagen-based nanofibers for skin regeneration and wound dressing applications," *Polymers (Basel)*, vol. 13, no. 24, p. 4368, 2021.

[330] Tripathi, D., Rastogi, K., Tyagi, P., Rawat, H., Mittal, G., Jamini, A., ... & Tyagi, A., "Comparative analysis of collagen and chitosan-based dressing for haemostatic and wound healing application," *AAPS PharmSciTech*, vol. 22, pp. 1–15, 2021.

[331] Sun, L., Li, L., Wang, Y., Li, M., Xu, S., & Zhang, C., "A collagen-based bi-layered composite dressing for accelerated wound healing," *J. Tissue Viability*, vol. 31, no. 1, pp. 180–189, 2022.

[332] Amirrah, I., Mohd Razip Wee, M. F., Tabata, Y., Bt Hj Idrus, R., Nordin, A., & Fauzi, M. B. N., "Antibacterial-integrated collagen wound dressing for diabetes-related foot ulcers: An evidence-based review of clinical studies," *Polymers (Basel)*, vol. 12, no. 9, p. 2168, 2020.

[333] Liao, W., Yang, D., Xu, Z., Zhao, L., Mu, C., Li, D., & Ge, L., "Antibacterial collagen-based nanocomposite dressings for promoting infected wound healing," *Adv. Healthc. Mater.*, p. 2203054, 2023.

[334] Chang, T., Yin, H., Yu, X., Wang, L., Fan, L., Xin, J. H., & Yu, H., "3D PCL/collagen nanofibrous medical dressing for one-time treatment of diabetic foot ulcers," *Colloids Surf. B Biointerfaces*, vol. 214, p. 112480, 2022.

[335] García-Hernández, A. B., Morales-Sánchez, E., Berdeja-Martínez, B. M., Escamilla-García, M., Salgado-Cruz, M. P., Rentería-Ortega, M., ... & Calderón-Domínguez, G., "PVA-based electrospun biomembranes with hydrolyzed collagen and ethanolic extract of Hypericum perforatum for potential use as wound dressing: Fabrication and characterization," *Polymers (Basel)*, vol. 14, no. 10, p. 1981, 2022.

[336] Wu, S. C., Hsu, H. C., Wang, H. F., Liou, S. P., & Ho, W. F., "Synthesis and characterization of nano-hydroxyapatite obtained from eggshell via the hydrothermal process and the precipitation method," *Molecules*, vol. 28, no. 13, p. 4926, 2023.

[337] Akram, W., Zahid, R., Usama, R. M., AlQahtani, S. A., Dahshan, M., Basit, M. A., & Yasir, M., "Enhancement of antibacterial properties, surface morphology and in vitro bioactivity of hydroxyapatite-zinc oxide nanocomposite coating by electrophoretic deposition technique," *Bioengineering*, vol. 10, no. 6, p. 693, 2023.

[338] Sugimoto, K., Zhou, Y., Galindo, T. G. P., Kimura, R., & Tagaya, M., "Investigation of surface layers on biological and synthetic hydroxyapatites based on bone mineralization process," *Biomimetics*, vol. 8, no. 2, p. 184, 2023.

[339] Bobrowska, K., Sadowska, K., Stolarczyk, K., Prześniak-Welenc, M., Golec, P., & Bilewicz, R., "Bovine serum albumin–hydroxyapatite nanoflowers as potential local drug delivery system of ciprofloxacin," *Int. J. Nanomed.*, pp. 6449–6467, 2023.

[340] Alinavaz, S., Mahdavinia, G. R., Jafari, H., Hazrati, M., & Akbari, A., "Hydroxyapatite (HA)-based hybrid bionanocomposite hydrogels: Ciprofloxacin delivery, release kinetics and antibacterial activity," *J. Mol. Struct.*, vol. 1225, p. 129095, 2021.

[341] Soriano-Souza, C., Valiense, H., Mavropoulos, E., Martinez-Zelaya, V., Costa, A. M., Alves, A. T., … & Calasans-Maia, M., "Doxycycline containing hydroxyapatite ceramic microspheres as a bone-targeting drug delivery system," *J. Biomed. Mater. Res. Part B Appl. Biomater.*, vol. 108, no. 4, pp. 1351–1362, 2020.

[342] Zha, L., Wang, B., Qian, J., Fletcher, B., Zhang, C., Dong, Q., … & Hong, L., "Preparation, characterization and preliminary pharmacokinetic study of pH-sensitive hydroxyapatite/zein nano-drug delivery system for doxorubicin hydrochloride," *J. Pharm. Pharmacol.*, vol. 72, no. 4, pp. 496–506, 2020.

[343] Guo, Q., Kong, F., Ma, C., & Cao, H., "Preparation of doxorubicin loaded poly (ethylene glycol)-poly (ε-caprolactone)-hydroxyapatite fibres as drug delivery systems," *Mater. Technol.*, vol. 35, no. 4, pp. 203–211, 2020.

[344] Li, X., Zeng, D., Chen, L., Ke, P., Tian, Y., & Wang, G., "Preparation and characterization of magnetic chitosan hydroxyapatite nanoparticles for protein drug delivery and antibacterial activity," *J. Mater. Res.*, vol. 36, pp. 4307–4316, 2021.

[345] Tut, T. A., Cesur, S., Ilhan, E., Sahin, A., Yildirim, O. S., & Gunduz, O., "Gentamicin-loaded polyvinyl alcohol/whey protein isolate/hydroxyapatite 3D composite scaffolds with drug delivery capability for bone tissue engineering applications," *Eur. Polym. J.*, vol. 179, p. 111580, 2022.

[346] Zhang, T., Li, J., Wang, Y., Han, W., Wei, Y., Hu, Y., … & Huang, D., "Hydroxyapatite/polyurethane scaffolds for bone tissue engineering," *Tissue Eng. Part B Rev.*, vol. 30, pp. 60–73, 2023.

[347] Aminatun, Suciati, T., Sari, Y. W., Sari, M., Alamsyah, K. A., Purnamasari, W., & Yusuf, Y., "Biopolymer-based polycaprolactone-hydroxyapatite scaffolds for bone tissue engineering," *Int. J. Polym. Mater. Polym. Biomater.*, vol. 72, no. 5, pp. 376–385, 2023.

[348] Gao, Y., Moshayedi, A. J., Sanatizadeh, E., Behfarnia, P., Kolamroudi, M. K., Semirumi, D. T., & Yusof, M. Y. P. M., "Analysis of amorphous structure with polycaprolactone-hydroxyapatite nanoparticles fabricated by 3D bioprinter technique for bone tissue engineering," *Ceram. Int.*, vol. 49, no. 10, pp. 16053–16060, 2023.

[349] Mehdizade, M., Eivani, A. R., Asgari, H., Naghshin, Y., & Jafarian, H. R., "Assessment of microstructure, biocompatibility and in-vitro biodegradation of a biomedical Mg-hydroxyapatite composite for bone tissue engineering," *J. Mater. Res. Technol.*, vol. 27, pp. 852–875, 2023.

[350] Shahgholi, M., Karimipour, A., Firouzi, P., Malekahmadi, O., Ghashang, M., Saadoon, N., … & Baghaei, S., "Fabrication and characterization of synthesized hydroxyapatite/ethanolamine for bone tissue engineering application," *Colloids Surf. A Physicochem. Eng. Asp.*, vol. 650, p. 129591, 2022.

[351] Allen, N. B., Abar, B., Johnson, L., Burbano, J., Danilkowicz, R. M., & Adams, S. B., "3D-bioprinted GelMA-gelatin-hydroxyapatite osteoblast-laden composite hydrogels for bone tissue engineering," *Bioprinting*, vol. 26, p. e00196, 2022.

2 Bionanocomposites in Wound Healing

Karimunnisa Shaikh, Ujwala Desai, Sangita Kale and Saniya Sameer Shaikh

2.1 INTRODUCTION

The treatment and management of various wound types, such as acute, chronic, and traumatic wounds, is the main focus of the quickly expanding global wound care market. The size of the global wound care market was forecast to be USD 22.25 billion in 2023, and from 2024 to 2030, it is anticipated to magnify at a compound annual growth rate (CAGR) of 4.17%. This market includes a broad range of goods and services, such as bioactive wound care products, innovative wound dressings, wound treatment devices, and software for managing wound care. Mounting cases of surgical operations, along with the high occurrence of chronic diseases, are driving the demand for wound care solutions. Moreover, one of the main drivers of market expansion is the rising prevalence of diabetes brought on by sedentary lifestyles [1–3].

This chapter throws light on this area of intense research of wound care solutions. More specifically, it discusses the perspective of bionanocomposites (BNCs) in wound healing. Before doing so, the chapter provides an overview of wounds and the process of wound healing.

2.2 WOUNDS AND PROCESS OF WOUND HEALING

A wound can be induced by physical, chemical, thermal, microbiological, or immunological assaults and is described as an interruption of the cellular, structural, and functional steadiness of living tissue. In another way, a wound is a breach of the integrity of the epithelium and may cause abnormalities in the normal tissue beneath it in terms of both structure and function. Skin, mucous membranes, and other tissues are susceptible to wounds [4].

2.2.1 Wound Healing Process

Acute wound healing proceeds physiologically in the following order: hemostasis, inflammation, proliferation, reepithelialization, and remodeling. These stages are depicted in Figures 2.1 and 2.2. As the wound heals, its appearance will also alter. Understanding the current stage of a wound's healing process and treating it appropriately are the objectives of wound management. The above-described wound healing process is actually a complex one that requires the synthesis of matrix components, biomolecular interactions, migration, proliferation, interaction, and differentiation of multiple cell types (such as dermal, epidermal, and infiltrating inflammatory cells), as well as a complex signaling network [4–7].

Hemostasis (occurs within the first few seconds): The primary part of wound healing is called hemostasis. The process of blood arteries narrowing to halt bleeding and generate blood clots happens in the initial few seconds. In hemostasis, clotting factors come into play and create a platelet knot that limits blood loss from the wounds. Growth factors such as

DOI: 10.1201/9781003650812-2

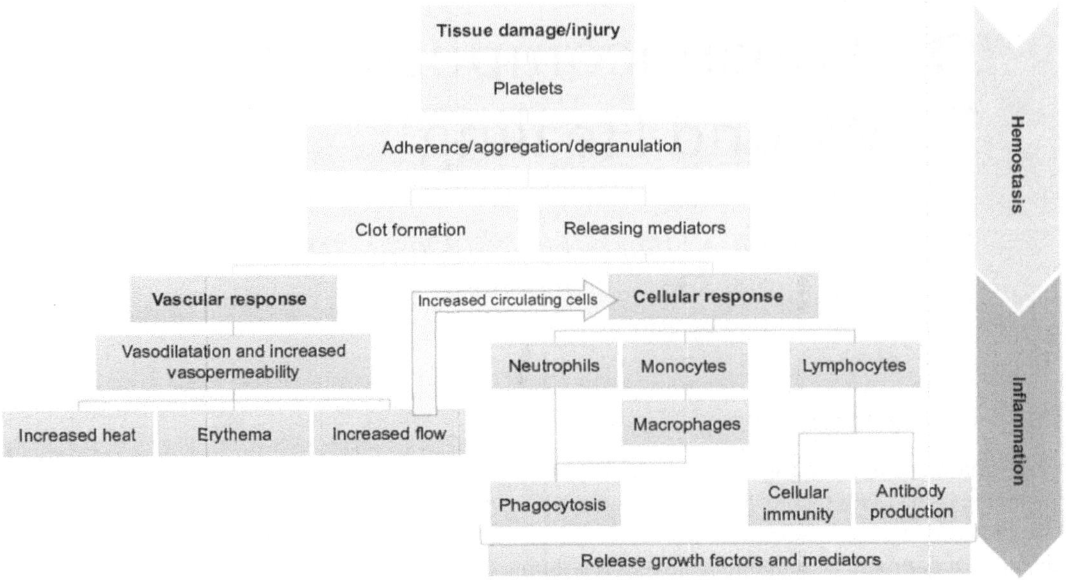

FIGURE 2.1 Hemostasis and inflammation stage of wound healing [8].

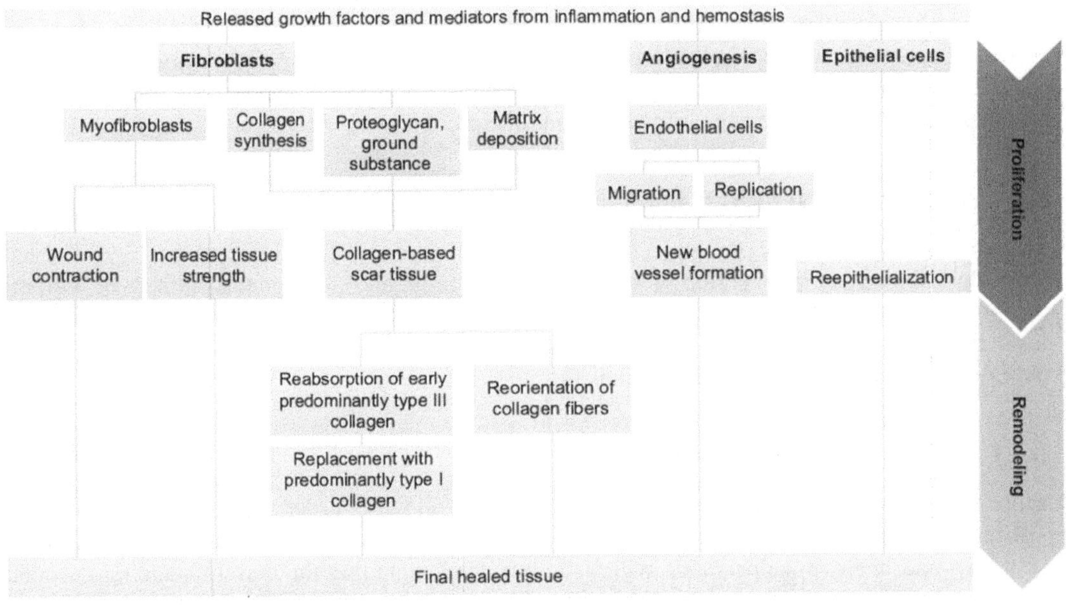

FIGURE 2.2 Proliferation and remodeling stage of wound healing [8].

cytokines, vascular endothelial growth factor (VEGF), and epithelial growth factor (EGF) are released while bleeding is under control. These factors help draw neutrophils, monocytes, and lymphocytes to the wounded tissue and advance the inflammatory stage. In this case, stopping the bleeding would be the aim of wound management [4–8].

Inflammation (0–4 days): Redness and swelling are among the symptoms and signs. In order to clear debris and stop infection, neutrophils and macrophages engage in a variety of reactions throughout the inflammatory stage. The cells help remove pathogens and debris from the body. They also release cytokines that aid in thrombolysis, viz., IL-6, as well as IL-1b in addition to tumor necrosis factor-a. Cleaning up debris and preventing infection would be the objectives of wound management in this case [4–8].

Proliferation (2–24 days): In order to rebuild the dermis and cause scarring, platelets and leukocytes trigger angiogenesis, fibroblast proliferation, collagen and elastin synthesis, and the release of cytokines during the third stage of proliferation. In order to encourage granulation and heal the wound, connective tissue is used to rebuild the wound. In this case, protecting the wound and encouraging tissue growth would be the objectives of wound treatment [4–8].

Reepithelialization: The re-establishment of intact epidermis over the freshly produced tissue is known as the reepithelialization stage. To improve the suppleness and stability of the skin, cells promote the creation of collagen and elastin. As extracellular matrix (ECM) is removed by proteases secreted by macrophages, keratocytes move into the wound site. Protecting the newly formed epithelial tissue would be the aim of wound care in this case [4–8].

Remodeling (24 days–1 year): Remodeling is known to be the concluding segment of the wound-healing proceeding. In this phase, the majority of fibroblasts and macrophages die, and recently produced capillaries recede. In a moist healing environment, epithelial tissue forms. Collagen cross-linking results in stronger skin in the wounded area. Once more, the aim of wound care is to safeguard newly formed epithelial tissue [4–8].

2.2.2 Classification of Wound

There are several ways of classifying wounds. One such is a simple classification as follows:

- **Acute Wound**: A wound that develops unpredictably and proceeds through the healing phases as planned.
- **Chronic Wound**: A chronic wound is one that either doesn't patch up at all or restores slowly over time. Healing takes more than four to six weeks.
- **Surgical Wound**: A wound resulting from a surgical procedure, such as a surgical drain or scalpel incision.
- **Non-surgical Wound**: A non-surgical wound is an injury, either acute or chronic, that does not result from surgery [6].

Based on the degree of infection and cleanliness of the wound, the Centers for Disease Control and Prevention divides wounds into four categories: (1) Clean wounds: sealed, devoid of inflammation and infection. (2) Clean-contaminated: not contaminated in an odd way. (3) Contaminated: new, visible, and devoid of purulent swelling. (4) Dirty-infected: These wounds are characterized by the presence of common microorganisms and are usually the consequence of trauma wounds that have not been properly cared for [9].

Another classification divides wounds into two types:

1. Acute Wounds: more prevalent, shorter-term injuries brought on by heat, radiation, electrical jolt, or mechanical harm;
2. Chronic Wounds: longer-term injuries that are frequently a side effect of long-term conditions like diabetes [9, 10].

2.2.2.1 Acute Wound Infection

Subject to the form, degree, and magnitude of damage; the patient's age; existing illnesses; and post-trauma care, the wounds of acute type often recuperate in 14 days. Infections occur in around 5–26% of the formed wounds, resulting in skin barrier vitiation and local microbial colonization.

The three most common types of wounds predisposed to infection are burns, surgical sites, and traumatic wounds.

Electricity, heat, flame, harmful chemicals, and exposure to radiation can all result in burn injuries. Numerous pathogens, including coagulase-negative *Staphylococci, Escherichia coli, Pseudomonas aeruginosa*, and many other aerobic and anaerobic microbes, were found to grow during the early acute period following burn injury [11].

Acute surgical site wound infections (SSWIs) can result from traumatic non-elective procedures as well as elective surgeries. Microorganisms on prostheses or sutures during surgery might cause both superficial and deep-seated infections. The pathogenic microbes identified are *Legionella pneumophila, P. aeruginosa, Mycobacterium chelonae, Clostridium perfringens, Mycobacterium fortuitum, Staphylococcus epidermidis, Acinetobacterbaumanii, Clostridium difficile, S. aureus, E. coli*, and the coagulase-negative *Staphylococci* [11].

Abrasions or laceration wounds involving significant damage to internal organs, bones, and tissue are considered traumatizing wounds. Two frequent bacteria associated with painful wound infections are Gram-negative and Gram-positive microbe [11].

2.2.2.2 Chronic Wound Infection

Chronic wounds are more difficult to heal than acute wounds because of their slower wound-healing ability. Patients with malnutrition, diabetes, chronic mechanical stress, obesity, vascular disease, or a combination of these and aging people are more likely to suffer from chronic wounds. Polymicrobial communities that have the ability to create biofilms inhabit the majority of chronic wounds, causing excessive inflammation and increased susceptibility to infections that greatly impede wound healing. Gram-negative bacteria, which make up 61% of all microbial isolates, are typically prevalent colonizing species in chronic wounds. P. aeruginosa is the organism that is most frequently discovered in chronic infections ahead of *S. aureus, A. baumanni, E. coli, Proteus mirabilis, and Klebsiella pneumoniae. Prevotella, Peptostreptococci, Anaerococcus, and Peptonipihlus* are among the anaerobic bacteria found in chronic wounds [11].

A wound form known as a diabetic foot ulcer is linked to persistent infection. It is a consequence of diabetes mellitus, especially in more advanced stages of the disease, such as diabetic neuropathy. The microorganisms causing the infection are coagulase-lacking *fungi, Prevotella spp., Poryphyromonas spp., Enterococcus spp., Corynebacterium spp., Bacteroidsfragilis, P. aeruginosa, Enterobacteriaceae, Gram-positive cocci, and Streptococcus streptococci* spp. [11].

Local damage to the skin as well as tissue beneath it, normally overhead the bony structures pooled with shear, especially while wounds are open to the fecal milieu, is what is referred to as a pressure ulcer. *Streptococcus haemolyticus*, MRSA, *P. aeruginosa*, and *S. aureus* are the microbes that flourish at the ulcer site [11].

Biofilms: Bacteria group together in biofilms, which are first formed during the local infection stage. Biofilms are organized, frequently multi-microbial, stick to wounds, and are encased by extracellular polymeric substances (EPS), as opposed to free-floating (planktonic) bacterial cells. Treatment of infected wounds is made more difficult by the presence of biofilms. On the one hand, the mechanical EPS barrier and antiphagocytic characteristics of the biofilm milieu make biofilm bacteria less vulnerable to the immune system. Biofilms, on the other hand, show a number of ways to become resistant to antibiotics. First, the EPS blocks the entry and activity of antimicrobial agents mechanically. Second, the biofilm environment fosters phenotypic alterations by facilitating bacterial communication. The creation of a diverse population of cells in various growth phases is facilitated by a tight progression arrangement and sluggish metabolic rates, which also add to the enhanced resistance to antimicrobial therapy. Consequently, biofilms have the ability to last for an extended length of time, promote chronification of a wound, and induce additional local or distant invasive infections by the dissemination of biofilm fragments, planktonic bacteria, and microcolonies of mature biofilms. Compared to planktonic bacteria, bacteria in biofilms can withstand standard antimicrobial treatments up to 1000 times better. Biofilms hinder appropriate therapy and hence extend the wound healing period because of these tolerances and resistances to antibiotics and biocides [12–16].

2.2.3 Factors Affecting Wound Healing [6]

Extrinsic as well as intrinsic factors influence wound healing. Addressing these issues is necessary for the best possible healing outcome.

Local or External Factors

- Moisture balance and wound management techniques (such as maceration or dehydration of the wound)
- Consistent temperature of about 37°C
- pH that is neutral or acidic to infection
- Location of the wound
- Mechanical strain, pressure, or friction
- Foreign body presence

Systemic or Intrinsic Factors

- Diet
- Chronic or underlying illness
- Reduced mobility
- Compromised perfusion
- Drugs (such as NSAIDs, immunotherapy, chemotherapy, or radiation)
- Mental well-being, encompassing stress, anxiety, and sadness
- The patient's age
- Knowledge, comprehension, or compliance by the patient

2.3 APPROACHES TO THE TREATMENT OF WOUND

2.3.1 Debridement

Debridement is the process of removing tissue that has lost vitality. Since the devitalized tissue in the wound bed acts as a physical barrier to healing and promotes bacterial development, speeding up this process improves healing efficiency. Excessive protease release can also occur from devitalized tissue. In modern clinical practice, debridement techniques include mechanical, biological, enzymatic, autolytic, and surgical [11].

2.3.2 Infection Control in Wounds

Healing may be hampered or delayed by bacterial bioburden. There are many levels of bacterial burden in wounds, including contamination, colonization, critical colonization, and infection. All chronic wounds contain bacteria, but only severe colonization and infection typically call for antibiotic intervention. The topical antimicrobials that are most commonly utilized in contemporary wound care practices include those that contain silver, povidone-iodine, and octenidine. Honey, hydrogen peroxide, and chlorhexidine are used less frequently [11].

2.3.3 Skin Substitutes Available for Wound Healing

Dermal grafts are readily usable because they are allogenic, cellular, or acellular in origin. The range of dressings for wound care has increased thanks to tissue engineering, which has produced multiple skin substitutes. For instance, the fibroblasts and keratinocytes in these products are cultured on collagen matrices. For the treatment of diabetic as well as venous ulcers, bioengineered skin, which is nothing but a bilayered, living skin buildup, has received approval. Additionally, a living dermal skin substitute for diabetic neuropathic ulcers was approved [11].

2.3.4 Growth Factors

Growth factors are important players in neovascularization, tissue development, reepithelialization, granulation, and local inflammation. They also produce ECM through a variety of processes and from different cell sources. Far-reaching research has been directed at the subject matter of exogenous wound healing. Based on the various findings, the kind of each wound is a crucial aspect in determining which growth factors to use.

Among the growth factors used to include human EGF, b-FGF, KGF-2, or repifermin, platelet-derived growth factor consisting of BB-homodimer, also known as becaplermin [11].

2.3.5 Moist Wound Treatment

Treatment of moist wounds has some advantages. The absence of scab formation during wet therapy lessens the chance of scarring. Essentially, growth factors and proteolytic enzymes need moisture to function. Additionally, it is essential for the effective distribution of nutrients and surface oxygen. Therefore, by enabling the cells to move over the wound surface and accelerating the pace of epithelization and angiogenesis, moisture enhances the courses of the migration as well as the proliferation phase. The protection and cushioning of the nerve terminals in a wet environment results in pain alleviation. Several techniques are used to treat wet wounds, such as absorbent dressings like foams and alginates and moisture-retentive dressings like occlusive films, hydrogels, and hydrocolloids [11].

2.3.6 Gene Therapy

With this method, a physical or biological vector is used to introduce the gene more willingly than the product (growth factor). For treating wounds which don't heal, it's believed to be more effective and less expensive. Gene introduction technology has been around for a while. Another method uses genetically altered cells to produce and distribute the required growth factor in a controlled manner [11].

2.3.7 Stem Cell Therapy

This method takes advantage of the possibility that body stem cells could reconstruct dermal, vascular, and other components needed in the course of wound healing. The administration of cultivated cells from autologous bone marrow directly could hasten the healing process. It is possible to use subsets of cultured cells taken from bone marrow or stem cells obtained from hair follicles [11].

2.4 WOUND DRESSINGS

Regardless of the size of the incision or cut, the wound needs to be properly cared for. This treatment includes the application of a dressing in contact near the wound. Conventional dressings for wounds, such as cotton wool, plasters, gauze, lint, and bandages, are available as dry primary/secondary dressings that keep the wound clean. Gauzes of cotton, rayon material, and fibers of synthetic polyester, both nonwoven and woven, offer some gradation of safeguard against bacterial contamination. Using the fibers in these dressings, certain sterile gauze pads are used to absorb liquids and exudates from an open wound. It is necessary to replace these dressings frequently so as to avert the soaking of healthy tissues. Gauze dressings are not as reasonable. Extreme drainage from wounds causes bandages to become wet and sticky, making removal rough and painful. Different purposes are aided when bandages are made of synthetic materials such as polyamide or natural cotton wool and cellulose [17].

Conventional dressings are typically used as secondary dressings or for clean, dry wounds which create low amounts of exudate. Recent dressings made from more refined formulas have replaced traditional dressings since the traditional dressings are unable to offer a damp milieu for the wound. Instead of just covering wounds, modern wound dressings are designed to help them function. The purpose of these dressings is to inhibit the drying out of the wound and support its healing. There are quite a lot of commercial products that can be picked based on the type and cause of the wound. The majority of contemporary wound dressings are prepared from synthetic polymers and fit into one of three categories: a) passive, b) interactive, or c) bioactive. The non-occluding passive constituents, including gauze and the tulle dressings, on application to the wound allowed it to heal and function again under the surface. Interactive dressings come in foam, films, hydrogel, and hydrocolloid forms and can be either occlusive or semi-occlusive. These dressings serve as a line of defense against microorganisms entering the wound environment [17].

Biomaterials are used to create bioactive dressings, decisive to the restorative process. These dressings, which are typically made from ingredients like collagen, alginate, elastin, hyaluronic acid, chitosan, and natural tissues, are renowned for their biocompatibility, biodegradability, and non-toxic qualities. Conditional to the type and nature of the wound, polymers of these materials can be unaccompanied or be in combination. Growth hormones and antibiotics usually speed up the healing process when added to biological dressings [17].

Additionally, pharmacologically active ingredients like antibiotics, non-steroidal anti-inflammatory, analgesic, and local anesthetic medications, as well as natural extracts with anti-inflammatory, epithelializing, antioxidant, and antibacterial qualities, may be present in contemporary wound dressings [5].

2.5 CHALLENGES IN THE TREATMENT OF WOUND/WOUND HEALING

A multitude of molecular factors (Figure 2.3), such as enzymes like matrix metalloproteinases (MMPs), tissue inhibitors of MMPs, seperinase, and growth factors and receptors like tumor necrosis alpha (TNFa), platelet-derived growth factor (PDGF), transforming growth factor-beta (TGF-ß), interleukin-1 (IL-1), and cytokines like fibroblast growth factor (FGF), frequently have manifold and overlying roles in the normal course of wound healing [18].

Inadequate blood supply, foreign particles that prevent tissue repair, persistent infection and microbes, wound dehiscence, impaired venous drainage, reduced macrophage activity, and elevated MMP levels are some of the systemic and local factors that affect wound healing [19–25]. It is common for chronic wounds to cease healing during the inflammatory phase. Despite the differences in the molecular etiology of chronic wounds, they all have specific traits such as high concentrations of senescent cells, reactive oxygen species (ROS); pro-inflammatory cytokines, proteases, and thriving infection coexistent with the absence of functional stem cells [26].

Following is the list of challenges faced during the wound healing process.

2.5.1 Biofilm Formation

It is quite difficult to eradicate the whole bacterial bioburden, especially in the event of biofilms, regardless of the type of debridement used. This is because the creation of biofilms is not restricted to the wound surface but also develops in deeper layers of the wound bed and because they are highly adhesive to the surrounding tissue. Whether single- or multi-microbial, biofilms complicate wound healing further by producing proteases that prevent keratinocyte migration and skin reepithelialization. Furthermore, repeated debridement is advised since mature films can regenerate in as little as 72 hours following debridement, depending on the current pathogens [27].

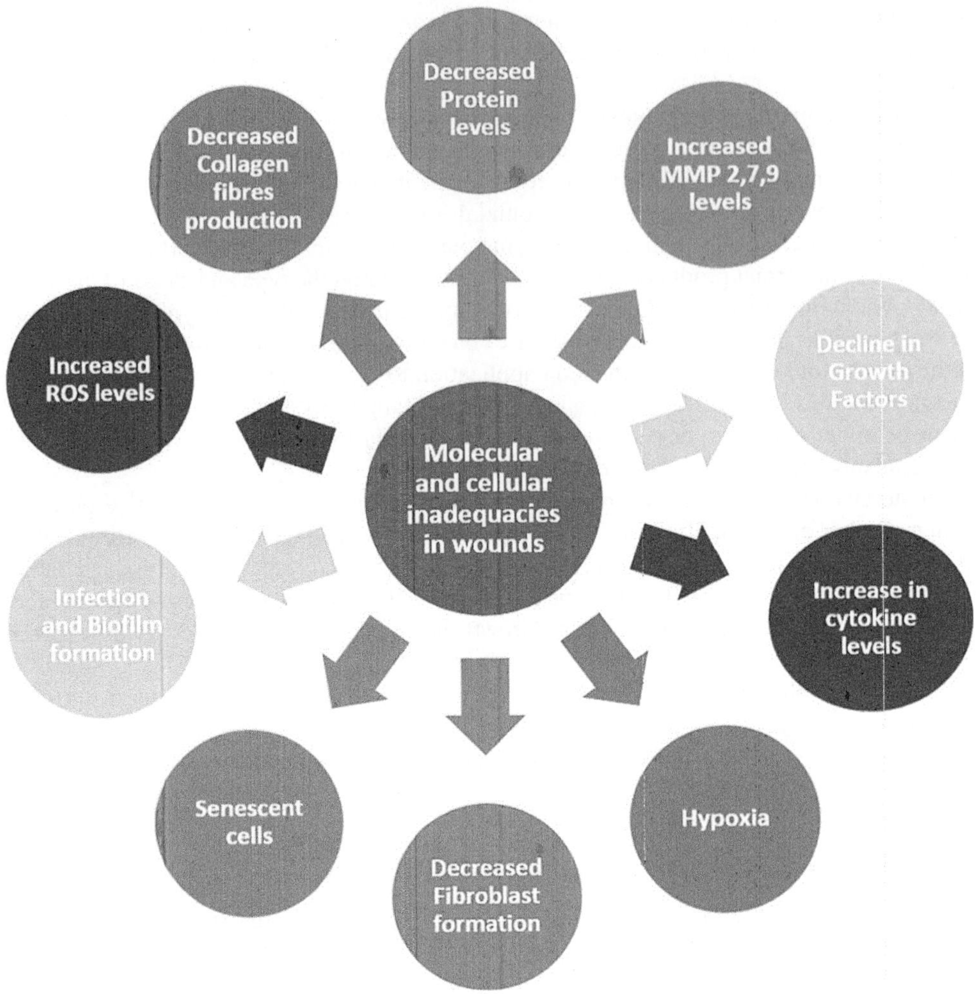

FIGURE 2.3 Molecular and cellular inadequacies in wounds.

2.5.2 High Levels of Proteases

Repeated tissue injury triggers an influx of immune cells that are sustained by microorganisms and platelet-derived factors like transforming growth factor-b (TGF-b)/ECM molecules. This prolongs and intensifies the pro-inflammatory cytokine cascade, which in turn increases the levels of proteases. These proteases are strictly controlled by their inhibitors in wounds of the acute type. When protease levels in chronic wounds surpass or counter their corresponding inhibitors, ECM is destroyed, and growth factors along with their receptors are broken down. In addition to keeping the lesion from making headway to the proliferative phase, the proteolytic breakdown of ECM draws additional inflammatory cells, intensifying the inflammatory cycle [28].

2.5.3 Reactive Oxygen Species (ROS) Production

ROS is a substance produced by immune cells that, in small amounts, offers protection against microbes. However, the predominantly inflammatory and hypoxic environment in chronic wounds enhances the generation of ROS, which breaks down ECM proteins and destroys cells. ROS have a key role in shielding against pathogenic microbes, but an excess can worsen oxidative stress, cause tissue damage, and cause an excessive amount of MMPs. Proteases and inflammatory cytokines are stimulated more intensely as a result of these occurrences [29].

2.5.4 Senescent Cell Populations

Moreover, senescent cell populations with compromised secretory and proliferative abilities, which make them insensitive to normal wound healing cues, are a hallmark of chronic wounds [30]. Fibroblasts from pus and veins have been described as senescent and with reduced capacity to proliferate. There is a direct correlation between this reduced ability to proliferate and a wound's inability to heal [31–33]. Compilation of evidence also suggests that endothelial cells, macrophages, fibroblasts, and senescent keratinocytes are present in chronic wounds [34–37]. Senescent phenotypic cells of chronic wounds are linked with aberrant metabolic fluctuations in diabetic individuals, creating problems in intracellular biochemical passageways, including the GSK-3b/Fyn/Nrf2 trail, or oxidative stress, which results in deoxyribonucleic acid damage causing cell cycle arrest [36].

In addition to this, many other factors or biological markers that significantly hinder the process of wound healing and can be targeted to improve the wound healing process are presented in Table 2.1.

TABLE 2.1
Targeting Biological Markers that are Clinically Significant Will Help to Improve the State of Chronic Wounds [27]

Biomarker	Features in Chronic Wound	Potential Fixes
Protein levels	A reduction in the amount of overall protein.	Boost your intake of protein in your diet.
Proteinase levels	Increased levels of metalloproteinases, including MMP-2, MMP-7, and MMP-9.	Raising the concentrations of MMP tissue inhibitors.
Bacterial levels in tissue	Elevated amounts of a wide variety of bacteria in the tissue. Enzymes that decrease growth factors are released by bacteria, and they also generate MMPs that break down the extracellular matrix. An elevated inflammatory reaction is noted.	By consistently eliminating the exudates, bacterial levels can be lowered, which lowers inflammation.
Growth factors	Decrease in the growth factors required for healing.	Boost the number and production of fibroblasts, which releases the essential growth factors.
Cytokine levels	Elevated levels of pro-inflammatory cytokines.	Treatment with vitamin D and an elemental diet can lower levels of pro-inflammatory cytokines.
Genes	Notable variations in the expression of a wide range of genes (which may exhibit up- or down-regulation).	Determine which genes to target for control with natural or artificial products.
pH	Compared to wounds with a pH near to neutral, the rate of wound healing was found to be decreased with increased alkaline pH.	Use topical pH-modifying chemicals to lower the pH in a more acidic environment.
Hypoxia	Partial pressure of oxygen of <30 mm Hg. It makes it more difficult for fibroblasts to proliferate and collagen to be produced, which slows down the healing of wounds by fostering the growth of harmful organisms like bacteria.	Negative pressure wound care using vacuum assistance, compression bandages, or clothing.
Poor nutrition	A wound's protracted inflammatory healing period is one of its characteristics. As long as the patient's low diet keeps them in a catabolic condition, less fibroblast production is seen.	Enhancing the patient's diet by giving them nourishing foods to eat or nutritional supplements.

Choosing the correct treatment modality or the drug delivery system is also a challenge that affects the success of the wound healing process. The current treatment options available for wound healing are listed in Table 2.2. Their deficiencies or incapabilities to assist the process of wound healing are also included therein. The table also provides remedies to overcome the deficiencies.

2.6 APPROACHES TO MEET THE CHALLENGES OF TREATMENT OF WOUNDS

For many years, a number of dressing materials have been investigated. Skin abnormalities were traditionally treated using bandages and gauze as wound dressings [38]. Table 2.2 enlisted current and widely used dressings and medicaments along with their limitations and remedies. These limitations and challenges in wound treatment discussed in the preceding section warranted the development of novel biocompatible modalities for quick and complete wound healing. The model dressing needs special ingredients with exceptional qualities in order to mimic the ECM for a moist environment, have antibacterial qualities, and promote cell growth and angiogenesis. These qualities are provided by nanomaterials. The market's enormous need for these resources has fueled the development of nanomaterial dressings [39].

Nanoparticles (NPs) have recently also been widely used in wound healing due to their improved adsorption capacity, antibacterial qualities, and medication loading [40].

Due to the unique physical, chemical, and biological features of NPs, their highly specific surface area also demonstrated prospective usage in wound dressings for the sustainable delivery and release of therapeutic medicines. Nanomaterials can provide multifunctional platforms with antibacterial properties, extended drug release, and bioactive molecule signaling delivery to optimize the wound healing practice. The capacity of NPs to enter microbial cells and pass through the extracellular polymer shell (EPS) of films has sparked a growing interest in them [41]. In addition, they have the ability to mimic the ECM, promote cell adhesion, migration, and proliferation, and alter signaling pathways related to tissue regeneration [42].

Establishing a platform for cell adhesion, cell migration, and cell proliferation—basically, a scaffold for cells—is necessary to repair tissue abnormalities in the wound area. A structure like this can also act as a platform for changing its functionality. Moreover, NPs can be used to create a smart dressing for wounds infected by microorganisms, which can be used to cure these infections depending on endogenous prompters like pH, wound temperature, present enzymes, and toxins released by the bacterium.

Recently, there has also been research on the integration of biodegradable polymeric NPs that can cargo, shield, and control the release of bioactive substances like proteins, growth factors, and medications [43]. Liposomes typically have a lesser loading capacity and a shorter drug release than polymeric systems. Solid lipid NPs and nanostructured lipid carriers were created to get over the drawbacks of liposomal architectures. Higher stability and encapsulation efficiency are offered by these formulations [44].

Usually, metal or metal oxide NPs are employed because of their inherent antibacterial properties. The primary mechanisms of their antibacterial activity are thought to be the discharge of responsive metal ions from the particle surface and the creation of ROS, which disrupts the pathogens' membranes [45]. The combination effect of surface adhesion and NP internalization into microbial cells is responsible for the improved efficacy of metal NPs as opposed to materials with larger sizes. Gold NPs' durability and anti-inflammatory qualities have drawn attention in a number of medication delivery applications [46]. Since inorganic materials do not include the proteins found in natural systems, they are often regarded as less immunogenic. Gold NPs have been utilized to transfer active substances like nucleic acids and antioxidants to wounds to aid in their healing. Research has demonstrated that gold NPs can momentarily open the stratum corneum, increasing the absorption of anti-inflammatory and antioxidant ingredients added to the mixture to hasten wound healing [47].

TABLE 2.2
Detailed Information on Current Treatment Options Regimens Along with Their Constraints [27]

Dressing Category	Treatment Options	Uses in Medical and Surgical Purposes	Constraints and Possible Remedies
Traditional dressings	Topical liquid formulations (povidone-iodine	Used as a bacterial load reducer in the early stages of wound healing; Debriding and de-sloughing agents.	**Constraints**: Short stays at the site of the wound, particularly in cases where there is a discernible level of suppuration (exudation) of the wound fluid. **Remedies**: Need for adhesive systems or long residence hydrogels.
	Semi-solid preparations (Silver nitrate ointment and silver sulfadiazine cream)	Treat bacterial infection.	**Constraints**: Being mobile, losing their rheological properties, and quickly absorbing fluid makes them less effective at staying on the wound site. **Remedies**: Hydrogel.
	Topical liquid formulations (saline solutions)	Wound cleansing agent; Irrigate dry wounds.	
	Gauze dressings	Antibacterial agent.	**Constraints**: When the dressing's outside is wet by wound exudates, bacterial protection is lost. As fluid production decreases, gauze dressings tend to stick to wounds more and become uncomfortable for patients to remove. **Remedies**: Semipermeable film dressings like calcium alginate dressings.
	Solid materials (wool, cotton, natural, or synthetic bandages and gauzes).	Used as primary or secondary dressings	**Constraints**: Since they are dry, they are unable to create a damp atmosphere. **Remedies**: Hydrating drug delivery system.
Modern dressings	Film dressings made up of nylon.	They offer a moist healing environment, encourage autolytic debridement, are flexible, and shield the 7 sites from bacterial invasion and mechanical damage.	**Constraints**: Restricted capacity to absorb adequate amounts of wound exudates, which causes surplus exudates to build up behind the dressing. **Remedies**: Calcium alginate dressing. **Constraints**: When removed from their packs, they have a tendency to wrinkle; they are too thin to be packed into deep or cavity wounds and are only appropriate for somewhat shallow wounds. **Remedies**: Iodoform gauze.
	Hydrocolloid dressings	Used for dry to moist wounds and light to moderately leaking wounds.	**Constraints**: Fibers get embedded in the wound and frequently need to be removed when changing the dressing. **Remedies**: Alginate dressings which absorb 20–30 times its weight fluid, fibers sticking can be prevented by moistening with saline of wound cleanser.

(Continued)

TABLE 2.2 (Continued)

Dressing Category	Treatment Options	Uses in Medical and Surgical Purposes	Constraints and Possible Remedies
	Biological dressings	Consists of natural tissue matrix components and decomposes biologically	Further studies with regular wound dressings as a comparison are necessary.
	Foam dressings	Keeps the area surrounding the incision wet; offers heat protection and is extremely absorbent.	**Constraints**: Not appropriate for dry scars or dry epithelializing wounds. **Remedies**: Gel dressings (solid gel sheets), hydrocolloid dressings, transparent adhesive dressings, nonadherent gauze/contact layers and zinc-oxide-based ointment.
	Tissue-engineered skin substitutes	Utilized to administer bioactive substances to a wound, such as growth factors and genetic materials.	**Constraints**: Its antigenicity, high expense, and carryover infection risk prevent it from replacing missing skin. **Remedies**: Use of biomaterial which reduces antigenicity, has a low risk of infection, and is biodegradable.
Medicated dressings	Supplements (vitamins and mineral supplements)	Encourage the body to heal wounds normally.	Limited information is available in the literature regarding the application of dressings to wounds to give nutrients.
	Antimicrobials	Treat infections	**Constraints**: Excessive dosages of antibiotics cause harmful side effects such as cumulative organ and cell damage. **Remedies**: Use of biomaterial and phytoconstituents having antimicrobial activity.
	Growth factors	Enhances the process of wound healing by promoting angiogenesis and cellular growth.	**Constraints**: Selecting a proper dressing that will allow for optimal release and activity at the wound site might be difficult. **Remedies**: Use of controlled drug delivery system.
Controlled drug delivery dressings	Polymeric drug delivery dressings	Act as conduits for the administration and release of medications to injury locations.	**Constraints**: Degradation of the polymer matrix after swelling and water diffusion in different dose forms. **Remedies**: Use of biodegradable polymers.

Another class of drug delivery vehicles that has drawn a lot of interest is mesoporous silica [48]. The high drug loading capacity of these particles can be greatly extended by the electrostatic interaction between the encapsulated compounds and the solid matrix [48, 49]. One drug carrier known to provide an approximately linear discharge profile is mesoporous NPs [50].

As instruments for drug delivery, carbon-based materials like graphene and carbon nanotubes (CNTs) have also been researched. Both materials bind well to active substances like nucleic acids. Examples of carbon-based systems for the management of chronic wounds exist [51].

In recent times, nanoneedles have surfaced as a valuable instrument capable of directly delivering plasmids into cell membranes [52, 53]. One such instance involved the successful engineering and testing of mesoporous silicon nanoneedles for the transport of many plasmids to cells in both in vitro and in vivo settings. In tests conducted on animals, the VEGF-165 gene was injected into the cells using a nanoneedle array, and the results indicate a considerable increase in vascularization when compared to animals who received the same gene via hypodermic injection [53]. The tellurium nanoneedles exhibited antibacterial and anti-inflammatory properties for bacteria-infected wound healing *in vivo* and were found to be safe in mice with no side effects [54].

Nano- to micrometer-diameter fibers are becoming more and more popular for use in wound-healing applications. Their fibrous arrangement is similar to the ECM of humans, which promotes cell adherence. At the same time, it permits gas exchange, prevents microbial infiltration, keeps the environment wet, and has a high mechanical stability [55]. Increasing the engineering structures' stickiness is another benefit of composite systems. Although the produced constructions gave adequate mechanical characteristics, their pore diameters were somewhat greater than those of the pure polymeric scaffolds. The structures exhibited remarkable efficacy against bacterial cultures while promoting keratinocyte proliferation [56]. Nano-scaffold systems are frequently employed in tissue engineering due to their superior biocompatibility, angiogenic capability, and biomimetic behavior to normal human skin [41].

Alongside the use of NPs, Tables 2.1 and 2.2 also point toward the use of a biodegradable wound-healing drug delivery system (to circumvent the frequent replacement of traditional dressings) and a biocompatible wound-healing drug delivery system (to avoid irritation and infection and improve patient compliance). These requisites can be fulfilled by the use of natural polymers. These natural polymers are capable of forming composites, which are known as biocomposites. These nanocomposites are frequently employed as wound-healing scaffolds, as previously mentioned. However, their utility for wound-healing applications has been hampered by certain undesirable aspects of their core constructions, such as their low mechanical strength, poor flexibility, and failure to allow for long-term drug release. Numerous investigations have demonstrated that they cannot ensure the protection of the wound spot and might malfunction when severe cyclic load is applied. Researchers have looked into the possibilities of adding NPs of metallic, ceramic, polymeric, and other types to the composite constructions in order to get around these issues [57, 58]. This possibility has greatly improved the role of biocomposites. This incorporation of nanostructures into biocomposite structures has given rise to the term "bionanocomposites." BNCs have revolutionized the treatment of wounds. The following sections describe BNCs and their application in wound healing.

2.7 BIONANOCOMPOSITES AND THEIR ADVANTAGES

As a result of people's constant need for increasingly advanced technology for healthcare development, a new class of materials known as nanocomposites is created when two distinct materials mix to create a completely new or very different material. We refer to these materials as composite materials. Currently, designing nanocomposites is essentially thought to include taking full advantage of the fascinating properties of NPs on a very large scale [59, 60]. First used by Komarneni [61], the term "nanocomposites," a type of material known as nanocomposites, is defined as having at least one phase with constituents in the nanometer (1 nm = 10–9 m) domain. There are two types of nanocomposites: those based on polymers and those that are not [62].

2.7.1 BIONANOCOMPOSITES

A distinct family of materials known as BNCs are nanocomposites that combine naturally occurring polymers, or biopolymers, with an inorganic nanomoiety. The term "bionanocomposite," also known as "Nanobiocomposites," "green composites," or, conversely, "biohybrids," was initially used in 2004 [63, 64]. As seen from Figure 2.4, BNCs are different from general composites in terms of reinforcement by Nps.

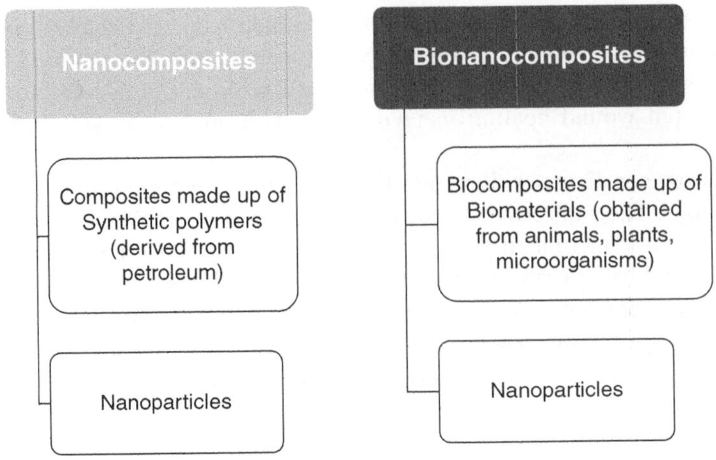

FIGURE 2.4 Difference between nanocomposites and bionanocomposites.

2.7.2 Advantages of Bionanocomposites

The most researched materials for the regeneration of damaged tissues are biocompatible materials containing biopolymers, such as collagen and PLA, which function as artificial scaffolds for cell growth. These bioresorbable scaffolds must meet the following criteria: they must be biocompatible, have appropriate mechanical qualities to prevent implant collapse, have enough macroporosity with connected pores to facilitate the passage of nutrients and metabolic wastes, and have controlled biodegradability; the rate of biodegradation must be balanced with the rate of tissue regeneration [65, 66].

Because they contain nanofiller components, BNCs weigh far less than ordinary composites. Additional advantages provided by BNCs include low density, transparency, compatibility with cells and tissues, good flow, improved surface qualities, and recyclability for packaging application [67].

Improved biocompatibility, mechanical characteristics (strength, elastic modules, dimensional stability, and thermal stability), permeability, and features such as biodegradability, swelling index, thermal stability, improved permeability, non-toxicity, cheapness, and easy availability are among the benefits of BNCs over other nano-formulations [68, 69]. BNCs are highly useful as drug delivery devices because of their decreased size and biocompatibility [70].

2.8 TYPICAL COMPONENTS OF BIONANOCOMPOSITES FOR WOUND HEALING

BNCs are made up of biomaterials from natural origins such as herbs, animals, or microorganisms. They are combined with NPs.

2.8.1 Biomaterial

The main and distinguishing constituent of BNCs is biomaterial, which separates it from other nano-formulations. The biomaterial is obtained from plants, animals, and microorganisms [64]. Examples of biomaterials used for the wound healing process include chitosan, silk, hyaluronic acid, carboxymethyl cellulose, guar gum, pectin, and gelatin [71–76].

2.8.2 Nanofillers

They are basically NPs and have a nanoscale size. There are spherical, tubular, and platy NPs. Large particles can grow into small particles with dimensions in the micro- or nano-size range [64]. They

TABLE 2.3
Types of Biomaterials Based on Their Origin

Category	Examples
Natural biomaterials	Chitosan, gelatin, agar, glucan, hyaluronic acid, collagen, silk fibroin, alginate, cellulose, starch, alginate, carrageenan, xanthan gum
Modified biomaterials	PEG-based nano-scaffold, alginate-polycaprolactone (PCL), electrospun membranes, polyurethane-based scaffold, microporous annealed particle scaffold, Polyglycolic acid, poly-l-lactic acid, polylactic acid (PLA), and poly e-caprolactone

can exist in different forms, such as CNTs, layered silicates, nanotubes, nanospheres, nanorods, nanoshells, quantum dots, nanowires, polyhedral oligomeric silsesquioxanes, dendrimers, metal oxides, and nanofibers [77, 78].

2.9 TYPES OF BIONANOCOMPOSITES

BNCs are categorized as different types on the basis of the origin of biomaterial and structure of BNCs.

2.9.1 Natural and Modified Bionanocomposites

Depending on the origin of the biomaterial, the BNCs can be classified (Table 2.3) as natural and modified biomaterials [69].

2.9.2 Particulate Bionanocomposites

Dimensional particles are frequently used in particulate BNCs, such as cement. The primary purpose of using such a sort of reinforcement is to upsurge fighting against flammability, diminish permeability, and lower the cost of composites [69].

2.9.3 Bionanocomposites with Elongated Particles

In such types of BNCs, elongated elements such as cellulose nanofibrils and CNTs provide fortification or reinforcement. The elevated aspect ratio of reinforcement in these BNCs contributes to their superior mechanical performance [69].

2.9.4 Particle-Reinforced Layered Nanocomposites

The particle-reinforced layered nanocomposites are made of biological materials. Based on how the particles are distributed throughout the matrix, layered particle-armored BNC, correspondingly identified as layered polymer nanocomposite, is divided into three subclasses [69].

1. Particle–particle interactions allow flocculated/phase-separated nanocomposites to form even when the partition is not sandwiched between the layers. This class of composites is sometimes referred to as microcomposites since the individual laminas are not separated. Functioning as tiny particles scattered throughout the polymeric matrix as a result.
2. Intercalated nanocomposites are created as polymer chains are inserted amid the stacked NP sheets.
3. Conversely, the production of exfoliated nanocomposites results from the partitioning of individual layers [79].

2.9.5 Composite Materials Hydrogel Nanocomposite

NP-loaded, hydrated, three-dimensional polymeric networks are known as nanocomposite hydrogels. These hydrogels swell after absorbing water, which increases in vivo cell viability by hydration. This allows nutrients and waste products to diffuse into a population of encapsulated cells in combination with a biomimetic milieu. Formulating a bioactive and mechanically stable hydrogel is difficult [80–82]. Additionally, bioactivity, electrical conductivity, and stimuli-responsiveness are included in nanocomposite hydrogels. To offer electrical conductivity, carbon-based nanomaterials, viz., graphene oxide and CNTs, are utilized. Utilizing inorganic NPs, viz., hydroxyapatite, bioglass, and silicates, allows for the acquisition of bioactive characteristics. NP of metals and their oxides have antimicrobial and magnetic characteristics. Polymeric NPss provide the organized release of biological indicators that can regulate cellular behavior. The physical and/or covalent interaction between polymers and NPs results in unique features. Nanocomposite hydrogels with varying functions are being used to assist in producing advanced biomaterials with biomedical and biotechnological applications. A number of fields, including immunomodulation, tissue engineering, stem cell therapy, cancer research, and cellular and molecular treatment, are looking into the application of nanocomposite hydrogels [83].

2.9.6 Bioinspired Metallic Nanoparticles

Using a green chemistry method, bioinspired metallic NPs are synthesized from different plant extracts or biological components. The reduction of metallic salt occurs during the synthesis process, either inside living cells or inside their constituent parts. Metallic NPs' catalytic activity has been employed as an antibacterial agent and for the catalytic breakdown of harmful dyes and pollutants that are not biodegradable. The surface plasmon resonance exhibited by silver NPs and gold NPs, for example, is a phenomenon of intonation of their optical characteristics at nanoscales that has broad applications in the detection of disease and its state [84].

2.9.7 Bioactive Silicate Assimilated Nanocomposites

Synthetic silicate nanomaterials are very useful and ultrathin, also known as two-dimensional. They network with biological objects in a varied positive way because of the huge surface-to-volume ratio [85, 86]. These nanomaterials have several biological and medicinal uses, including diagnostics for diseases, imaging, and treatments. Because of these NPs' potent bioactive properties, several musculoskeletal tissue engineering applications have been suggested for them [87].

2.9.8 Bioinspired Hydroxyapatite Nanocomposites

Hard tissue contains a naturally occurring material called nano-hydroxyapatite (nHAp), which has a bioinspired nanofiller inserted into it. Because of its reduced fracture strength and lasting qualities, nHAp can only be used as a biomaterial in non-stressed structural areas in clinical orthopedic and dental applications. Accordingly, nHAp polymeric hydrogel linkage is explored for non-load-bearing applications [88].

2.9.9 Bioinspired Rosette Nanotube Composites

Synthetic DNA bases are assembled to create bioinspired rosette nanotube composites. Typically, guanine and cytosine hydrogen bonding arrays are employed. They are used in regenerative medicine [89, 90]. The structure's base composition resembles the collagen fibers found in ECM. To increase the scaffold's bioactivity and cell adherence, more amino acids and peptide sequences were added.

2.9.10 Graphene-Enhanced Polymeric Nanocomposites

Three-dimensional structures are created by self-assembling graphene oxide sheets interacting non-covalently with single-strand DNA [91]. The ensuing biomimetic hierarchical structure keeps graphene's mechanical forte besides the electrical conductivity. In tissue engineering, it is utilized. Gene delivery is facilitated by the biomolecule filling and cell-internalization capabilities of graphene oxide nanosheets.

2.9.11 Polymeric Nanocomposites Bearing Metallic Nanoparticles

The incorporation of metal-based constituents into polymeric systems offers distinct avenues for the regeneration of functional tissue. So as to mend the regenerative performance of implanted devices, it has been reported that the reorganized molecular structures are formed through interactions between solid inorganic surfaces and peptides. These surfaces might be contrived to heighten bioactivity and auxiliary functionality using synthetic ingredients. Metallic NP conductivity in a polymeric matrix (nanofiber) embedded within renders them worthwhile for regenerative processes [92].

2.10 APPLICATIONS OF BIONANOCOMPOSITES FOR WOUND HEALING

BNCs contain two major components, viz., the biomaterial or the biopolymer and the NP counterpart. Hence, the applications of BNCs in wound healing have been described components-wise. The following dedicated sections explain applications of the biomaterials and NPs in BNCs for wound healing.

2.10.1 Biomaterials

Biopolymers or biomaterials are materials that are flexible, elastic, or fibrous coming from bioresources such as herbs, animals, microbes, or other living things. Among the natural polymers that are frequently utilized in wound dressing applications are proteins and polysaccharides. These polymers can be employed for a variety of therapeutic applications because of their intrinsic biocompatibility, low immunogenicity, non-toxicity, and biodegradable qualities [93]. Numerous studies proved the ability of various polymers to speed up the healing process. Examples of polymers reported include poly(ε-caprolactone), chitosan, gelatin collagen, hydroxypropyl methylcellulose, maltodextrin, zein, polydatin, sodium alginate, calcium alginate, fibrin, keratin, and hyaluronic acid [94–105]. Furthermore, the skin's cellular backdrop and natural ECM structural components can be replaced with naturally derived polymers [106, 107].

2.10.1.1 Hyaluronic Acid

Hyaluronic acid (HA) is a non-sulfated glycosaminoglycan compilation of repeat units of D-disaccharide, viz., glucuronic acid along with N-acetyl-D-glucosamine held by the glucuronidic bond, that is, a β (1→3) bond. This polymer is anionic with a linear architecture. It is present in connective tissue and dermis and is present in all living things [108]. HA, whether in solution or hydrogel form, possesses biochemical and physical properties that enhance bodily healing [109]. In order to promote good healing rates with thick epidermal wounds and production of skin appendages, researchers devised a decellularized framework of HA laden with epidermal growth factor [110]. Nanocomposites based on HA are thought to be very effective at accelerating wound curing. HA is non-toxic, bioconvenient, degradable in the body, hemostatic, and resistant to the adhesion of bacteria. HA-based nanocomposites support wound healing. Because of its special biological properties, HA can operate as a growth factor, an antibiotic, and a medication, all of which work together to quicken the healing process. Applications for HA nanocomposites loaded with metal or their oxides NPs have been reported for wound healing [111].

2.10.1.2 Dextran

Dextran polysaccharide is obtained by several bacterial strains; it is hydrophilic. It has linear chains of D-glucopyranose units linked by α-1, 6 linkages. Phagocytosis is the mechanism by which this polymer is broken down. It has a lot of hydroxyl groups readily conjugated with medicines or proteins via direct addition or via a linker [112, 113]. To increase cell adhesion and improve biocompatibility, researchers have endeavored to modify the characteristics of dextran hydrogels [114]. In order to increase the dextran's functioning as a scaffold for burn wound curing [115], researchers modified the degradation profile of dextran by treating it with glycocidyl methacrylate [116]. Using a mouse model, they investigated a cellular dextran hydrogel in the treatment of full-thickness burns. This investigation showed that the hydrogel that has been created promotes skin regeneration and angiogenesis [117].

2.10.1.3 Egg White

Egg white has been mentioned in traditional medicine. The muscle may readily absorb the protein found in egg whites. Egg white contains proteins and vitamins along with amino acids. In addition to their great nutritional value, eggs offer functional, immunogenic, and medicinal qualities. Eggs may produce immunogenicity and antibacterial qualities [118]. Wang et al. reported hydrogel wound dressing formulated using egg white. The resulting hydrogel dressing has direct 3D printability, good cytocompatibility, and interconnectivity of microporous channels with intrinsic biomolecules to promote cell activities. Adipose-derived stem cells can adhere to and multiply within the egg white hydrogel, which is 3D printed without any discernible cytotoxicity. Furthermore, the adipose-derived stem cells together with this integrated hydrogel platform promote angiogenesis, fibroblast proliferation, and collagen rearrangement, all of which hasten the healing process. With its low cost, accessible availability, quick manufacture, and sophisticated therapeutic impact, egg white hydrogel offers an efficient wound care solution that can also be used to heal chronic or other difficult wounds [119].

2.10.1.4 Alginate

This polymer is obtained from sources like kelp, brown algae, and certain microorganisms. The units of mannuronic acid and guluronic acid combine to form alginate, a linear anionic polymer. For many years, skin regeneration has been achieved with the application of alginate [120]. In order to achieve cell proliferation, antibacterial activity, and improved wound healing, a simple method has been described for creating biocomposite dressing material by means of interpolymeric fixation of fibrous chitosan-alginate abridged with NPs of calcium phosphate and NPs of zinc oxide by solvent casting process using sodium tripolyphosphate as a crosslinking agent. The biocomposite's biocompatibility testing was conducted using Vero BHK-cell cultures, which had a considerable increase in cell density, while BHK-21 fibroblast cells were devoid of mammalian cell toxicity. Using an experimental full-thickness wound model on mice, the biocomposite's wound-healing efficacy was evaluated. Within 10 days, results showed that the wound was filled with new epithelium, with no noticeable adverse effects in comparison to 30% closure with standard bandage dressing. Thus the formulated biocomposite was shown to be a viable option for efficient wound closure based on the in vivo data [121].

A study reported a biocompatible nanostructured composite with two distinct uses: it was to promote wound healing and ensure local antibiotic delivery. The biopolymers were sodium alginate and chitin. The commercial antibiotics, cefuroxime or cefepime, were loaded into the composite. With their proven biocompatibility and antibacterial qualities, the sodium alginate and chitin-based materials synthesized in this study appeared to have potential for use in the control of wound healing.

Moreover, this polymer possesses conformability, little toxicity, sufficient water absorption, antibacterial qualities, and an ideal water vapor transmission level, all of which are essential qualities for wound dressings [122, 123]. Because of its advantageous qualities, alginate can also be utilized to make scaffolds for tissue engineering. In fact, scaffolds that replicate the skin microenvironment and exhibit enhanced biocompatibility have been used as skin substitutes. These scaffolds include any combination of alginate and/or chitosan and/or chito-oligosaccharides and/or collagen [124].

2.10.1.5 Scleroglucan

Halleck initially described scleroglucan, an extracellular polymer, from the fungus Sclerotium glucanicum. The non-ionic, water-soluble homopolysaccharide scleroglucan is made up of a linear chain of glucopyranosyl and glucopyranosyl groups with D-(1-3) and D-(1-6) groups. [125]. Bozoğlan reported thermosensitive chitosan/carboxymethylcellulose/scleroglucan/montmorillonite (CHT/CMC/SGL/MMT) nanocomposite hydrogels for pharmaceutical applications. This study reported evaluation by rheology, FTIR, and SEM study. Other evaluation studies were TEM, TGA, X-ray diffraction, and swelling capacities to characterize the formulated nanocomposite hydrogels. The study's findings suggested that thermosensitive CHT/CMC/SGL/MMT BNC could find use in tissue engineering, medication delivery, and wound dressing [126].

2.10.1.6 Cellulose

One intriguing property of bacterial cellulose is that it possesses a skin-like porous structure. Since a wound needs to be kept moist, the material's high hydrophilicity is a crucial characteristic of a wound dressing [127]. Cellulose can also be linked to other elements to intensify its effects. It was observed that the mechanical and antibacterial qualities of the wound dressing were enhanced when they blended cellulose with zinc oxide NPs. The strong attachment of keratinocytes and fibroblasts to electrospun nanofibers made of collagen from healthy skin allows the extra support that the ECM provides for their migration through the wound bed, regeneration, and repair of the damaged cells [128]. Because it may be mixed with other copolymers and is a malleable, bioresorbable, non-toxic, antimitogenic, and highly biocompatible biomaterial, cellulose is an excellent choice for use in nanofibers [129].

2.10.1.7 Hydroxyapatite

Hydroxyapatite (HAP) is highly biocompatible; it has a great potential for wound healing, having sufficient angiogenic potential. However, conventional HAP materials' excessive brittleness and subpar mechanical qualities make them unsuitable for wound dressing. In order to overcome this obstacle, Gao et al. created a unique wound treatment composed of biopaper based on flexible, ultralong HAP nanowires. These nanowire-based biopapers successfully stimulated the production of additional angiogenic factors in rat skin tissue and human umbilical vein endothelial cells (HUVECs) facing hypoxia, according to experiments conducted both in vitro and in vivo. Additionally, the as-prepared biopaper promoted HUVEC migration, proliferation, and in vitro angiogenesis. Furthermore, the biopaper facilitated the development of new blood vessels, thicker skin, and reepithelialization in rats, all of which aided in the wound's healing process [130].

2.10.1.8 Silk

A naturally occurring fibrous protein derived from Lepidoptera larvae, silk is made up of two essential proteins: a water-soluble protein called sericin and a fibrous protein [131, 132]. The silk fiber is a great option for biomedical applications since it is biocompatible and biodegradable, produces minimal inflammatory responses, and offers enough oxygen. The silk fibroin-based nanofibers have potential properties in wound healing and skin regeneration treatment [133]. Researchers examined the synergistic effects of silver oxide NPs and silk fibroin on wound healing. Through the use of in vitro scratch assay, the produced biomaterial displayed a striking antibacterial action against both pathogenic and non-pathogenic bacteria. Additionally, the 3T3 fibroblast cells swiftly moved to the scratch region, covering the entire area within 24 hours. Using a cytotoxicity experiment, this work additionally verified the scaffold's biocompatibility and demonstrated its prospect in wound therapy [134].

2.10.1.9 Elastin

Another hydrophobic and insoluble ECM protein is elastin. It can create biomaterials incorporating repeats of synthetic peptide sequences, soluble elastin after hydrolysis, elastin fibers and their copolymers, recombinant tropoelastin, and in combination with other polymers [135, 136]. A unique collagen-elastin scaffold was reported to offer a dermal replacement for burn injuries involving full-thickness skin [137].

2.10.1.10 Starch

Starch is a polysaccharide with intriguing qualities such as biodegradability, non-cytotoxicity, and renewability. Additionally, starch may be readily altered chemically, which makes it useful for tissue engineering and medication administration [138]. Starch-based scaffolds can function as a substrate for cell adhesion and have a decent rate of biodegradation [139]. Researchers have demonstrated the probability of these frameworks in wound curative applications by demonstrating a low-toxicity rise in mouse fibroblast cells, their growth, and proliferation [140]. The creation of starch-gelatin platforms for particularly wound-curative applications was described by Chhabra et al. (2020). This study demonstrated how the scaffold might encourage tissue remodeling and reorganization while hastening wound healing [141].

2.10.1.11 Collagen

According to Sherman et al. (2015), collagen is a part of ECM and also the most prevalent protein in the human body. It is the primary structural protein in the dermis and plays a crucial part in the healing of wounds [142]. Collagen has therefore been used in the creation of a number of skin scaffolds [143]. Type I collagen is the most employed kind of collagen in skin scaffolds [108]. Using a casting approach, Natarajan and colleagues assessed the impact of a tannic acid-linked collagen scaffold [143]. A collagen/chitosan composite scaffold bearing L-glutamic acid was created to help diabetic wounds heal more quickly. The scaffolds demonstrated greater rates and showed no toxicity [144].

2.10.1.12 Chondroitin Sulfate

Zou et al. investigated the role of chondroitin sulfate in extracted and cultivated rabbit palatal fibroblasts following surgical correction of cleft palate. Treatment with this biomaterial increased cell adhesion and cell proliferation in a dose-dependent manner; however, after chondroitin sulfate was broken down by chondroitinase, the opposite effects were observed. The presence and orientation of sulfate groups seem to affect the biological effects of chondroitin sulfate. Reductions in cell adhesion and proliferation as well as a relaxed level of wound healing were observed in vitro when glycosaminoglycan sulfation was inhibited by chlorate treatment. Additionally, chondroitin-4-sulfate exposure demonstrated a dose-dependent decrease in cell adhesion. All of these findings point to chondroitin sulfate's effective part in the healing of palatal injuries [145].

2.10.1.13 Gelatin

It is a derivative of collagen, known for being less antigenic, biocompatible, and biodegradable to the highest degree [146]. Compared to other polymers, this one has a great degree of structural flexibility since it contains both basic and acidic groups. Due to its gelation properties and ease of processing, gelatin can be formulated as injectable hydrogels, sponges, and microspheres [147]. Furthermore, gelatin can be modified to include additional peptides and cell adhesion molecules in order to use it in various tissue engineering techniques [148]. By freeze-drying porous gelatin/zeolite scaffolds, researchers demonstrated their cytocompatibility, antibacterial activity, and capacity to accelerate Sprague Dawley rat wound healing [149].

2.10.1.14 Chitosan/Chitin

Chitosan is a polysaccharide that is produced when chitin is deacetylated. Crustaceans' or fungi exoskeletons' structural component is chitin [108, 150]. Rezaii et al. created a chitosan-collagen scaffold by adding curcumin NPs. On a Wistar rat model, this structure allowed full-thickness punch wounds to heal successfully [151]. According to research, chitosan can enhance how well inflammatory cells work while a wound heals [152]. Wound healing uses the bilayered electrospun nanofiber scaffolds of hyaluronic acid and chitosan combined with natural or synthetic polymers [153, 154]. As a wound dressing, the bacterial cellulose-chitosan composite-created films incorporating nanodiamonds displayed flexibility and biocompatibility [155]. The hydrogel wound dressing containing chitosan-ZnONPs exhibits appropriate antibacterial activity while posing little hazard [156]. Due to their low mechanical qualities, chitosan pristine fibers have few biological uses; however, chitosan composite structures involving synthetic polymers performed superiorly. Chitosan-based gold nanocomposites exhibited a total bactericidal effect against antibiotic-resistant strains (*S. aureus* and *P. aeruginosa*), which are responsible for biofilm formation with reduced toxicity [157]. The nanocomposite crafted from TiO_2- chitosan and backed with collagen artificial skin maintained a modest TNF-α level, indicating its anti-inflammatory effect. [158].

2.10.1.15 Fibronectin

A high molecular weight glycoprotein derived from plasma from humans and cows, fibronectin can be employed as a scaffold to help cells adhere to surfaces and migrate, hence controlling the proliferation and differentiation of cells [159, 160]. For use in wound healing, researchers created platforms built on nanofibronectin fibers. The collected results showed that this scaffold can promote tissue repair and reclamation of dermal and epidermal structures, adipose tissue, and skin appendages, in addition to speeding wound healing [161].

2.10.1.16 Agar

Agar is a polymer that has been shown to be highly immunogenic and biocompatible [162]. It may be used to create a gel that bears a resemblance to the physical properties of the ECM and can be used to transfer cell progression factors to injured tissues and organs [163]. Nayak and Gupta (2015) showed that a binary combination of keratin and agar is safe to employ in wound curing and skin rejuvenation since it promotes cell proliferation and is non-toxic [164]. In order to address wound healing, researchers synthesized fumaric acid incorporated in the hydrogel of agar-silver composite. This hydrogel demonstrated increased collagen deposition and angiogenesis, as well as a synergistic antibacterial impact against microorganisms and a faster pace of wound healing [165].

2.10.1.17 Fibrin

The proteolytic thrombin, which is triggered by tissue damage, cleaves soluble fibrinogen to produce fibrin, an insoluble protein. It makes sense that fibrin would form a fibrous mesh because of its capacity to function as a blood-clotting agent. Many studies have been conducted on this polymer for applications related to wound healing [108]. By electrospinning a fibrous framework composed of polycaprolactone, keratin, and platelet-rich fibrin, Mirhaj et al. (2022) showed the scaffold's angiogenic potential and its capacity to hasten wound restoration, collagen deposition, and creation of skin components [166].

2.10.1.18 Keratin

Found in skin, nails, and hair, keratin is a fibrous protein. It possesses intriguing characteristics such as biocompatibility to the highest degree and self-organizational ability that coordinates cellular recognition and cell behavior [167, 168]. More antibacterial activity was shown in a study that involved lyophilizing a porous keratin/chitosan scaffold by lyophilization exposing superior antibacterial action and cell proliferation rates, emphasizing its potential application as a bandage for wounds [169]. Research on the development of an in situ forming keratin hydrogel and its use as a drug depot for wound repair revealed that the deferoxamine-loaded scaffold increased angiogenesis and neovascularization in wounds, accelerating healing in the full-thickness wounds of streptozotocin-induced diabetic rats [170].

2.10.2 Nanomaterials for Wound Healing

Natural nanomaterials and nano-sized drug carriers are ideal for cellular responses, penetrability, and active drug supply in wound healing due to their nanosize and elevated surface area-to-volume ratios [171, 172]. Nanocomposites, of both inorganic and organic types, find a place in the treatment of wounds. Because of their nature, the ratio of inorganic to organic materials, and the size and distribution of the inorganic NPs in the polymer matrix, inorganic/organic nanocomposites have been able to meet the growing needs of wound healing [173]. For instance, in vivo activity against multidrug-resistant (MDR) bacteria has been demonstrated for intermediate-modified gold nanoparticles (AuNPs) in combination with polycaprolactone (PCL)/gelatin nanofibers [174]. In vivo electrospun scaffolds of copper sulfide (Cu_2S) NPs with polylactic acid (PLA)/PCL polymers significantly induce angiogenesis and cure diabetic full-thickness skin lesions [175]. Natural polymers show uncontrolled degradability and lack strength, despite being biocompatible and enzymatically biodegradable.

A variety of purely inorganic nanomaterials, including carbon-based NPs, metals and NPs of their oxides, and ceramic NPs, are assimilated into visually appealing BNCs. These nanomaterials have promising bioactive, mechanical, and antibacterial properties that can hasten wound healing [176]. Similarly, purely organic nanomaterials such as liposomes are also incorporated in BNCs. Nevertheless, the hybrid type incorporating inorganic and organic types is gaining popularity.

Following are different types of nanomaterials used in BNCs for the wound healing process.

2.10.2.1 Carbon-Based Nanomaterials

The four stages of wound healing use carbon-originated nanomaterials, such as graphene, CNTs, fullerene, nanodiamonds, and diamond-like carbon. These materials can supply growth factors, antibiotics, antioxidants, or stem cells [177–181]. Because of their enormous surface area and favorable physicochemical properties, carbon-based nanomaterials find applications in skin care, targeted medication delivery, and tissue engineering [182, 183]. The intrinsic antibacterial activity of carbon nanomaterials is caused by the generation of ROS in addition to their hydrophobic properties [184–190].

2.10.2.2 Graphene

Excellent antibacterial properties are exhibited by grapheme, its oxide, graphite, its oxide, and reduced graphene oxide as nanofilms [185]. When in contact with bacteria, graphene and graphene oxide significantly cause ROS-independent oxidative damage [186–188]. In vitro and in vivo healing of incurable bacterial wound infections was markedly accelerated by biocompatible graphene oxide or copper-incorporated composites crafted from chitosan with hyaluronic acid. [189]. Chitosan-polyvinyl alcohol (PVA) nanofibers containing graphene disrupted the genetic material of mice and rabbits, preventing the growth of E. coli as well as Agrobacterium cells [190].

2.10.2.3 Carbon Nanotubes

Dermal fibroblasts' ability to heal wounds is impacted by exposure to CNTs, which changes their motility, adhesion, spreading, and viability [191]. Through ROS and heavy metal residues, single-walled nanocarbon tubes and multiple-walled nanocarbon tubes significantly impact bacterial membrane's structural integrity, metabolic process, and morphology [192–197]. Higher antibacterial effects were seen when CNTs were combined with silver and titanium dioxide NPs [198–199].

2.10.2.4 Fullerenes

By lowering inflammation, battling bacteria, modifying the discharge of harmful factors from cells, promoting cell migration, and quickening the healing of injuries, fullerenes and their derivatives may be able to treat difficult-to-heal wounds [200]. The most researched fullerene, buckminsterfullerene (C), is slightly water soluble and highly hydrophobic [201]. In vivo wound healing was accelerated by the C-(ethylenediamine) type of fullerene derivative, which also expressively suppressed *E. coli* and regulated immunological response and growth factor production [202].

2.10.2.5 Nanodiamonds

Additionally, while shielding healthy cells and tissues, nanodiamonds quicken the healing process [203]. In vitro doxorubicin concentrations were higher, and the cytotoxicity was decreased in a membrane made of carboxylated nanodiamond-cellulose nanocomposite loaded with doxorubicin [204]. As a wound dressing, the chitosan/bacterial cellulose composite films, which included nanodiamonds, were flexible and biocompatible [205].

2.10.2.6 Diamond Carbon Looks Alike

Because diamond-like carbon films are hydrophobic, which changes the cell membrane and kills bacteria, they are chemically steady and have higher mechanical, biocompatible, and antibacterial efficacious qualities [206]. Diamond-like carbon inhibits the attachment and growth of bacteria, improves bioactivity characteristics and cell adhesion, and regulates inflammation [207]. Methicillin-resistant *S. aureus* (MRSA) and nearly all other bacterial strains were eliminated by the bandage of synthetic silk tissue covered with diamond-like carbon nanoparticles (AgNPs) [208]. Because of the quick Ag ion release from these NPs, angiogenesis was stimulated and microbial colonization of *S. aureus* and *S. epidermidis* was inhibited, enabling longstanding tissue rejuvenation in vitro [209].

2.10.2.7 Metals and Metal Oxide Nanomaterials

The effectiveness of metals in biological applications is influenced by their nanosize and shape, surface characteristics, porosity, and resistance to breakdown in aqueous solutions [210–212].

2.10.2.8 Silver Nanoparticles (AgNPs)

The unique physicochemical, antibacterial, and anti-inflammatory properties of silver NPs have sparked a great deal of attention for their perspective in wound-healing applications [213]. By lowering the release of cytokine growth factor, mast cell infiltrators, and lymphocytic cells, silver NPs improve wound healing [214, 215]. The development of *E. coli, Staphylococcus, and Pseudomonas species* was inhibited by the poly(methyl methacrylate-co-dopamine methacrylamide)-AgNPs wound dressings. Within two weeks of using the MADO-AgNPs wound dressing, rats' skin wounds completely healed and their epithelialization increased [216, 217]. Because AgNPs have anti-inflammatory and antioxidant qualities, reduced graphene oxide/silver-silver chloride NPs hastened injury closing; improved reepithelialization was achieved in mice following burn injury [218, 219].

2.10.2.9 Gold Nanoparticles (AuNPs)

By halting the production of ROS, gold NPs, which are antioxidants, promote wound healing [220]. The transcutaneous distribution of various medications in vivo was made easier by gold NPs, which penetrated the subcutaneous layer of skin and extended across the epidermis layer [221]. AuNPs' biocompatibility and biodegradability are enhanced by crosslinking with collagen, gelatin, and chitosan, which also boosts their ability to scavenge free radicals [222, 223]. In comparison to chitosan alone, the chitosan-AuNPs composite enhanced both hemostasis and the development of epithelial tissue in injured rats. Applying AuNPs-cryopreserved human fibroblasts topically decreased inflammation and accelerated the time at which burn wounds heal overall [224, 225].

2.10.2.10 Zinc Oxide Nanoparticles

Because they promote collagen formation and have bacteriostatic and bactericidal effects by disturbing the structure of cell membranes, ROS and NPs of zinc oxide are common inorganic ingredients used in burn wounds [226–229]. One of the most crucial trace elements, zinc, controls the activity of enzymes such as ribonuclease, thymidine kinase, and DNA and RNA polymerases, which in turn controls burns and wounds that heal slowly [230]. In comparison to AuNPs and AgNPs, constant valent zinc oxide NPs exhibited higher aggregate stability, decreased toxicity, and high permeability in skin [231, 232].

2.10.2.11 Copper Nanoparticles

By promoting keratinocytic cells, fibroblast cells' proliferation, epithelialization step, collagen synthesis, ECM remodeling step, and angiogenesis step in rats, copper NPs expedited wound termination [233, 234]. By creating key signal proteins that elicit a role in wound healing in diabetic mice, such as TGF-β, HIF-1α, MMP-2, and VEGF, copper oxide NP dressings promoted wound restoration [235]. Metal copper nanocomposites built on chitosan demonstrated antifungal and antibacterial characteristics, boosted VEGF, TGF-β1, interleukin-10 (IL-10), and TNF-α, improving wound remedy in mice [236].

2.10.2.12 Silica Nanoparticles

By facilitating the proliferation and dissemination of skin fibroblast cells over the injured region, silica NPs (SiNPs) enhanced topical wound healing in vitro by releasing silicic acid [237]. In wound dressings, SiNP-collagen hydrogel nanocomposites enhanced the harmonized result of collagen and SiNPs, decreased fibroblast toxicity, and strengthened the mechanical powers and durability against degradation [238]. Similarly, the migration and reepithelialization were increased by silicon dioxide NPs and polyvinylpyrrolidone as a carrier, confirming the involvement of silica-based nanomaterials in wound healing [239].

2.10.2.13 Titanium Dioxide Nanoparticles (TiONP)

By producing and secreting monocyte chemoattractant protein-1, PDGF, macrophage inflammatory protein-1-α, MIP-1-β, IL-8, and VEGF in union with contact system (FXII) activation, titanium dioxide NPs enhanced wound healing [240]. TiONP wound dressings encapsulated with chitosan and pectin have intriguing wound-healing characteristics in addition to antimicrobial qualities [241]. The collagen-artificial skin nanocomposite containing nano-TiO-chitosan maintained a modest level of TNF-α, indicating its anti-inflammatory properties [242].

2.10.2.14 Superparamagnetic Iron Oxide Nanoparticles (SPIONs)

The use of superparamagnetic iron oxide nanoparticles (SPIONs) as medication delivery vehicles and wound-healing agents seems promising. Iron oxide cores with or without nickel, cobalt, manganese, or copper make up SPIONs, tiny forms of magnetic NPs [243]. Higher toxicity plus strong penetration of bacterial biofilms are demonstrated by gold-coated SPIONs. By extending the half-life of thrombin in human plasma relative to free thrombin, SPION conjugated with iron oxide NP-thrombin improved skin flexibility while improving thrombin's ability to repair wounds [244, 245].

2.10.2.15 Ceramic Nanoparticles

Ceramic NPs, which can be compact, crystalline, amorphous, hollow, or porous, are inorganic and non-metallic solids that are synthesized by cooling-heating cycles [246–249]. By encouraging cell proliferation and the production of cytokines like HIF-1 and VEGF, bioactive glass promotes angiogenesis by gradually releasing silicon and Ca ions at the injured sites [250, 251]. Bioactive glass produces silicon ions that shield endothelial cells from low oxygen levels and promote angiogenesis [252].

2.10.2.16 Lipid-Based Nanomaterials

Nanolipidic drug delivery is based on lipid-based NPs such as liposomes [253, 254]. Lipid-based NPs are a promising treatment option for vascular disorders and limb ischemia [255]. Compared to liposomes, solid lipid NPs stabilize medications and prolong their release. Moreover, they are safer since they don't use organic solvents during their manufacturing process [256, 257]. In a human-based three-dimensional wound restorative model, dermal morphine encapsulated solid lipid NPs decreased toxicity and irritation, expedited wound closure, improved reepithelialization, and permitted keratinocytes to proliferate throughout the dermis [258].

2.10.2.17 Nanofibers

Nanofibers are unique in the field of wound soothing due to their nanosize, exceptional mechanical and physical properties, high packing capability, and regulated discharge of drugs. The proliferation, motility, differentiation, and ECM deposition of cells are all regulated by electrospun nanofibers, permitting their production into skin substitutes, wound dressings, wound-healing sutures, and engineered skin tissues [259]. In order to create innovative scaffolds of natural polymers that transport bioactive compounds, nanoelectrospun fibers are highly porous and have a significant surface area-to-volume value [260, 261]. To produce nanomaterials, electrospinning increases the number of nanofibers in the three-dimensional setup [262]. Electrospun nanofibers replicate the biological and mechanical characteristics of the skin in part because of the thoughtful selection of nanofiber components [263, 264]. These properties render them suitable for application in drug delivery, tissue engineering scaffolds, intelligent fabrics and clothing, and biosensors [265].

2.10.2.18 Green Synthesized Nanoparticles

TiO_2NPs, AgNPs, AuNPs, and CuONPs produced via green synthesis improve wound healing and reduce or eliminate infections and negative effects from treatment [266–268]. When combined with phytoextracts, green-synthesized NPs like AgNPs are economical, environmentally benign, and have antibacterial and antifungal qualities that aid in wound healing [269, 270]. The Sprague Dawley rats with multiple-strain diseased wounds were successfully treated by the manufacture of stable AgNPs utilizing the fungus Orchid anthachinensis [271]. AgNPs that were created reduced the number of scars, reepithelialized the epidermis, sped up wound healing and the pace at which wounds contracted, and decreased the levels of TNF-α, IL-1β, and IL-6 [272]. When crosslinked with chitosan, PEG, and AgNPs, genipin—a chemical made from geniposide, which is derived from the slow-developing fungus Penicillium nigricans—heightened wound healing with superior antibacterial activity [273].

2.10.2.19 Nitric Oxide-Releasing Nanoparticles

Nitric oxide regulates the growth of keratinocytes and skin homeostasis. It also promotes angiogenesis and ECM protein deposition during wound curing. Because inducible nitric oxide synthase levels are dysregulated in psoriasis and systemic lupus erythematosus (SLE), nitric oxide has a role in both conditions [274, 275]. Biomaterials such as chitosan and L-arginine with coatings that release nitric oxide reduce the incidence of infections linked to biomaterials. S. aureus and other pathogen biofilms were eliminated in vitro using monofilament polypropylene mesh backed by coatings based on carbon that release nitric oxide [276].

2.10.2.20 Antibiotic-Loaded Nanoparticles (Nanobiotics)

The recent breakthrough known as nanobiotics enhances the effectiveness of traditional antibiotics in treating wounds by countering multidrug-resistant bacterial growth. Vancomycin-modified NPs demonstrated broad-spectrum in vitro efficacy [277]. Antibiotics conjugated with polyacrylate NP and poly(butyl acrylate-styrene) NP-N-thiolated β-lactam conjugates demonstrated significant action and reduced toxicity against MRSA, which causes serious infections in many body sections [278, 279]. A gelatin/chitosan/epigallocatechin gallate NP dressing, which was combined with activated carbon fibers and antibiotic gentamicin, slowed the development of bacteria and enhanced both in-vitro and in-vivo reepithelialization [280].

2.10.2.21 Polymer Nanoparticles

The worth of biocompatible polymeric NPs is underlined by the field of biomedicine and the field of bioengineering [281]. Most polymeric NPs have been developed utilizing poly lactic-co-glycolic acid, chitosan, gelatin, alginate, and other polymeric combinations [282, 283]. Drugs are stabilized against proteases by conjugation with polymeric NPs, which also makes regulated drug release easier and lowers dosage frequency. Effective biomolecules for delivering genes, growth factors, and antibiotics are polymeric NPs [284, 285]. Growth factors, FGF2 and EGF, are indispensable for wound curing; however, the wound microenvironment contains a proteolytic enzyme, matrix metalloproteinase, which significantly shortens the half-life of these growth factors [286]. Interesting nanocarriers like poly-L-lactic acid can carry proteins and medications that are very hydrophobic and poorly soluble in the right amount. When PLLA NPs were used instead of the unencapsulated version of curcumin-bortezomib, the toxic effects were lessened [287]. Adapalene is a topical retinoid used to promote wound healing; its encapsulation efficiency was also enhanced by the use of PLA-PEG NPs [288].

2.11 METHODS OF PREPARATION OF BIONANOCOMPOSITES

Nanomaterials are intended to be inserted into biomaterial matrices to produce BNCs in order to further benefit from their wide range of uses. Numerous techniques, including intercalation, sol-gel transformation, in-situ method of polymerization, and direct polymer mixing with nanofillers, can be used to produce them [289]. Following are some common methods used for the production of BNCs.

2.11.1 In Situ Polymerization

As low-molecular-weight possessing monomer permeates the different layers, in situ polymerization causes swelling of filler in liquid monomer or monomer solution [290]. According to a reported method, polymerization can commence by means of heat application, radiation exposure, initiator diffusion, an organic catalyst, or initiator fixation by cation exchange. After that, the monomers polymerize within the strata of layers and generate exfoliated or intercalated nanocomposites [291]. When compared to other methods, this strategy has the benefit of better exfoliation. The formation of an exfoliated nanocomposite under polymerization circumstances is achieved by dispersing the substance to be incorporated into polymer monomer, as depicted in Figure 2.5, which shows the synthesis of nanocomposite by in situ polymerization [292].

2.11.2 Melt Extrusion

In the melt extrusion technique, no solvent is required; hence, this approach offers a significant advantage over the others. On the other hand, the amount of NPs that need to be distributed is crucial. Due to their agglomeration tendency, the NPs in this approach need to be closely monitored during their dispersion. The same equipment is utilized to process polymers without the utilization

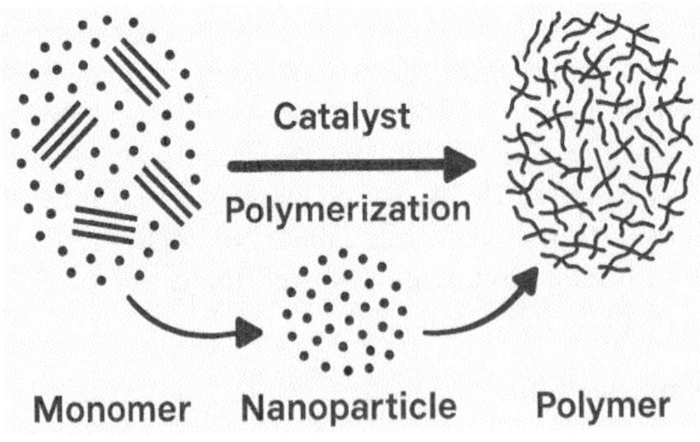

FIGURE 2.5 In situ polymerization technique for the synthesis of bionanocomposites [293].

of NPs. As a result, the temperature at which the polymer is extruded must be carefully monitored by the researcher, as must the amount of time required for the NPs to spread evenly. The degradation and melting temperatures of natural polymers and a small number of biopolymers are extremely near [294–296]. Figure 2.6 illustrates a scheme of synthesis of BNCs by melt extrusion technique using a standard extruder. It shows an example of a twin-screw extruder that is commonly used in industry to distribute CNTs within a thermoplastic biopolymer matrix. After PNC has been extruded, it can be put into an injection molding machine to create the final product that has the necessary geometric shape. In hot melt extrusion (HME), materials are melted, mixed, and pushed together with different solids at high pressures and temperatures [297].

2.11.3 Melt Intercalation

It is the standard procedure used to create thermoplastic polymer nanocomposites. The method encompasses adding a filler to polymer matrices heated at high temperatures to fabricate the composite and kneading the formed composite to obtain an even distribution, as shown in Figure 2.7. The absence of solvent usage confers an environmentally favorable advantage. Furthermore, it is believed to be compatible with industrial procedures of extrusion and procedures of injection molding, which increases its usability and, consequently, lowers its cost. Nevertheless, the filler's surface modification may be harmed by the process's high temperatures. For instance, alkyl ammonium-modified organo clays often breakdown at temperatures above 140°C; yet, melt intercalation processing temperatures range from 190°C to 220°C [292, 298, 299].

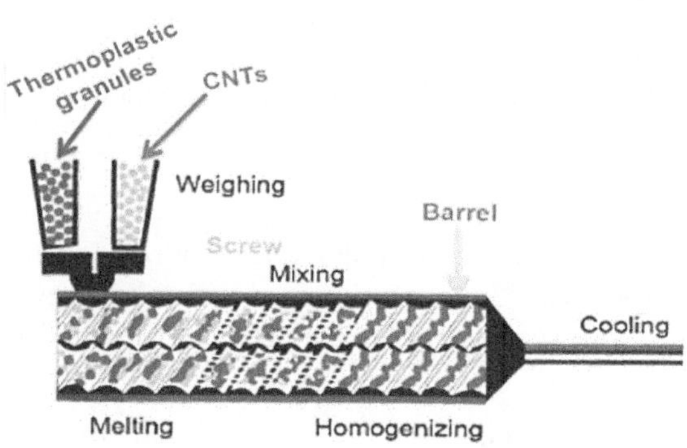

FIGURE 2.6 Synthesis of polymer nanocomposites by melt extrusion [293].

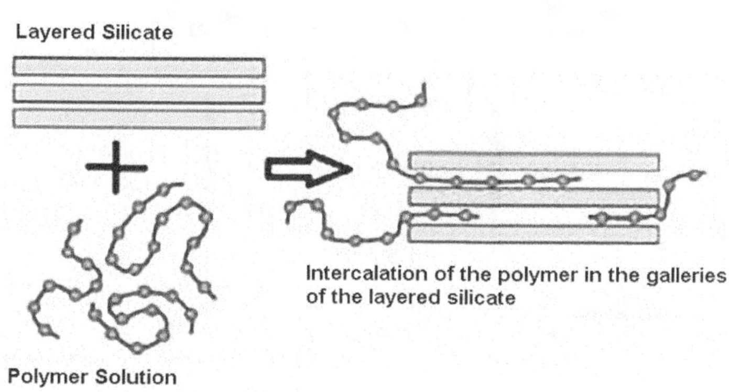

FIGURE 2.7 Melt intercalation [293].

2.11.4 Method of Solution

Another way to create nanocomposites is the solution method, which involves dissolving hydrophobic NPs in a polymer solution and then casting or coating the mixture onto substrates to create composite sheets or films when the solvent evaporates. With this approach, producing high-quality nanocomposites is considerably easier. With the favorable interaction vis-à-vis the solvent and polymer, varied quantities of NPs can be distributed. The solvent must be handled carefully because it needs to be eliminated entirely in the end [300–303]. The equipment used in this process is shown in Figure 2.8. Combining solution dispersion with spray drying is one intriguing technique. The material is dried into a powder by injecting the dispersion containing the NPs in the polymer solution into the spray dryer after it has had some time to homogenize. The ultimate yield of the material is the main disadvantage of this process. However, once all parameters are set and the finished product exhibits good dispersion and dispersal, this process just takes place in one phase. Drugs and nanosystems can be injected simultaneously in this approach to provide targeted or controlled distribution [304].

2.11.5 Exfoliation Adsorption Process

The exfoliation adsorption technique relies on a solvent which can imbibe the prepolymer or polymer. It is also known as polymer or prepolymer intercalation from solution. For example, before admixture with the polymeric solution (see Figure 2.9), the multilayer silicate is inflated and dissolved in the solvent. After that, the solvent inside the silicate interlayers is displaced by the polymer chains intercalating. As the solvent is eventually removed, the sheets eventually reassemble and create a multilayer structure that traps the polymer chains [306–308].

Clay particle-reinforced starch-based nanocomposites are shown in Figure 2.9. A unique nanocomposite material is formed as a result of this specific combination.

2.11.6 Electrospinning

By delivering a high-magnitude voltage to a polymeric solution via a micro-syringe pump, electrospinning is an effective, somewhat easy, and inexpensive technology that may be used to create continuous nanofibers on a wide scale. The fiber diameter can be varied from nanometers to microns.

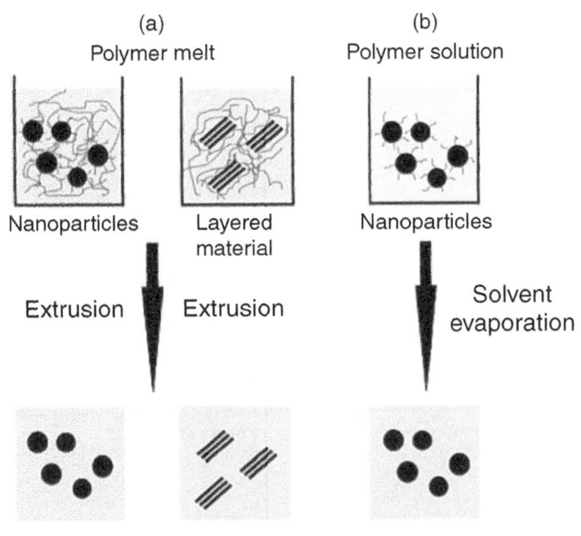

FIGURE 2.8 Synthesis of nanocomposites by solvent method or method of solutions [305].

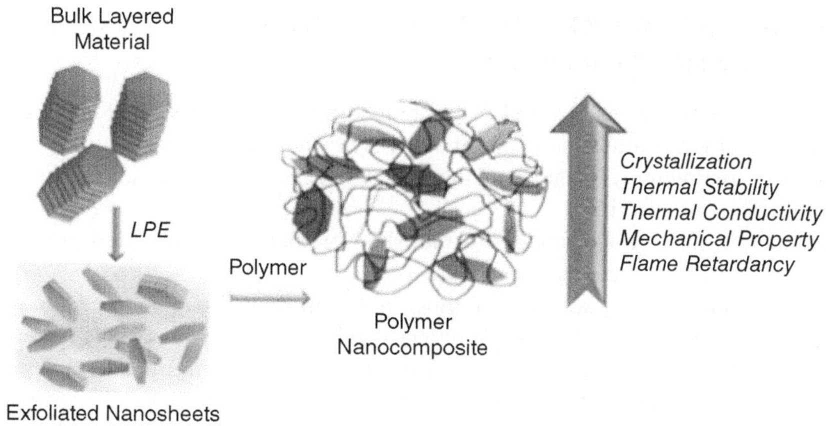

FIGURE 2.9 Synthesis of bionanocomposites by exfoliation-adsorption process way [309].

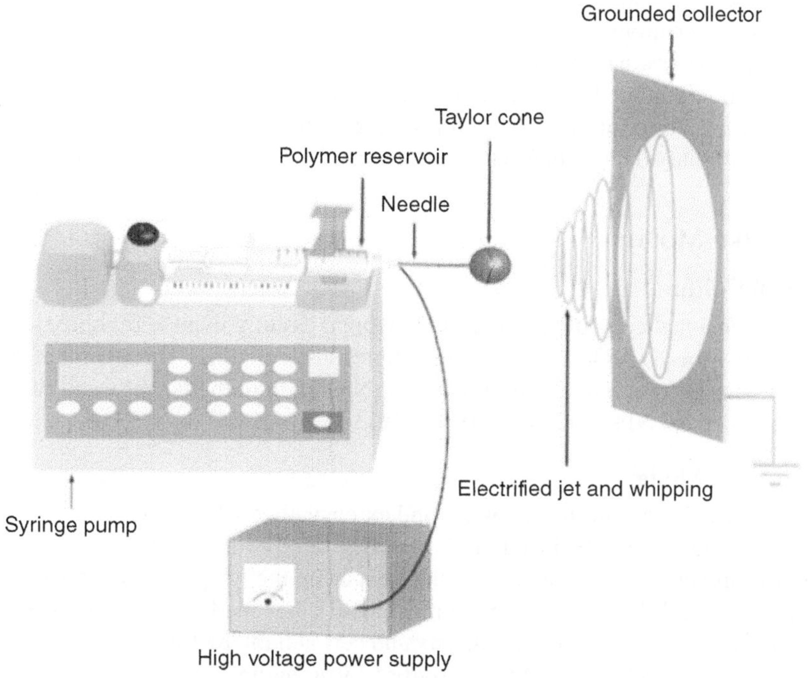

FIGURE 2.10 The schematic diagram of an electrospinning device for the production of nanofibers [312].

Electrospun polymer nanofibers possess specific surface areas that are roughly two or three orders of magnitude grander than those of flat films. This makes them the most promising option for use in energy storage, release control, wound healing, filtration, and tissue scaffold engineering [310]. A nonwoven web of micro- or nanofibers is produced during the electrospinning process. This method involves applying high-magnitude electricity to the polymeric liquid solution, enabling the solution to extrude via a nozzle and create a jet. Fibers formed in the created jet as it dried and settled on the collector. One easy and flexible way to prepare micro- or nanopolymer fibers is by electrospinning. Another method for creating inorganic fibers is by electrospinning polymers that are present in the precursor solution (Figure 2.10). The electrospinning process depends on the viscosity, conductivity, surface tension, and other properties of the electrospinning solution, all of which can be affected by the presence of polymers) [311].

2.12 ASSESSMENT OF WOUND HEALING ACTIVITY OF BIONANOCOMPOSITES

Periodic wound assessment, as covered in the preceding sections, will increase the likelihood of giving the patient a more suitable course of therapy. The medical team may be able to determine the optimal course of treatment by considering the wound's features, etiology, and other medical history in addition to routine monitoring.

However, the ability of both new and established biomaterials, NPs, and medication delivery methods to promote wound healing needs to be assessed.

Researchers should take into account a number of design-related factors when conducting wound-healing inquiry studies, such as the study's objectives, the wound type, sample appearances or features and accessibility, costs, schedule, and available facilities. Combining several wound assessment techniques would also improve the validity and reliability of the findings and advance our knowledge of the mechanisms behind tissue repair. Additionally, if a suitable wound healing model is selected early on in the testing of a new product, less time and resources will be required for the experiments, which will save costs and increase the value of the finished product [4]. The many instruments, models, and approaches for assessing wound healing at the preclinical stage are covered in the following sections.

In an attempt to assess new treatment modalities and get a deeper understanding of the tissue repair process, numerous models of experimental wound restoration have been developed. These models are either in vitro or animal (sometimes referred to as in vivo or preclinical).

Important preliminary data from in vitro models can be used in the design of later in vivo studies.

2.12.1 In Vitro Models

2.12.1.1 Cell Culture

In-vitro two-dimensional cell culture models for wound healing include (a) chronic-wound-derived fibroblasts and (b) the hTERT chronic wound fibroblast cell line. Three-dimensional techniques include (a) fibroblasts from diabetic foot ulcers or NKs or endothelial cells and (b) patient-derived (type 2 diabetes) dermal NFs, NKs, and HUVECs [313, 314].

2.12.1.2 Scratch Model

In vitro scratch assay is an easy, inexpensive, and extensively studied mode for assessing cell migration in vitro. Creating a "scratch" in a monolayer of cultured cells, sealing the scratch, taking photos at the beginning and end of cell migration, and comparing the images are the basic steps in figuring out how quickly the cells are migrating. Compared to other methods, the in vitro scratch assay is particularly useful for studying how cell-matrix and cell-cell interactions affect migration. If needed, it can also be used to track intracellular activities by imaging living cells during migration. This method has been applied not only to follow the migration of homogeneous cell groups but also to evaluate the immigration of cells in the leading edge of the scratch. If one is merely thinking about the time needed for cell transfection, an in vitro scratch experiment can take anywhere from a few hours to an entire night [314, 315].

2.12.1.3 Skin Explant Culture

In actuality, skin explants are ex vivo treatments. Skin tissue following an excision is processed to create skin explants. The tissue is cleansed of contaminants and subcutaneous fat, after which it is cultivated. Such processed tissue is devoid of both nerve and blood supply. The experimental model that most nearly mimics both healthy and pathological skin physiology is skin explants. This kind of model includes every type of native skin cell, such as keratinocytes, melanocytes, and Langerhans cells, in addition to a dermal matrix made up of fibroblasts, collagen, elastin, glycosaminoglycans, and so forth [316, 317].

2.12.2 In Vivo Models

In vivo models entail inflicting wounds on lab animals and tracking the healing process. Modifications to the wound environment that are physical, chemical, or biological can also be included. They provide a genuine depiction of the wound milieu, encompassing varied cell types, signals, and paracrine interactions. Experiments on cutaneous wounds are conducted on a variety of animals, including pigs, rabbits, and rodents (rats or mice). It is quite easy to genetically modify certain small mammals to create a model that approximates human diseases, including diabetes, immunological deficits, and obesity. When choosing a model, considerations such as the lesion's exact reproducibility, the capacity to collect multiple biopsy samples, the potential for multiple investigations, compatibility with animal facilities, handling convenience, and the time required to get meaningful results should be taken into account. Small animal trials usually endure for days, as opposed to the weeks or months that human research usually lasts, because they heal more quickly than humans. Although the physiology and structure of mouse and human skin differ, investigations on wound healing that account for these differences can provide valuable translational insights. For research purposes, a vast variety of rodents are available, and rats are simple to house, handle, and maintain. The skin of rodents is distinct from human skin in that it has a thin muscular layer called the panniculus carnosus, which is only present in the platysma of the neck and causes fast wound contraction after damage. Comparatively, human wounds recover through the production of granulation tissue and reepithelialization, which are significant distinctions to take into account when evaluating the translational significance of rodent studies. When designing the studies, it is important to take into account the variations in skin structure and physiology across genders. For instance, female skin is thinner than male skin. These models have had an extensive influence on our understanding of skin pathophysiology, despite these disparities. Rats are generally seen to be a better option than mice. The mice's small size and the differences in skin tone between individuals are a couple of the causes. Compared to rat skin, mouse skin is thinner and has fewer keratinocyte layers. Wounds on mice heal in approximately 7 days; however, recovery in rats can take up to 12–14 days to assess. Because the size of a wound should match the size of the animal, mice's wounds are smaller than rats' and heal more quickly. However, investigations requiring small sample sizes for analysis could be better off using mice. Since an animal can sustain many wounds, larger animals like rats or rabbits are more suited when a greater sample size is required.

The rabbit ear excisional wound model is a wound-healing model that has been used on rabbits for many years. A biopsy punch causes wounds that involve damage to the cartilage, dermis, and epidermis. Unlike in murine models, there is no contraction, and the repair happens from the margin inward. One benefit of this concept is that injuries will heal by reepithelialization. Additionally, this methodology makes it possible to use fewer animals while still producing sufficient data for within-animal duplicates; for instance, up to six wounds per ear can be produced.

Pig skin is believed to be the most similar, from an anatomical and physiological point of view, to human skin, despite the fact that models have been employed in investigational dermatological research. Pigs and humans have comparable structural dermal-epidermal thickness ratios and epidermal thickness. They have human-like dermal hair follicles and a stable subcutaneous layer, yet their skin is comparatively hairless. Compared to other lab animals, pigs have skin that is more biochemically similar to humans in terms of dermal collagen and elastic content. Pigs react to different growth factors in a similar way on a molecular and physical level. Molecular reagents are frequently not approved for use with pig tissues and thus are more costly to house and maintain. Additionally, they are more susceptible to infection. Overall, in vivo wound models are beneficial. They make it possible to inflict multiple wounds on an animal, examine how the immune system functions, look into various facets of the healing process, examine different cell populations and the interactions between bodily systems during repair, and model different wounds or types of injury such as crushing, burns, and surgery. On the other hand, there are disadvantages to using in vivo models, including the fact that they can be expensive and that the intricacy of the whole animal makes it challenging to identify the many roles that different tissues and cells play during the healing process; the immune response of animals may differ from that of humans, the size, depth, and dimensions of wounds may be difficult to control, and there is currently no repeatable and reliable chronic wound model representation. Animal skin does not imitate human skin completely [4, 318–324].

Both incisional and excisional wound models can be made using the mentioned animals.

2.12.2.1 Incisional Wound Model

Studies examining the mechanical characteristics of surgical incision materials, such as the tensile strength assessment and the degradation of various suture threads, can benefit from the use of this model. Wounds of incisional type can be considered as either primary or secondary, and they can be sutured either right away or not. Attributable to the small amount of wound healing activity, primary closure or initial intention is a poor model for histologic calculation of cure, tissue biochemistry, and epithelialization. However, it is a great model for biomechanical analysis of wound strength. Investigating scarring at late times (more than 65 days after incision) can be aided by using the secondary closure model of incisional wounds, also known as second intention.

Incisional wound healing can be assessed using mice, rats, rabbits, and pigs as models. A number of experimental animal models, including incisional injuries to mice's backs that permit tensile strength measurements using tensiometry, were described by Reid et al. to study healing. The method was employed by Januszyk et al. to assess stress in pig surgical incisions. Additionally, Most et al. employed knockout iNOS mice in an incisional paradigm to elucidate the molecular process underlying wound healing [4, 325].

2.12.2.2 Excisional Wound Model

A well-accepted model for wound healing is the excisional wound, which is thought to mimic acute clinical wounds that need healing without the borders of the skin being sewn together. The surgical removal of the animal's whole skin layer, including the dermis, epidermis, and subcutaneous fat, is what causes these wounds. The study of the hemorrhage stage, inflammation stage, granulation stage, tissue development, reepithelialization, angiogenesis stage, and remodeling is made possible by this model. The area of the wound can be tracked over time by taking regular photos, and the wound closure rate is determined by comparing the size of the wound to its initial measurements. Animals can be put to sleep (mice, rats, etc.) or given a local anesthetic (rabbit ear model, etc.) before biopsies are taken, processed, and analyzed for histological analysis. These biopsies are then analyzed for the following characteristics: collagen organization, recruited cell numbers, the extent of vascularity, and changes in matrix alterations, as well as the epithelial gap. Using this model requires a few readily available, rather easy materials and techniques. It is simple to smear topical agents (such as medications, cells, biomaterials, and wound dressings) on the wound bed and examine how they affect the healing process. Animals, including mice, rats, rabbits, and pigs, can be employed, and each species may sustain a different number of wounds. For example, it is possible to inflict four wounds in rats, four or more in pigs, up to two excisional wounds in mice, and six wounds in rabbits. The type of excision used and the diameter of the biopsy punch will determine how many wounds each animal has. Remarkably, a significant portion of wound closure in many of the traditional excisional models—mice, in particular—is attributed to contraction-induced wound healing. One of the biggest drawbacks of modeling human wounds in loose-skinned animals is wound contraction. A few strategies to get around this include selecting anatomical locations (like a rabbit ear) where the dermis and subcutaneous tissue are securely linked or mechanically fixing the skin with splints or other devices. It has been suggested and considered to employ a splinted wound model in order to prevent skin contraction and improve the murine model's applicability to human wound healing. Using this method, two full-thickness incisions are made in the mouse dorsum's panniculus carnosus. The silicone splints are then positioned, centered, and secured to the skin using nylon sutures and instant-bonding adhesive. The splinting ring in the mouse excisional splinted wound model firmly sticks to the skin surrounding the wound to prevent contraction. As a result, the wound will heal similarly to how humans heal—through the creation of granulation tissue and reepithelialization [4, 325–327].

2.12.2.3 Burn Wounds Model

Burn wound healing models can be produced by thermal injury or by scorching the skin with water. Blisters are produced in the model by subjecting an immobile patch of skin to boiling water, while in another model, the skin is directly heated by a hot metal plate. It is possible to de-roof a blister in both models, exposing the dermis and opening up the wound. Subject to the depth of the burn, these wounds caused by thermal injury provide the measurement of reepithelialization, the extent of granulation, the extent of tissue development, the level of angiogenesis, the level of contraction, scarring, and the revelation of wound tissue biochemistry. The objectives and the time needed to monitor the results of an experimental therapy will determine how far the burned area can be extended. A tiny area won't take long to recover and might not be the best place to collect adequate information. In order to assess the prospect of xenogeneic mesenchymal stromal-type cells in treatment for severe burns, some authors discussed the use of a severe burn wound model in rats mimicking third-degree burns in humans. The animal's dorsal region was subjected to gentle pressure from a metal plate maintained at 200°C for 25 seconds, resulting in large burn wounds measuring 2 cm by 3 cm and impacting all three layers of skin. Digital photos of the wounds taken over time, myeloperoxidase assay (MPO), and histological investigations were used to evaluate the healing process. The models mentioned above are inadequate for studying chronic wounds and developing viable therapies. Therefore, it is common practice to use damaged wound models that imitate the chronicity of non-healing wound situations. By employing these models, the pathology—such as diabetes or conditions related to nutrition—associated with chronic wounds as shown in people is to be mimicked. There are various methods for obtaining models of damaged wounds. Notably, most models of defective acute wound healing are not thought to be real chronic wound models, but they can offer helpful insights into delayed wound healing [4, 326].

2.12.2.4 Diabetes Wound Model

Diabetic wound healing is impaired due to a complex process that impacts multiple processes required for the healing process. It has been demonstrated that in comparison to non-diabetic wounds, diabetic wounds in humans and lab animals have an erratic inflammatory response and impaired neovascularization. The mice are first given a diabetes induction medication, after which they get experimental wound care (excisional or incisional). By using chemicals, surgical procedures, or alterations such as diabetes/diabetes (db/db) and alteration such as obese/obese (ob/ob) mice, animal models can be made diabetic. Type 1 diabetes that is chemically induced is typically acquired through the use of medications like streptozotocin or alloxan. Since its discovery in 1943, β-cell necrosis induced by the chemical alloxan has been utilized to produce diabetes. This medication causes hyperglycemia, insulin insufficiency, and ketosis by destroying the pancreatic β islets. Similar to alloxan, streptozotocin mostly induces hyperglycemia by its cytotoxic effect on the β type of cells of the pancreas. Similar to type 1 diabetes in humans, it causes insulinopenic diabetes in vulnerable mice, where immunological damage is a contributing factor. There is data that suggests chemically induced diabetes may not be a perfect representation of genuine diabetes while offering a straightforward and reasonably inexpensive diabetic model. However, without the possible negative consequences of pharmaceutical treatment, genetic models enable the study of the endogenous pathways underlying diabetes. Type 2 diabetes models like db/db and ob/ob are similar to the human condition since they naturally acquire hyperglycemia as a result of obesity and show many of the same symptoms as people with the disease. Specifically, the db/db mice demonstrate progressive hyperglycemia as a result of beta-cell loss, becoming hyperinsulinemic at about two weeks of age and developing insulin resistance. Patients who present with diabetes and insulin resistance are at a significantly greater threat of mounting cardiac and vascular disease and developing cutaneous ulcers. As a result of hyperglycemia and diabetes, oxidative stress is anticipated to be the cause of microvascular problems, such as retinopathy problems, nephron, and neuron-related problems [4, 328, 329].

2.12.2.5 Malnutrition Wound Model

As damaged tissues begin to regain their structural and functional integrity, there is a rise in the metabolic demand for nutrients during the healing process. Protein-energy malnutrition (PEM) has an impact on the skin, leading to notable morphological and functional alterations that make it more vulnerable to injury (ulceration), which impedes healing. Malnutrition alters the immunity built up, tissue repair, and cascade of inflammatory response, which surges the levels of pro-inflammatory cytokines, slows down the healing course, and increases the threat of infection. Researchers delved into the trophic skin alterations that take place in group rats used in an experimental model that mimicked PEM marasmus. Participating rodents were observed for two months after being randomly allocated to consume either 50% of the daily food (named as a malnourished group) or rat chow ad libitum (named as a well-nourished group). According to histological findings, the animals who were malnourished had considerably thinner dermis and a smaller amount of collagen in their bodies than the animals that were fed well. In order to assess how well wounds heal, animals who are underweight are utilized as models for malnutrition wounds [4, 330].

2.12.2.6 Metabolic Syndrome/Obesity Wound Model

ROS concentrations are raised by variables, such as metabolic disorders, which can modify the course of wound healing. Under these circumstances, the inflammatory phase experiences protracted disruptions in the angiogenesis procedure, granulation tissue decrease, and delayed epithelialization. Furthermore, oxidative stress is brought on by modifications to the cellular redox environment, which can result in significant alterations to the cell. A high-calorie diet may be the cause of metabolic illnesses, and numerous studies have mimicked these changes in human metabolism in animals fed a high-fat diet [4, 331].

2.12.3 Methods/Techniques of Evaluation

In addition to choosing a suitable wound model, it is critical to ascertain the techniques that would work best with a given model. In order to track the progress of wound healing, wounds created in the appropriate model are processed, inspected, or statistically assessed. Numerous methods, each evaluating certain data, can be used to evaluate the progressive changes in wounds as they heal. Understanding the pathophysiology of healing, the variables that impede the process, and the ideal circumstances needed at the bed of injury to promote restoration and efficacy are all necessary for conducting an appropriate wound evaluation. It is crucial that, during follow-up, a thorough examination of the injury and its surrounding tissue's healing progression be carried out and recorded. In general, measurements of wound healing pertain to the size of the wound, the features of the bed of injury and their potential correlation with tissue development, the degree of scarring, degree of numerous causal vascular alongside the pathophysiological problems that could be impeding the restorative process. Both qualitative and quantifiable protocols might be followed in order to assess the wound's course till the tissue has healed [4, 332–334].

2.12.3.1 Wound Healing Rate

Complete and permanent closure of the wound is the endpoint of a successful course of treatment. The wound healing rate is defined as the rate at which the surface area of the wound changes. There are numerous methods for calculating surface area, from using a ruler to measure length and width to using image processing algorithms. A technique that was put forth involved the use of live mice that had been genetically induced to express the GFP fusion protein of histone H2B, which is driven by the keratin 14 promoter. These mice, known as K14-H2BGFP mice, would be used to monitor wound repair in real-time. Anesthesia was used to generate and film a rounded, full-thickness injury in live mice on the mouse ear, which was chosen for imaging due to its ease of use and resemblance to other mouse skin locations in terms of epithelial functions. Imaging software was utilized to ascertain the rates of migration and proliferation (reepithelialization). The formula for calculating wound healing rate (denoted as WHR) index or ulcer healing rate (denoted as UHR) index is [(Ai – Af)/Ai]. Herein, Ai denotes the original wound area. Af denotes the final area. WHR can be expressed in a range of -1.0 to 1.0. The same can be expressed as percentage closure on multiplication by a value of 100. Values equal to 1% or 100% indicate total reepithelialization. In the wound tracing method, using a permanent marker, the wound perimeter is traced and the surface area is calculated. Various image software can be utilized to determine the wound parameters by taking digital images of the wound surface [4, 335–337].

2.12.3.2 Wound Image Analysis

Throughout the course of wound healing, photographic images might offer crucial facts on morphological alterations, color deviations, and other related topics. Epithelial progression at the wound or injury margins can be easily identified by high-resolution pictures [4].

2.12.3.3 Image Analysis by Software

Once the computer has the image of the wound, a number of software programs can compute and analyze the wound's dimensions, viz., surface area and volume. These programs can also provide facts about the clinical facets of the wound restoration process by using colorimetric analyses to track recessions in the surface area of the tissues according to their corresponding colors, such as necrosis (black), fibrin/sphacelus (yellow), and granulation tissue (red). In addition, a plethora of software is available to support histological, immunohistochemical, enzymatic, and fluorescence techniques, ranging from tissue biopsies on slides to collagen analysis and cell counting (e.g., fibroblasts and blood vessels). ImageJ, Sigma-pro® image, DigiSkinTM, and LEICA QWin Image are some of the software available [4].

2.12.3.4 Biophysical Assessment of Wound Healing

Biophysical methods, including diffuse near-infrared spectroscopy (DNIRS), confocal laser scanning microscopy, and optical coherence tomography (OCT), quantify the wound healing course and diagnose and monitor inflammatory dermatological conditions. These methods also produce high-resolution and real-time images of the cutaneous architecture [4].

2.12.3.5 Histopathological Analysis

Histopathology can track the course of healing, provide insight into the etiology of non-healing injuries, estimate morphological alterations, and also support diagnosis. In terms of clinical practice, the border at the injury is ideal for a biopsy since it allows for a comparison between the normal and injured skin. After that, the tissue will go through a number of histological processing procedures, such as sectioning, embedding, and staining with trichromes, immunohistochemical markers, and either hematoxylin and eosin (H&E) or a different stain. Quantification of white blood cells (macrophage type, mast cell type, lymphocyte type, and neutrophil type) to assess the inflammatory phase, blood vessels to assess angiogenesis stage, fibroblast activity, and collagen level are typically included in the histopathological investigation of wounds [4].

2.12.3.6 Immunological Methods

Several methods, including ELISA and immunohistochemistry (IHC), identify and quantify signaling chemicals such as growth factors and cytokines, cytokeratins, vimentin, and collagen (including types I, III, and IV), along with IL-1β, IL-10, IL-17, and all other pro-inflammatory cytokines can be quantified. Similarly, anti-inflammatory cytokines, for example, EGF and TGF-β1, can be quantified by ELISA [4, 338–342].

2.12.3.7 Biochemical Methods

Several methods, including ELISA and immunohistochemistry (IHC), can identify and quantify signaling chemicals such as growth factors and cytokines, cytokeratins, vimentin, and collagen (including types I, III, and IV). To track the development of the wound-healing progression, a number of biochemical techniques can be used, including the hydroxyproline assay to measure collagen turnover, the myeloperoxidase assay (MPO) to measure neutrophil levels, the N-acetylglucosaminidase (NAG) to measure N-acetylglucosaminidase levels, and the oxidative stress profile to measure malondialdehyde (MDA) and hydrogen peroxide levels, which reflect ROS and NO levels [4, 343–345].

2.12.3.8 Flow Cytometry

Another method that can be used to gather data for studies on how cells are recruited in response to wound management techniques is flow cytometry. Endothelial progenitor cells, endothelial cells, macrophages, T cells, and B cells are the most often employed human markers in research [4].

2.12.3.9 Macrophage Polarization

Techniques, including immunohistochemistry examination, Western blotting technique, and the technique of real-time PCR, can be used to identify particular cell surface indicators, the release of cytokine factors, and chemokine factors in order to study the phenotypes and subclasses of macrophages [4].

2.12.3.10 In Vitro Antimicrobial Activity

The viable cell count assay is the typically used in vitro test in order to assess the antibacterial and anti-adherent capabilities of the BNCs. Generally, it is performed against two clinically relevant bacterial strains, *Escherichia coli* and *Staphylococcus aureus*. Depending on the kind of wound, different specialized microorganisms may be employed [4].

2.13 CONCLUSION

BNCs are intensely exploited for wound-healing applications. In this context, the traditional approaches have been compared to advanced wound dressings. The manner in which BNCs address the challenges of wound treatment has been discussed. Recent advances in BNCs have been provided. The methods for assessing the wound-healing efficacy of biomaterials and nanomaterials have been elaborated. The information provided should assist a formulation scientist in the development of natural and nanoparticulate materials and BNC technology for wound-healing purposes.

ABBREVIATIONS

°C	degree Celsius or degree Centigrade
3D	3 dimensional
3T3	mouse embryonic fibroblasts cell lines
Af	final wound area after healing
AgNPs	silver nanoparticles
Ai	original wound area
AuNPs	gold nanoparticles
B cells	B type of lymphocytes: coming from bone marrow
b-FGF	basic fibroblast growth factor
BHK-21	Baby hamster kidney cells
BNCs	bionanocomposites
CAGR	compound annual growth rate
CHT	chitosan
CLSM	confocal laser scanning microscopy

CMC	carboxymethylcellulose
CNT	carbon nanotubes
db/db	diabetes/diabetes
DNA	deoxyribonucleic acid
DNIRS	diffuse near-infrared spectroscopy
ECM	extra cellular matrix
EGF	epithelial growth factor
ELISA	enzyme-linked immunosorbent assay
EPS	extracellular polymeric substances
FGF	fibroblast growth factor
FGF2	fibroblast growth factor 2
FTIR	Fourier transform infra-red
Fyn	proto-oncogene tyrosine-protein kinase
GFP	green fluorescent protein
GSK-3b	glycogen synthase kinase 3 beta
H2B	histone 2B
HA	hyaluronic acid
HAP	hydroxyapatite
HIF	hypoxia-inducible factor
HME	hot melt extrusion
hTERT	human telomerase reverse transcriptase
HUVEC	human umbilical vein endothelial cells
IHC	immune histo chemistry
IL-1	interleukin-1
IL-1b	interleukin-1b
IL-6	interleukin-6
iNOS	inducible nitric oxide synthase
K14-H2BGFP	keratin-14 promoter histone 2b–green fluorescent protein
KGF-2	keratinocyte growth factor-2
MADO-AgNPs	poly (methyl methacrylate-co-dopamine methacrylamide)-silver nanoparticles
MDA	malon di aldehyde
MDR	multidrug-resistant
MIP-1-β	macrophage inflammatory protein-1 beta
MMP-2	matrix metalloproteinase-2
MMP-7	matrix metalloproteinase-7
MMP-9	matrix metalloproteinase-9
MMPs	matrix metalloproteinases
MMT	montmorillonite
MPO	myeloperoxidase assay
MRSA	methicillin-resistant *Staphylococcus aureus*
NAG	N-acetylglucosaminidase
NF	normal human fibroblasts
nHAp	nano-hydroxyapatite
NK	natural killer cells
NP	nanoparticle
Nrf2	nuclear factor erythroid 2-related factor 2
NSAID	non-steroidal anti-inflammatory drugs
ob/ob	obese/obese
OCT	optical coherence tomography
PCL	poly capro lactone
PDGF	platelet-derived growth factor

PEG	polyethylene glycol
PEM	protein energy malnutrition
PLA	poly lactic acid
PLLA	poly-l-lactic acid
PNC	polymeric nanocomposites
PVA	polyvinyl alcohol
RNA	ribonucleic acid
ROS	reactive oxygen species
SEM	scanning electron microscope
SGL	scleroglucan
SiNPs	silica nanoparticle
SLE	systemic lupus erythematosus
SPIONs	super paramagnetic iron oxide nanoparticles
SSWIs	surgical site wound infections
T cells	T type of lymphocytes; coming from thymus
TGA	thermogravimetric analysis
TGF	tumor growth factor
TGF-b	transforming growth factor-beta
TGF-ß	transforming growth factor-beta
TGF-β1	transforming growth factor-beta-1
TiO2NPs	titanium dioxide nanoparticles
TiONP	titanium dioxide nanoparticles
TNF	tumor necrosis factor
TNF-a	tumor necrosis factor alpha
UHR	ulcer healing rate
USD	United States Dollar
VEGF	vascular endothelial growth factor
WHR	wound healing rate
ZnONPs	zinc oxide nanoparticles

REFERENCES

[1] "Biggest players in the global wound care market," *NS Medical Devices*, Mar. 24, 2023. https://www.nsmedicaldevices.com/analysis/biggest-players-in-the-global-wound-care-market/

[2] "Wound care market size, share analysis report, 2021–2028," *www.grandviewresearch.com*. https://www.grandviewresearch.com/industry-analysis/wound-care-market

[3] H. Nosrati, et al., "Nanocomposite scaffolds for accelerating chronic wound healing by enhancing angiogenesis," *Journal of Nanobiotechnology*, vol. 19, no. 1, Jan. 2021. https://doi.org/10.1186/s12951-020-00755-7

[4] D. S. Masson-Meyers, et al., "Experimental models and methods for cutaneous wound healing assessment," *International Journal of Experimental Pathology*, vol. 101, no. 1–2, pp. 21–37, Feb. 2020. https://doi.org/10.1111/iep.12346

[5] H. Minh Nguyen, T. T. N. Le, A. Thanh Nguyen, H. N. T. Le, and T. Tan Pham, "Biomedical materials for wound dressing: Recent advances and applications," *RSC Advances*, vol. 13, no. 8, pp. 5509–5528, 2023. https://doi.org/10.1039/D2RA07673J

[6] The Royal Children's Hospital Melbourne, "Clinical guidelines (nursing): Wound assessment and management," *The Royal Children's Hospital Melbourne*, Feb. 2023. https://www.rch.org.au/rchcpg/hospital_clinical_guideline_index/Wound_Assessment_and_Management/

[7] L. Jaldin-Crespo, N. Silva, and J. Martínez, "Nanomaterials based on honey and propolis for wound healing—A mini-review," *Nanomaterials*, vol. 12, no. 24, p. 4409, Dec. 2022. https://doi.org/10.3390/nano12244409

[8] J. Hunckler and A. de Mel, "A current affair: Electrotherapy in wound healing," *Journal of Multidisciplinary Healthcare*, vol. 10, no. 10, pp. 179–194, Apr. 2017. https://doi.org/10.2147/jmdh.s127207

[9] A. Pormohammad, N. K. Monych, S. Ghosh, D. L. Turner, and R. J. Turner, "Nanomaterials in wound healing and infection control," *Antibiotics*, vol. 10, no. 5, p. 473, May 2021. https://doi.org/10.3390/antibiotics10050473

[10] C. Shi, et al., "Selection of appropriate wound dressing for various wounds," *Frontiers in Bioengineering and Biotechnology*, vol. 8, no. 8, pp. 1–17, Mar. 2020. https://doi.org/10.3389/fbioe.2020.00182

[11] X. Ding, et al., "Challenges and innovations in treating chronic and acute wound infections: From basic science to clinical practice," *Burns & Trauma*, vol. 10, Jan. 2022. https://doi.org/10.1093/burnst/tkac014

[12] P. Kaiser, J. Wächter, and M. Windbergs, "Therapy of infected wounds: Overcoming clinical challenges by advanced drug delivery systems," *Drug Delivery and Translational Research*, vol. 11, no. 4, pp. 1545–1567, Feb. 2021. https://doi.org/10.1007/s13346-021-00932-7

[13] A. R. Siddiqui and J. M. Bernstein, "Chronic wound infection: Facts and controversies," *Clinics in Dermatology*, vol. 28, no. 5, pp. 519–526, Sep. 2010. https://doi.org/10.1016/j.clindermatol.2010.03.009

[14] L. Hall-Stoodley, J. W. Costerton, and P. Stoodley, "Bacterial biofilms: From the natural environment to infectious diseases," *Nature Reviews Microbiology*, vol. 2, no. 2, pp. 95–108, Feb. 2004. https://doi.org/10.1038/nrmicro821

[15] C. de la Fuente-Núñez, F. Reffuveille, L. Fernández, and R. E. Hancock, "Bacterial biofilm development as a multicellular adaptation: Antibiotic resistance and new therapeutic strategies," *Current Opinion in Microbiology*, vol. 16, no. 5, pp. 580–589, Oct. 2013. https://doi.org/10.1016/j.mib.2013.06.013

[16] J. W. Costerton, "Bacterial biofilms: A common cause of persistent infections," *Science*, vol. 284, no. 5418, pp. 1318–1322, May 1999. https://doi.org/10.1126/science.284.5418.1318

[17] S. Dhivya, V. V. Padma, and E. Santhini, "Wound dressings–a review," *BioMedicine*, vol. 5, no. 4, Nov. 2015. https://doi.org/10.7603/s40681-015-0022-9

[18] R. Blakytny and E. B. Jude, "Altered molecular mechanisms of diabetic foot ulcers," *The International Journal of Lower Extremity Wounds*, vol. 8, no. 2, pp. 95–104, May 2009. https://doi.org/10.1177/1534734609337151

[19] S.-N. Park, J. K. Kim, and H. Suh, "Evaluation of antibiotic-loaded collagen-hyaluronic acid matrix as a skin substitute," *Biomaterials*, vol. 25, no. 17, pp. 3689–3698, Aug. 2004. https://doi.org/10.1016/j.biomaterials.2003.10.072

[20] M. N. Khan and C. G. Davies, "Advances in the management of leg ulcers – The potential role of growth factors," *International Wound Journal*, vol. 3, no. 2, pp. 113–122, Jul. 2006. https://doi.org/10.1111/j.1742-4801.2006.00211.x

[21] B. N. Patrick, M. P. Rivey, and D. R. Allington, "Acute renal failure associated with Vancomycin- and Tobramycin-Laden cement in total hip arthroplasty," *Annals of Pharmacotherapy*, vol. 40, no. 11, pp. 2037–2042, Nov. 2006. https://doi.org/10.1345/aph.1h173

[22] H. Chu, et al., "Aminoglycoside ototoxicity in three murine strains and effects on NKCC1 of stria vascularis," *Chinese Medical Journal*, vol. 119, no. 12, pp. 980–985, Jun. 2006. https://doi.org/10.1097/00029330-200606020-00003

[23] M. Kietzmann and M. Braun, "Effects of the zinc oxide and cod liver oil containing ointment Zincojecol in an animal model of wound healing,"*Dtsch Tierarztl Wochenschr*, vol. 113, no. 9, pp. 331–334, Sep. 2006.

[24] K. H. Flanigan, "Nutritional aspects of wound healing," *Advances in Wound Care: The Journal for Prevention and Healing*, vol. 10, no. 3, pp. 48–52, 1997.

[25] H. P. Ehrlich, H. Tarver, and T. K. Hunt, "Effects of vitamin A and glucocorticoids upon inflammation and collagen synthesis," *Annals of Surgery*, vol. 177, no. 2, pp. 222–227, Feb. 1973. https://doi.org/10.1097/00000658-197302000-00017

[26] P. Monika, M. N. Chandraprabha, A. Rangarajan, P. V. Waiker, and K. N. Chidambara Murthy, "Challenges in healing wound: Role of complementary and alternative medicine," *Frontiers in Nutrition*, vol. 8. 2296–861X, Jan. 2022. https://doi.org/10.3389/fnut.2021.791899

[27] R. G. Frykberg and J. Banks, "Challenges in the treatment of chronic wounds," *Advances in Wound Care*, vol. 4, no. 9, pp. 560–582, Sep. 2015. https://doi.org/10.1089/wound.2015.0635

[28] S. M. McCarty and S. L. Percival, "Proteases and delayed wound healing," *Advances in Wound Care*, vol. 2, no. 8, pp. 438–447, Oct. 2013. https://doi.org/10.1089/wound.2012.0370

[29] S. Schreml, R. M. Szeimies, L. Prantl, S. Karrer, M. Landthaler, and P. Babilas, "Oxygen in acute and chronic wound healing," *British Journal of Dermatology*, vol. 163, no. 2, pp. 257–268, Apr. 2010. https://doi.org/10.1111/j.1365-2133.2010.09804.x

[30] G. S. Schultz, et al., "Wound bed preparation: A systematic approach to wound management," *Wound Repair and Regeneration*, vol. 11, no. s1, pp. S1–S28, Mar. 2003. https://doi.org/10.1046/j.1524-475x.11.s2.1.x

[31] A. Stanley and T. Osler, "Senescence and the healing rates of venous ulcers," *Journal of Vascular Surgery*, vol. 33, no. 6, pp. 1206–1211, Jun. 2001. https://doi.org/10.1067/mva.2001.115379

[32] R. Lobmann, A. Ambrosch, G. Schultz, K. Waldmann, S. Schiweck, and H. Lehnert, "Expression of matrix-metalloproteinases and their inhibitors in the wounds of diabetic and non-diabetic patients," *Diabetologia*, vol. 45, no. 7, pp. 1011–1016, Jun. 2002. https://doi.org/10.1007/s00125-002-0868-8

[33] E. Tsourdi, A. Barthel, H. Rietzsch, A. Reichel, and S. R. Bornstein, "Current aspects in the pathophysiology and treatment of chronic wounds in diabetes mellitus," *BioMed Research International*, vol. 2013, no. 2314–6133, pp. 1–6, 2013. https://doi.org/10.1155/2013/385641

[34] L. Y. W. Bourguignon, "Matrix hyaluronan-activated CD44 signaling promotes keratinocyte activities and improves abnormal epidermal functions," *The American Journal of Pathology*, vol. 184, no. 7, pp. 1912–1919, Jul. 2014. https://doi.org/10.1016/j.ajpath.2014.03.010

[35] H. Cook, P. J. Stephens, K. J. Davies, D. W. Thomas, and K. Harding, "Defective extracellular matrix reorganization by chronic wound fibroblasts is associated with alterations in TIMP-1, TIMP-2, and MMP-2 activity," *Journal of Investigative Dermatology*, vol. 115, no. 2, pp. 225–233, Aug. 2000. https://doi.org/10.1046/j.1523-1747.2000.00044.x

[36] D. Telgenhoff and B. Shroot, "Cellular senescence mechanisms in chronic wound healing," *Cell Death & Differentiation*, vol. 12, no. 7, pp. 695–698, Apr. 2005. https://doi.org/10.1038/sj.cdd.4401632

[37] I. B. Wall, et al., "Fibroblast dysfunction is a key factor in the non-healing of chronic venous leg ulcers," *Journal of Investigative Dermatology*, vol. 128, no. 10, pp. 2526–2540, Oct. 2008, https://doi.org/10.1038/jid.2008.114

[38] A. Sood, M. S. Granick, and N. L. Tomaselli, "Wound dressings and comparative effectiveness data," *Advances in Wound Care*, vol. 3, no. 8, pp. 511–529, Aug. 2014. https://doi.org/10.1089/wound.2012.0401

[39] G. Han and R. Ceilley, "Chronic wound healing: A review of current management and treatments," *Advances in Therapy*, vol. 34, no. 3, pp. 599–610, 2017. https://doi.org/10.1007/s12325-017-0478-y

[40] M. Berthet, Y. Gauthier, C. Lacroix, B. Verrier, and C. Monge, "Nanoparticle-based dressing: The future of wound treatment?," *Trends in Biotechnology*, vol. 35, no. 8, pp. 770–784, Aug. 2017. https://doi.org/10.1016/j.tibtech.2017.05.005

[41] A. Kushwaha, L. Goswami, and B. S. Kim, "Nanomaterial-based therapy for wound healing," *Nanomaterials*, vol. 12, no. 4, p. 618, Feb. 2022. https://doi.org/10.3390/nano12040618

[42] J. Nandhini, E. Karthikeyan, and S. Rajeshkumar, "Nanomaterials for wound healing: Current status and futuristic frontier," *Biomedical Technology*, vol. 6, pp. 26–45, 2024. https://doi.org/10.1016/j.bmt.2023.10.001

[43] S. S. Behera, U. Das, A. Kumar, A. Bissoyi, and A. K. Singh, "Chitosan/TiO_2 composite membrane improves proliferation and survival of L929 fibroblast cells: Application in wound dressing and skin regeneration," *International Journal of Biological Macromolecules*, vol. 98, pp. 329–340, May 2017. https://doi.org/10.1016/j.ijbiomac.2017.02.017

[44] R. H. Müller, M. Radtke, and S. A. Wissing, "Solid lipid nanoparticles (SLN) and nanostructured lipid carriers (NLC) in cosmetic and dermatological preparations," *Advanced Drug Delivery Reviews*, vol. 54, pp. S131–S155, Nov. 2002. https://doi.org/10.1016/s0169-409x(02)00118-7

[45] S. M. Dizaj, F. Lotfipour, M. Barzegar-Jalali, M. H. Zarrintan, and K. Adibkia, "Antimicrobial activity of the metals and metal oxide nanoparticles," *Materials Science and Engineering: C*, vol. 44, pp. 278–284, Nov. 2014. https://doi.org/10.1016/j.msec.2014.08.031

[46] P. Ghosh, G. Han, M. De, C. Kim, and V. Rotello, "Gold nanoparticles in delivery applications☆," *Advanced Drug Delivery Reviews*, vol. 60, no. 11, pp. 1307–1315, Aug. 2008. https://doi.org/10.1016/j.addr.2008.03.016

[47] J. Leu, et al., "The effects of gold nanoparticles in wound healing with antioxidant epigallocatechin gallate and α-lipoic acid," *Nanomedicine: Nanotechnology, Biology and Medicine*, vol. 8, no. 5, pp. 767–775, Jul. 2012. https://doi.org/10.1016/j.nano.2011.08.013

[48] I. Slowing, J. Viveroescoto, C. Wu, and V. Lin, "Mesoporous silica nanoparticles as controlled release drug delivery and gene transfection carriers," *Advanced Drug Delivery Reviews*, vol. 60, no. 11, pp. 1278–1288, Aug. 2008. https://doi.org/10.1016/j.addr.2008.03.012
[49] A. Tamayol, et al., "Flexible pH-sensing hydrogel fibers for epidermal applications," *Advanced Healthcare Materials*, vol. 5, no. 6, pp. 711–719, Jan. 2016. https://doi.org/10.1002/adhm.201500553
[50] N. Gargiulo, et al. "Confined mesoporous silica membranes for albumin zero-order release," *Microporous and Mesoporous Materials*, vol. 167, pp. 71–75, Feb. 2013. https://doi.org/10.1016/j.micromeso.2012.04.003
[51] Z. Fan, B. Liu, J. Wang, S. Zhang, Q. Lin, P. Gong, L. Ma, and S. Yang, "A novel wound dressing based on Ag/graphene polymer hydrogel: Effectively kill bacteria and accelerate wound healing," *Advanced Functional Materials*, vol. 24, pp. 3933–3943, Mar. 2014. https://doi.org/10.1002/adfm.201304202
[52] C. Chiappini, J. O. Martinez, E. De Rosa, C. S. Almeida, E. Tasciotti, and M. M. Stevens, "Biodegradable nanoneedles for localized delivery of nanoparticles in vivo: Exploring the biointerface," *ACS Nano*, vol. 9, no. 5, pp. 5500–5509, May 2015. https://doi.org/10.1021/acsnano.5b01490
[53] C. Chiappini, et al., "Biodegradable silicon nanoneedles delivering nucleic acids intracellularly induce localized in vivo neovascularization," *Nature Materials*, vol. 14, no. 5, pp. 532–539, May 2015. https://doi.org/10.1038/nmat4249
[54] L. Huang, et al., "Biocompatible tellurium nanoneedles with long-term stable antibacterial activity for accelerated wound healing," *Materials Today Bio*, vol. 15, pp. 100271–100271, Jun. 2022. https://doi.org/10.1016/j.mtbio.2022.100271
[55] J. Wang and M. Windbergs, "Functional electrospun fibers for the treatment of human skin wounds," *European Journal of Pharmaceutics and Biopharmaceutics*, vol. 119, pp. 283–299, Oct. 2017. https://doi.org/10.1016/j.ejpb.2017.07.001
[56] A. Nasajpour, et al., "Nanostructured fibrous membranes with rose spike-like architecture," *Nano Letters*, vol. 17, no. 10, pp. 6235–6240, Sep. 2017. https://doi.org/10.1021/acs.nanolett.7b02929
[57] M. Kokabi, M. Sirousazar, and Z. M. Hassan, "PVA–clay nanocomposite hydrogels for wound dressing," *European Polymer Journal*, vol. 43, no. 3, pp. 773–781, Mar. 2007. https://doi.org/10.1016/j.eurpolymj.2006.11.030
[58] P. Rujitanaroj, N. Pimpha, and P. Supaphol, "Wound-dressing materials with antibacterial activity from electrospun gelatin fiber mats containing silver nanoparticles," *Polymer*, vol. 49, no. 21, pp. 4723–4732, Oct. 2008. https://doi.org/10.1016/j.polymer.2008.08.021
[59] S. Cho, J. S. Lee, J. Jun, S. G. Kim, and J. Jang, "Fabrication of water-dispersible and highly conductive PSS-doped PANI/graphene nanocomposites using a high-molecular weight PSS dopant and their application in H_2S detection," *Nanoscale*, vol. 6, no. 24, pp. 15181–15195, Nov. 2014. https://doi.org/10.1039/c4nr04413d
[60] K. Kandiah, V. Rajendran, C. Wang, S. Valiyaveettil, and K. Ganesan, "In vitro and preliminary in vivo toxicity screening of high-surface-area TiO_2–chondroitin-4-sulfate nanocomposites for bone regeneration application," *Colloids and Surfaces B: Biointerfaces*, vol. 128, pp. 347–356, Apr. 2015. https://doi.org/10.1016/j.colsurfb.2015.02.027
[61] M. M. Harriott and M. C. Noverr, "Candida albicans and Staphylococcus aureus form polymicrobial biofilms: Effects on antimicrobial resistance," *Antimicrobial Agents and Chemotherapy*, vol. 53, no. 9, pp. 3914–3922, Jun. 2009. https://doi.org/10.1128/aac.00657-09
[62] A. Varma, et al., "The role of nanocomposites against biofilm infections in humans," *Frontiers in Cellular and Infection Microbiology*, vol. 13, Feb. 2023. https://doi.org/10.3389/fcimb.2023.1104615
[63] A. Khan, et al., "Carrageenan based bionanocomposites as drug delivery tool with special emphasis on the influence of ferromagnetic nanoparticles," *Oxidative Medicine and Cellular Longevity*, vol. 2017, pp. 1–13, 2017. https://doi.org/10.1155/2017/8158315
[64] V. Pande and V. Sanklecha."Bionanocomposite: A review,"*Austin Journalof Nanomedicine and Nanotechnology*. vol 5, no. 1, pp. 1045, Dec. 2017.
[65] V. Thomas, D. Dean, and Y. Vohra. "Nanostructured biomaterials for regenerative medicine,"*Current Nanoscience*. vol 2 no. 3, pp. 155–177, Aug. 2006.
[66] C. W. Patrick, A. G. Mikos, and L. V. McIntire, *Frontiers in Tissue Engineering*. Elsevier, 1998.
[67] R. Saini, A. Bhajpal, and E. Jain, "Fundamentals of bionanocomposites, biodegradable and biocompatible polymer composites," *Biodegradable and Biocompatible Polymer Composites*, pp. 351–377, 2017. https://doi.org/10.1016/B978-0-08-100970-3.00012-2

[68] S. Mondal, "Polymer nano-composite membranes," *Journal of Membrane Science & Technology*, vol. 05, no. 01, 2015. https://doi.org/10.4172/2155-9589.1000134

[69] S. D. Wani and A. S. Mundada, "A review: Emerging trends in bionanocomposites," *International Journal of Pharmacy Research and Technology*, vol. 11, no. 1, pp. 1–8, Mar. 2023. https://doi.org/10.31838/ijprt/11.01.01

[70] N. Sreenivasulu, P. Kumari, and P. Reddy, "Growing importance of bionanocomposites," *International Journal of Advance Research in Science and Engineering*, vol. 5, no. 1, pp. 378–381, Feb. 2016.

[71] R. Mala, M. Rani, N. Prasath, and A Celsia, "Nano composite material of chitosan for wound healing: A review," *AIP Conference Proceeding*, May. 2019. https://doi.org/10.1063/1.5100698

[72] D. Chouhan and B. B. Mandal, "Silk biomaterials in wound healing and skin regeneration therapeutics: From bench to bedside," *Acta Biomaterialia*, vol. 103, pp. 24–51, Feb. 2020, https://doi.org/10.1016/j.actbio.2019.11.050

[73] B. S. Anisha, R. Biswas, K. P. Chennazhi, and R. Jayakumar, "Chitosan–hyaluronic acid/nano silver composite sponges for drug resistant bacteria infected diabetic wounds," *International Journal of Biological Macromolecules*, vol. 62, pp. 310–320, Nov. 2013. https://doi.org/10.1016/j.ijbiomac.2013.09.011

[74] P. Orsu and S. Matta, "Fabrication and characterization of carboxymethyl guar gum nanocomposite for application of wound healing," *International Journal of Biological Macromolecules*, vol. 164, pp. 2267–2276, Dec. 2020. https://doi.org/10.1016/j.ijbiomac.2020.07.322

[75] A. K. Kodoth, V. M. Ghate, S. A. Lewis, B. Prakash, and V. Badalamoole, "Pectin-based silver nanocomposite film for transdermal delivery of Donepezil," *International Journal of Biological Macromolecules*, vol. 134, pp. 269–279, Aug. 2019. https://doi.org/10.1016/j.ijbiomac.2019.04.191

[76] J. M. Galdopórpora, M. F. Morcillo, A. Ibar, C. J. Pérez, M. V. Tuttolomondo, and M. F. Desimone, "Development of silver nanoparticles/gelatin thermoresponsive nanocomposites: Characterization and antimicrobial activity," *Current Pharmaceutical Design*, vol. 25, no. 38, pp. 4121–4129, Dec. 2019. https://doi.org/10.2174/1381612825666191007163152

[77] J. Njuguna, F. Ansari, S. Sachse, H. Zhu, and V. M. Rodriguez, "Nanomaterials, nanofillers, and nanocomposites: Types and properties," *Elsevier eBooks*, pp. 3–27, Jan. 2014. https://doi.org/10.1533/9780857096678.1.3

[78] N. H. Al-Mutairi, A. H. Mehdi, and B. J. Kadhim, "Nanocomposites materials definitions, types and some of their applications: A review," *European Journal of Research Development and Sustainability*, vol. 3, no. 2, pp. 102–108, Feb. 2022.

[79] C. Bastioli, *Handbook of Biodegradable Polymers*. Smithers Rapra Technology Limited, 2005.

[80] O. Z. Fisher, A. Khademhosseini, R. Langer, and N. A. Peppas, "Bioinspired materials for controlling stem cell fate," *Accounts of Chemical Research*, vol. 43, no. 3, pp. 419–428, Dec. 2009. https://doi.org/10.1021/ar900226q

[81] B. V. Slaughter, S. S. Khurshid, O. Z. Fisher, A. Khademhosseini, and N. A. Peppas, "Hydrogels in regenerative medicine," *Advanced Materials*, vol. 21, no. 32–33, pp. 3307–3329, Sep. 2009. https://doi.org/10.1002/adma.200802106

[82] A. M. Kloxin, C. J. Kloxin, C. N. Bowman, and K. S. Anseth, "Mechanical properties of cellularly responsive hydrogels and their experimental determination," *Advanced Materials*, vol. 22, no. 31, pp. 3484–3494, May 2010. https://doi.org/10.1002/adma.200904179

[83] S. Mishra, et al., "Bioinspired nanocomposites: Applications in disease diagnosis and treatment," *Pharmaceutical Nanotechnology*, vol. 7, no. 3, pp. 206–219, Aug. 2019. https://doi.org/10.2174/2211738507666190425121509

[84] M. S. Alam, et al., "Gum ghatti mediated, one pot green synthesis of optimized gold nanoparticles: Investigation of process-variables impact using Box-Behnken based statistical design," *International Journal of Biological Macromolecules*, vol. 104, pp. 758–767, Nov. 2017. https://doi.org/10.1016/j.ijbiomac.2017.05.129

[85] Y. Xia, "Nanomaterials at work in biomedical research," *Nature Materials*, vol. 7, no. 10, pp. 758–760, Oct. 2008. https://doi.org/10.1038/nmat2277

[86] R. Cingolani, "The road ahead," *Nature Nanotechnology*, vol. 8, no. 11, pp. 792–793, Nov. 2013. https://doi.org/10.1038/nnano.2013.238

[87] H. Zreiqat, et al., "Mechanisms of magnesium-stimulated adhesion of osteoblastic cells to commonly used orthopaedic implants," *Journal of Biomedical Materials Research*, vol. 62, no. 2, pp. 175–184, Aug. 2002. https://doi.org/10.1002/jbm.10270

[88] A. K. Gaharwar, S. A. Dammu, J. M. Canter, C.-J. Wu, and G. Schmidt, "Highly extensible, tough, and elastomeric nanocomposite hydrogels from poly(ethylene glycol) and hydroxyapatite nanoparticles," *Biomacromolecules*, vol. 12, no. 5, pp. 1641–1650, May 2011. https://doi.org/10.1021/bm200027z

[89] A. Childs, U. D. Hemraz, N. J. Castro, H. Fenniri, and L. G. Zhang, "Novel biologically-inspired rosette nanotube PLLA scaffolds for improving human mesenchymal stem cell chondrogenic differentiation," *Biomedical Materials*, vol. 8, no. 6, p. 065003, Nov. 2013. https://doi.org/10.1088/1748-6041/8/6/065003

[90] M.-H. You, et al., "Synergistically enhanced osteogenic differentiation of human mesenchymal stem cells by culture on nanostructured surfaces with induction media," *Biomacromolecules*, vol. 11, no. 7, pp. 1856–1862, Jul. 2010. https://doi.org/10.1021/bm100374n

[91] X.-Y. Xu, et al., "The behaviour of neural stem cells on polyhydroxyalkanoate nanofiber scaffolds," *Biomaterials*, vol. 31, no. 14, pp. 3967–3975, May 2010. https://doi.org/10.1016/j.biomaterials.2010.01.132

[92] C. Tamerler and M. Sarikaya, "Molecular biomimetics: Utilizing nature's molecular ways in practical engineering," *Acta Biomaterialia*, vol. 3, no. 3, pp. 289–299, May 2007. https://doi.org/10.1016/j.actbio.2006.10.009

[93] I. Negut, G. Dorcioman, and V. Grumezescu, "Scaffolds for wound healing applications," *Polymers*, vol. 12, no. 9, p. 2010, Sep. 2020. https://doi.org/10.3390/polym12092010

[94] P. Chandika, F. Nawaz Khan, S.-Y. Heo, Y. Kim, M. Yi, and W. Jung, "Enhanced wound-healing capability with inherent antimicrobial activities of usnic acid incorporated poly(ε-caprolactone)/decellularized extracellular matrix nanofibrous scaffold," *Biomaterials advances*, vol. 140, pp. 213046–213046, Sep. 2022. https://doi.org/10.1016/j.bioadv.2022.213046

[95] K. Zhou, et al., "Hybrid Ag nanoparticles/polyoxometalate-polydopaminenano-flowers loaded chitosan/gelatin hydrogel scaffolds with synergistic photothermal/chemodynamic/Ag+ anti-bacterial action for accelerated wound healing," *International Journal of Biological Macromolecules*, vol. 221, pp. 135–148, Nov. 2022. https://doi.org/10.1016/j.ijbiomac.2022.08.151

[96] S. Kumar, et al., "Fabrication of hybrid povidone-iodine impregnated collagen-hydroxypropyl methylcellulose composite scaffolds for wound-healing application," *Journal of Drug Delivery Science and Technology*, vol. 70, pp. 103247–103247, Apr. 2022. https://doi.org/10.1016/j.jddst.2022.103247

[97] S. Barzegar, et al., "Core-shell chitosan/PVA-based nanofibrous scaffolds loaded with Saturejamutica or Oliveriadecumbens essential oils as enhanced antimicrobial wound dressing," *International Journal of Pharmaceutics*, vol. 597, p. 120288, Mar. 2021. https://doi.org/10.1016/j.ijpharm.2021.120288

[98] M. Ghorbani, P. Nezhad-Mokhtari, and S. Ramazani, "Aloe vera-loaded nanofibrous scaffold based on zein/polycaprolactone/collagen for wound healing," *International Journal of Biological Macromolecules*, vol. 153, p. 921–930. Mar. 2020. https://doi.org/10.1016/j.ijbiomac.2020.03.036

[99] G. Selvakumar and S. Lonchin, "Bioactive functional collagen-oxidized pullulan scaffold loaded with polydatin for treating chronic wounds," *Biomaterials Advances*, vol. 140, p. 213078, Sep. 2022. https://doi.org/10.1016/j.bioadv.2022.213078

[100] C.-H. Lee, et al., "Augmentation of diabetic wound healing and enhancement of collagen content using nanofibrous glucophage-loaded collagen/PLGA scaffold membranes," *Journal of Colloid and Interface Science*, vol. 439, pp. 88–97, Feb. 2015. https://doi.org/10.1016/j.jcis.2014.10.028

[101] H. Yu, et al., "The efficacy of a paeoniflorin-sodium alginate-gelatin skin scaffold for the treatment of diabetic wound: An in vivo study in a rat model," *Biomedicine & Pharmacotherapy*, vol. 151, p. 113165, Jul. 2022. https://doi.org/10.1016/j.biopha.2022.113165

[102] P. S. Mohamadi, A. Hivechi, S. H. Bahrami, S. Nezari, P. B. Milan, and M. Amoupour, "Fabrication and investigating in vivo wound healing property of coconut oil loaded nanofiber/hydrogel hybrid scaffold," *Biomaterials Advances*, p. 213139, Oct. 2022. https://doi.org/10.1016/j.bioadv.2022.213139

[103] A. Koyuncu, S. Koç, Ö. E. Akdere, A. S. Çakmak, and M. Gümüşderelíoğlu, "Investigation of the synergistic effect of platelet-rich plasma and polychromatic light on human dermal fibroblasts seeded chitosan/gelatin scaffolds for wound healing," *Journal of Photochemistry and Photobiology B: Biology*, vol. 232, pp. 112476–112476, Jul. 2022. https://doi.org/10.1016/j.jphotobiol.2022.112476

[104] S. Sivakumar, et al., "Ferulic acid loaded microspheres reinforced in 3D hybrid scaffold for antimicrobial wound dressing," *International Journal of Biological Macromolecules*, vol. 177, pp. 463–473, Apr. 2021. https://doi.org/10.1016/j.ijbiomac.2021.02.124

[105] L. Huang, et al., "Silver doped-silica nanoparticles reinforced poly (ethylene glycol) diacrylate/hyaluronic acid hydrogel dressings for synergistically accelerating bacterial-infected wound healing," *Carbohydrate Polymers*, vol. 304, p. 120450, Mar. 2023. https://doi.org/10.1016/j.carbpol.2022.120450

[106] Y. Yu, B. Yang, D. Tian, J. Liu, A. Yu, and Y. Wan, "Thiolated hyaluronic acid/silk fibroin dual-network hydrogel incorporated with bioglass nanoparticles for wound healing," *Carbohydrate Polymers*, vol. 288, p. 119334, Jul. 2022. https://doi.org/10.1016/j.carbpol.2022.119334

[107] M. H. Teaima, M. K. Elasaly, S. A. Omar, M. A. El-Nabarawi, and K. R. Shoueir, "Wound healing activities of polyurethane modified chitosan nanofibers loaded with different concentrations of linezolid in an experimental model of diabetes," *Journal of Drug Delivery Science and Technology*, vol. 67, p. 102982, Jan. 2022. https://doi.org/10.1016/j.jddst.2021.102982

[108] B. ter Horst, N. S. Moiemen, and L. M. Grover, "Natural polymers," *Biomaterials for Skin Repair and Regeneration*, pp. 151–192, 2019. https://doi.org/10.1016/b978-0-08-102546-8.00006-6

[109] M. N. Collins and C. Birkinshaw, "Hyaluronic acid based scaffolds for tissue engineering—A review," *Carbohydrate Polymers*, vol. 92, no. 2, pp. 1262–1279, Feb. 2013. https://doi.org/10.1016/j.carbpol.2012.10.028

[110] Z. Su, et al., "Enhancement of skin wound healing with decellularized scaffolds loaded with hyaluronic acid and epidermal growth factor," *Materials Science and Engineering: C*, vol. 44, pp. 440–448, Nov. 2014. https://doi.org/10.1016/j.msec.2014.07.039

[111] K. Sudhakar, S. M. Ji, M. R. Kummara, and S. S. Han, "Recent progress on hyaluronan-based products for wound healing applications," *Pharmaceutics*, vol. 14, no. 10, p. 2235, Oct. 2022. https://doi.org/10.3390/pharmaceutics14102235

[112] E. Rostami, *Carbohydrate-Based Materials in Tissue Engineering Applications*, pp. 1–31, Dec. 2021. https://doi.org/10.1002/9783527832095.ch18

[113] R. Mehvar, "Dextrans for targeted and sustained delivery of therapeutic and imaging agents," *Journal of Controlled Release*, vol. 69, no. 1, pp. 1–25, Oct. 2000. https://doi.org/10.1016/s0168-3659(00)00302-3

[114] S. P. Massia and J. Stark, "Immobilized RGD peptides on surface-grafted dextran promote biospecific cell attachment," *Journal of biomedical Material and Research*, vol. 56, no. 3, pp. 390–399 Sep. 2001. https://doi.org/10.1002/1097-4636(20010905)56:3<390::aid-jbm1108>3.0.co;2-l

[115] S. Moller, J. Weisser, S. Bischoff, and M. Schnabelrauch, "Dextran and hyaluronan methacrylate based hydrogels as matrices for soft tissue reconstruction," *Biomolecular Engineering*, vol. 24, no. 5, pp. 496–504, Nov. 2007. https://doi.org/10.1016/j.bioeng.2007.08.014

[116] G. Sun, Y.-I. Shen, C. C. Ho, S. Kusuma, and S. Gerecht, "Functional groups affect physical and biological properties of dextran-based hydrogels," *Journal of Biomedical Materials Research Part A*, vol. 9999A, 2009. https://doi.org/10.1002/jbm.a.32604

[117] G. Sun, et al., "Dextran hydrogel scaffolds enhance angiogenic responses and promote complete skin regeneration during burn wound healing," *Proceedings of the National Academy of Sciences*, vol. 108, no. 52, pp. 20976–20981, Dec. 2011. https://doi.org/10.1073/pnas.1115973108

[118] S. Jahani, H. Ashrafizadeh, K. Babai, A. Siahpoosh, and B. Cheraghian, "Effect of ointment-based egg white on healing of second- degree wound in burn patients: A triple-blind randomized clinical trial study," *Avicenna Journal of Phytomedicine*, vol. 9, no. 3, pp. 260–270, 2019.

[119] X. Wang, et al., "Direct three-dimensional printed egg white hydrogel wound dressing promotes wound healing with hitching adipose stem cells," *Frontiers in Bioengineering and Biotechnology*, vol. 10, Aug. 2022. https://doi.org/10.3389/fbioe.2022.930551

[120] A. Barbu, B. Neamtu, M. Zăhan, G. M. Iancu, C. Bacila, and V. Mireşan, "Current trends in advanced alginate-based wound dressings for chronic wounds," *Journal of Personalized Medicine*, vol. 11, no. 9, p. 890, Sep. 2021. https://doi.org/10.3390/jpm11090890

[121] M. Ashiqur Rahman, et al., "Calcium ion mediated rapid wound healing by nano-ZnO doped calcium phosphate-chitosan-alginate biocomposites," *Materialia*, vol. 13, pp. 100839–100839, Sep. 2020. https://doi.org/10.1016/j.mtla.2020.100839

[122] M. Rădulescu, et al., "Fabrication, characterization, and evaluation of bionanocomposites based on natural polymers and antibiotics for wound healing applications," *Molecules*, vol. 21, no. 6, p. 761, Jun. 2016. https://doi.org/10.3390/molecules21060761

[123] B. A. Aderibigbe and B. Buyana, "Alginate in wound dressings," *Pharmaceutics*, vol. 10, no. 2, p. 42, Apr. 2018. https://doi.org/10.3390/pharmaceutics10020042

[124] S. E. Barnett and S. J. Varley, "The effects of calcium alginate on wound healing," *Annals of the Royal College of Surgeons of England*, vol. 69, no. 4, pp. 153–155, 1987.

[125] S.A. Survase, et al., "Fermentative production of scleroglucan," *Food Technology and Biotechnology, vol.* 45, no. 2, pp. 107–118, 2007.

[126] B. K. Bozoğlan, O. Duman, and S. Tunç, "Preparation and characterization of thermosensitive chitosan/carboxymethylcellulose/scleroglucannanocomposite hydrogels," *International Journal of Biological Macromolecules*, vol. 162, pp. 781–797, Nov. 2020. https://doi.org/10.1016/j.ijbiomac.2020.06.087

[127] J. Kucińska-Lipka, I. Gubanska, and H. Janik, "Bacterial cellulose in the field of wound healing and regenerative medicine of skin: Recent trends and future prospectives," *Polymer Bulletin*, vol. 72, no. 9, pp. 2399–2419, Jun. 2015. https://doi.org/10.1007/s00289-015-1407-3

[128] M. Alavi and A. Nokhodchi, "An overview on antimicrobial and wound healing properties of ZnO nanobiofilms, hydrogels, and bionanocomposites based on cellulose, chitosan, and alginate polymers," *Carbohydrate Polymers*, vol. 227, p. 115349, Jan. 2020. https://doi.org/10.1016/j.carbpol.2019.115349

[129] J. Ahmed, M. Gultekinoglu, and M. Edirisinghe, "Bacterial cellulose micro-nano fibres for wound healing applications," *Biotechnology Advances*, vol. 41, p. 107549, Jul. 2020. https://doi.org/10.1016/j.biotechadv.2020.107549

[130] J. Gao, et al., "Biopaper based on ultralong hydroxyapatite nanowires and cellulose fibers promotes skin wound healing by inducing angiogenesis," *Coatings*, vol. 12, no. 4, p. 479, Apr. 2022. https://doi.org/10.3390/coatings12040479

[131] P. P. Patil, M. R. Reagan, and R. A. Bohara, "Silk fibroin and silk-based biomaterial derivatives for ideal wound dressings," *International Journal of Biological Macromolecules*, vol. 164, pp. 4613–4627, Dec. 2020. https://doi.org/10.1016/j.ijbiomac.2020.08.041

[132] M. S. B. Reddy, D. Ponnamma, R. Choudhary, and K. K. Sadasivuni, "A comparative review of natural and synthetic biopolymer composite scaffolds," *Polymers*, vol. 13, no. 7, p. 1105, Mar. 2021. https://doi.org/10.3390/polym13071105

[133] G. Sabarees, et al., "Emerging trends in silk fibroin based nanofibers for impaired wound healing," *Journal of Drug Delivery Science and Technology*, vol. 79, pp. 103994–103994, Nov. 2022. https://doi.org/10.1016/j.jddst.2022.103994

[134] P. J. Babu, M. Doble, and A. M. Raichur, "Silver oxide nanoparticles embedded silk fibroin spuns: Microwave mediated preparation, characterization and their synergistic wound healing and anti-bacterial activity," *Journal of Colloid and Interface Science*, vol. 513, pp. 62–71, Mar. 2018. https://doi.org/10.1016/j.jcis.2017.11.001

[135] J. C. Rodríguez-Cabello, I. González de Torre, A. Ibañez-Fonseca, and M. Alonso, "Bioactive scaffolds based on elastin-like materials for wound healing," *Advanced Drug Delivery Reviews*, vol. 129, pp. 118–133, Apr. 2018. https://doi.org/10.1016/j.addr.2018.03.003

[136] B. K. H. L. Boekema, et al., "Effect of pore size and cross-linking of a novel collagen-elastin dermal substitute on wound healing," *Journal of Materials Science: Materials in Medicine*, vol. 25, no. 2, pp. 423–433, Nov. 2013. https://doi.org/10.1007/s10856-013-5075-2

[137] W. Daamen, J. Veerkamp, J. Vanhest, and T. Vankuppevelt, "Elastin as a biomaterial for tissue engineering," *Biomaterials*, vol. 28, no. 30, pp. 4378–4398, Oct. 2007. https://doi.org/10.1016/j.biomaterials.2007.06.025

[138] S. Kawabata, et al., "The development of a novel wound healing material, silk-elastin sponge," *Journal of Biomaterials Science, Polymer Edition*, vol. 28, no. 18, pp. 2143–2153, Sep. 2017. https://doi.org/10.1080/09205063.2017.1382829

[139] M. R. Roslan, N. F. M. Nasir, E. M. Cheng, and N. A. M. Amin, "Tissue engineering scaffold based on starch: A review," *2016 International Conference on Electrical, Electronics, and Optimization Techniques (ICEEOT)*, Mar. 2016. https://doi.org/10.1109/iceeot.2016.7755010

[140] V. S. Waghmare, P. R. Wadke, S. Dyawanapelly, A. Deshpande, R. Jain, and P. Dandekar, "Starch based nanofibrous scaffolds for wound healing applications," *Bioactive Materials*, vol. 3, no. 3, pp. 255–266, Sep. 2018. https://doi.org/10.1016/j.bioactmat.2017.11.006

[141] R. Chhabra, et al., "*In vivo* studies of 3D starch–gelatin scaffolds for full-thickness wound healing," *ACS Applied Bio Materials*, vol. 3, no. 5, pp. 2920–2929, Mar. 2020. https://doi.org/10.1021/acsabm.9b01139

[142] V. R. Sherman, W. Yang, and M. A. Meyers, "The materials science of collagen," *Journal of the Mechanical Behavior of Biomedical Materials*, vol. 52, pp. 22–50, Dec. 2015. https://doi.org/10.1016/j.jmbbm.2015.05.023

[143] S. Chattopadhyay and R. T. Raines, "Review collagen-based biomaterials for wound healing," *Biopolymers*, vol. 101, no. 8, pp. 821–833, May 2014. https://doi.org/10.1002/bip.22486

[144] V. Natarajan, N. Krithica, B. Madhan, and P. K. Sehgal, "Preparation and properties of tannic acid cross-linked collagen scaffold and its application in wound healing," *Journal of Biomedical Materials Research Part B: Applied Biomaterials*, vol. 101B, no. 4, pp. 560–567, Dec. 2012. https://doi.org/10.1002/jbm.b.32856

[145] S.-B. Park, E. Lih, K.-S. Park, Y. K. Joung, and D. K. Han, "Biopolymer-based functional composites for medical applications," *Progress in Polymer Science*, vol. 68, pp. 77–105, May 2017. https://doi.org/10.1016/j.progpolymsci.2016.12.003

[146] B. Kumar Reddy Sanapalli, et al., "L-glutamic acid loaded collagen chitosan composite scaffold as regenerative medicine for the accelerated healing of diabetic wounds," *Arabian Journal of Chemistry*, vol. 15, no. 6, p. 103841, Jun. 2022. https://doi.org/10.1016/j.arabjc.2022.103841

[147] X. H. Zou, K. Weng, T. Cao, B. Bay, H. Ouyang, and G. W. Yip, "Chondroitin sulfate in palatal wound healing," *Journal of Dental Research*, vol. 83, no. 11, pp. 880–885, Nov. 2004. https://doi.org/10.1177/154405910408301111

[148] P. B. Malafaya, G. A. Silva, and R. L. Reis, "Natural–origin polymers as carriers and scaffolds for biomolecules and cell delivery in tissue engineering applications," *Advanced Drug Delivery Reviews*, vol. 59, no. 4–5, pp. 207–233, May 2007. https://doi.org/10.1016/j.addr.2007.03.012

[149] A. Ito, et al., "Transglutaminase-mediated gelatin matrices incorporating cell adhesion factors as a biomaterial for tissue engineering," *Journal of Bioscience and Bioengineering*, vol. 95, no. 2, pp. 196–199, Jan. 2003. https://doi.org/10.1016/s1389-1723(03)80129-9

[150] N. Ninan, et al., "Antibacterial and wound healing analysis of gelatin/zeolite scaffolds," *Colloids and Surfaces B: Biointerfaces*, vol. 115, pp. 244–252, Mar. 2014. https://doi.org/10.1016/j.colsurfb.2013.11.048

[151] F. Ahmadi, Z. Oveisi, S. M. Samani, Z. Amoozgar, "Chitosan based hydrogels: Characteristics and pharmaceutical applications," *Research in Pharmaceutical Sciences*, vol. 10, no. 1, pp. 1–16, Feb. 2015.

[152] M. Rezaii, S. Oryan, and A. Javeri, "Curcumin nanoparticles incorporated collagen-chitosan scaffold promotes cutaneous wound healing through regulation of TGF-β1/Smad7 gene expression," *Materials Science and Engineering: C*, vol. 98, pp. 347–357, May 2019. https://doi.org/10.1016/j.msec.2018.12.143

[153] P. Feng, et al., "Chitosan-based functional materials for skin wound repair: Mechanisms and applications," *Frontiers in Bioengineering and Biotechnology*, vol. 9, Feb. 2021. https://doi.org/10.3389/fbioe.2021.650598

[154] A. Chanda, et al., "Electrospun chitosan/polycaprolactone-hyaluronic acid bilayered scaffold for potential wound healing applications," *International Journal of Biological Macromolecules*, vol. 116, pp. 774–785, Sep. 2018. https://doi.org/10.1016/j.ijbiomac.2018.05.099

[155] D. R. Figueira, S. P. Miguel, K. D. de Sá, and I. J. Correia, "Production and characterization of polycaprolactone- hyaluronic acid/chitosan- zeinelectrospun bilayer nanofibrous membrane for tissue regeneration," *International Journal of Biological Macromolecules*, vol. 93, pp. 1100–1110, Dec. 2016. https://doi.org/10.1016/j.ijbiomac.2016.09.080

[156] R. Jayakumar, M. Prabaharan, P. T. Sudheesh Kumar, S. V. Nair, and H. Tamura, "Biomaterials based on chitin and chitosan in wound dressing applications," *Biotechnology Advances*, vol. 29, no. 3, pp. 322–337, May 2011. https://doi.org/10.1016/j.biotechadv.2011.01.005

[157] P. T. Sudheesh Kumar, et al., "Flexible and microporous chitosan hydrogel/nanoZNO composite bandages for wound dressing: In vitro and in vivo evaluation," *ACS Applied Materials & Interfaces*, vol. 4, no. 5, pp. 2618–2629, Apr. 2012. https://doi.org/10.1021/am300292v

[158] A. Regiel-Futyra, et al., "Development of noncytotoxic chitosan–gold nanocomposites as efficient antibacterial materials," *ACS Applied Materials & Interfaces*, vol. 7, no. 2, pp. 1087–1099, Jan. 2015. https://doi.org/10.1021/am508094e

[159] L. M. Anaya-Esparza, et al., "Chitosan-TiO_2: A versatile hybrid composite," *Materials*, vol. 13, no. 4, p. 811, Feb. 2020. https://doi.org/10.3390/ma13040811

[160] F. Grinnell, "Fibronectin and wound healing," *Journal of Cellular Biochemistry*, vol. 26, no. 2, pp. 107–116, 1984. https://doi.org/10.1002/jcb.240260206

[161] R. Pankov, "Fibronectin at a glance," *Journal of Cell Science*, vol. 115, no. 20, pp. 3861–3863, Oct. 2002. https://doi.org/10.1242/jcs.00059

[162] C. O. Chantre, et al., "Production-scale fibronectin nanofibers promote wound closure and tissue repair in a dermal mouse model," *Biomaterials*, vol. 166, pp. 96–108, Jun. 2018. https://doi.org/10.1016/j.biomaterials.2018.03.006

[163] P. Zarrintaj, et al., "Agarose-based biomaterials for tissue engineering," *Carbohydrate Polymers*, vol. 187, pp. 66–84, May 2018. https://doi.org/10.1016/j.carbpol.2018.01.060

[164] D. Y. Lewitus, et al., "Biohybrid carbon nanotube/agarose fibers for neural tissue engineering," *Advanced Functional Materials*, vol. 21, no. 14, pp. 2624–2632, May 2011. https://doi.org/10.1002/adfm.201002429

[165] K. K. Nayak and P. Gupta, "In vitro biocompatibility study of keratin/agar scaffold for tissue engineering," *International Journal of Biological Macromolecules*, vol. 81, pp. 1–10, Nov. 2015. https://doi.org/10.1016/j.ijbiomac.2015.07.025

[166] S. I. Basha, et al., "Fumaric acid incorporated Ag/agar-agar hybrid hydrogel: A multifunctional avenue to tackle wound healing," *Materials Science and Engineering: C*, vol. 111, p. 110743, Jun. 2020. https://doi.org/10.1016/j.msec.2020.110743

[167] M. Tavakoli, et al., "Coaxial electrospun angiogenic nanofiber wound dressing containing advanced platelet rich-fibrin," *International Journal of Biological Macromolecules*, vol. 222, pp. 1605–1618, Dec. 2022. https://doi.org/10.1016/j.ijbiomac.2022.09.109

[168] H. H. Bragulla and D. G. Homberger, "Structure and functions of keratin proteins in simple, stratified, keratinized and cornified epithelia," *Journal of anatomy*, vol. 214, no. 4, pp. 516–559, 2009. https://doi.org/10.1111/j.1469-7580.2009.01066.x

[169] J. G. Rouse and M. E. Van Dyke, "A review of keratin-based biomaterials for biomedical applications," *Materials*, vol. 3, no. 2, pp. 999–1014, Feb. 2010. https://doi.org/10.3390/ma3020999

[170] H. Tan, et al., "Fabrication and evaluation of porous keratin/chitosan (KCS) scaffolds for effectively accelerating wound healing," *PubMed*, vol. 28, no. 3, pp. 178–189, Mar. 2015. https://doi.org/10.3967/bes2015.024

[171] Y. Chen, et al., "Glucose-triggered in situ forming keratin hydrogel for the treatment of diabetic wounds," *Acta Biomaterialia*, vol. 125, pp. 208–218, Apr. 2021. https://doi.org/10.1016/j.actbio.2021.02.035

[172] S. Hamdan, et al., "Nanotechnology-driven therapeutic interventions in wound healing: Potential uses and applications," *ACS Central Science*, vol. 3, no. 3, pp. 163–175, Feb. 2017. https://doi.org/10.1021/acscentsci.6b00371

[173] M. M. Mihai, M. B. Dima, B. Dima, and A. M. Holban, "Nanomaterials for wound healing and infection control," *Materials*, vol. 12, no. 13, p. 2176, Jul. 2019. https://doi.org/10.3390/ma12132176

[174] X. Wang, C. Yang, and C. Wu, "Bioactive inorganic/organic nanocomposites for wound healing," *Applied Materials Today*, vol. 11, pp. 308–319, Jun. 2018. https://doi.org/10.1016/j.apmt.2018.03.001

[175] X. Yang, et al., "Pharmaceutical intermediate-modified gold nanoparticles: Against multidrug-resistant bacteria and wound-healing application via an electrospun scaffold," *ACS Nano*, vol. 11, no. 6, pp. 5737–5745, May 2017. https://doi.org/10.1021/acsnano.7b01240

[176] M. A. Shalaby, M. M. Anwar, H. Saeed, "Nanomaterials for application in wound healing: Current state-of-the-art and future perspectives," *Journal of Polymer Research*, vol. 29, no. 91, 2022. https://doi.org/10.1007/s10965-021-02870-x

[177] I. Khan, K. Saeed, and I. Khan, "Nanoparticles: Properties, applications and toxicities," *Arabian Journal of Chemistry*, vol. 12, no. 7, pp. 908–931, May 2017. https://doi.org/10.1016/j.arabjc.2017.05.011

[178] M. Maas, "Carbon nanomaterials as antibacterial colloids," *Materials*, vol. 9, no. 8, p. 617, Jul. 2016. https://doi.org/10.3390/ma9080617

[179] P. Singh, K. R. B. Singh, A. K. Yadav, J. Singh, P. R. Solanki, and R. P. Singh, "Carbon-based nanostructured materials for effective strategy in wound management," *Elsevier eBooks*, pp. 193–218, Jan. 2024. https://doi.org/10.1016/b978-0-323-99165-0.00013-7

[180] N. Kumar and S. Kumbhat, *Essentials in Nanoscience and Nanotechnology*, Apr. 2016. https://doi.org/10.1002/9781119096122

[181] M. Triesscheijn, M. Ruevekamp, M. Aalders, P. Baas, and F. A. Stewart, "Outcome of mTHPC mediated photodynamic therapy is primarily determined by the vascular response," *Photochemistry and Photobiology*, vol. 81, no. 5, p. 1161, 2005. https://doi.org/10.1562/2005-04-04-ra-474

[182] F. Salimi and F. Mohammadipanah, "Nanomaterials versus the microbial compounds with wound healing property," *Frontiers in Nanotechnology*, vol. 2, Jan. 2021. https://doi.org/10.3389/fnano.2020.584489

[183] N. A. Monteiro-Riviere, R. J. Nemanich, A. O. Inman, Y. Y. Wang, J. E. Riviere, "Multi-walled carbon nanotube interactions with human epidermal keratinocytes," *Toxicology Letters*, vol. 155, no. 3, pp. 377–384, 2005. https://doi.org/10.1186/s12989-018-0285-x

[184] N. R. Jacobsen, G. Pojana, P. White, P. Moller, C. A. Cohn, S. Korsholm, et al., "Genotoxicity, cytotoxicity, and reactive oxygen species induced by single-walled carbon nanotubes and C60 fullerenes in the FE1-MutaTMMouse lung epithelial cells," *Environmental and Molecular Mutagenesis*, vol. 49, no. 6, pp. 476–487, 2008. https://doi.org/10.1002/em.20406

[185] P. Sundaram and H. Abrahamse, "Phototherapy combined with carbon nanomaterials (1D and 2D) and their applications in cancer therapy," *Materials*, vol. 13, no. 21, p. 4830, Oct. 2020. https://doi.org/10.3390/ma13214830

[186] S. Liu, et al., "Antibacterial activity of graphite, graphite oxide, graphene oxide, and reduced graphene oxide: Membrane and oxidative stress," *ACS Nano*, vol. 5, no. 9, pp. 6971–6980, Aug. 2011. https://doi.org/10.1021/nn202451x

[187] K. Yang, Y. Li, X. Tan, R. Peng, and Z. Liu, "Behavior and toxicity of graphene and its functionalized derivatives in biological systems," *Small*, vol. 9, no. 9–10, pp. 1492–1503, Sept. 2012. https://doi.org/10.1002/smll.201201417

[188] S. Gurunathan, J. W. Han, A. A. Dayem, V. Eppakayala, and J. H. Kim, "Oxidative stress-mediated antibacterial activity of grapheme oxide and reduced graphene oxide in Pseudomonas aeruginosa," *International Journal of Nanomedicine*, vol. 7, pp. 5901–5914, 2012. https://doi.org/10.2147/IJN.S37397

[189] K. Krishnamoorthy, N. Umasuthan, R. Mohan, J. Lee, and S.-J. Kim, "Antibacterial activity of graphene oxide nanosheets," *Science of Advanced Materials*, vol. 4, no. 11, pp. 1111–1117, Nov. 2012. https://doi.org/10.1098/rsos.200640

[190] Y. Yang, et al., "Graphene oxide/copper nanoderivatives-modified chitosan/hyaluronic acid dressings for facilitating wound healing in infected full-thickness skin defects," *International Journal of Nanomedicine*, vol. 15, pp. 8231–8247, Oct. 2020. https://doi.org/10.2147/IJN.S278631

[191] B. Lu, T. Li, H. Zhao, X. Li, C. Gao, S. Zhang, et al. "Graphene-based composite materials beneficial to wound healing," *Nanoscale*, vol. 4, no. 9, pp. 2978–2982, 2012. https://doi.org/10.1039/c2nr11958g

[192] S. Luanpitpong, L. Wang, and Y. Rojanasakul, "The effects of carbon nanotubes on lung and dermal cellular behaviors," *Nanomedicine (London, England)*, vol. 9, no. 6, pp. 895–912, May 2014. https://doi.org/10.2217/nnm.14.42

[193] C. A. Poland, et al., "Carbon nanotubes introduced into the abdominal cavity of mice show asbestos-like pathogenicity in a pilot study," *Nature Nanotechnology*, vol. 3, no. 7, pp. 423–428, May 2008. https://doi.org/10.1038/nnano.2008.111

[194] A. E. Porter, M. Gass, K. Muller, J. N. Skepper, P. A. Midgley, and M. E. Welland, "Direct imaging of single-walled carbon nanotubes in cells," *Nature Nanotechnology* vol. 2, no. 11, pp. 713–717, Nov. 2007. https://doi.org/10.1038/nnano.2007.347

[195] B. K. Rada, "Dual role of phagocytic NADPH oxidase in bacterial killing," *Blood*, vol. 104, no. 9, pp. 2947–2953, Nov. 2004. https://doi.org/10.1182/blood-2004-03-1005

[196] S. Kang, M. Herzberg, D. F. Rodrigues, and M. Elimelech, "Antibacterial effects of carbon nanotubes: Size does matter," *Langmuir*, vol. 24, no. 13, pp. 6409–6413, Jul. 2008. https://doi.org/10.1021/la800951v

[197] A. O. Oyelami and K. T. Semple, "Impact of carbon nanomaterials on microbial activity in soil," *Soil Biology and Biochemistry*, vol. 86, pp. 172–180, Jul. 2015. https://doi.org/10.1016/j.soilbio.2015.03.029

[198] N. Kittana, et al., "Enhancement of wound healing by single-wall/multi-wall carbon nanotubes complexed with chitosan," *International Journal of Nanomedicine*, vol. 13, pp. 7195–7206, Nov. 2018. https://doi.org/10.2147/IJN.S183342

[199] A. Niu, Y. Han, J. Wu, N. Yu, and Q. Xu, "Synthesis of one-dimensional carbon nanomaterials wrapped by silver nanoparticles and their antibacterial behavior," *Journal of Physical Chemistry C*, vol. 114, no. 29, pp. 12728–12735, Jul. 2010. https://doi.org/10.1021/jp104720w

[200] O. Akhavan, M. Abdolahad, Y. Abdi, and S. Mohajerzadeh, "Synthesis of titania/carbon nanotube heterojunction arrays for photoinactivation of E. coli in visible light irradiation," *Carbon*, vol. 47, no. 14, pp. 3280–3287, Nov. 2009. https://doi.org/10.1016/j.carbon.2009.07.046

[201] Z. Zhou, et al., "A novel class of compounds with cutaneous wound healing properties," *Journal of Biomedical Nanotechnology*, vol. 6, no. 5, pp. 605–611, Oct. 2010. https://doi.org/10.1166/jbn.2010.1157

[202] D. Y. Lyon, J. D. Fortner, C. M. Sayes, V. L. Colvin, J. B. Hughes, "Bacterial cell association and antimicrobial activity of a C60 water suspension," *Environmental and Toxicological Chemistry*, vol. 24, no. 11, pp. 2757–2762, 2005. https://doi.org/10.1897/04-649r.1

[203] J. Zhang, et al., "Designing an amino-fullerene derivative C_{70}–$(EDA)_8$ to fight superbacteria," *ACS Applied Materials & Interfaces*, vol. 11, no. 16, pp. 14597–14607, Apr. 2019. https://doi.org/10.1021/acsami.9b01483

[204] S. A. Ansari, R. Satar, M. A. Jafri, M. Rasool, W. Ahmad, and S. Kashif Zaidi, "Role of nanodiamonds in drug delivery and stem cell therapy," *Iranian Journal of Biotechnology*, vol. 14, no. 3, pp. 130–141, Sep. 2016. https://doi.org/10.15171/ijb.1320

[205] X. Luo, H. Zhang, Z. Cao, N. Cai, Y. Xue, and F. Yu, "A simple route to develop transparent doxorubicin-loaded nanodiamonds/cellulose nanocomposite membranes as potential wound dressings," *Carbohydrate Polymers*, vol. 143, pp. 231–238, Jun. 2016. https://doi.org/10.1016/j.carbpol.2016.01.076

[206] F. Ostadhossein, et al., "Development of chitosan/bacterial cellulose composite films containing nanodiamonds as a potential flexible platform for wound dressing," *Materials*, vol. 8, no. 9, pp. 6401–6418, Sep. 2015. https://doi.org/10.3390/ma8095309

[207] J. Robertson, "Diamond-like amorphous carbon," *Materials Science and Engineering: R: Reports*, vol. 37, no. 4–6, pp. 129–281, May 2002. https://doi.org/10.1016/s0927-796x(02)00005-0

[208] F. S. Lopes, et al., "Biomineralized diamond-like carbon films with incorporated titanium dioxide nanoparticles improved bioactivity properties and reduced biofilm formation," *Materials Science and Engineering: C*, vol. 81, pp. 373–379, Dec. 2017. https://doi.org/10.1016/j.msec.2017.07.043

[209] T. Juknius, et al., "Antimicrobial properties of diamond-like carbon/silver nanocomposite thin films deposited on textiles: Towards smart bandages," *Materials*, vol. 9, no. 5, p. 371, May 2016. https://doi.org/10.3390/ma9050371

[210] C. Gorzelanny, et al., "Silver nanoparticle-enriched diamond-like carbon implant modification as a mammalian cell compatible surface with antimicrobial properties," *Scientific Reports*, vol. 6, no. 1, Mar. 2016. https://doi.org/10.1038/srep22849

[211] N. K. Rajendran, S. S. D. Kumar, N. N. Houreld, and H. Abrahamse, "A review on nanoparticle based treatment for wound healing," *Journal of Drug Delivery Science and Technology*, vol. 44, pp. 421–430, Apr. 2018. https://doi.org/10.1016/j.jddst.2018.01.009

[212] M. Jiao, et al., "Recent advancements in biocompatible inorganic nanoparticles towards biomedical applications," *Biomaterials Science*, vol. 6, no. 4, pp. 726–745, 2018. https://doi.org/10.1039/c7bm01020f

[213] A. Naskar and K. Kim, "Black phosphorus nanomaterials as multi-potent and emerging platforms against bacterial infections," *Microbial Pathogenesis*, vol. 137, pp. 103800–103800, Dec. 2019. https://doi.org/10.1016/j.micpath.2019.103800

[214] T. Gunasekaran, T. Nigusse, and M. D. Dhanaraju, "Silver nanoparticles as real topical bullets for wound healing," *The Journal of the American College of Clinical Wound Specialists*, vol. 3, no. 4, pp. 82–96, Dec. 2011. https://doi.org/10.1016/j.jcws.2012.05.001

[215] G. Thirumurugan, V. S. Veni, S. Ramachandran, J. V. L. N. Seshagiri Rao, and M. D. Dhanaraju, "Superior wound healing effect of topically delivered silver nanoparticle formulation using eco-friendly potato plant pathogenic fungus: Synthesis and characterization," *Journal of Biomedical Nanotechnology*, vol. 7, no. 5, pp. 659–666, Oct. 2011. https://doi.org/10.1166/jbn.2011.1336

[216] W. Boucher, et al., "Intravesical nanocrystalline silver decreases experimental bladder inflammation," *The Journal of Urology*, vol. 179, no. 4, pp. 1598–1602, Apr. 2008. https://doi.org/10.1016/j.juro.2007.11.037

[217] A. Ghavami Nejad, et al., "Mussel-inspired electrospun nanofibers functionalized with size-controlled silver nanoparticles for wound dressing application," *ACS Applied Materials & Interfaces*, vol. 7, no. 22, pp. 12176–12183, May 2015. https://doi.org/10.1021/acsami.5b02542

[218] J. Liu, D. A. Sonshine, S. Shervani, and R. H. Hurt, "Controlled release of biologically active silver from nanosilver surfaces," *ACS Nano*, vol. 4, no. 11, pp. 6903–6913, Oct. 2010. https://doi.org/10.1021/nn102272n

[219] Y. Zhou, et al., "Biomedical potential of ultrafine Ag/AgCl nanoparticles coated on graphene with special reference to antimicrobial performances and burn wound healing," *ACS applied materials & interfaces*, vol. 8, no. 24, pp. 15067–15075, Jun. 2016. https://doi.org/10.1021/acsami.6b03021

[220] M. R. El-Aassar, O. M. Ibrahim, M. M. G. Fouda, N. G. El-Beheri, and M. M. Agwa, "Wound healing of nanofiber comprising polygalacturonic/hyaluronic acid embedded silver nanoparticles: In-vitro and in-vivo studies," *Carbohydrate Polymers*, vol. 238, p. 116175, Jun. 2020. https://doi.org/10.1016/j.carbpol.2020.116175

[221] V. Vijayakumar, S. K. Samal, S. Mohanty, and S. K. Nayak, "Recent advancements in biopolymer and metal nanoparticle-based materials in diabetic wound healing management," *International Journal of Biological Macromolecules*, vol. 122, pp. 137–148, Feb. 2019. https://doi.org/10.1016/j.ijbiomac.2018.10.120

[222] Y. Huang, et al., "Co-administration of protein drugs with gold nanoparticles to enable percutaneous delivery," *Biomaterials*, vol. 31, no. 34, pp. 9086–9091, Dec. 2010. https://doi.org/10.1016/j.biomaterials.2010.08.046

[223] N. R. Kolarijani, et al., "Nanofibrous polycaprolactone/gelatin scaffold containing gold nanoparticles: Physicochemical and biological characterization for wound healing," *Wound Repair and Regeneration*, vol. 31, no. 6, pp. 804–815, Nov. 2023. https://doi.org/10.1111/wrr.13126

[224] S. Hsu, Y.-B. Chang, C.-L. Tsai, K.-Y. Fu, S.-H. Wang, and H.-J. Tseng, "Characterization and biocompatibility of chitosan nanocomposites," *Colloids and Surfaces B: Biointerfaces*, vol. 85, no. 2, pp. 198–206, Jul. 2011. https://doi.org/10.1016/j.colsurfb.2011.02.029

[225] M. A. Sherwani, S. Tufail, A. A. Khan, M. Owais, "Gold nanoparticle-photosensitizer conjugate based photodynamic inactivation of biofilm producing cells: Potential for treatment of C. albicans infection in BALB/c mice," *PLoS One*, vol. 10, no. 7, pp. e0131684, 2015. https://doi.org/10.1371/journal.pone.0131684

[226] N. Volkova, M. Yukhta, O. Pavlovich, and A. Goltsev, "Application of cryopreserved fibroblast culture with Au nanoparticles to treat burns," *Nanoscale Research Letters*, vol. 11, no. 1, Jan. 2016. https://doi.org/10.1186/s11671-016-1242-y

[227] A. Naskar, H. Khan, R. Sarkar, S. Kumar, D. Halder, S. Jana, "Anti-biofilm activity and food packaging application of room temperature solution process based polyethylene glycol capped Ag-ZnO graphene nanocomposite," *Material Science and Engineering: C*, vol. 91, pp. 743–753, 2018. https://doi.org/10.1016/j.msec.2018.06.009

[228] M. S. Khan, M. L. Bhaisare, J. Gopal, H. F. Wu, "Highly efficient gold nanorods assisted laser phototherapy for rapid treatment on mice wound infected by pathogenic bacteria," *Journal of Industrial and Engineering Chemistry*, vol. 36, pp. 49–58, 2016. https://doi.org/10.1016/j.jiec.2015.12.011

[229] M. Gupta, V. K. Mahajan, K. S. Mehta, and P. S. Chauhan, "Zinc therapy in dermatology: A review," *Dermatology Research and Practice*, vol. 2014, no. 1, pp. 1–11, 2014. https://doi.org/10.1155/2014/709152

[230] K. S. Siddiqi, A. Rahman, and A. Husen, "Properties of zinc oxide nanoparticles and their activity against microbes," *Nanoscale Research Letters*, vol. 13, no. 1, May 2018. https://doi.org/10.1186/s11671-018-2532-3

[231] I. Wessels, M. Maywald, L. Rink, "Zinc as a gatekeeper of immune function," *Nutrients, vol.* 9, no. 12, pp. 1286, 2017. https://doi.org/10.3390/nu9121286

[232] J. Jiang, J. Pi, and J. Cai, "The advancing of zinc oxide nanoparticles for biomedical applications," *Bioinorganic Chemistry and Applications*, vol. 2018, 2018. https://doi.org/10.1155/2018/1062562

[233] P. K. Mishra, H. Mishra, A. Ekielski, S. Talegaonkar, and B. Vaidya, "Zinc oxide nanoparticles: A promising nanomaterial for biomedical applications," *Drug Discovery Today*, vol. 22, no. 12, pp. 1825–1834, Dec. 2017. https://doi.org/10.1016/j.drudis.2017.08.006

[234] M. Tiwari, K. Narayanan, M. B. Thakar, H. V. Jagani, and J. Venkata Rao, "Biosynthesis and wound healing activity of copper nanoparticles," *IET Nanobiotechnology*, vol. 8, no. 4, pp. 230–237, Dec. 2014. https://doi.org/10.1049/iet-nbt.2013.0052

[235] G. Borkow, et al., "Molecular mechanisms of enhanced wound healing by copper oxide-impregnated dressings," *Wound Repair and Regeneration*, vol. 18, no. 2, pp. 266–275, Mar. 2010. https://doi.org/10.1111/j.1524-475x.2010.00573.x

[236] X. Ma, S. Zhou, X. Xu, and Q. Du, "Copper-containing nanoparticles: Mechanism of antimicrobial effect and application in dentistry-a narrative review," *Frontiers in Surgery*, vol. 9, Aug. 2022. https://doi.org/10.3389/fsurg.2022.905892

[237] A. Gopal, V. Kant, A. Gopalakrishnan, S. K. Tandan, and D. Kumar, "Chitosan-based copper nanocomposite accelerates healing in excision wound model in rats," *European Journal of Pharmacology*, vol. 731, pp. 8–19, May 2014. https://doi.org/10.1016/j.ejphar.2014.02.033

[238] S. Quignard, T. Coradin, J. J. Powell, and R. Jugdaohsingh, "Silica nanoparticles as sources of silicic acid favoring wound healing in vitro," *Colloids and Surfaces. B, Biointerfaces* vol. 155, pp. 530–537, Jul. 2017. https://doi.org/10.1016/j.colsurfb.2017.04.049

[239] G. S. Alvarez, C. Hélary, A. M. Mebert, X. Wang, T. Coradin, and M. F. Desimone, "Antibiotic-loaded silica nanoparticle–collagen composite hydrogels with prolonged antimicrobial activity for wound infection prevention," *Journal of Materials Chemistry B*, vol. 2, no. 29, p. 4660, 2014. https://doi.org/10.1039/c4tb00327f

[240] F. Öri, et al., "Silicon-dioxide–polyvinylpyrrolidone as a wound dressing for skin defects in a murine model," *Journal of Cranio-Maxillofacial Surgery*, vol. 45, no. 1, pp. 99–107, Jan. 2017. https://doi.org/10.1016/j.jcms.2016.10.002

[241] G. A. Seisenbaeva, et al., "Dispersion of TiO_2 nanoparticles improves burn wound healing and tissue regeneration through specific interaction with blood serum proteins," *Scientific Reports*, vol. 7, no. 1, Nov. 2017. https://doi.org/10.1038/s41598-017-15792-w

[242] D. Archana, J. Dutta, and P. K. Dutta, "Evaluation of chitosan nano dressing for wound healing: Characterization, in vitro and in vivo studies," *International Journal of Biological Macromolecules*, vol. 57, pp. 193–203, Jun. 2013. https://doi.org/10.1016/j.ijbiomac.2013.03.002

[243] C. C. Peng, et al., "Composite nano-titanium oxide-chitosan artificial skin exhibits strong wound-healing effect-an approach with anti-inflammatory and bactericidal kinetics," *Macromolecular Bioscience*, vol. 8, no. 4, pp. 316–327, Dec. 2007. https://doi.org/10.1002/mabi.200700188

[244] N. Wahajuddin and S. Arora, "Superparamagnetic iron oxide nanoparticles: Magnetic nanoplatforms as drug carriers," *International Journal of Nanomedicine*, p. 3445, Jul. 2012. https://doi.org/10.2147/ijn.s30320

[245] M. Arakha, et al., "Antimicrobial activity of iron oxide nanoparticle upon modulation of nanoparticle-bacteria interface," *Scientific Reports*, vol. 5, Oct. 2015. https://doi.org/10.1038/srep14813

[246] O. Ziv-Polat, M. Topaz, T. Brosh, and S. Margel, "Enhancement of incisional wound healing by thrombin conjugated iron oxide nanoparticles," *Biomaterials*, vol. 31, no. 4, pp. 741–747, Feb. 2010. https://doi.org/10.1016/j.biomaterials.2009.09.093

[247] N. Kamaly, Z. Xiao, P. M. Valencia, A. F. Radovic-Moreno, and O. C. Farokhzad, "Targeted polymeric therapeutic nanoparticles: Design, development and clinical translation," *Chemical Society Reviews*, vol. 41, no. 7, pp. 2971–3010, Apr. 2012. https://doi.org/10.1039/c2cs15344k

[248] D. Jong, "Drug delivery and nanoparticles: Applications and hazards," *International Journal of Nanomedicine*, vol. 3, no. 2, p. 133, Jun. 2008. https://doi.org/10.2147/ijn.s596

[249] E. Blanco, A. Hsiao, A. P. Mann, M. G. Landry, F. Meric-Bernstam, and M. Ferrari, "Nanomedicine in cancer therapy: Innovative trends and prospects," *Cancer Science*, vol. 102, no. 7, pp. 1247–1252, May 2011. https://doi.org/10.1111/j.1349-7006.2011.01941.x

[250] W. Sigmund, et al., "Processing and structure relationships in electrospinning of ceramic fiber systems," *Journal of the American Ceramic Society*, vol. 89, no. 2, pp. 395–407, Feb. 2006. https://doi.org/10.1111/j.1551-2916.2005.00807.x

[251] C. Vichery and J.-M. Nedelec, "Bioactive glass nanoparticles: From synthesis to materials design for biomedical applications," *Materials*, vol. 9, no. 4, p. 288, Apr. 2016. https://doi.org/10.3390/ma9040288

[252] C. Wu, et al., "Hypoxia-mimicking mesoporous bioactive glass scaffolds with controllable cobalt ion release for bone tissue engineering," *Biomaterials*, vol. 33, no. 7, pp. 2076–2085, Mar. 2012. https://doi.org/10.1016/j.biomaterials.2011.11.042

[253] K. Zhang, et al., "Bioglass promotes wound healing by inhibiting endothelial cell pyroptosis through regulation of the connexin 43/reactive oxygen species (ROS) signaling pathway," *Laboratory Investigation*, vol. 102, no. 1, pp. 90–101, Jan. 2022. https://doi.org/10.1038/s41374-021-00675-6

[254] S. Mashaghi, T. Jadidi, G. Koenderink, and A. Mashaghi, "Lipid nanotechnology," *International Journal of Molecular Sciences*, vol. 14, no. 2, pp. 4242–4282, Feb. 2013. https://doi.org/10.3390/ijms14024242

[255] C. R. Safinya and K. K. Ewert, "Liposomes derived from molecular vases," *Nature*, vol. 489, no. 7416, pp. 372–374, Sep. 2012. https://doi.org/10.1038/489372b

[256] N. Naseri, H. Valizadeh, and P. Zakeri-Milani, "Solid lipid nanoparticles and nanostructured lipid carriers: Structure, preparation and application," *Advanced Pharmaceutical Bulletin*, vol. 5, no. 3, pp. 305–313, Sep. 2015. https://doi.org/10.15171/apb.2015.043

[257] V. T. Arantes, et al., "Retinoic acid-loaded solid lipid nanoparticles surrounded by chitosan film support diabetic wound healing in in vivo study," *Colloids and Surfaces B: Biointerfaces*, vol. 188, p. 110749, Apr. 2020. https://doi.org/10.1016/j.colsurfb.2019.110749

[258] S. Kuchler, et al, "3D-Wound healing model: Influence of morphine and solid lipid nanoparticles," *Journal of Biotechnology*, vol. 148, no. 1, pp. 24–30, Jul. 2010. https://doi.org/10.1016/j.jbiotec.2010.01.001

[259] S. Chen, B. Liu, M. A. Carlson, A. F. Gombart, D. A. Reilly, and J. Xie, "Recent advances in electrospun nanofibers for wound healing," *Nanomedicine*, vol. 12, no. 11, pp. 1335–1352, Jun. 2017. https://doi.org/10.2217/nnm-2017-0017

[260] G. Ajith, et al., "Recent developments in electrospun nanofibers as delivery of phytoconstituents for wound healing," *Drugs and Drug Candidates*, vol. 2, no. 1, pp. 148–171, Mar. 2023. https://doi.org/10.3390/ddc2010010

[261] D. S. Katti, K. W. Robinson, F. K. Ko, and C. T. Laurencin, "Bioresorbablenanofiber-based systems for wound healing and drug delivery: Optimization of fabrication parameters," *Journal of Biomedical Materials Research*, vol. 70B, no. 2, pp. 286–296, 2004. https://doi.org/10.1002/jbm.b.30041

[262] A. Keirouz, M. Chung, J. Kwon, G. Fortunato, and N. Radacsi, "2D and 3D electrospinning technologies for the fabrication of nanofibrous scaffolds for skin tissue engineering: A review," *WIREs Nanomedicine and Nanobiotechnology*, vol. 12, no. 4, Mar. 2020. https://doi.org/10.1002/wnan.1626

[263] K. Ma, C. K. Chan, S. Liao, W. Y. K. Hwang, Q. Feng, and S. Ramakrishna, "Electrospun nanofiber scaffolds for rapid and rich capture of bone marrow-derived hematopoietic stem cells," *Biomaterials*, vol. 29, no. 13, pp. 2096–2103, May 2008. https://doi.org/10.1016/j.biomaterials.2008.01.024

[264] M. Gümüşderelioğlu, S. Dalkıranoğlu, R. Aydın, and S. Çakmak, "A novel dermal substitute based on biofunctionalized electrospun PCL nanofibrous matrix," *Journal of Biomedical Materials Research Part A*, vol. 98A, no. 3, pp. 461–472, Sep. 2011. https://doi.org/10.1002/jbm.a.33143

[265] B. Veleirinho, F. V. Berti, P. F. Dias, M. Maraschin, R. M. Ribeiro-do-Valle, and J. A. Lopes-da-Silva, "Manipulation of chemical composition and architecture of non-biodegradable poly(ethylene terephthalate)/chitosan fibrous scaffolds and their effects on L929 cell behavior," *Materials Science and Engineering: C*, vol. 33, no. 1, pp. 37–46, Jan. 2013. https://doi.org/10.1016/j.msec.2012.07.047

[266] V. V. Makarov, et al., "'Green' nanotechnologies: Synthesis of metal nanoparticles using plants," *Acta Naturae*, vol. 6, no. 1, pp. 35–44, Jan. 2014. Accessed: Jan. 11, 2024. [Online]. Available: https://pubmed.ncbi.nlm.nih.gov/24772325

[267] P. Kuppusamy, M. M. Yusoff, G. P. Maniam, and N. Govindan, "Biosynthesis of metallic nanoparticles using plant derivatives and their new avenues in pharmacological applications – An updated report," *Saudi Pharmaceutical Journal*, vol. 24, no. 4, pp. 473–484, Jul. 2016. https://doi.org/10.1016/j.jsps.2014.11.013

[268] S. Naraginti, P. L. Kumari, R. K. Das, A. Sivakumar, S. Patil, and V. V. Andhalkar, "Amelioration of excision wounds by topical application of green synthesized, formulated silver and gold nanoparticles in albino Wistar rats," *Materials Science and Engineering: C*, vol. 62, pp. 293–300, May 2016. https://doi.org/10.1016/j.msec.2016.01.069

[269] A. Gibała, et al., "Antibacterial and antifungal properties of silver nanoparticles—effect of a surface-stabilizing agent," *Biomolecules*, vol. 11, no. 10, p. 1481, Oct. 2021. https://doi.org/10.3390/biom11101481

[270] Y. Liu, W. Chen, and H.-I. Kim, "Antibacterial activity of pH-sensitive genipin cross-linked chitosan/poly(ethylene glycol)/silver nanocomposites," *Polymers for Advanced Technologies*, vol. 23, no. 1, pp. 8–14, Nov. 2010. https://doi.org/10.1002/pat.1818

[271] G. Chen, L. Wen, P. Zeng, L. Zhang, W. Huang, and H. Wang, "Symbiosis theory-directed green synthesis of silver nanoparticles and their application in infected wound healing," *International Journal of Nanomedicine*, p. 2757, Jun. 2016. https://doi.org/10.2147/ijn.s106662

[272] K. Zhang, V. C. H. Lui, Y. Chen, C. N. Lok, and K. K. Y. Wong, "Delayed application of silver nanoparticles reveals the role of early inflammation in burn wound healing," *Scientific Reports*, vol. 10, no. 1, Apr. 2020. https://doi.org/10.1038/s41598-020-63464-z

[273] M. Arteche Pujana, L. Pérez-Álvarez, L. C. Cesteros Iturbe, and I. Katime, "Biodegradable chitosan nanogels crosslinked with genipin," *Carbohydrate Polymers*, vol. 94, no. 2, pp. 836–842, May 2013. https://doi.org/10.1016/j.carbpol.2013.01.082

[274] B. Stallmeyer, H. Kämpfer, N. Kolb, J. Pfeilschifter, and S. Frank, "The function of nitric oxide in wound repair: Inhibition of inducible nitric oxide-synthase severely impairs wound reepithelialization," *Journal of Investigative Dermatology*, vol. 113, no. 6, pp. 1090–1098, Dec. 1999. https://doi.org/10.1046/j.1523-1747.1999.00784.x

[275] R. B. Weller, "Nitric oxide–containing nanoparticles as an antimicrobial agent and enhancer of wound healing," *Journal of Investigative Dermatology*, vol. 129, no. 10, pp. 2335–2337, Oct. 2009. https://doi.org/10.1038/jid.2009.149

[276] A. F. Engelsman, B. P. Krom, H. J. Busscher, G. M. van Dam, R. J. Ploeg, and H. C. van der Mei, "Antimicrobial effects of an NO-releasing poly(ethylene vinylacetate) coating on soft-tissue implants in vitro and in a murine model," *Acta Biomaterialia*, vol. 5, no. 6, pp. 1905–1910, Jul. 2009. https://doi.org/10.1016/j.actbio.2009.01.041

[277] A. J. Kell, et al., "Vancomycin-modified nanoparticles for efficient targeting and preconcentration of Gram-positive and Gram-negative bacteria," *ACS Nano*, vol. 2, no. 9, pp. 1777–1788, Sep. 2008. https://doi.org/10.1021/nn700183g

[278] E. Turos, et al., "Antibiotic-conjugated polyacrylate nanoparticles: New opportunities for development of anti-MRSA agents," *Bioorganic & Medicinal Chemistry Letters*, vol. 17, no. 1, pp. 53–56, Jan. 2007. https://doi.org/10.1016/j.bmcl.2006.09.098

[279] J. C. Garay-Jimenez, D. Gergeres, A. Young, D. V. Lim, and E. Turos, "Physical properties and biological activity of poly(butyl acrylate–styrene) nanoparticle emulsions prepared with conventional and polymerizable surfactants," *Nanomedicine: Nanotechnology, Biology and Medicine*, vol. 5, no. 4, pp. 443–451, Dec. 2009. https://doi.org/10.1016/j.nano.2009.01.015

[280] Y. H. Lin, et al., "Dressing with epigallocatechin gallate nanoparticles for wound regeneration," *Wound Repair and Regeneration*, vol. 24, no. 2, pp. 287–301, Dec. 2015. https://doi.org/10.1111/wrr.12372

[281] S. Huang and X. Fu, "Naturally derived materials-based cell and drug delivery systems in skin regeneration," *Journal of Controlled Release*, vol. 142, no. 2, pp. 149–159, Mar. 2010. https://doi.org/10.1016/j.jconrel.2009.10.018

[282] M. Ye, S. Kim, and K. Park, "Issues in long-term protein delivery using biodegradable microparticles," *Journal of Controlled Release*, vol. 146, no. 2, pp. 241–260, Sep. 2010. https://doi.org/10.1016/j.jconrel.2010.05.011

[283] G. Gainza, J. Aguirre, J. L. Pedraz, R. M. Hernandez, and M. Igartua, "rhEGF-loaded PLGA-alginate microspheres enhance the healing of full-thickness excisional wounds in diabetised Wistar rats," *European Journal of Pharmaceutical Sciences*, vol. 50, no. 3–4, pp. 243–252, Nov. 2013. https://doi.org/10.1016/j.ejps.2013.07.003

[284] Y. H. Yun, D. J. Goetz, P. Yellen, and W. Chen, "Hyaluronan microspheres for sustained gene delivery and site-specific targeting," *Biomaterials*, vol. 25, no. 1, pp. 147–157, Jan. 2004. https://doi.org/10.1016/s0142-9612(03)00467-8

[285] Y. Chu, D. Yu, P. Wang, J. Xu, D. Li, and M. Ding, "Nanotechnology promotes the full-thickness diabetic wound healing effect of recombinant human epidermal growth factor in diabetic rats," *Wound Repair and Regeneration*, vol. 18, no. 5, pp. 499–505, Sep. 2010. https://doi.org/10.1111/j.1524-475x.2010.00612.x

[286] G. Murphy and H. Nagase, "Progress in matrix metalloproteinase research," *Molecular Aspects of Medicine*, vol. 29, no. 5, pp. 290–308, Oct. 2008. https://doi.org/10.1016/j.mam.2008.05.002

[287] S. Medel, et al., "Curcumin-bortezomib loaded polymeric nanoparticles for synergistic cancer therapy," *European Polymer Journal*, vol. 93, pp. 116–131, Aug. 2017. https://doi.org/10.1016/j.eurpolymj.2017.05.036

[288] D. X. Medina, E. P. Chung, R. Bowser, and R. W. Sirianni, "Lipid and polymer blended polyester nanoparticles loaded with adapalene for activation of retinoid signaling in the CNS following intravenous administration," *Journal of Drug Delivery Science and Technology*, vol. 52, pp. 927–933, Aug. 2019. https://doi.org/10.1016/j.jddst.2019.04.013

[289] C. M. Hussain and S. Thomas, *Handbook of Polymer and Ceramic Nanotechnology*. Springer, 2021.

[290] V. Mittal, "Polymer layered silicate nanocomposites: A review," *Materials*, vol. 2, no. 3, pp. 992–1057, Aug. 2009. https://doi.org/10.3390/ma2030992

[291] M. Alexandre and P. Dubois, "Polymer-layered silicate nanocomposites: Preparation, properties and uses of a new class of materials," *Materials Science and Engineering: R: Reports*, vol. 28, no. 1–2, pp. 1–63, Jun. 2000. https://doi.org/10.1016/s0927-796x(00)00012-7

[292] S. Abedi and M. Abdouss, "A review of clay-supported Ziegler–Natta catalysts for production of polyolefin/clay nanocomposites through in situ polymerization," *Applied Catalysis A: General*, vol. 475, pp. 386–409, Apr. 2014. https://doi.org/10.1016/j.apcata.2014.01.028

[293] A. Hiremath, A. A. Murthy, S. Thipperudrappa, and K. N. Bharath, "Nanoparticles filled polymer nanocomposites: A technological review," *Cogent Engineering*, vol. 8, no. 1, Jan. 2021. https://doi.org/10.1080/23311916.2021.1991229

[294] K. Dean, L. Yu, and D. Y. Wu, "Preparation and characterization of melt-extruded thermoplastic starch/clay nanocomposites," *Composites Science and Technology*, vol. 67, no. 3–4, pp. 413–421, Mar. 2007. https://doi.org/10.1016/j.compscitech.2006.09.003

[295] A. C. S. Valentim, M. I. B. Tavares, and E. O. da Silva, "The effect of the Nb_2O_5 dispersion on ethylene vinyl acetate to obtain ethylene vinyl acetate/Nb_2O_5 nanostructured materials," *Journal of Nanoscience and Nanotechnology*, vol. 13, no. 6, pp. 4427–4432, Jun. 2013. https://doi.org/10.1166/jnn.2013.7162

[296] M. R. Tavares, et al., "Polymeric nanoparticles assembled with microfluidics for drug delivery across the blood-brain barrier," *The European Physical Journal Special Topics*, vol. 225, no. 4, pp. 779–795, Jul. 2016. https://doi.org/10.1140/epjst/e2015-50266-2

[297] M. Vasilaki, U. Zafar, I. S. Fragkopoulos, and I. K. Kookos, "Efficient 1D modelling of hot melt extrusion process for pharmaceutical applications," *Computer-aided Chemical Engineering*, pp. 553–559, Jan. 2023. https://doi.org/10.1016/b978-0-443-15274-0.50088-3

[298] R. A. Vaia and E. P. Giannelis, "Polymer melt intercalation in organically-modified layered silicates: Model predictions and experiment," *Macromolecules*, vol. 30, no. 25, pp. 8000–8009, Dec. 1997. https://doi.org/10.1021/ma9603488

[299] N. N. Nassar, L. A. Utracki, and M. R. Kamal, "Melt intercalation in montmorillonite/polystyrene nanocomposites," *International Polymer Processing*, vol. 20, no. 4, pp. 423–431, Aug. 2005. https://doi.org/10.1515/ipp-2005-0071

[300] P. S. R. C. da Silva and M. I. B. Tavares, "Solvent effect on the morphology of lamellar nanocomposites based on HIPS," *Materials Research*, vol. 18, no. 1, pp. 191–195, Feb. 2015. https://doi.org/10.1590/1516-1439.307314

[301] M. S. S. B. Monteiro, C. L. Rodrigues, R. P. C. Neto, and M. I. B. Tavares, "The Structure of Polycaprolactone-Clay Nanocomposites Investigated by $_1$H NMR Relaxometry," *Journal of Nanoscience and Nanotechnology*, vol. 12, no. 9, pp. 7307–7313, Sep. 2012. https://doi.org/10.1166/jnn.2012.6431

[302] I. L. Soares, J. P. Chimanowsky, L. Luetkmeyer, E. O. D. Silva, D. D. H. S. Souza, and M. I. B. Tavares, "Evaluation of the influence of modified TiO_2 particles on polypropylene composites," *Journal of Nanoscience and Nanotechnology*, vol. 15, no. 8, pp. 5723–5732, Aug. 2015. https://doi.org/10.1166/jnn.2015.10041

[303] A. D. P. C. B. Cunha, M. I. B. Tavares, E. O. Silva, and S. Zaioncz, "The effect of montmorillonite clay on the crystallinity of poly(vinyl alcohol) nanocomposites obtained by solution intercalation and in situ polymerization," *Journal of Nanoscience and Nanotechnology*, vol. 15, no. 4, pp. 2814–2820, Apr. 2015. https://doi.org/10.1166/jnn.2015.9233

[304] M. I. B. Tavares and P. S. R. C. Da Silva, "Intercalaçãopor Solução de Poliestireno de Alto Impactoem Montmorilonita OrganofílicaObtenção e Caracterização," *Polímeros Ciência e Tecnologia*, vol. 23, no. 5, pp. 644–648, 2013. https://doi.org/10.4322/polimeros.2013.047

[305] S. Li, M. Meng Lin, M. S. Toprak, D. K. Kim, and M. Muhammed, "Nanocomposites of polymer and inorganic nanoparticles for optical and magnetic applications," *Nano Reviews*, vol. 1, no. 1, p. 5214, Jan. 2010. https://doi.org/10.3402/nano.v1i0.5214

[306] S. Sinha Ray and M. Okamoto, "Polymer/layered silicate nanocomposites: A review from preparation to processing," *Progress in Polymer Science*, vol. 28, no. 11, pp. 1539–1641, Nov. 2003. https://doi.org/10.1016/j.progpolymsci.2003.08.002

[307] J. Zhao, Z. Wang, Q. Zhao, and B. Xing, "Adsorption of phenanthrene on multilayer graphene as affected by surfactant and exfoliation," *Environmental Science & Technology*, vol. 48, no. 1, pp. 331–339, Dec. 2013. https://doi.org/10.1021/es403873r

[308] B. Li, Y. Hu, J. Liu, Z. Chen, and W. Fan, "Preparation of poly (methyl methacrylate)/LDH nanocomposite by exfoliation-adsorption process," *Colloid & Polymer Science*, vol. 281, no. 10, pp. 998–1001, Oct. 2003. https://doi.org/10.1007/s00396-003-0874-5

[309] S. Suresh, V. G. Krishnan, A. George, C. V. Baku Nagendra S. Rosely, and E. Bhoje Gowd, "Liquid phase exfoliated nanosheets as multifunctional fillers to semicrystalline polymers," *Journal of Macromolecular Science, Part A: Pure and Applied Chemistry*, vol. 59, no. 4, pp. 257–270, Feb. 2022. https://doi.org/10.1080/10601325.2022.2039068

[310] H. Abdali and A. Ajji, "Preparation of electrospun nanocomposite nanofibers of polyaniline/poly(methyl methacrylate) with amino-functionalized graphene," *Polymers*, vol. 9, no. 12, p. 453, Sep. 2017. https://doi.org/10.3390/polym9090453

[311] M. Fazeli, F. Fazeli, T. Nuge, O. Abdoli, and S. Moghaddam, "Study on the preparation and properties of polyamide/chitosan nanocomposite fabricated by electrospinning method," *Journal of Polymers and the Environment*, vol. 30, no. 2, pp. 644–652, Jul. 2021. https://doi.org/10.1007/s10924-021-02229-9

[312] A. Eatemadi, H. Daraee, N. Zarghami, H. MelatYar, and A. Akbarzadeh, "Nanofiber: Synthesis and biomedical applications," *Artificial Cells, Nanomedicine, and Biotechnology*, vol. 44, no. 1, pp. 111–121, Jun. 2014. https://doi.org/10.3109/21691401.2014.922568

[313] S. R. Bolla, et al., "In vitro wound healing potency of methanolic leaf extract of Aristolochia saccata is possibly mediated by its stimulatory effect on collagen-1 expression," *Heliyon*, vol. 5, no. 5, p. e01648, May 2019. https://doi.org/10.1016/j.heliyon.2019.e01648

[314] E. Hofmann, et al., "Human in vitro skin models for wound healing and wound healing disorders," *Biomedicines*, vol. 11, no. 4, p. 1056, Mar. 2023. https://doi.org/10.3390/biomedicines11041056

[315] C.-C. Liang, A. Y. Park, and J.-L. Guan, "In vitro scratch assay: A convenient and inexpensive method for analysis of cell migration in vitro," *Nature Protocols*, vol. 2, no. 2, pp. 329–333, Feb. 2007. https://doi.org/10.1038/nprot.2007.30

[316] J. Shannon, S. Kirchner, and J. Zhang, “Human skin explant preparation and culture,” *Bio-Protocol*, vol. 12, no. 18, 2022. https://doi.org/10.21769/bioprotoc.4514

[317] J. E. Neil, M. B. Brown, and A. C. Williams, “Human skin explant model for the investigation of topical therapeutics,” *Scientific Reports*, vol. 10, no. 1, Dec. 2020. https://doi.org/10.1038/s41598-020-78292-4

[318] D. S. Masson-Meyers, A. Moretti, M. N. Leite, and M. Andrey, “Cytotoxicity and wound healing properties of Copaifera langsdorffii oleoresin in rabbits,” *International Journal of Natural Product Science*, vol. 3, no. 3, pp. 10–20, Jan. 2013.

[319] V. W. Wong, M. Sorkin, J. P. Glotzbach, M. T. Longaker, and G. C. Gurtner, “Surgical approaches to create murine models of human wound healing,” *Journal of Biomedicine and Biotechnology*, vol. 2011, no. 2011, pp. 1–8, 2011. https://doi.org/10.1155/2011/969618

[320] F. Gottrup, M. S. Ågren, and T. Karlsmark, “Models for use in wound healing research: A survey focusing on in vitro and in vivo adult soft tissue,” *Wound Repair and Regeneration*, vol. 8, no. 2, pp. 83–96, Apr. 2000. https://doi.org/10.1046/j.1524-475x.2000.00083.x

[321] D. J. Geer, D. D. Swartz, and S. T. Andreadis, “In vivo model of wound healing based on transplanted tissue-engineered skin,” *Tissue Engineering*, vol. 10, no. 7–8, pp. 1006–1017, Jul. 2004. https://doi.org/10.1089/ten.2004.10.1006

[322] T. P. Sullivan, W. H. Eaglstein, S. C. Davis, and P. Mertz, “The pig as a model for human wound healing,” *Wound Repair and Regeneration*, vol. 9, no. 2, pp. 66–76, Mar. 2001. https://doi.org/10.1046/j.1524-475x.2001.00066.x

[323] A. Abdullahi, S. Amini-Nik, and M. G. Jeschke, “Animal models in burn research,” *Cellular and Molecular Life Sciences*, vol. 71, no. 17, pp. 3241–3255, Apr. 2014. https://doi.org/10.1007/s00018-014-1612-5

[324] T. A. Mustoe, G. F. Pierce, C. Morishima, and T. F. Deuel, “Growth factor-induced acceleration of tissue repair through direct and inductive activities in a rabbit dermal ulcer model,” *Journal of Clinical Investigation*, vol. 87, no. 2, pp. 694–703, Feb. 1991. https://doi.org/10.1172/jci115048

[325] H. E. Koschwanez and E. Broadbent, “The use of wound healing assessment methods in psychological studies: A review and recommendations,” *British Journal of Health Psychology*, vol. 16, no. 1, pp. 1–32, Jan. 2011. https://doi.org/10.1348/135910710x524633

[326] P. Stephens, M. Caley, and M. Peake, “Alternatives for animal wound model systems,” in: Gourdie, R., Myers, T. (eds.) *Wound Regeneration and Repair. Methods in Molecular Biology*, vol 1037. Humana Press, 2013. https://doi.org/10.1007/978-1-62703-505-7_10

[327] P. V. Peplow, T.-Y. Chung, and G. David Baxter, “Laser photobiomodulation of proliferation of cells in culture: A review of human and animal studies,” *Photomedicine and Laser Surgery*, vol. 28, no. S1, p. S40, Aug. 2010. https://doi.org/10.1089/pho.2010.2771

[328] E. P. K. Mensah-Brown, S. Stosic Grujicic, D. Maksimovic, A. Jasima, A. Shahin, and M. L. Lukic, “Downregulation of apoptosis in the target tissue prevents low-dose streptozotocin-induced autoimmune diabetes,” *Molecular Immunology*, vol. 38, no. 12–13, pp. 941–946, May 2002. https://doi.org/10.1016/s0161-5890(02)00021-4

[329] Z. Yang, M. Chen, L. B. Fialkow, J. D. Ellett, R. Wu, and J. L. Nadler, “The novel anti-inflammatory compound, lisofylline, prevents diabetes in multiple low-dose streptozotocin-treated mice,” *Pancreas*, vol. 26, no. 4, pp. e99–e104, May 2003. https://doi.org/10.1097/00006676-200305000-00021

[330] S. N. Leite, A. A. Jordão Júnior, T. A. M. de Andrade, D. dos S. Masson, and M. A. C. Frade, “Experimental models of malnutrition and its effect on skin trophism,” *Anais Brasileiros de Dermatologia*, vol. 86, no. 4, pp. 681–688, Aug. 2011. https://doi.org/10.1590/s0365-05962011000400009

[331] M. S. D. M. Henriques, J. A. Leite, M. D. F. F. D. M. Diniz, and M. S. T. D. Araújo, “Immunohistochemistry pattern of hepatic inflammatory and insulin resistance markers in experimental model of nonalcoholic steatohepatitis,” *Jornal Brasileiro De Patologia E Medicina Laboratorial*, vol. 50, no. 2, Jan. 2014. https://doi.org/10.5935/1676-2444.20140007

[332] J. E. Grey, S. Enoch, and K. G. Harding, “Wound assessment,” *British Medical Journal*, vol. 332, no. 7536, pp. 285–288, Feb. 2006. https://doi.org/10.1136/bmj.332.7536.285

[333] M. C. Robson and A. Barbul, “Guidelines for the best care of chronic wounds,” *Wound Repair and Regeneration*, vol. 14, no. 6, pp. 647–648, Nov. 2006. https://doi.org/10.1111/j.1524-475x.2006.00173.x

[334] V. Falanga, “Wound healing and its impairment in the diabetic foot,” *The Lancet*, vol. 366, no. 9498, pp. 1736–1743, Nov. 2005. https://doi.org/10.1016/s0140-6736(05)67700-8

[335] K. S. Caetano, M. A. C. Frade, D. G. Minatel, L. Á. Santana, and C. S. Enwemeka, “Phototherapy improves healing of chronic venous ulcers,” *Photomedicine and Laser Surgery*, vol. 27, no. 1, pp. 111–118, Feb. 2009. https://doi.org/10.1089/pho.2008.2398

[336] L. de Ávila Santana, et al., "Clinical and immunohistopathological aspects of venous ulcers treatment by low-intensity pulsed ultrasound (LIPUS)," *Ultrasonics*, vol. 53, no. 4, pp. 870–879, Apr. 2013. https://doi.org/10.1016/j.ultras.2012.12.009

[337] D. G. Minatel, C. S. Enwemeka, S. C. França, and M. A. C. Frade, "Phototherapy (LEDs 660/890nm) in the treatment of leg ulcers in diabetic patients: Case study," *Anais Brasileiros de Dermatologia*, vol. 84, no. 3, pp. 279–283, Jul. 2009. https://doi.org/10.1590/s0365-05962009000300011

[338] S. Aydin, "A short history, principles, and types of ELISA, and our laboratory experience with peptide/protein analyses using ELISA," *Peptides*, vol. 72, no. 1, pp. 4–15, 2015. https://doi.org/10.1016/j.peptides.2015.04.012

[339] M. A. Carlson and M. T. Longaker, "The fibroblast-populated collagen matrix as a model of wound healing: A review of the evidence," *Wound Repair and Regeneration*, vol. 12, no. 2, pp. 134–147, Mar. 2004. https://doi.org/10.1111/j.1067-1927.2004.012208.x

[340] G. C. E. Keustermans, S. B. E. Hoeks, Jenny M. Meerding, B. J. Prakken, and W. de Jager, "Cytokine assays: An assessment of the preparation and treatment of blood and tissue samples," *Methods*, vol. 61, no. 1, pp. 10–17, May 2013. https://doi.org/10.1016/j.ymeth.2013.04.005

[341] S. Y. Toh, M. Citartan, S. C. B. Gopinath, and T.-H. Tang, "Aptamers as a replacement for antibodies in enzyme-linked immunosorbent assay," *Biosensors and Bioelectronics*, vol. 64, pp. 392–403, Feb. 2015. https://doi.org/10.1016/j.bios.2014.09.026

[342] S. Watabe, et al., "Ultrasensitive detection of proteins and sugars at single-cell level," *Communicative & Integrative Biology*, vol. 9, no. 1, p. e1124201, Jan. 2016. https://doi.org/10.1080/19420889.2015.1124201

[343] E. Amirthalingam, et al., "Macrocyclic imidazolium-based amphiphiles for the synthesis of gold nanoparticles and delivery of anionic drugs," *Journal of Colloid Interface Science*, vol. 437, no. 1, pp. 132–139, Jan. 2015. https://doi.org/10.1016/j.jcis.2014.09.026

[344] A. Leite, P. Rogério, and J. B. Calixto, "The role of ETA and ETB receptor antagonists in acute and allergic inflammation in mice," *Peptides*, vol. 29, no. 8, pp. 1329–1337, Aug. 2008. https://doi.org/10.1016/j.peptides.2008.03.008

[345] T. Guaratini, M. H. G. Medeiros, and P. Colepicolo, "Antioxidants in the skin: Applications and evaluation of their efficacy," *Química Nova*, vol. 30, no. 1, pp. 206–213, Feb. 2007. https://doi.org/10.1590/s0100-40422007000100033

3 Bionanocomposites in Bone Tissue Engineering

Pınar Terzioğlu, Büşra Mutlu and Şeyma Duman

3.1 INTRODUCTION

Bone is an important organ providing various essential functions as well as playing supporting roles in critical organs [1]. Therefore, comprehending the structure and function of natural bone is crucial. It has a hierarchical structure, and the extracellular matrix (ECM) plays a fundamental role in its composition and function. The ECM of bone consists of both organic and inorganic components that ensure its mechanical and functional properties [2]. Bone is a dynamic, complex, and highly vascularized tissue composed of minerals (mainly hydroxyapatite and carbonated apatite), collagen fibers (type 1, approximately 85–90% of total bone protein), and various cells, primarily osteoblasts and osteoclasts [3].

Bone has a self-healing property which can provide renewal and restoration of its structure by continuous remodeling [3]. This process ensures that bone tissue remains healthy, strong, and capable of supporting the body's mechanical and metabolic needs throughout life. Unfortunately, remodeling of the bone process may not be sufficient to repair large traumatic injuries. When bones are severely damaged due to traumatic injuries such as fractures, there are limitations to the body's ability to completely regenerate and heal the bone tissue on its own, especially when the injury or disease involves significant bone loss or fragmentation [1]. In such cases, surgical interventions are often necessary to facilitate the healing process and restore the bone's structural integrity. Autografts, allografts, and xenografts are used in the field of transplantation and tissue grafting [4]. However, there are some limitations of existing treatments, including improper devices, infection, and longer recovery time [5].

Bone tissue engineering is an interdisciplinary field that combines principles of biology, chemistry, materials science, and engineering to develop technologies and materials for regenerating and repairing damaged or lost bone tissue. This area of research and development aims to provide solutions for bone defects resulting from injuries, diseases, or congenital conditions by combating the limitations of conventional treatments. Annually, numerous bone transplants are performed around the world [6]. While bone transplantation techniques and materials have evolved and continue to improve, there are ongoing research and development efforts to enhance the field further. Researchers are investigating methods to reduce complications for patients by developing innovative biomaterials.

Bionanocomposites are a class of advanced materials that combine biodegradable matrix with nanodimensional reinforcements or additives. They have gained significant attention in various fields, especially bone tissue engineering, regarding their applicability in the biomedical field (Figure 3.1). Different types of materials (polymers, bioceramics, etc.), nanofillers (carbon-based, polymeric, ceramic, metal, and hybrid nanoparticles), and combinations have been shown to be promising candidates for developing bionanocomposites. Additionally, the development of biomaterials for bone tissue engineering is often complemented by the incorporation of cells and biologically active molecules to create functional and regenerative tissue constructs. On the other hand, the bionanocomposites can be developed in various forms, such as aerogels, hydrogels, foams, nanofibers, sponges, and other formats. Hence, it is critical to consider the selection of proper materials

DOI: 10.1201/9781003650812-3

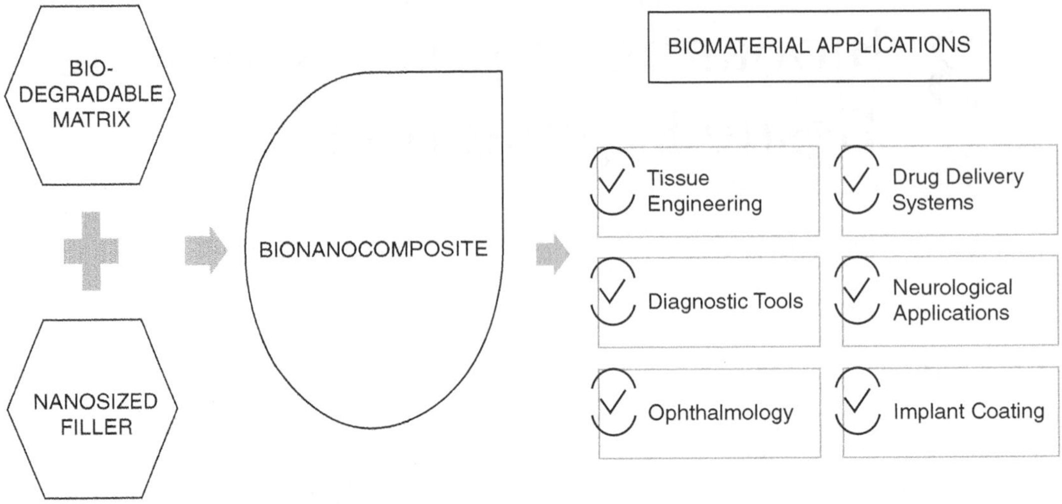

FIGURE 3.1 Some of the biomaterial applications of bionanocomposites.

and designs for bionanocomposites for the success of the application. This chapter gives the details of the reported recent studies to develop bionanocomposites for bone tissue engineering applications. The most widely evaluated nanofillers with several benefits to fabricate bionanocomposites as bone tissue engineering materials will be summarized.

3.2 NANOMATERIALS FOR BIONANOCOMPOSITES

3.2.1 Carbon-Based Nanoparticles

Carbon materials are emerging stars of the current scientific revolution of bionanomaterials in tissue engineering. Several carbon-based materials incorporated into bionanocomposites have been proposed for tissue engineering purposes. This section summarizes the bone tissue engineering applications of bionanocomposites containing various types of carbon nanostructures (Figure 3.2), which can be classified as zero-dimensional (0D: carbon dots, fullerene, and nanodiamonds), one-dimensional (1D: carbon nanotubes), and two-dimensional (2D: graphene, graphene oxide, and reduced graphene oxide).

3.2.1.1 Carbon Dots

Carbon dots (CDs) are the zero-dimensional nanocarbons with sizes of approximately 10 nm [7]. CDs with special properties such as abundant functional groups, biocompatibility, cellular uptake, high water dispersibility, low toxicity, low-cost fabrication, photoluminescence features, tunable

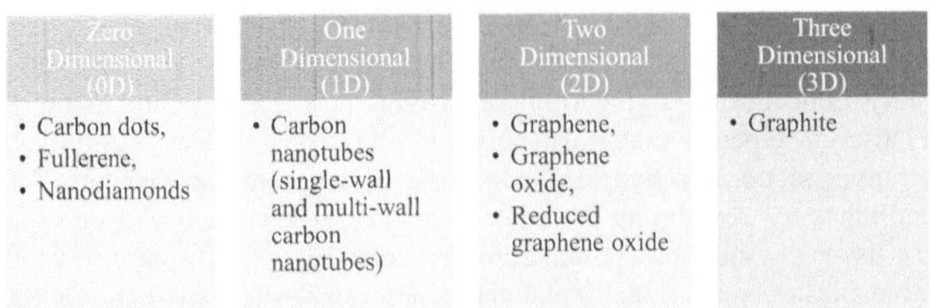

FIGURE 3.2 Examples for dimensional classification of carbon-based nanoparticles.

TABLE 3.1
Carbon Dot Incorporated Bionanocomposites for Bone Tissue Engineering Applications

Nanomaterial	Polymer Matrix	Form	General Results	Ref.
Nitrogen-doped carbon dots	Oxidized alginate/ gelatin	Hydrogel	Higher mechanical properties	[12]
Pectin microparticles loaded carbon dots conjugated with BMP-2	Elastin/hyaluronic acid/gelatin	Hydrogel	Promising bioimaging agents for growth factor delivery	[8]
Carbon quantum dots	Captopril-loaded polycaprolactone	Electrospun nanocomposite	Increase in the proliferation of cells and ALP activity	[13]
Carboxylic carbon quantum dot	PLA	3D-printed scaffolds	Enhanced osteoblast differentiation and bone mineralization	[14]
Graphene quantum dots	Bacterial cellulose	Hydrogel	High level of singlet oxygen production	[15]

surfaces, and ultra-small sizes are emerging nanomaterials in the field of biomedical applications [7–9]. CDs are generally classified as carbon quantum dots, graphene quantum dots, and carbonized polymeric dots [10].

In recent years, CDs have been evaluated in drug delivery, bioimaging, and tissue engineering applications. The biological application of CDs provides new opportunities in bone tissue engineering scaffolds (Table 3.1).

Carbon quantum dots are especially preferred as a nano-additive due to their hydrophilicity [11]. It was demonstrated that when blue-emissive and water-soluble CDs were used for physicochemical modification of polycaprolactone (PCL), the wettability and biocompatibility of electrospun scaffolds were increased [9].

An injectable hydrogel design for cartilage tissue repair based on the oxidized alginate/gelatin/nitrogen-doped CDs developed by Ghanbari et al. [12]. The obtained nanocomposite mimicked the natural ECM with porous architecture and stability properties. The increased amount of nitrogen-doped CDs in the composite provided higher mechanical properties.

Additionally, the fluorescence and remarkable photoluminescence properties of CDs make them highly useful in bioimaging applications besides bone tissue regeneration. To integrate both advantages, a controlled delivery system was designed based on elastin-hyaluronic acid-gelatin freeze-dried composite scaffolds containing pectin microparticles loaded with bone morphogenetic protein-2 (BMP-2)-CDs. Sustained growth factor delivery, pro-osteogenic effect, and improved biological properties showed that the composites were ideal for tissue regeneration [8].

3.2.1.2 Fullerene

Among various allotropes of carbon, fullerenes (C_n) are the third allotropic form after diamond and graphite that exhibit structures with several shapes (ellipsoid, hollow sphere, etc.) [16, 17]. The spherical fullerene with the formula C_{60}, known as buckminsterfullerene (buckyballs or bucky onion), is convenient for forming fullerene derivatives and high-performance nanocomposites [17]. The buckyballs are the most representative compounds that have recently been evaluated internationally for many applications in nanomedicine. The fullerenes have excellent electrical, chemical, physical, and mechanical properties as well as good thermal stability and stiffness [18]. However, the major weak point of fullerene for biological uses is its insolubility in polar solvents [19]. Fortunately, this drawback could be solved by derivatization strategies [20]. For example, PEG (polyethylene glycol)-functionalized C_{60} fullerene derivative was synthesized by Piotrowski et al. [21]. The water-soluble and non-toxic final product is suggested as a polymer-based bone scaffold for potential applications of tissue engineering.

In current studies, fullerenes were investigated as interesting nanoparticles for bone tissue regeneration, as they can enhance cell adhesion and growth [18, 21]. Tovar et al. [22] reported that multilayer fullerenes (oxidized carbon nano-onions) are powerful candidates to enhance the properties of chitosan/polyvinyl alcohol-based biodegradable scaffolds for potential biomedical applications.

On the other hand, there is an increasing interest in developing bone graft substitute materials with osteogenic activity and antibacterial ability as a local drug delivery agent to treat infected bone defects [23]. Ribeiro et al. [18] prepared a hybrid nanocomposite composed of nanohydroxyapatite (nHA), poly(3-hydroxybutyrate-co-3-hydroxyvalerate) (PHBHV), fullerene (C_{60}), and antibiotic (vancomycin) to develop a local antibiotic release material as a solution for osteomyelitis. In this study, fullerene was specially selected due to its suitability for sustained drug release. The results showed that nanocomposite had a mechanical behavior and structure favorable for cortical bone filling. It also demonstrated no cytotoxicity to macrophage cells as well as enhanced cell adhesion and proliferation compared to pure PHBHV. The developed bone-filling composite will be highly useful for the treatment of bone infections through the controlled release of vancomycin for 14 days. Sukhodub et al. [24] also developed bioactive composite beads as bone fillers consisting of chitosan matrix and inorganic nanoparticles such as hydroxyapatite and C_{60} fullerene. This composite was proposed as a suitable system for prolonged release of hydrophobic Anesthesinum drug for up to 18 days. In another research, C_{60} fullerene and whitlockite were loaded to alginate to obtain microspheres. The consequences showed that the resultant hybrid biocomposites were ideal candidates for bone therapy due to inhibiting the growth of pathogenic bacteria (*Staphylococcus aureus*) [25].

3.2.1.3 Nanodiamonds

Nanodiamonds or diamond nanoparticles are a novel type of semiconductor nanosized carbon materials [7, 26]. Nanodiamonds have impressive properties that make them favorable materials in drug delivery and especially hard tissue engineering applications. Their average particle size is about 4–5 nm [27]. They have chemical stability, electrical resistance, fluorescence resistance, high biocompatibility, high surface area, low or no cytotoxicity, thermal conductivity, and tunable surface structures [7, 26–29]. They can enhance cellular interactions such as cellular adhesion and cell proliferation [30]. Nanodiamonds have good mechanical properties, such as prominent hardness and rigidity [18], which make them ideal candidates to provide mechanical benefits in biodegradable polymer composites.

Fox et al. [30] examined the effect of detonation nanodiamond addition to a PCL matrix to fabricate a biodegradable biocomposite scaffold with better cellular interactions for bone regeneration, such as in maxillofacial surgical implants. The findings indicated that high loading of nanodiamonds in PCL altered the physicochemical features of the composite. The nanodiamond addition led to an increase in the hydrophilicity, surface roughness, and biodegradation of the composite. The osteoblast adhesion also increased with higher loading of nanodiamonds when compared to pure PCL.

Another advantage of nanodiamonds is easy surface functionalization, which allows researchers to obtain products with better properties due to improved interactions between the polymer matrix and nanofiller. Therefore, the agglomeration problem of nanodiamonds can be solved. Ribeiro et al. [31] verified that nanodiamonds functionalized with amino groups in a PHBHV matrix had a reinforcement effect and led to an increase in the flexural elastic modulus of pure polymer (30%), similar to human bones. The nanocomposite was found to be appropriate for bone tissue regeneration and bone-filling defect applications because it was non-cytotoxic and non-cytostatic as well as induced adhesion and growth of cells. In another study, phospholipid was used to modify nanodiamonds to assist its dispersion in poly-l-lactic acid (PLLA). The PLLA/nanodiamond-phospholipid scaffolds showed better mechanical properties, including compressive modulus, compressive strength, and Vickers hardness, than the unmodified scaffolds. The composites exhibited good cytocompatibility in terms of cell adhesion, differentiation, and proliferation, which may open new avenues in applications of bone tissue engineering [32].

To overcome the agglomeration of nanodiamonds without surface functionalization, the particles were embedded into molybdenum disulfide (MoS_2) nanosheets and then loaded into PHBHV bone scaffolds by Feng et al. [33]. The addition of both nanofillers remarkably improved the tensile strength of the neat PHBHV scaffold. Additionally, according to the in vitro cell culture experiments, the scaffold showed favorable cytocompatibility for cell growth, adhesion, and spreading with increased mineral deposition.

3.2.1.4 Carbon Nanotubes

Carbon nanotube (CNT) is an sp^2 nanocarbon material which is based on rolled-up 2D graphene sheets to form a cylindrical shape [34, 35]. CNTs, characterized by their hollow cylinder structure, possess a large surface area, exceptional electrical conductivity, high mechanical strength, and optical properties, rendering them well-suited for a diverse array of biomedical applications. However, the cytocompatibility of CNTs is still a challenge for clinical orthopedic applications [36]. CNTs are mostly evaluated as a strengthening phase in composites for applications as load-bearing material [36, 37]. The mechanical strength of the hydrogels was increased from kPa to MPa by incorporating single-wall CNTs into a chitosan/collagen injectable matrix [37].

In previous studies [38–40], CNTs-incorporated bionanocomposites have indeed shown promise for bone repair and regeneration applications. In the regeneration of large bone defects, porous scaffolds that can promote osteoblast migration and proliferation play a crucial role [41]. Lan et al. [38] constructed a novel porous bone scaffold based on polyvinyl alcohol/biphasic calcium phosphate/CNT using a freeze-thawing and freeze-drying method. The outcome displayed that CNT reinforcement positively influenced the compressive strength of the scaffolds (81 ± 6 kPa) when compared to neat hydrogels (48 ± 2 kPa). The hydrogels containing 0.25 CNT showed good cytocompatibility, confirming that they could be utilized as a beneficent candidate for bone tissue regeneration. Similarly, CNT's addition enhanced the stiffness of polyethylene glycol hydrogels and the initial cell viability of L929 fibroblasts provided the fabrication of a cytocompatible nanocomposite [42]. In another study [43], chitosan/gelatin composite scaffolds were functionalized with multi-wall carbon nanotubes (MWCNTs) by freeze-drying method. The MWCNTs improved the in vitro proliferation, adhesion, and osteogenesis differentiation and mineralization of MC3T3-E1 cells, which could support bone replacement and growth.

There are some studies reported on the evaluation of CNTs to enhance the biological and mechanical properties of electrospun scaffolds [44–47]. Tohidlou et al. [44] achieved a significant enhancement in the bioactivity and degradation rate of PCL electrospun scaffolds with amine-functionalized single-walled CNT addition. The incorporation of CNTs into scaffolds improved the adhesion, proliferation, and differentiation of mesenchymal stem cells from rat bone marrow but also provided an increase in the alkaline phosphatase (ALP) activity. These findings suggested that single-walled CNTs can be used to design bioactive nanocomposites. Similarly, Wang et al. [45] developed a steroidal drug (dexamethasone)-loaded composite nanofibrous scaffold by electrospinning method to promote regeneration of bone tissue. MWCNTs were used as fillers to strengthen polylactic acid (PLA) fiber, while polyethylene glycol (PEG) was added to modulate drug release behavior. Results showed that the mechanical performances of nanofibers containing slight MWCNTs were higher when compared to the pristine PLA nanofibers. The enhanced osteogenesis of rat bone marrow stromal cells and mineralization with the continuous dexamethasone release from drug-incorporated PLA/MWCNTs/PEG nanofibers were examined, which was promising for their usage in bone regeneration areas. Following this investigation, Mirmursavi et al. [46] also found out that MWCNTs incorporation into PCL/chitosan nanocomposite scaffolds could increase the crystallinity, resulting in an enhanced bioactivity and stability in phosphate-buffered saline (PBS) proportional to natural cartilage healing rate. The electrospun scaffold containing 0.5% wt. MWCNTs is suggested for high load-bearing long-term bone healing applications such as articular cartilage due to tensile strength (30 MPa) and no cytotoxicity of composite.

The functionalization of 3D-printed scaffolds with conductive CNTs is an innovative approach with a wide range of potential applications, especially in tissue engineering and regenerative medicine. Liu et al. [39] developed 3D-printed poly(propylene fumarate) scaffolds containing CNTs. To enhance the cytocompatibility of biomaterial, the conductive CNTs were functionalized with water-soluble single-stranded deoxyribonucleic acid (ssDNA). The influence of CNT functionalization on the morphology, biocompatibility, cell differentiation, and proliferation of 3D-printed scaffolds. The authors found that scaffolds functionalized with ssDNA-CNT nano-complex improved ALP activity, osteocalcin amount, and the Runx2 gene expression in pre-osteoblast cells, thus verifying cellular osteogenic differentiation. It was reported that electrical stimulation also enhanced the compatibility and impressively promoted proliferation and differentiation of pre-osteoblast cells. Furthermore, Huang et al. [48] 3D printed PCL-based hierarchical scaffolds containing aligned MWCNTs and nano-hydroxyapatite (nHA), mimicking the bone composition and structure. The MWCNTs were chosen as additives to mimic the highly aligned fibril collagens. The addition of both nanofillers positively influenced the mechanical features and cellular activities. The results demonstrated that MWCNTs had a significant effect on the enhancement of osteogenic differentiation by the promotion of ALP, collagen, and osteocalcin expressions.

A bionanocomposite based on poly(3-hydroxybutyrate)/chitosan containing MWCNTs was applied as a coating on nano-bioglass-titania scaffolds. MWCNTs showed a dominant effect on the improvement of electrical conductivity and mechanical properties of scaffolds. The bioactivity tests of coated scaffolds showed that more proliferation, MG-63 cell viability, and ALP secretion occurred as compared to pure ones [49].

In addition, there are reports on the favorable *in vivo* results of CNT-containing bionanocomposite scaffolds paving the way for commercialization and future clinical applications [50–53].

3.2.1.5 Graphene

Graphene is indeed a remarkable and relatively new material with unique properties. Comprising a two-dimensional honeycomb lattice structure, it consists of a solitary layer of carbon atoms bonded through sp^2 hybridization [54]. It is one of the thinnest and strongest materials known to humankind [55]. Graphene's special two-dimensional lattice structure plays a pivotal role in determining its remarkable properties such as exceptional mechanical strength, ease of functionalization, excellent thermal and electrical conductivity, and its potential for applications in the biomedical field. Particularly, its good biocompatibility and osteogenic abilities along with its outstanding Young's modulus and high fracture strength make it a favorable filler candidate for bone regeneration composites [54, 56]. In addition, one of the advantages of graphene and graphene-based materials is their large specific surface area, which allows for interactions with biomolecules [55]. It is worth mentioning that graphene also shows antibacterial properties by exhibiting electrostatic interactions with bacterial cell walls, which can disrupt the cell membrane and lead to bacterial degradation [57]. Stevanovic et al. [58] assessed graphene's potential to develop an antibacterial drug-eluting composite coating for titanium that consisted of chitosan, hydroxyapatite, and an antibiotic (gentamicin). Large specific areas of graphene provided good interactions and strong bonding with the polymer matrix. The final composite could be suitable to prevent implant-associated infections in hard tissue engineering applications.

The choice of convenient materials for the development of 3D porous scaffolds is a critical and fundamental aspect of bone tissue engineering. An experiment conducted by Huang and coworkers [59] demonstrated that graphene enhanced the mechanical characteristics of the PCL porous scaffold. The presence of graphene changed the hydrophobic surface of the biocomposite to hydrophilic. Graphene, especially when loaded at higher ratios, increased the attachment and proliferation of osteoblast-like MG-63 cells on scaffolds, according to the in vitro results of MTT and ALP assays, respectively.

Exploring the integration of electrical stimulation with 3D-printed scaffolds made from graphene for bone regeneration represents an exciting area of research. The combination of graphene-based

3D-printed scaffolds and electrical stimulation holds the potential to accelerate bone regeneration in cases of bone defects, fractures, or other orthopedic conditions. For this purpose, Wang et al. [60] investigated the in vitro and in vivo properties of 3D-printed scaffolds based on PCL and graphene. The in vitro studies highlighted that the prepared osteoconductive grafts could stimulate cell proliferation and reduce immune response. The results of the in vivo studies focused on treating a critical-size calvaria defect in a rat model with and without microelectrical stimulation and also showed that PCL/graphene-based composites improved the formation of new tissue as well as modulated bone remodeling phase, resulting in well-organized tissue deposition. A follow-up study by Wang et al. [61] reported the evaluation of nitrogen-doped graphene for the fabrication of 3D PCL-based electro-active scaffolds. Nitrogen-doped graphene was selected due to having superior electrical conductivity and better surface hydrophilicity compared to neat graphene, which leads to higher biological performance, enhancement of cell-cell signaling, and cell-material interactions. The results were encouraging because better cell attachment and cell spreading were achieved for lower nitrogen-doped graphene-added scaffolds, which could minimize the dose-dependent cytotoxicity of graphene.

3.2.1.6 Graphene Oxide

Graphene oxide (GO) is a derivative of graphene that is primarily composed of carbon, oxygen, and hydrogen atoms. It is produced by the oxidation of graphite, resulting in the introduction of various oxygen-containing functional groups to the graphene structure. These functional groups can include epoxide (C-O-C), hydroxyl (OH), carboxyl (COOH), carbonyl (C=O), ketone, and diol groups [62, 63]. The presence of these functional groups in the graphene oxide structure leads to its enhanced reactivity, solubility in water, potential for functionalization, and matrix-filler phase interactions. Graphene oxide is preferred in the design of scaffolds for bone tissue engineering applications due to its unique characteristics, including the capability of osteoconduction and osteoinduction that can provide a scaffold for bone ingrowth and promote the formation of new bone tissue [62, 64]. The large specific surface area and oxygen-containing functional groups in GO can be leveraged to improve the biomineralization process [64].

Various studies showed the potential of GO-incorporated polymeric scaffolds for bone tissue engineering applications. GO was evaluated in chitosan [65–68], chitosan methacrylate [69], collagen [70], fibrin [71], gellan gum [72], poly(propylene fumarate) [73], PCL [74–76], silk fibroin [77, 78], agarose/chitosan [79], chitosan/oxidized hyaluronic acid [80], gelatin/alginate [63], and polyhydroxybutyrate/chitosan-based [64] bionanocomposites for potential bone regeneration applications. It was revealed that the incorporation of GO improved the mechanical properties in terms of compressive modulus [70, 74, 76], tensile strength [64, 66, 68], Young's modulus [64, 68], thermal stability [64, 68, 78], hydrophilicity [63, 64, 75], cell viability [75, 76, 80], cell attachment [63, 64, 72, 78, 79], cell proliferation [63, 64, 66, 72, 78, 79], and osteogenic differentiation [70, 74, 75, 80] in comparison with net polymeric scaffolds. Furthermore, some of the GO-incorporated bionanocomposites were found to be biocompatible [67, 69–71, 79].

Furthermore, some recent studies on bone tissue engineering have focused on the synergistic effect of different fillers to find a solution for treating bone and bone-related diseases. Chitosan/polyvinyl alcohol/GO/HA/gold polymeric films were developed by Prakash et al. [62]. The composite film served better mechanical and good antibacterial properties against gram-positive and gram-negative bacteria. The ALP activity results showed the potential of biofilms for bone regeneration applications. In the literature [81], GO and montmorillonite have also been highlighted as beneficial filler candidates for the development of chitosan/gelatin porous scaffolds. Simultaneous incorporation of GO and montmorillonite into the polymer matrix resulted in higher mechanical properties as well as cell viability when compared to only GO-incorporated samples.

Smart scaffolds with drug-release ability have the potential to revolutionize the field of bone tissue engineering by providing precise control over the delivery of therapeutic agents, which can enhance tissue repair and regeneration. These advanced materials are an exciting area of research and development, offering promising solutions for a wide range of medical conditions. Mahdavi et al. [82] have fabricated gelatin/HA/GO scaffolds with the ability to release vitamin D for potential orthopedic applications. The increase in the GO amount led to interconnected porosities. The acceptable mechanical properties and in vitro biological responses of scaffolds according to ALP activity and MTT assay showed that the nanocomposites fulfilled many needs for bone tissue engineering applications. Another similar study [83] has reported the preparation of an osteoinductive drug (dexamethasone) and GO-loaded sodium alginate microspheres as a potential bone graft substitute. *In vitro* analysis revealed that the microspheres showed cell biocompatibility tested using osteoblast-like MG-63 cells. Excellent apatite formation was reported for both alginate/GO and alginate/GO/dexamethasone composites.

3.2.1.7 Reduced Graphene Oxide

Reduced graphene oxide (rGO) is a 2D nanomaterial that is derived from GO through a reduction process in order to lower the oxygen content. rGO is being explored for various biomedical applications, including as a component in scaffolds for bone tissue engineering. Its unique properties, such as its electrical conductivity, mechanical strength, and biocompatibility, make it a promising filler for creating suitable microenvironments to support living cells and promote their growth and differentiation [84].

Piezoelectricity is considered a key functionality in scaffolds that can enhance bone tissue regeneration [85]. Therefore, improving the electrical features of scaffolds is of great importance [86]. Researchers are continually exploring and developing biomaterials that exhibit piezoelectricity as well as many other properties, including antibacterial activity, biocompatibility, and biodegradability, to optimize their effectiveness in bone tissue regeneration. Some literature surveys have been focused on the design of rGO-incorporated gelatin [87], PCL [88], polyhydroxybutyrate [85], silk fibroin [86], and silk fibroin/chitosan-based [89] hybrid biomaterials for bone tissue engineering. The use of rGO in the drug delivery systems for the treatment of osteoporosis [90]-related bone tissue applications has also been noted in the literature. The results were found to be encouraging to use these scaffolds as potential clinical candidates for bone tissue engineering.

3.2.2 Polymeric Nanoparticles

Polymeric nanoparticles have promising potential in the development of bionanocomposites for bone tissue engineering. Researchers are actively exploring various ways to utilize these nanoparticles to enhance bone regeneration.

Among the polymeric nanoparticles, lignin [91, 92] nanoparticles have been evaluated to prepare different bionanocomposites promising functional biomaterials for bone tissue regeneration. Lignin has gained attention in recent years due to its various beneficial properties: high hydrophilicity, favorable mechanical properties, amorphous structure, adhesiveness, antioxidant properties, inherent antibacterial activity, biodegradability, and biocompatibility [91, 93]. The study of Mohammadalipour et al. [91] has pointed to the significant influence of lignin on the performance of PHB/lignin electrospun scaffolds. The results of antioxidant activity, bioactivity, biomineralization, degradation, cell viability, and proliferation verify the potential of nanocomposite as a biomaterial.

Cellulose serves similar characteristics as lignin, including availability, biodegradability, biocompatibility, mechanical properties, sustainability, and cost-effectiveness [94]. Cellulose-based [94–99] nanofillers for the same purposes have sparked widespread attention. The outputs of the studies confirm that these bio-scaffolds are suitable for potential bone tissue engineering applications.

3.2.3 Ceramic Nanoparticles

In ancient times, humans discovered that they could preserve grains by turning clay into ceramic pots, leading to a settled agricultural society [100]. Over the years, revolutions in the human way of life have taken place with the evolution of operational ceramics such as dielectrics, semiconductors, piezoelectrics, and superconductors. In the last 50 years, bioceramic materials have emerged with the use of innovative ceramics for the restoration or regeneration of defective components of the body.

Generally, ceramics are inorganic materials combining ionic and covalent bonds [101]. Biocompatible ceramic materials, "bioceramics," that are in contact with living tissue in the body are significant bionanocomposite sources for applications in bone tissue engineering [101–105]. Bioceramics can be classified as first-, second-, and third-generation. The first generation of bioceramics is biologically inert and does not react with surrounding tissues and organs, such as aluminum oxide and zirconium oxide. Calcium phosphate, calcium silicate-based bioceramics, and bioactive glass are bioactive ceramics, meaning that provide a strong bond between material and tissue, which were introduced as second-generation bioceramics. The category of third-generation bioceramics consists of mesoporous silica-based materials and organic-inorganic hybrids incorporated with biologically active substances [101]. More detailed explanations of these bioceramics are given under the relevant title.

3.2.3.1 Calcium Phosphates

One of the subcategories of bioceramics, calcium phosphates, has a great resemblance to the mineral compound of the biological calcified tissues of mammals, such as bones, teeth, and horns [106, 107]. This similarity is indicative of the *biocompatibility* of calcium phosphates. Biocompatibility is defined as the capability to present with an optimal tissue response without evoking any reject local or systemic effects. More significantly, some calcium phosphate ceramics stimulate new bone formation by triggering immature cells to differentiate into preosteoblasts. This indicates that the calcium phosphates are capable of *osteointegration*. Furthermore, calcium phosphates also exhibit *osteoconductive properties*, which promote cell proliferation and enable the generation of the three-dimensional structure of bone [108].

Calcium phosphates can be grouped as different parameters. In regards to anion phosphate, classified as ortho (PO_4^{3-}), meta (PO_3^-), pyro ($P_2O_7^{4-}$), and poly $(PO_3)_n^{n-}$, although calcium phosphates are generally used as ortho type. Calcium orthophosphates, which are typically used in the application of bone tissue, their Ca/P molar ratio, solubility, and pH are given in Table 3.2.

In terms of reactivity with living tissues, calcium phosphates are divided into bioinert, bioactive, and biodegradable. Bioactive calcium phosphates slightly dissolve under physiological conditions, increasing the content of Ca^{2+} and orthophosphate in the surrounding fluid. Crystalline and/or amorphous CaP solution precipitates on the nanocomposite and forms a mineralized layer on the surface. Under in vitro conditions, this layer indicates that the material has a bioactivity able to form a direct bond with bone tissue. Also, the process proceeds as a series of complicated biological reactions such as ion exchange at the material and tissue interface, deposition of organic phase, cell differentiation, attachment, proliferation, and ECM formation under in vivo conditions [101]. The mechanism of bioactivity is schematized in Figure 3.3.

Among the calcium orthophosphates, *hydroxyapatite (HA)* is one of the most remarkable for its chemical and structural similarities to the inorganic components of native bone [110–112]. Owing to this feature, HA is extraordinarily biocompatible [113]. The biocompatibility of HA is owing to its chemical composition, which enables it to establish a strong electrostatic interaction with the surface of the protein [113]. In addition, it has high osteoconductive and osteoinductive properties and is the most stable calcium phosphate with regard to temperature, pH, and intravascular fluid composition [114]. HA, which is found in two forms, natural and synthetic, has phosphate groups instead of carbonate groups in its synthetic form. It enables a suitable structure for angiogenesis, less inflammation and antigenic effect, as well as high chemical stability. These unique features of HA make it a significant reinforcement for use in bionanocomposites. According to research, nanocomposites of HA nanoparticles (nHA) promote attachment and proliferation of the cells [113]. Besides cellular activity, nHA provides numerous benefits to nanocomposites in terms of mechanical

TABLE 3.2
Summary of Calcium Phosphates Which Have Been Listed with Respect to General Properties [109]

Compound	Formula	Molar Ratio (Ca/P)	Solubility at 25°C (g.l^{-1})	pH Stability Range in Aqueous Solutions at 25°C
Calcium-deficient hydroxyapatite	$Ca_{10-x}(HPO_4)_x(PO_4)_{6-x}(OH)_{2-x}$ $(0 < x < 1)$	1.67 to 1.5	0.0094	6.5–9.5
Dicalcium phosphate anhydrous	$CaHPO_4$	1.0	0.048	Stable at temperatures above 100°C
Dicalcium phosphate dihydrate	$CaHPO_4*2H_2O$	1.0	0.088	2.0–6.0
Fluorapatite	$Ca_{10}(PO_4)_6(F)_2$	1.67	0.0002	7–12
Hydroxyapatite	$Ca_{10}(PO_4)_6(OH)_2$	1.67	0.0003	9.5–12
Monocalcium phosphate anhydrous	$Ca(H_2PO_4)_2$	0.5	17	*
Monocalcium phosphate monohydrate	$(Ca(H_2PO_4)_2*H_2O)$	0.5	18	0.0–2.0
Octacalcium phosphate	$Ca_8(HPO_4)_2(PO_4)_4{\cdot}5H_2O$	1.33	0.0081	5.5–7.0
Tetracalcium phosphate	$Ca_4(PO_4)_2O$	2.0	0.0007	**
α-Tricalcium phosphate	α-$Ca_3(PO_4)_2$	1.5	0.0025	**
β-Tricalcium phosphate	β-$Ca_3(PO_4)_2$	1.5	0.0005	**

* Stable at temperatures exceeding 100°C.

** Precipitating these compounds from aqueous solutions is not feasible.

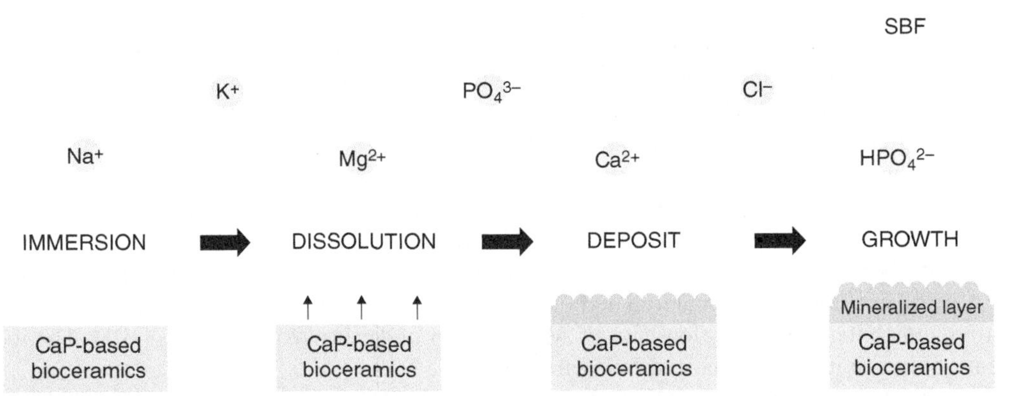

FIGURE 3.3 Schematic representation of bioactivity mechanism.

properties. In a work conducted by Nazeer et al. [115], CS/HA nanocomposites were fabricated by solution casting method, incorporating HA nanoparticles (nHA) synthesized by the sol-gel technique into CS. SEM micrographs confirmed the layered morphology of the composites containing 10% and 20% by weight nHA compared to the smooth surface of the composite containing 5% nHA. The increase in nHA content displayed an enhancement in the roughness, hardness, and mechanical strength of the scaffold. It has been reported that the presence of disk-shaped uniform nHA particles on the surface of the composites can prevent inflammatory reactions, with their similarity to the regular structural features of native bone apatite. Lu et al. [116] also prepared bioactive nHA/hydroxypropyl chitosan (HPCS) nanocomposite scaffolds and hydrogels by doping the nHA into HPCS solution and cross-linking the nHA/HPCS with genipin. In addition, fucoidan (FD), which has osteoconductive and osteogenic potential, was adsorbed to the scaffolds. It was observed that the presence of nHA decreased the hydrophilicity and biodegradability of the scaffolds while increasing the mechanical strength. Also, it was found that doping of nHA and adsorption of FD to the scaffolds enhanced ALP activity in 7F2 osteoblast cells. Mondal et al. [113] studied the effect of three-dimensional printing on the mechanical properties of PLA scaffolds modified with nHA. The results demonstrated that the compressive strength of porous PLA scaffolds with improved surface activity incorporating nHA increased by up to 47.16%. Additionally, HA has been reported to affect the cellular activities of composite scaffolds, such as cell attachment, proliferation, and differentiation. Chaves et al. [117] manufactured magnetite (Fe_3O_4) and HA-incorporated chitosan composite scaffolds functionalized with oleic acid and simvastatin by freeze-drying method. It has been reported that Fe_3O_4-HA nanoparticles with average sizes of 15 and 23 nm increase the thermal stability; however, the presence of HA does not affect the magnetic structure of the nanocomposite scaffolds. SEM analysis showed that the scaffolds had high porosity with very pronounced voids that ensured the functionality of bone growth.

Another calcium phosphate-based bioceramic, tricalcium phosphate (TCP; $Ca_3(PO_4)_2$), which resorbs faster than HA, exists in alpha (α-TCP) and beta (β-TCP) crystal forms [118–120]. β-tricalcium phosphate (β-TCP, β-$Ca_3(PO_4)_2$) stands out with its excellent chemical stability and consistent bioresorption rate [121]. Furthermore, β-TCP is widely used for its properties such as superior biodegradability, bioactivity, and osteoconductivity in nanocomposites [106, 118, 122, 123]. In the study conducted on the β-TCP-incorporated nanocomposites, Baheiraei et al. [124] prepared a collagen/β-TCP scaffold by freeze-drying technique. The results showed that the presence of β-TCP could provide the differentiation of mesenchymal stem cells to osteoblasts with higher ALP activity and mechanical strength of the scaffold. Also, the scaffolds promoted vascularization with good integration with the surrounding tissue. Ghaffari et al. [123] prepared porous composite hydrogels consisting of different amounts of β-TCP nanoparticles (n β-TCP) and dextran by the chemical crosslinking reaction. It was found that the presence of nβ-TCP, which is homogeneously distributed through the hydrogel matrix, affects the pore size and structure as well as porosity and swelling capacity. In vitro cell culture assays showed that the hybrid hydrogels had good biocompatibility. Some calcium phosphate bioceramics, their forms, and general properties frequently used in bionanocomposites for bone tissue applications are summarized in Table 3.3.

Although bionanocomposites containing calcium phosphates such as HA and β-TCP are potential candidates for use in bone tissue engineering applications, these ceramics generally exhibit low compressive strength and fracture toughness. Moreover, the low degradation rate of calcium phosphates is associated with low resorption kinetics. In order to overcome the limitations of calcium phosphate-based materials, calcium silicate-based materials are being investigated as an alternative to these materials.

3.2.3.2 Calcium Silicates

Calcium silicate-based bioceramics have been widely investigated in their application to bone tissue engineering [129]. Calcium silicates stimulate bone regeneration by releasing the Ca^{2+} and Si^{4+} ions. Ca^{2+} ions are the main component of newly formed bones, while Si^{4+} ions play a vital role in bone tissue growth and skeletal development [130]. Additionally, Si^{4+} ions promote the bone marrow mesenchymal stromal cells' differentiation and osteoblasts, accelerating new bone deposition [129, 131, 132].

Calcium silicates are classified as monocalcium silicate ($CaSiO_3$), dicalcium silicate (Ca_2SiO_4) and tricalcium silicate (Ca_3SiO_5) compounds, depending on their Ca/Si ratio. Among them, monocalcium silicate has received significant attention for bone tissue applications with its superior biofunctional properties [133]. *Wollastonite* is a mineral of monocalcium silicate, which is the basic component of calcium silicates. Wollastonite, whose main chemical composition is 48.38% calcium oxide (CaO) and 51.78% silicon dioxide (SiO_2), also contains small amounts of various ions such as

TABLE 3.3
Overview of the Recent Studies Performed on Calcium Phosphates-Incorporated Bionanocomposites, Which Have Been Listed with Respect to the Bioceramic Used

Composite	Bioceramic	Form	General Results	Reference
nHA/chitosan	nHA	Scaffold	Scaffolds included nHA incorporated chitosan showed high mechanical strength	[115]
Dexamethasone (DEX)-loaded BCP/collagen	nBCP	Scaffold	Scaffolds showed interconnected pore structures, high mechanical strength, good biocompatibility, and osteogenic differentiation	[125]
BCP-incorporated chitosan/gelatin hydrogels	nBCP	Hydrogel	Hydrogels showed good biodegradability, osteogenic capability and cytocompatibility. Incorporation of nBCP effect porosity, swelling ratio, compressive strength, and degradation rate	[126]
nβ-TCP coated with poly(3-hydroxybutyrate) (PHB) scaffold	nβ-TCP	Scaffold	Porous scaffolds containing 50 wt.% of nβ-TCP showed good bioactivity and significant increase in cell proliferation	[106]
nβ-TCP incorporated poly(vinyl alcohol) (PVA), polycaprolactone (PCL) nanofibrous scaffold	nβ-TCP	Nanofiber scaffold	Scaffolds containing TCP, PVA, and PCL had ultrafine nanofibrous structures and proper porosity. The incorporation of TCP improved the thermal stability of nanocomposite scaffolds	[121]
nβ-TCP incorporated thermoplastic starch nanocomposites	nβ-TCP	Scaffold	Incorporation of β-TCP provided an increase in the tensile modulus and ultimate tensile strength while a decrease in its deformation and toughness. Nanocomposites showed good bioactivity, excellent biocompatibility, and no negative effect on cytotoxicity	[119]
PCL/PVP and PVA/β-TCP hybrid nanofiber scaffolds	β-TCP	Nanofiber scaffold	Hybrid nanofibers containing PCL, PVP, and B-TCP demonstrated interconnected networks. The presence of β-TCP provided desired mechanical properties and more uniformly biodegradability. Nanofibers showed cell viability without a cytotoxic effect	[120]
nHA and β-TCP loaded gelatin/carboxymethyl chitosan	nHA and β-TCP	Scaffold	Hybrid scaffolds consisting of nHA and β-TCP had a macroporous structure with high porosity and pore connectivity. The scaffolds showed good biodegradation and proper swelling ratio. Increasing the nHA and β-TCP content of nanocomposite scaffolds enhanced the osteoinduction and osteoconduction	[127]
Zoledronic acid (ZA) drug loaded β-TCP/gelatin nanocomposite scaffold	β-TCP	Scaffold	Scaffold consisting of zoledronic acid loaded with gelatin/β-TCP had spherical morphology with interconnected pores and desired porosity. Also, the scaffolds showed biocompatibility without cytotoxicity. Incorporation of the higher nβ-TCP amount increased the rate of cell proliferation. The in vivo evaluation revealed the formation of cancellous bone	[128]

Fe^{2+}, Mg^{2+}, and Mn^{2+} [134, 135]. It is divided into two polymorphic forms depending on the change of temperature: high-temperature phase (pseudowollastonite, α-$CaSiO_3$) and low-temperature phase (beta wollastonite, β-$CaSiO_3$). α-$CaSiO_3$ forms at high temperatures exceeding 1125–1436°C, while β-$CaSiO_3$ forms at low temperatures not exceeding 1125°C [135].

On the other hand, calcium silicates with further improved performance are being investigated by doping trace elements such as Mg (magnesium), Zn (zinc), and Zr (zirconium) into the crystal structure of the calcium silicate system [136]. The most commonly used trace elements incorporated in silicate-based bioceramics are akermanite, baghdadite, bredigite, diopside, hardystonite, merwinite, and monticellite [137].

Mg, along with Ca and Si, which are important for the mammalian body, affects skeletal metabolism by stimulating cell growth and proliferation. Additionally, Mg is responsible for the capability of scaffolds to generate bone-like apatite [138, 139].

Calcium magnesium silicate ceramics have a promoting effect that lets the osteoblast cells adhere and proliferate [130, 140, 141]. The stimulation effect occurs through the release of Ca, Mg, and Si ions. However, Si and Mg ions have a more positive effect on the differentiation of cells than Ca ions. Moreover, calcium magnesium silicates exhibit enhanced mechanical strength and a slower dissolution rate than the other calcium silicates. This is occasioned by the difference between Mg-O and Ca-O bond energies. Ceramics with high bond energy exhibit a more stable crystal structure, slower degradation, and improved mechanical properties [133].

Diopside ($CaMgSi_2O_6$), a member of calcium magnesium silicates, shows greater mechanical properties compared to HA and other silicate minerals [133, 142–144]. Shemshad et al. reported that bending strength and fracture toughness of diopside are importantly higher than HA [138]. In this context, the incorporation of diopside into HA can lead to improvement in the low mechanical strength of HA [142]. Hosseini et al. have shown that the inclusion of various amounts of diopside nanopowder in PCL, not only notably improved tensile strength and elastic modulus but also significantly increased proliferation and spreading of SAOS-II cells on bioactive nanocomposite scaffolds [145]. Ba et al. [146] fabricated porous composite scaffolds containing diopside bioglass (nDPB) and gliadins (GL) by solution compressing and particle leaching methods. The outcomes demonstrated that the incorporation of 30 wt % of nanoporous nDPB improved biocompatibility and new bone formation ability.

Another calcium magnesium silicate ceramic, *akermanite* ($Ca_2MgSi_2O_7$), shows good stability regarding the degradation rate, and controllable and superior mechanical properties [130, 147–149]. The releasing of Mg, Si, and Ca ions in akermanite allows for the differentiation of stem cells to osteoblasts and enhances the proliferation and osteogenic phenotype maintenance of mature osteoblasts [140]. In a study conducted on in vitro biological properties of akermanite incorporated in the nanocomposite scaffold, an increase in the concentrations of akermanite nanoparticles enhanced the proliferation, growth, and viability of the MG-63 cell line. Moreover, it is stated that the presence of akermanite in the scaffold was important to increase the activity of ALP and calcium deposition [140]. Furthermore, it is found that doping akermanite nanoparticles to the PLA matrix allows for an enhancement in the mechanical strength of the nanocomposite scaffolds [150]. Arastouei et al. [151] produced PLA-based nanocomposite scaffolds using FDM technology with akermanite nanoparticles. Mechanical test results showed that the compressive strength of the nanocomposite scaffold containing 20% akermanite by weight increased to 33.8 MPa compared to the compressive strength of the pure PLA scaffold, which was 24.9 MPa. The scaffolds with interconnected pores that would be suitable for the penetration of oxygen and nutrients and the removal of wastes from the tissue were confirmed by SEM analysis. Furthermore, the bioactivity of the nanocomposite scaffolds determined by soaking in Simulated Body Fluid (SBF) for approximately 1 month confirmed that the addition of akermanite nanoparticles increased the bioactivity.

Similarly, *monticellite* has the biological properties, for instance, ability to form apatite in SBF, proliferation and adhesion of osteoblast, and superior mechanical strength. Askari et al. [152] reported that the nanocomposite powders containing akermanite and monticellite showed that cell viability of 1.5 times the control value as a result of biological characterizations. They also stated that particles with crystallite sizes of 58 and 49 nm increased by 4 and 2 times the control value of nanocomposite powders, respectively, according to the ALP activity results obtained under 2- and 3-dimensional conditions. Other calcium magnesium silicates consisting of bredigite and merwinite ceramics have also been investigated.

On the other hand, zinc (Zn), as well as Ca, Si, and Mg, is a significant trace element in the human body [133, 137]. Zn plays a vital role in bone growth, and it has a positive effect on osteoblast proliferation and ALP activity [133]. *Hardystonite* ($Ca_2ZnSi_2O_7$), formed by adding Zn into the Ca-Si system, is a calcium zinc silicate mineral. Hardystonite has high potential for nanocomposites used in bone tissue applications due to its favorable mechanical properties, degradation rate, and good bioactivity. Dehghanpour et al. [153] reported that the presence of the hardystonite particles significantly affects the porosity volume, hydrophilicity, biodegradability, cellular behavior, and mechanical properties of the PCL/hardystonite nanocomposite fibrous scaffolds. Hadisi et al. [154] showed that the addition of hardystonite into the silk fibroin/gentamicin nanofibrous mats improved the cell attachment and proliferation in osteoblast cell lines.

Baghdadite ($Ca_3ZrSi_2O_9$) is a calcium silicate ceramic containing zirconium that is suitable for building nanocomposites for bone tissue engineering applications. Compared to HA, this material shows promise due to its outstanding mechanical features, bioactivity both in vitro and in vivo, biocompatibility, resorbability, and enhanced cell interaction [152]. Some calcium silicate bioceramics, their forms, and general properties frequently used in bionanocomposites for bone tissue applications are summarized in Table 3.4.

3.2.3.3 Bioactive Glass

Among the inorganic bioactive ceramics, bioactive glass is a suitable reinforcement that can be added to the matrix to generate bionanocomposites for bone tissue applications [162]. Bioactive glass is named 45S5 and denominated by its commercial name, Bioglass®, which was discovered by Hench in 1969 [163]. It contains a SiO_2–CaO–P_2O_5 network [163, 164]. The key compositional characteristics of the bioactivity of this ceramic are low SiO_2, high Na_2O, CaO content, and high CaO/P_2O_5 ratio in this network. The mechanism of bioactivity of bioglass has been ascribed to the generation of a carbonate-substituted hydroxyapatite-like layer on the surface to be in touch with the body fluid, as with other bioactive ceramics [165]. Bioactive glass exhibits biodegradable, osteoinductive, and osteoconductive properties as well as the capability to improve strong interfacial bonds with the surrounding tissues [166–168] Furthermore, it has enhanced bioactivity and stimulates bone regeneration compared to CaP-based bioceramics [162, 167–169]. Moreira et al. [170] studied the in vitro and in vivo biological properties of nanocomposite hydrogels containing bioactive glass-incorporated chitosan/gelatin. In vitro analyses showed that the bioactive glass content of hydrogels increased the viability of encapsulated rat bone marrow mesenchymal stem cells. The presence of bioglass revealed the formation of an apatite layer, indicating bioactivity. Moreover, nanocomposites have been shown to be promising for use in 3D cultures of bone tissue cells in in vivo applications [170]. Kazemi et al. [166] evaluated the osteogenic potential of nanocomposite scaffolds containing different amounts of strontium (Sr) substituted β-TCP and bioactive glass (BG). The chosen sample of 50Sr-TCP/50BG exhibited better in vitro osteoinductive properties and in vivo bone formation capability [166]. Recent studies on bioactive glass ceramics-containing bionanocomposites are given in Table 3.5.

3.2.4 Metal and Metal Oxide Nanoparticles

In recent decades, nanoparticles made of gold, silver, and nickel have gained significant attention for their potential applications in wound drug delivery, biosensors, dressings, bio-imaging, cellular targeting, and tissue engineering, particularly for bone [182–186]. Unique properties of gold nanoparticles, such as ease of synthesis and handling, high X-ray absorption, high thiol, disulfide, and amine

TABLE 3.4
Overview of the Recent Studies Performed on Calcium Silicates Incorporated-Bionanocomposites Which Have Been Listed with Respect to the Bioceramic Used

Composite	Bioceramic	Form	General Results	Reference
Magnetic nanoparticles (MNPs) loaded Bioglass/Wollastonite	Wollastonite	Scaffold	Scaffolds containing 10 wt % MNPs offer a better apatite formation in SBF while those containing 15 wt % had the best mechanical properties. The pore structure is similar to the native bone increasing to 180 μm as the amount of MNPs increases	[155]
Graphene nanosheets doped wollastonite/ sodium alginate	Wollastonite	Scaffold	Scaffolds containing 1 wt % graphene nanosheet exhibited suitable mechanical and biological characteristics	[156]
Magnetite NPs-doped bredigite	Bredigite	Scaffold	Scaffolds containing a lower amount of CuO-NP were degraded, while the higher amount of CuO-NP had better chemical stability	[157]
Akermanite and monticellite nanocomposite powder	Akermanite, monticellite	Powder	Bionanocomposite powder containing akermanite and monticellite shows G-292 cell viability 1.5 times the control value, increased ECM expression, and increased ALP activity	[152]
Akermanite-coated electroconductive PLA scaffold	Akermanite	Scaffold	Composite scaffold containing 10 wt % akermanite had better mechanical strength and a favorable porosity for cell attachment	[158]
HA/diopside scaffolds	Diopside	Scaffold	The optimal scaffold which contains 20 wt % of diopside shows high porosity and compressive strength	[139]
Hardystonite-diopside porous scaffolds modified by polycaporolacton fumarate coating	Hardystonite-diopside	Scaffold	Scaffolds composed of hardystonite with 15 wt % diopside and 6 w/v % polymer polycaprolacton fumarate (PCLF) exhibit noteworthy bioactivity. Good biocompatibility mean pore size, porosity, and mechanical features are in the appropriate range for trabecular bone	[159]
Hardystonite and diopside (HT-Di) scaffolds	Hardystonite and diopside	Scaffold	Scaffold containing 12.5 wt % of diopside demonstrated commendable mechanical properties, exceptional bioactivity, and biocompatibility	[144]
Natural HA- nano-diopside/forstrite	Diopside/ forsterite	Coating (film)	Scaffold has a highly porous structure, interconnected porosity, highly mechanical properties, and excellent bioactivity	[143]
Magnesium-aluminum-zinc alloy (AZ91) coated with diopside, bredigite, and fluoridated hydroxyapatite (FHA)	Diopside, bredigite	Coating (film)	Nanocomposite coating significantly reduced the corrosion rate and improved the bioactivity of the biodegradable AZ91 Mg implant	[160]
Diopside/HA biocomposite scaffolds	Diopside	Scaffold	Scaffolds show enhanced mechanical strength, good bioactivity, and an acceptable degradation rate	[142]
Hardystonite/BCP scaffold	Hardystonite	Scaffold	Increasing the hardystonite content enhanced the mechanical properties, bioactivity, and biodegradability. The scaffolds containing 30 wt % of hardystonite had cellular activity compared to the BCP scaffold.	[137]
Hardystonite/fluorapatite nanocomposite scaffold	Hardystonite	Scaffold	Scaffolds had a porous structure with interconnected pores, desirable mechanical properties, and proper bioactivity	[161]

TABLE 3.5
Overview of Recent Studies Performed on Bioactive Glass Ceramics-Incorporated Bionanocomposites, Which Have Been Listed with Respect to the Bioceramic Used

Composite	Bioceramic	Form	General Results	Reference
Soluble starch-coated silver and bioactive glass particles incorporated gelatin Gt/Ag-NPs/BG electrospun nanocomposite membranes	Bioactive glass	Membrane	Optimized nanocomposite membrane has a similar fiber size of bone tissue extracellular matrix of 557 nm	[171]
Amine-functionalized copper (Cu)-doped mesoporous bioactive glass nanoparticles (ACuMBGNs)-incorporated alginate dialdehyde-gelatin (AG) hydrogel	Mesoporous bioactive glass	Hydrogel	Incorporation of bioactive glass nanoparticles significantly endowed superior bioactivity and long-term stability. Nanocomposite hydrogel with ACuMBGNs showed osteogenic and angiogenic effects. It had a controllable degradation behavior	[172]
Bioactive glass nanoparticles incorporated dextran (dex) hydrogels	Bioactive glass	Hydrogel	Composite scaffolds consist of a porous 3D microstructure, favorable physicochemical, and bioactivity properties. Increasing bioactive glass content up to 16 wt % showed improved human osteoblasts proliferation and ALP activity	[173]
Strontium substituted-bioactive glass /PCL scaffolds	Bioactive glass	Scaffold	Optimum scaffold containing 15 wt % bioactive glass nanoparticles showed acceptable degradation, wettable surface, bioactivity, ALP activity, and cell attachment without cytotoxicity	[164]
Three-dimensional (3D) 45S5 BG /β-tricalcium phosphate (TCP) nanocomposite scaffold	Bioactive glass	Scaffold	3D nanocomposite (BG/β-TCP) scaffold shows hierarchical structure with interconnected porosity and extraordinary mechanical strength. The scaffolds displayed cytocompatibility, proper cellular attachment, and a high level of bioactivity	[174]
Bioactive glass/halloysite nanotubes (HNTs) (BG@HNT) incorporated polyacrylamide/poly (vinyl alcohol) (PMPV) based nanocomposite hydrogels.	Bioactive glass	Hydrogel	Nanocomposite hydrogel containing PMPV/BG40@HNT10 showed higher mechanical strength and stiffness values. Incorporating bioactive glass into the matrix, in-vitro biomineralization ability increased while the swelling ratio (%) and degradation (%) reduced. The hydrogels demonstrated enhanced adhesion and growth of human bone osteoblast cells from 3 to 14 days	[175]
Nano bioactive glass/nano zinc-incorporated chitosan (C)/poly(vinyl alcohol) (P) scaffolds	Bioactive glass	Film	Bionanocomposites was non-toxic to the human body and rough and interconnected porous structure. Incorporation of nano bioactive glass and nano ZnO, demonstrated an increase in tensile strength and apparent density while a decrease in the porosity and swelling compared to the control sample	[162]

(Continued)

TABLE 3.5 (Continued)

Composite	Bioceramic	Form	General Results	Reference
HA/bioactive glass and fluorapatite/bioactive glass nanocomposite foams	Bioactive glass	Foam	Nanocomposite foams containing HA/BG and FA/BG, show the ability to have antimicrobial properties and proper biocompatibility	[176]
Chitosan/gelatin/bioactive glass hydrogel	Bioactive glass	Hydrogel	Incorporation of gelatin and bioactive glass increased mechanical properties and cell viability.	[177]
PLA/bioactive glass/ magnesium oxide electrospun scaffold	Bioactive glass	Scaffold	Hybrid scaffold containing PLA/bioactive glass/MgO shows interconnected porous 3D structure. The presence of the nanoparticles affected the thermal properties. Incorporation of nanoparticles increased bioactivity ALP expression as compared with pure PLA	[178]
Starch/aluminum oxide/ bioactive glass/nHA composite scaffold	Bioactive glass	Scaffold	Composite scaffold containing starch, aluminum oxide, bioactive glass, and HA exhibited enhanced mechanical properties, with compressive and tensile strength, and porosity. The presence of bioglass and HA increased the biocompatibility and osteoconductivity of the scaffold. The scaffold showed superior cellular attachment and proliferation on its surface without any toxic effects on the MG-63 cell lines	[179]
Nano-bioactive glass and nano-β-TCP incorporated 1,4-butanediamin-modified poly(lactide-co-glycolide) (BMPLGA)	Bioactive glass	Scaffold	Hybrid scaffolds containing BMPLGA/ bioactive glass -β-TCP showed a network of interconnected pores. The incorporation of nanobioactive glass improved the mechanical properties and hydrophilic ability of the hybrid scaffolds. The cell proliferation of fibroblast was significantly improved	[180]
HA/bioactive glass and fluorapatite (FA)/bioactive glass nanocomposite foams	Bioactive glass	Foam	Nanocomposite containing FA and bioactive glass has acceptable in vitro biocompatibility	[181]
Fluorapatite and 45S5 bioactive glass nanocomposite powders	Bioactive glass	Powder	Nanocomposites exhibited non-cytotoxicity and excellent bioactivity	[167]
58S BAG nanoparticles incorporated poly (3-hydroxybutyrate) (P3HB) electrospun scaffolds	Bioactive glass	Electrospun scaffold	Nanocomposite scaffolds have interconnected porosity. Incorporation of bioactive glass (7.5%wt.) had a higher amount of tensile strength and good bioactivity	[168]

affinities, unique tunable spectroscopy, and distinct electronic characteristics, make them highly promising for a great number of applications [187–189]. AuNPs' antibacterial properties in scaffold surroundings, reduced toxicity, and increased biocompatibility make them a preferred choice for bone tissue engineering. It was revealed in the literature that the AuNPs have good biocompatibility. A study by Pooja et al. [190] showed that xanthan gum-modified AuNPs were not cytotoxic against human lung cancer cells for 48 hours. Yang and Li prepared gold nanoparticles using chitosan oligosaccharide as both a capping and reducing agent and also investigated the in vitro cytotoxic effects on human fibroblast cells [191]. They showed that chitosan AuNPs exhibited concentration-dependent cytotoxicity against human fibroblasts, with cell viability decreasing above 62.5 g/ml. In vitro studies demonstrated that gold nanorods coated with gellan gum were non-toxic, as they had no effect on the viability of cells after 14 days. Vieira et al. [192] further modified the surface of the AuNRs with an non-toxic and biodegradable heteropolysaccharide, gellan gum. In vitro studies have shown that cell viability was not affected even after 14 days of exposure to gold nanorods coated with gellan gum. This demonstrates that these NRs are non-toxic. The impact of gold nanorods coated with gellan gum on osteogenic differentiation was evaluated through the measurement of mineral deposition. It was shown that gellan gum-coated gold nanorods increased the mineralization of osteoblast-like cells, despite a reduction in ALP activity [192]. Besides, gold nanorods (AuNRs) can be used in personalized cancer therapy by combining therapeutic hyperthermia with diagnostic properties, according to Varvara et al. [193]. Gold nanorods coated with gellan gum and lipoic acid were prepared and found to be the most promising for further in vivo photothermal cancer therapy.

To enhance the antibacterial activity of the implant, silver (Ag) is used as an additive in the form of metal or metal alkoxide. A proposed mechanism for silver's antibacterial activity is that the Ag ion penetrates the bacterial cell walls, is incorporated into the cell, and then converts the DNA into an intensified form, which inhibits growth and kills the microorganisms [194–197]. Ag-based scaffolds are materials with higher cell adhesion and spreading high proliferative activity, improved osteogenesis, favorable antibacterial activity, higher cytocompatibility, osteoconductivity, higher osteoblast proliferation rate, ability to bind between oxygen molecules, and finally satisfactory mechanical strength. Even above a certain threshold, Ag is cytotoxic, so it is possible to achieve antibacterial activity without harming the body by adding the right amount of Ag to implants that are capable of controlled release [185, 197]. Controlled release is necessary to avoid overdosage because the balance of toxicity and therapeutic effect is concentration-dependent. Ag is inert as a metal, but it is ionized by reaction with fluid in the wound and moisture in the skin. The binding of Ag to tissue proteins leads to structural variances in the cell wall of bacteria, leading to cell destruction and bacterial mortality. In this respect, nanosized silver metal ions hold great promise as antimicrobial species that, after coupling with calcium apatite, enhance the disinfectant properties of the entire biomaterial with little or no cytotoxic effect on mammalian cells [198]. Due to these characteristics, they are a suitable choice for producing scaffolds in bone tissue engineering. Trace amounts of zirconium (Zr) are among the natural elements used in bone formation. As a trace element, zirconium is considered a biocompatible material with osteoinductive properties. Additionally, zirconium possesses notable characteristics such as lower cytotoxicity, higher mechanical strength, optimal corrosion resistance, and magnetic sensitivity [199–201]. Consequently, this material has potential for use in biomedical applications. In a study, a degradable bionanocomposite composed of chitosan (CS), wollastonite (WS), hydroxyapatite (HA), and zirconium nanoparticles (ZrNPs) was designed and produced by freeze-drying [202]. In this work, biodegradable nanocomposite scaffolds containing different weight percentages of ZrNPs were analyzed from various perspectives. SEM images revealed porous and interconnected structures in the bionanocomposite scaffolds, and it was observed that an increase in ZrNP concentration increased the porosity of these scaffolds. The designed nanostructures had suitable pore sizes for bone cell growth. After mechanical tests were conducted, it was found that integrating ZrNPs into the structure of the bionanocomposite scaffolds (up to 20% by weight) could enhance their mechanical properties. Scaffold samples containing 10% and 20% ZrNPs reached the desired level of bioactivity and biodegradability in PBS solution. The MTT assay results indicate that the prepared scaffold samples do not exhibit cytotoxicity. Furthermore, an efficient and optimized scaffold for bone tissue engineering is the bionanocomposite scaffold containing 10% ZrNPs. Zirconium compounds have recently been found to be effective for dental and medical implants. Zirconium-based implants have excellent osseointegrating properties; furthermore, zirconium-containing materials and coatings have been found to be usable for bone implants due to their chemical stability and ability to form apatite structures [203, 204]. Baghdadite ($Ca_3ZrSi_2O_9$) nanoparticles were synthesized using the sol-gel method from a study conducted by Doostmohammadi et al. [205]. Baghdadite nanoparticles showed acceptable bioactivity properties according to the results obtained. These nanoparticles, which are non-toxic, resulted in significant expansion of bone marrow mesenchymal stem cells, which increased after 96 hours in culture. Furthermore, based on the histopathological results obtained after six weeks, it was found that the bagdadite nanoparticles facilitated the complete regeneration of the bone defects. Doostmohammadi et al. [205] reported that $Ca_3ZrSi_2O_9$ nanoparticles have potential for bone tissue engineering because of their regenerative properties [205]. Zirconia (ZrO_2), one of the ceramic materials, is also a qualifying biomaterial, as are zirconium nanoparticles. Due to its higher mechanical strength, biocompatibility, fracture toughness, and perfect chemical stability, zirconia is becoming a highly desirable material in regenerative medicine strategies, especially in tissue engineering [206]. In bone tissue engineering, osteoblast cells have been found to proliferate and differentiate on this zirconia material without adverse effects [207–209]. ZrO_2 may be preferred as an osteoinductive material, according to biological evaluations of the Sakthiabirami et al. study [208, 209].

Researchers developed a hybrid composite material consisting of chitosan, poly(ethylene glycol), nanohydroxyapatite, and zirconium oxide nanoparticles (ZrO_2 NPs) with both organic and inorganic properties [206]. In this study, differences in the chemical and physical properties of the chitosan-nanohydroxyapatite-poly(ethylene glycol) (CS-HA-PEG) composite were observed and quantified upon incorporation of varying amounts of ZrO_2 nanoparticles (0.1 to 0.3 wt %). Based on the results, a nanocomposite scaffold ideal for bone tissue engineering can be produced by incorporating 15 wt % HA-ZrO_2 with CS-PEG (55:30 wt %). Similarity to the cancellous bone of humans was observed in the mechanical strength and porosity of the composite samples. Antibacterial activity was clearly shown against both gram-negative and gram-positive bacteria. Furthermore, its non-toxicity and high compatibility with human body blood and pH are confirmed by the demonstration of less than 5% hemolysis and positive human osteoblastic MG-63 cells MTT assay results and in vitro cell proliferation. When designing a scaffold for bone grafting, it is important to consider several factors. These factors include mechanical strength to support tissue growth and a well-connected, porous structure to allow for nutrient diffusion. The use of a suitable biomaterial can greatly enhance the stability and functionality of the scaffold, helping to ensure seamless regeneration of bone tissue [206–208].

Electrospinning polymer nanofibers have potential applications in tissue engineering; however, they show a limited ability to facilitate cellular infiltration into scaffolds and are difficult to manufacture. Poly(D, L-lactic acid) (PDLLA) composite nanofiber scaffolds containing zirconia-modified amorphous calcium phosphate (Zr/ACP) were successfully produced by airbrushing to form nanofiber scaffolds [210]. For the production of open-structured nanofiber scaffolds, airbrushing is a new and fast technique. In this study, researchers used airbrush techniques to create bone graft scaffolds made from poly(methyl methacrylate) (PMMA), PDLLA, and PCL. The airbrushed scaffolds were significantly superior to traditional electrospun meshes in terms of cell penetration. A positive correlation between osteocalcin protein levels and higher levels of Zr/ACP was observed in cell proliferation on Zr/ACP in PDLLA fibers [210].

One of the most important trace elements for the human body, copper (Cu), is essential for a wide range of biochemical and physiological functions, including the production of enzyme-active copper proteins, the regulation of bone metabolism, and the regulation of the nervous system. Cu has aroused great interest in bone tissue engineering due to its specific and unique properties, including industrial catalysis, antifungal and antibacterial activity, and the stimulation of collagen fiber deposition and angiogenesis [182, 211, 212]. Cu element can induce mesenchyme cells to differentiate into osteogenic lines [211, 213]. Cu is required for lysyl oxidase catalytic activity. This Cu-requiring enzyme is capable of mediating the final biosynthetic step of keratin, collagen, and elastin, and normalizing bone calcium and phosphorus deposition [214]. Research on Cu supplementation has shown that dietary Cu deficiency leads to a reduction in bone mass and mechanical strength, resulting in fractures. Functional defects in osteoblast cells have been implicated as a possible mechanism for these changes. Thus, adequate Cu supplementation should accompany the bone formation process. As a new alternative, the use of Cu nanoparticles has emerged recently. Due to their high physical activity, copper dosage can be reduced [214]. They have also been shown to have a positive effect on bone mineralization, osteoblastic cell adhesion and proliferation, and finally bone formation [215]. Copper metals (nitrate salts and nanoparticles) have also been observed to have anticancer properties [216–219]. Although copper nanoparticles have potential for biomedical applications, there have been reports of cellular toxicity and intense inflammatory responses induced by them [220]. Additionally, in vivo toxicity of copper nanoparticles has also been reported [217]. Studies conducted in vitro and in vivo have shown that the toxicity of Cu nanoparticles can be influenced by various parameters, such as size, concentration, solubility, and biodistribution. It is important to note that these studies have only demonstrated the potential for toxicity, and further research is required to fully understand the effects of Cu nanoparticles [221]. Sahmani et al. [157] prepared a novel bionanocomposite scaffold consisting of natural hydroxyapatite and cupric oxide (CuO) nanoparticles with different weight proportions and coated them with an ibuprofen-loaded gelled polymer. The material's mechanical and biomechanical properties were evaluated for potential use in drug delivery and tissue engineering applications. According to the mechanical evaluation results, a nonlinear mechanical behavior was predicted based on the mechanical properties. All scaffolds exhibited a thin layer of apatite in terms of cell survival and electrical conductivity. However, the scaffold with a higher concentration of CuO nanoparticles demonstrated a significant increase in apatite formation, a lower degradation rate, and improved chemical stability. In addition, for the lower proportion by weight of the CuO nanoparticles (5 wt %), the release of ibuprofen in PBS solution became significant [157].

Nickel occurs naturally in human blood. Nickel has been found to be present in the serum of normal individuals at levels of approximately 0.25 μg/L, although it was previously thought to be harmful to the health of humans. Nickel toxicity has been found to be concentration-dependent and has presently been added to a list of materials which can be used for tissue engineering, particularly bone [183, 222]. Compared to traditional scaffold materials, nickel alloys have several advantages. These include its multi-functionality, high recovery later loading, comparatively low Young modulus, higher strength, shape memory effect, and super-flexibility. Presumably, the porosity, shape, size, and surface chemical composition of the scaffold surroundings can be controlled through the shape memory effect of Ni-based NPs [183].

Aluminum is a bio-inert metal which gives materials used in biological settings mechanical strength and resistance against breakage. Modified alumina materials, particularly porous ceramic-coated materials, show better osteointegrative properties and are less susceptible to long-term implant failure. Alumina and ionized forms have been used in bone tissue engineering through different chemical production approaches; for example, the biodegradable $Ca_2Al_2SiO_7$ material with reduced cytotoxicity supports cell proliferation and multi-nucleated osteoclast cells (OC) [185, 223]. Cell viability is sometimes compromised by the reduction of pore size from the microscale to the nanoscale. This means that nanopores promote cell proliferation as the pore size increases from microns to 200 nm. In contrast, a study by Karunakaran et al. [224] of cytotoxicity of nanoscale SiO_2 and Al_2O_3 against NIH 3T3 Swiss albino cells found that nanoscale SiO_2 and Al_2O_3 exhibited greater antioxidant activity than microscale SiO_2 and Al_2O_3.

Platinum nanoparticles (PtNPs) are presently used in a variety of catalysts and in the biotechnology, nanomedical, and pharmacological industries. Due to their unique large specific surface area, the use of PtNPs is widespread [225–227]. Furthermore, its alloys are attractive catalytic candidates and have multiple industrial applications [228].

Iron is a transition metal and the fourth most abundant element in the Earth's crust. Nanoparticles of iron oxide are classified as ferromagnets due to their magnetic properties. Nowadays, magnetic nanoparticles in general are very important, and iron is a fundamental magnet used in a lot of applications, especially in biomedical, life sciences, agricultural, and environmental. Lately, iron nanoparticles are increasingly being applied due to their unequaled properties, including surface/volume ratios, simple separation methods, superparamagnetism, and large surface areas [229, 230].

Zinc has been used for many decades because it is highly biocompatible and has unique physical and chemical properties. It is used to alleviate itching and pain in industrial outputs, such as paints, ointments, and cosmetics. Zinc is an essential element for the human body because it plays a crucial role in many enzymes, including carbonic anhydrase and carboxypeptidase. Zinc oxide nanoparticles are being considered for use in various biomedical applications, such as bioimaging, drug delivery, biosensing, and biocatalysis, due to their high biodegradability, low toxicity, and high biocompatibility [231, 232].

3.3 CONCLUSION

In this chapter, an overview of bionanocomposites has been summarized to introduce the advances in bone tissue engineering applications. Bionanocomposites, which combine multiple functions within a single system, are a cutting-edge approach in the tissue engineering field. The chapter presented an understanding of the evaluation of different types of nanofiller-incorporated composites to provide a perspective of their usability in the bone repair and regeneration field. These advanced materials have the potential to significantly enhance patient expectations, reduce complications, and broaden the scope of applications in tissue engineering. However, there is still a need to overcome many challenges, including biodistribution, biotransformation, dose-dependent cytotoxicity, and immune response. It is important to consider that while the reported findings are promising, biomedical applications are a subject of ongoing research, and the safety and potential long-term effects of each bionanocomposite must be carefully evaluated to ensure their suitability for clinical use.

REFERENCES

[1] J. R. Porter, T. T. Ruckh, and K. C. Popat, "Bone tissue engineering: A review in bone biomimetics and drug delivery strategies," *Biotechnol. Prog.*, vol. 25, no. 6, pp. 1539–1560, 2009.

[2] M. M. Stevens, "Biomaterials for bone tissue engineering," *Mater. Today*, vol. 11, no. 5, pp. 18–25, 2008.

[3] L. Guo, Z. Liang, L. Yang, W. Du, T. Yu, H. Tang, C. Li, and H. Qiu, "The role of natural polymers in bone tissue engineering," *J. Control. Release*, vol. 338, pp. 571–582, 2021.

[4] Y. Li, C. Liao, and S. C. Tjong, "Synthetic biodegradable aliphatic polyester nanocomposites reinforced with nanohydroxyapatite and/or graphene oxide for bone tissue engineering applications," *Nanomaterials*, vol. 9, no. 4, pp. 590, April 2019.

[5] M. S. Enayati, T. Behzad, P. Sajkiewicz, M. Rafienia, R. Bagheri, L. Ghasemi-Mobarakeh, D. Kolbuk, Z Pahlevanneshan, and S. H. Bonakdar, "Development of electrospun poly (vinyl alcohol)-based bionanocomposite scaffolds for bone tissue engineering," *J. Biomed. Mater. Res.*, vol. 106, no. 4, pp. 1111–1120, 2018.

[6] S. Yue, H. He, B. Li, and T. Hou, "Hydrogel as a biomaterial for bone tissue engineering: A review," *Nanomaterials*, vol. 10, no. 8, pp. 1511, July 2020.

[7] R. Eivazzadeh-Keihan, A. Maleki, M. de la Guardia, M. S. Bani, K. K. Chenab, P. Pashazadeh-Panahi, B. Baradaran, A. Mokhtarzadeh, and M. R. Hamblin, "Carbon based nanomaterials for tissue engineering of bone: Building new bone on small black scaffolds: A review," *J. Adv. Res.*, vol. 18, 185–201, 2019.

[8] A. R. Keleshteri, F. Moztarzadeh, M. Farokhi, A. A. Mehrizi, H. Basiri, and S. S. Mohseni, "Preparation of microfluidic-based peçtin microparticles loaded carbon dots conjugated with BMP-2 embedded in gelatin-elastin-hyaluronic acid hydrogel scaffold for bone tissue engineering application," *Int. J. Biol. Macromol.*, vol. 184, pp. 29–41, 2021.

[9] H. Ehtesabi and F. Massah, "Improvement of hydrophilicity and cell attachment of polycaprolactone scaffolds using green synthesized carbon dots," *Mater. Today Sustain.*, vol. 13, p. 100075, 2021.

[10] N. Farshidfar, S. Fooladi, M. H. Nematollahi, and S. Iravani, "Carbon dots with tissue engineering and regenerative medicine applications," *RSC Adv.*, vol. 13, pp. 14517–14529, 2023.

[11] S. Kanagasubbulakshmi, K. Lakshmi, and K. Kadirvelu, "Carbon quantum dots-embedded electrospu-nantimicrobial and fluorescent scaffold for reepithelialization inalbino wistar rats," *J. Biomed. Mater. Res.*, vol. 109, pp. 637–648, 2021.

[12] M. Ghanbari, M. Salavati-Niasari, and F. Mohandes, "Thermosensitive alginate–gelatin–nitrogen-doped carbon dots scaffolds as potential injectable hydrogels for cartilage tissue engineering applications," *RSC Adv.*, vol. 11, p. 18423, 2021.

[13] M. Ghorghi, M. Rafienia, V. Nasirian, F. S. Bitaraf, A. M. Gharravi, and A. Zarrabi, "Electrospun captopril-loaded PCL-carbon quantum dots nanocomposite scaffold: Fabrication, characterization, and in vitro studies," *Polym. Adv. Technol.*, vol. 31, pp. 3302–3315, 2020.

[14] K. Dave and V. G. Gomes, "Bioresorbable poly(lactic acid) and organic quantum dot-based nanocomposites: Luminescent scaffolds for enhanced osteogenesis and real-time monitoring," *J. Nanostruct. Chem.*, vol. 12, pp. 951–962, 2022.

[15] Z. M. Markovic, D. Z. Zmejkoski, M. D. Budimir, N. Bugarova, A. Kleinova, S. B. Kuzman, Z. Špitalský, V. D. Pavlovic, D. D. Milivojevic, and B. M. Todorovic-Markovic, "Photoactive graphene quantum dots/bacterial cellulose hydrogels: Structural, mechanical, and pro-oxidant study," *J. Appl. Polym. Sci.*, vol. 139, no. 16, p. 51996, 2022.

[16] B. Poulomi and B. Bhavna, "Fullerene and its applications: A review," *J. Indian Acad. Oral Med. Radiol.*, vol. 32, no. 2, pp. 159–163, April–June 2020.

[17] M. Azizi-Lalabadi, H. Hashemi, J. Feng, and S. M. Jafari, "Carbon nanomaterials against pathogens; the antimicrobial activity of carbon nanotubes, graphene/graphene oxide, fullerenes, and their nanocomposites," *Adv. Colloid Interface Sci.*, vol. 284, p. 102250, 2020.

[18] M. E. A. Ribeiro, N. R. C. Huaman, M. M. Folly, J. G. C. Gomez, and R. J. S. Rodríguez, "A potential hybrid nanocomposite of poly(3-hydroxybutyrate-co-3-hydroxyvalerate) and fullerene for bone tissue regeneration and sustained drug release against bone infections," *Int. J. Biol. Macromol.*, vol. 251, p. 126531, 2023.

[19] S. Bosi, T. Da Ros, G. Spalluto, and M. Prato, "Fullerene derivatives: An attractive tool for biological applications," *Eur. J. Med. Chem.*, vol. 38, no. 11–12, pp. 913–923, 2003.

[20] L. Tanzi, M. Terreni, and Y. Zhang, "Synthesis and biological application of glyco- and peptide derivatives of fullerene C60," *Eur. J. Med. Chem.*, vol. 230, p. 114104, 2022.

[21] P. Piotrowski, K. Klimek, G. Ginalska, and A. Kaim, "Beneficial influence of water-soluble PEG-functionalized C60 fullerene on human osteoblast growth in vitro," *Materials*, vol. 14, no. 6, pp. 1566, March 2021.

[22] C. D. G. Tovar, J. I. Castro, C. H. Valencia, D. P. N. Porras, J. H. M. Hernandez, M. E. Valencia, J. D. Velásquez, and M. N. Chaur, "Preparation of chitosan/poly(vinyl alcohol) nanocomposite films incorporated with oxidized carbon nano-onions (multi-layer fullerenes) for tissue-engineering applications," *Biomolecules*, vol. 9, no. 11, pp. 684, 2019.

[23] M. Chen, Y. Li, W. X. Hou, D. Y. Peng, J. K. Li, and H. X. Zhang, "The antibacterial effect, biocompatibility, and osteogenesis of vancomycin-nanodiamond composite scaffold for infected bone defects," *Int. J. Nanomed.*, vol. 18, pp. 1365–1380, 2023.

[24] L. B. Sukhodub, L. F. Sukhodub, M. O. Kumeda, S. V. Prylutska, V. Deineka, Y. I. Prylutskyy, and U. Ritter, "C60 fullerene loaded hydroxyapatite-chitosan beads as a promising system for prolonged drug release," *Carbohydr. Polym.*, vol. 223, p. 115067, 2019.

[25] N. Y. Strutynska, I. I. Grynyuk, O. M. Vasyliuk, S. V. Prylutska, L. L. Vovchenko, I. A. Kraievska, N. S. Slobodyanik, U. Ritter, and Y. I. Prylutskyy, "Novel whitlockite/alginate/C_{60} fullerene composites: Synthesis, characterization and properties for medical application," *Arab. J. Sci. Eng.*, vol. 47, pp. 7093–7104, 2022.

[26] E. Aram and S. Mehdipour-Ataei, "Carbon-based nanostructured composites for tissue engineering and drug delivery," *Int. J. Polym. Mater.*, vol. 70 no. 16, pp. 1167–1188, 2021.

[27] S. Chauhan, N. Jain, and U. Nagaich, "Nanodiamonds with powerful ability for drug delivery and biomedical applications: Recent updates on in vivo study and patents," *J. Pharm. Anal.*, vol. 10, no. 1, pp. 1–12, 2020.

[28] A. Şelaru, D. M. Drăguşin, E. Olăreţ, A. Serafim, D. Steinmüller-Nethl, E. Vasile, H. Iovu, I. C. Stancu, M. Costache, and S. Dinescu, "Fabrication and biocompatibility evaluation of nanodiamonds-gelatin electrospun materials designed for prospective tissue regeneration applications," *Materials*, vol. 12, no. 18, pp. 2933, September 2019.

[29] F. Pan, M. Khan, A. H. Ragab, E. Javed, H. A. Alsalmah, I. Khan, T. Lei, A. Hussain, A. Mohamed, A. Zada, and M. Z. Ansari, "Recent advances in the structure and biomedical applications of nanodiamonds and their future perspectives," *Mater. Des.*, vol. 233, p. 112179, 2023.
[30] K. Fox, R. Ratwatte, M. A. Booth, H. M. Tran, and P. A. Tran, "High nanodiamond content-PCL composite for tissue engineering scaffolds," *Nanomaterials*, vol. 10, no. 5, p. 948, May 2020.
[31] M. E. A. Ribeiro, N. R. C. Huaman, J. G. C. Gomez, and R. J. S. Rodríguez, "Poly(3-hydroxybutyrate-co-3-hydroxyvalerate) and amino-functionalized nanodiamond bionanocomposites for bone tissue defect repair," *Int. J. Biol. Macromol.*, vol. 226, pp. 1041–1053, 2023.
[32] C. Shuai, Y. Li, G. Wang, W. Yang, S. Peng, and P. Feng, "Surface modification of nanodiamond: Toward the dispersion of reinforced phase in poly-l-lactic acid scaffolds," *Int. J. Biol. Macromol.*, vol. 126, pp. 1116–1124, 2019.
[33] P. Feng, Y. Kong, L. Yu, Y. Li, C. Gao, S. Peng, H. Pan, Z. Zhao, and C. Shuai, "Molybdenum disulfide nanosheets embedded with nanodiamond particles: Co-dispersion nanostructures as reinforcements for polymer scaffolds," *Appl. Mater. Today*, vol. 17, pp. 216–226, 2019.
[34] V. R. Raphey, T. K. Henna, K. P. Nivitha, P. Mufeedha, C. Sabu, and K. Pramod, "Advanced biomedical applications of carbon nanotube," *Mater. Sci. Eng. C*, vol. 100, pp. 616–630, 2019.
[35] N. Anzar, R. Hasan, M. Tyagi, N. Yadav, and J. Narang, "Carbon nanotube – A review on synthesis, properties and plethora of applications in the field of biomedical science," *Sens. Int.*, vol. 1, p. 100003, 2020.
[36] K. S. Munir, C. Wen, and L. Yuncang, "Carbon nanotubes and graphene as nanoreinforcements in metallic biomaterials: A review," *Adv. Biosys.*, vol. 3 no. 3, p. 1800212, 2019.
[37] K. Kaur, S. Sa' Paiva, D. Caffrey, B. L. Cavanagh, and C. M. Murphy, "Injectable chitosan/collagen hydrogels nano-engineered with functionalized single wall carbon nanotubes for minimally invasive applications in bone," *Mater. Sci. Eng. C*, vol. 128, p. 112340, 2021.
[38] W. Lan, X. Zhang, M. Xu, L. Zhao, D. Huang, X. Wei, and W. Chen, "Carbon nanotube reinforced polyvinyl alcohol/biphasic calcium phosphate scaffold for bone tissue engineering," *RSC Adv.*, vol. 9, pp. 38998–39010, 2019.
[39] X. Liu, M. N. George, S. Park, A. L. Miller II, B. Gaihre, L. Li, B. E. Waletzki, A. Terzic, M. J. Yaszemski, and L. Lu, "3D-printed scaffolds with carbon nanotubes for bone tissue engineering: Fast and homogeneous one-step functionalization," *Acta Biomater.*, vol. 111, pp. 129–140, 2020.
[40] R. Lemos, F. R. Maia, V. P. Ribeiro, J. B. Costa, P. J. G. Coutinho, R. L. Reis, and J. M. Oliveira, "Carbon nanotube-reinforced cell-derived matrix-silk fibroin hierarchical scaffolds for bone tissue engineering applications," *J. Mater. Chem. B*, vol. 9, pp. 9561–9574, 2021.
[41] N. Wang, S. T. Dheen, J. Y. H. Fuh, and A. S. Kumar, "A review of multi-functional ceramic nanoparticles in 3D printed bone tissue engineering," *Bioprinting*, vol. 23, p. e00146, 2021.
[42] L. Van den Broeck, S. Piluso, A. H. Soultan, M. De Volder, and J. Patterson, "Cytocompatible carbon nanotube reinforced polyethylene glycol composite hydrogels for tissue engineering," *Mater. Sci. Eng. C.*, vol. 98, pp. 1133–1144, 2019.
[43] J. Xu, X. Hu, S. Jiang, Y. Wang, R. Parungao, S. Zheng, Y. Nie, T. Liu, and K. Song, "The application of multi-walled carbon nanotubes in bone tissue repair hybrid scaffolds and the effect on cell growth in vitro," *Polymers*, vol. 11, no. 2, pp. 230, February 2019.
[44] H. Tohidlou, S. S. Shafiei, S. Abbasi, M. Asadi-Eydivand, and M. Fathi-Roudsari, "Amine-functionalized single-walled carbon nanotube/polycaprolactone electrospun scaffold for bone tissue engineering: In vitro study," *Fibers Polym.*, vol. 20, pp. 1869–1882, 2019.
[45] S. F. Wang, Y. C. Wu, Y. C. Cheng, and W. W. Hu, "The development of polylactic acid/multi-wall carbon nanotubes/polyethylene glycol scaffolds for bone tissue regeneration application," *Polymers*, vol. 13, no. 11, pp. 1740, May 2021.
[46] M. H. Mirmusavi, M. Ahmadian, and S. Karbasi, "Polycaprolactone-chitosan/multi-walled carbon nanotube: A highly strengthened electrospun nanocomposite scaffold for cartilage tissue engineering," *Int. J. Biol. Macromol.*, vol. 209, Part B, pp. 1801–1814, 2022.
[47] P. Zadehnajar, B. Akbari, S. Karbasi, and M. H. Mirmusavi, "Preparation and characterization of poly ε-caprolactone-gelatin/multi-walled carbon nanotubes electrospun scaffolds for cartilage tissue engineering applications," *Int. J. Polym. Mater.*, vol. 69, no. 5, pp. 326–337, 2020.
[48] B. Huang, C. Vyas, J. J. Byun, M. El-Newehy, Z. Huang, and P. Bártolo, "Aligned multi-walled carbon nanotubes with nanohydroxyapatite in a 3D printed polycaprolactone scaffold stimulates osteogenic differentiation," *Mater. Sci. Eng. C.*, vol. 108, p. 110374, 2020.

[49] M. Parvizifard and S. Karbasi, "Physical, mechanical and biological performance of PHB-Chitosan/MWCNTs nanocomposite coating deposited on bioglass based scaffold: Potential application in bone tissue engineering," *Int. J. Biol. Macromol.*, vol. 152, pp. 645–662, 2020.
[50] M. Zarei, S. Karbasi, F. Sari Aslani, S. Zare, O. Koohi-Hosseinabad, and N. Tanideh, "In vitro and in vivo evaluation of poly (3-hydroxybutyrate)/carbon nanotubes electrospun scaffolds for periodontal ligament tissue engineering," *J. Dent. (Shiraz)*, vol. 21, no. 1, pp. 18–30, 2020.
[51] L. Liu, B. Yang, L. Q. Wang, J. P. Huang, W. Y. Chen, Q. Ban, Y. Zhang, R. You, L. Yin, and Y. Q. Guan, "Biomimetic bone tissue engineering hydrogel scaffolds constructed using ordered CNTs and HA induce the proliferation and differentiation of BMSCs," *J. Mater. Chem. B*, vol. 8, no. 3, pp. 558–567, 2020.
[52] Z. Gan, Y. Zhao, Y. Wu, W. Yang, Z. Zhao, and L. Zhao, "Three-dimensional, biomimetic electrospun scaffolds reinforced with carbon nanotubes for temporomandibular joint disc regeneration," *Acta Biomater.*, vol. 147, pp. 221–234, 2022.
[53] E. P. E. Silva, B. Huang, J. V. Helaehil, P. R. L. Nalesso, L. Bagne, M. A. de Oliveira, G. C. C. Albiazetti, A. Aldalbahi, M. El-Newehy, M. Santamaria Jr, F. A. S. Mendonça, P. Bartolo, and G. F. Caetano, "In vivo study of conductive 3D printed PCL/MWCNTs scaffolds with electrical stimulation for bone tissue engineering," *Bio-Des. Manuf.*, vol. 4, pp. 190–202, 2021.
[54] M. Wu, L. Zou, L. Jiang, Z. Zhao, and J. Liu, "Osteoinductive and antimicrobial mechanisms of graphene-based materials for enhancing bone tissue engineering," *J. Tissue Eng. Regen. Med.*, vol. 15, no. 11, pp. 915–935, 2021.
[55] K. Ghosal, P. Mondal, S. Bera, and S. Ghosh, "Graphene family nanomaterials- opportunities and challenges in tissue engineering applications," *FlatChem*, vol. 30, p. 100315, 2021.
[56] J. Cheng, J. Liu, B. Wu, Z. Liu, M. Li, X. Wang, P. Tang, and Z. Wang, "Graphene and its derivatives for bone tissue engineering: In vitro and in vivo evaluation of graphene-based scaffolds, membranes and coatings," *Front. Bioeng. Biotechnol.*, vol. 9, p. 734688, 2021.
[57] H. Maleki-Ghaleh, M. H. Siadati, A. Fallah, B. Koc, M. Kavanlouei, P. Khademi-Azandehi, E. Moradpur-Tari, Y. Omidi, J. Barar, Y. Beygi-Khosrowshahi, A. P. Kumar, and K. Adibkia, "Antibacterial and cellular behaviors of novel zinc-doped hydroxyapatite/graphene nanocomposite for bone tissue engineering," *Int. J. Mol. Sci.*, vol. 22, no. 17, p. 9564, September 2021.
[58] M. Stevanovic, M. Djošic, A. Jankovic, V. Kojić, M. Vukašinović-Sekulić, J. Stojanović, J. Odović, M. C. Sakač, R. K. Yop, and V. Mišković-Stanković, "Antibacterial graphene-based hydroxyapatite/chitosan coating with gentamicin for potential applications in bone tissue engineering," *J. Biomed. Mater. Res.*, vol. 108, pp. 2175–2189, 2020.
[59] H. Y. Huang, F. Y. Fan, Y. K. Shen, C. H. Wang, Y. T. Huang, M. J. Chern, Y. H. Wang, and L. Wang, "3D poly-ε-caprolactone/graphene porous scaffolds for bone tissue engineering," *Colloids Surf. A: Physicochem. Eng. Asp.*, vol. 606, p. 125393, 2020.
[60] W. Wang, J. R. P. Junior, P. R. L. Nalesso, D. Musson, J. Cornish, F. Mendonça, G. F. Caetano, and P. Bártolo, "Engineered 3D printed poly(ε-caprolactone)/graphene scaffolds for bone tissue engineering," *Mater. Sci. Eng. C*, vol. 100, pp. 759–770, 2019.
[61] W. Wang, J. X. Chen, Y. Hou, P. Bartolo, and W. H. Chiang, "Investigations of graphene and nitrogen-doped graphene enhanced polycaprolactone 3D scaffolds for bone tissue engineering," *Nanomaterials*, vol. 11, no. 4, pp. 929, April 2021.
[62] J. Prakash, D. Prema, K. S. Venkataprasanna, K. Balagangadharan, N. Selvamurugan, and G. Devanand Venkatasubbu, "Nanocomposite chitosan film containing graphene oxide/hydroxyapatite/gold for bone tissue engineering," *Int. J. Biol. Macromol.*, vol. 154, pp. 62–71, 2020.
[63] S. D. Purohit, R. Bhaskar, H. Singh, I. Yadav, M. K. Gupta, and N. C. Mishra, "Development of a nanocomposite scaffold of gelatin–alginate–graphene oxide for bone tissue engineering," *Int. J. Biol. Macromol.*, vol. 133, 592–602, 2019.
[64] E. S. Motiee, S. Karbasi, E. Bidram, and M. Sheikholeslam, "Investigation of physical, mechanical and biological properties of polyhydroxybutyrate-chitosan/graphene oxide nanocomposite scaffolds for bone tissue engineering applications," *Int. J. Biol. Macromol.*, vol. 247, p. 125593, 2023.
[65] S. Dinescu, M. Ionita, S. R. Ignat, M. Costache, and A. Hermenean, "Graphene oxide enhances chitosan-based 3D scaffold properties for bone tissue engineering," *Int. J. Mol. Sci.*, vol. 20, no. 20, pp. 5077, Oct. 2019.
[66] M. A. Shamekhi, H. Mirzadeh, H. Mahdavi, A. Rabiee, D. Mohebbi-Kalhori, and M. B. Eslaminejad, "Graphene oxide containing chitosan scaffolds for cartilage tissue engineering," *Int. J. Biol. Macromol.*, vol. 127, pp. 396–405, 2019.

[67] H. P. Zhang, B. Yang, Z. M. Wang, C. Xie, P. Tang, L. Bian, F. Dong, and Y. Tang, "Porous graphene oxide/chitosan nanocomposites based on interfacial chemical interactions," *Eur. Polym. J.*, vol. 119, pp. 114–119, 2019.

[68] M. Tavakoli, S. Karbasi, and S. S. E. Bakhtiari, "Evaluation of physical, mechanical, and biodegradation of chitosan/graphene oxide composite as bone substitutes," *Polym.-Plast. Technol. Mater.*, vol. 59, no. 4, pp. 430–440, 2020.

[69] D. N. Céspedes-Valenzuela, S. Sánchez-Rentería, J. Cifuentes, M. Gantiva-Diaz, J. A. Serna, L. H. Reyes, C. Ostos, C. Cifuentes-De la Portilla, C. Muñoz-Camargo, and J. C. Cruz, "Preparation and characterization of an injectable and photo-responsive chitosan methacrylate/graphene oxide hydrogel: Potential applications in bone tissue adhesion and repair," *Polymers*, vol. 14, no. 1, pp. 126, December 2021.

[70] S. Liu, C. Zhou, S. Mou, J. Li, M. Zhou, Y. Zeng, C. Luo, J. Sun, Z. Wang, W. Xu, "Biocompatible graphene oxide–collagen composite aerogel for enhanced stiffness and in situ bone regeneration," *Mater. Sci. Eng. C*, vol. 105, p. 110137, 2019.

[71] S. P. Mtech, P. Periyathambi, and S. K. Anandasadagopan, "Fibrin hydrogel incorporated with graphene oxide functionalized nanocomposite scaffolds for bone repair – In vitro and in vivo study," *Nanomed.: Nanotechnol. Biol. Med.*, vol. 29, p. 102251, 2020.

[72] S. Zhu, L. Yao, C. Pan, J. Tian, L. Li, B. Luo, C. Zhou, and L. Lu, "3D printed gellan gum/graphene oxide scaffold for tumor therapy and bone reconstruction," *Compos. Sci. Technol.*, vol. 208, p. 108763, 2021.

[73] B. Farshid, G. Lalwani, M. S. Mohammadi, J. S. Sankaran, S. Patel, S. Judex, J. Simonsen, and B. Sitharaman, "Two-dimensional graphene oxide-reinforced porous biodegradablepolymeric nanocomposites for bone tissue engineering," *J. Biomed. Mater. Res. A*, vol. 107, no. 6, pp. 1143–1153, 2019.

[74] J. M. Unagolla and A. C. Jayasuriya, "Enhanced cell functions on graphene oxide incorporated 3D printed polycaprolactone scaffolds," *Mater. Sci. Eng. C*, vol. 102, pp. 1–11, 2019.

[75] F. Rostami, E. Tamjid, and M. Behmanesh, "Drug-eluting PCL/graphene oxide nanocomposite scaffolds for enhanced osteogenic differentiation of mesenchymal stem cells," *Mater. Sci. Eng. C*, vol. 115, p. 111102, 2020.

[76] D. Dias, A. C. Vale, E. P. F. Cunha, M. C. Paiva, R. L. Reis, C. Vaquette, and N. M. Alves, "3D-printed cryomilled poly(ε-caprolactone)/graphenecomposite scaffolds for bone tissue regeneration," *J. Biomed. Mater. Res.*, vol. 109, pp. 961–972, 2021.

[77] L. Wang, R. Lu, J. Hou, X. Nan, Y. Xia, Y. Guo, K. Meng, C. Xu, X. Wang, and B. Zhao, "Application of injectable silk fibroin/graphene oxide hydrogel combined with bone marrow mesenchymal stem cells in bone tissue engineering," *Colloids Surf. A: Physicochem. Eng. Asp.*, vol. 604, p. 125318, 2020.

[78] M. Narimani, A. Teimouri, and Z. Shahbazarab, "Synthesis, characterization and biocompatible properties of novel silk fibroin/graphene oxide nanocomposite scaffolds for bone tissue engineering application," *Polym. Bull.*, vol. 76, pp. 725–745, 2019.

[79] P. R. Sivashankari and M. Prabaharan, "Three-dimensional porous scaffolds based on agarose/chitosan/graphene oxide composite for tissue engineering," *Int. J. Biol. Macromol.*, vol. 146, pp. 222–231, 2020.

[80] S. J. Lee, H. Nah, D. N. Heo, K. H. Kim, J. M. Seok, M. Heo, H. J. Moon, D. Lee, J. S. Lee, S. Y. An, Y. S. Hwang, W. K. Ko, S. J. Kim, S. Sohn, S. A. Park, S. Y. Park, and I. K. Kwon, "Induction of osteogenic differentiation in a rat calvarial bone defect model using an In situ forming graphene oxide incorporated glycol chitosan/oxidized hyaluronic acid injectable hydrogel," *Carbon*, vol. 168, pp. 264–277, 2020.

[81] A. Olad, H. B. K. Hagh, A. Mirmohseni, and F. F. Azhar, "Graphene oxide and montmorillonite enriched natural polymeric scaffold for bone tissue engineering," *Ceram. Int.*, vol. 45, no. 12, pp. 15609–15619, 2019.

[82] R. Mahdavi, G. Belgheisi, M. Haghbin-Nazarpak, M. Omidi, A. Khojasteh, and M. Solati-Hashjin, "Bone tissue engineering gelatin–hydroxyapatite/graphene oxide scaffolds with the ability to release vitamin D: Fabrication, characterization, and in vitro study," *J. Mater. Sci. Mater. Med.*, vol. 31, pp. 97, 2020.

[83] G. V. Yashaswini Devi, A. Prabhu, S. Anil, and J. Venkatesan, "Preparation and characterization of dexamethasone loaded sodium alginate-graphene oxide microspheres for bone tissue engineering," *J. Drug Deliv. Sci. Technol.*, vol. 64, p. 102624, 2021.

[84] A. Raslan, L. S. del Burgo, J. Ciriza, and J. L. Pedraz, "Graphene oxide and reduced graphene oxide-based scaffolds in regenerative medicine," *Int. J. Pharm.*, vol. 580, p. 119226, 2020.

[85] R. V. Chernozem, K. N. Romanyuk, I. Grubova, P. V. Chernozem, M. A. Surmeneva, Y. R. Mukhortova, M. Wilhelm, T. Ludwig, S. Mathur, A. L. Kholkin, E. Neyts, B. Parakhonskiy, A. G. Skirtach, and R. A. Surmenev, "Enhanced piezoresponse and surface electric potential of hybrid biodegradable polyhydroxybutyrate scaffolds functionalized with reduced graphene oxide for tissue engineering," *Nano Energy*, vol. 89, Part B, p. 106473, 2021.

[86] C. Zhang, X. Wang, S. Fan, P. Lan, C. Cao, and Y. Zhang, "Silk fibroin/reduced graphene oxide composite mats with enhanced mechanical properties and conductivity for tissue engineering," *Colloids Surf., B Biointerfaces*, vol. 197, p. 111444, 2021.

[87] D. Jiao, A. Zheng, Y. Liu, X. Zhang, X. Wang, J. Wu, W. She, K. Lv, L. Cao, and X. Jiang, "Bidirectional differentiation of BMSCs induced by a biomimetic procallus based on a gelatin-reduced graphene oxide reinforced hydrogel for rapid bone regeneration," *Bioact. Mater.*, vol. 6, no. 7, pp. 2011–2028, 2021.

[88] P. H. M. Gohari, M. H. Nazarpak, and M. Solati-Hashjin, "The effect of adding reduced graphene oxide to electrospun polycaprolactone scaffolds on MG-63 cells activity," *Mater. Today Commun.*, vol. 27, p. 102287, 2021.

[89] F. Jabbari, S. Hesaraki, and B. Houshmand, "The physical, mechanical, and biological properties of silk fibroin/chitosan/reduced graphene oxide composite membranes for guided bone regeneration," *J. Biomater. Sci. Polym. Ed.*, vol. 30, no. 18, pp. 1779–1802, 2019.

[90] X. Wang, W. Guo, L. Li, F. Yu, J. Li, L. Liu, B. Fang, and L. Xia, "Photothermally triggered biomimetic drug delivery of Teriparatide via reduced graphene oxide loaded chitosan hydrogel for osteoporotic bone regeneration," *Chem. Eng. J.*, vol. 413, p. 127413, 2021.

[91] M. Mohammadalipour, T. Behzad, S. Karbasi, and Z. Mohammadalipour, "Optimization and characterization of polyhydroxybutyrate/lignin electro-spun scaffolds for tissue engineering applications," *Int. J. Biol. Macromol.*, vol. 218, pp. 317–334, 2022.

[92] Md. K. Haider, D. Kharaghani, L. Sun, S. Ullah, M. N. Sarwar, A. Ullah, M. Khatri, Y. Yoshiko, M. Gopiraman, and I. S. Kim, "Synthesized bioactive lignin nanoparticles/polycaprolactone nanofibers: A novel nanobiocomposite for bone tissue engineering," *Biomater. Adv.*, vol. 144, p. 213203, 2023.

[93] P. Terzioğlu, F. N. Parın, and Y. Sıcak, "Lignin composites for biomedical applications: Status, challenges and perspectives," in *Lignin*, 1st ed., S. Sharma, A. Kumar, Eds. Springer Series on Polymer and Composite Materials. Springer. 2020, pp. 253–273.

[94] S. Iswarya, T. Theivasanthi, and S. C. B. Gopinath, "Sodium alginate/hydroxyapatite/nanocellulose composites: Synthesis and potentials for bone tissue engineering," *J. Mech. Behav. Biomed. Mater.*, vol. 148, p. 106189, 2023.

[95] B. Maharjan, J. Park, V. K. Kaliannagounder, G. P. Awasthi, M. K. Joshi, C. H. Park, and C. S. Kim, "Regenerated cellulose nanofiber reinforced chitosan hydrogel scaffolds for bone tissue engineering," *Carbohydr. Polym.*, vol. 251, p. 117023, 2021.

[96] I. E. Carlström, A. Rashad, E. Campodoni, M. Sandri, K. Syverud, A. I. Bolstad, and K. Mustafa, "Cross-linked gelatin-nanocellulose scaffolds for bone tissue engineering," *Mater. Lett.*, vol. 264, p. 127326, 2020.

[97] A. V. Stanzani, A. Giubilini, M. Checchi, F. Bondioli, M. Messori, and C. Palumbo, "Eco-sustainable approaches in bone tissue engineering: Evaluating the angiogenic potential of different poly(3-hydroxybutyrate-Co-3-hydroxyhexanoate)–nanocellulose composites with the chorioallantoic membrane," *Adv. Eng. Mater.*, vol. 25, p. 2200934, 2023.

[98] A. Ali, A. Hasan, and Y. S. Negi, "Effect of cellulose nanocrystals on xylan/chitosan/nanoβ-TCP composite matrix for bone tissue engineering," *Cellulose*, vol. 29, pp. 5689–5709, 2022.

[99] A. Ali, S. Bano, S. Poojary, A. Chaudhary, D. Kumar, and Y. S. Negi, "Effect of cellulose nanocrystals on chitosan/PVA/nano β-TCP composite scaffold for bone tissue engineering application," *J. Biomater. Sci. Polym. Ed.*, vol. 33, no. 1, p. 1–19, 2022.

[100] L. L. Hench, "Bioceramics: From concept to clinic," *J. Am. Ceram. Soc.*, vol. 74, no. 7, pp. 1487–1510, 1991.

[101] M. Vallet-Regi, *Bio-ceramics With Clinical Applications*. John Wiley & Sons, 2014.

[102] M. Vallet-Regí and A. J. Salinas, "Ceramics as bone repair materials," in *Bone Repair Biomaterials*, Elsevier, 2019, pp. 141–178.

[103] F. Baino, "Ceramics for bone replacement: Commercial products and clinical use," in *Advances in Ceramic Biomaterials*, Elsevier, 2017, pp. 249–278.

[104] M.-P. Ginebra, M. Espanol, Y. Maazouz, V. Bergez, and D. Pastorino, "Bioceramics and bone healing," *EFORT Open Rev.*, vol. 3, no. 5, pp. 173–183, 2018.

[105] A. J. Salinas, M. Vallet-Regi, and J. Heikkilä, "Use of bioactive glasses as bone substitutes in orthopedics and traumatology," in *Bioactive Glasses*, Elsevier, 2018, pp. 337–364.

[106] S. Shahi, S. Karbasi, T. Ahmadi, F. Naeimi, V. Goodarzi, and S. Ebrahimi-Barough, "Evaluation of physical, mechanical and biological properties of β-tri-calcium phosphate/poly-3-hydroxybutyrate nano composite scaffold for bone tissue engineering application," *Mater. Technol.*, vol. 36, no. 4, pp. 237–249, 2021.

[107] M. Matinfar, A. S. Mesgar, and Z. Mohammadi, "Evaluation of physicochemical, mechanical and biological properties of chitosan/carboxymethyl cellulose reinforced with multiphasic calcium phosphate whisker-like fibers for bone tissue engineering," *Mater. Sci. Eng. C*, vol. 100, pp. 341–353, 2019.

[108] R. Mala and A. S. R. Celsia, "Bioceramics in orthopaedics: A review," *Fundam. Biomater. Ceram.*, pp. 195–221, 2018.

[109] S. V. Dorozhkin, "Functionalized calcium orthophosphates ($CaPO_4$) and their biomedical applications," *J. Mater. Chem. B*, vol. 7, no. 47, pp. 7471–7489, 2019.

[110] T. J. Levingstone, S. Herbaj, and N. J. Dunne, "Calcium phosphate nanoparticles for therapeutic applications in bone regeneration," *Nanomaterials*, vol. 9, no. 11, pp. 1–22, 2019.

[111] P. Terzioğlu, H. Öğüt, and A. Kalemtaş, "Natural calcium phosphates from fish bones and their potential biomedical applications," *Mater. Sci. Eng. C*, vol. 91, pp. 899–911, 2018.

[112] B. Mutlu, S. Çaylak, and Ş. Duman, "Incorporation of cerium oxide into hydroxyapatite/chitosan composite scaffolds for bone repair," *Process. Appl. Ceram.*, vol. 16, no. 3, pp. 207–217, 2022.

[113] S. Mondal, T. P. Nguyen, V. H. Pham, G. Hoang, P. Manivasagan, M. H. Kim, S. Y. Nam, and J. Oh, "Hydroxyapatite nano bioceramics optimized 3D printed poly lactic acid scaffold for bone tissue engineering application," *Ceram. Int.*, vol. 46, no. 3, pp. 3443–3455, 2020.

[114] R. M. Kavasi, C. C. Coelho, V. Platania, P. A. Quadros, and M. Chatzinikolaidou, "In vitro biocompatibility assessment of nano-hydroxyapatite," *Nanomaterials*, vol. 11, no. 5, pp. 1–15, 2021. https://doi.org/10.3390/nano11051152

[115] M. A. Nazeer, E. Yilgör, and I. Yilgör, "Intercalated chitosan/hydroxyapatite nanocomposites: Promising materials for bone tissue engineering applications," *Carbohydr. Polym.*, vol. 175, pp. 38–46, 2017.

[116] H.-T. Lu, T.-W. Lu, C.-H. Chen, and F.-L. Mi, "Development of genipin-crosslinked and fucoidan-adsorbed nano-hydroxyapatite/hydroxypropyl chitosan composite scaffolds for bone tissue engineering," *Int. J. Biol. Macromol.*, vol. 128, pp. 973–984, 2019.

[117] A. V. Chaves, R. M. Freire, V. P. Feitosa, N. M. P. S. Ricardo, J. C. Denardin, D. M. A. Neto, and P. B. A. Fechine, "Hydroxyapatite-based magnetic bionanocomposite as pharmaceuticals carriers in chitosan scaffolds," *J. Compos. Sci.*, vol. 5, no. 2, p. 37, 2021.

[118] H. Goodarzi, S. Hashemi-Najafabadi, N. Baheiraei, and F. Bagheri, "Preparation and characterization of nanocomposite scaffolds (collagen/β-TCP/SrO) for bone tissue engineering," *Tissue Eng. Regen. Med.*, vol. 16, pp. 237–251, 2019.

[119] M. Taherimehr, R. Bagheri, and M. Taherimehr, "In-vitro evaluation of thermoplastic starch/beta-tricalcium phosphate nano-biocomposite in bone tissue engineering," *Ceram. Int.*, vol. 47, no. 11, pp. 15458–15463, 2021.

[120] M. Sohrabi, M. Abbasi, M. M. Ansar, and B. Soltani Tehrani, "Evaluation of electrospun nanofibers fabricated using PCL/PVP and PVA/β-TCP as potential scaffolds for bone tissue engineering," *Polym. Bull.*, pp. 1–17, 2021.

[121] S. U. Maheshwari, K. Govindan, M. Raja, A. Raja, M. B. Pravin, and S. V. Kumar, "Synthesis and characterization of calcium phosphate ceramic/(poly (vinyl alcohol)–polycaprolactone) bilayer nanocomposites-A bone tissue regeneration scaffold," *J. Nanosci. Nanotechnol.*, vol. 18, no. 3, pp. 1548–1556, 2018.

[122] M. R. Rad, F. Fahimipour, E. Dashtimoghadam, H. Nokhbatolfoghahaei, L. Tayebi, and A. Khojasteh, "Osteogenic differentiation of adipose-derived mesenchymal stem cells using 3D-Printed PDLLA/β-TCP nanocomposite scaffolds," *Bioprinting*, vol. 21, p. e00117, 2021.

[123] R. Ghaffari, H. Salimi-Kenari, F. Fahimipour, S. M. Rabiee, H. Adeli, and E. Dashtimoghadam, "Fabrication and characterization of dextran/nanocrystalline β-tricalcium phosphate nanocomposite hydrogel scaffolds," *Int. J. Biol. Macromol.*, vol. 148, pp. 434–448, 2020.

[124] N. Baheiraei, M. R. Nourani, S. M. J. Mortazavi, M. Movahedin, H. Eyni, F. Bagheri, and M. H. Norahan, "Development of a bioactive porous collagen/β-tricalcium phosphate bone graft assisting rapid vascularization for bone tissue engineering applications," *J. Biomed. Mater. Res. Part A*, vol. 106, no. 1, pp. 73–85, 2018.

[125] Y. Chen, N. Kawazoe, and G. Chen, "Preparation of dexamethasone-loaded biphasic calcium phosphate nanoparticles/collagen porous composite scaffolds for bone tissue engineering," *Acta Biomater.*, vol. 67, pp. 341–353, 2018. https://doi.org/10.1016/j.actbio.2017.12.004

[126] L. Nie, Q. Wu, H. Long, K. Hu, P. Li, C. Wang, M. Sun, J. Dong, X. Wei, J. Suo, D. Hua, S. Liu, H. Yuan, and S. Yang, "Development of chitosan/gelatin hydrogels incorporation of biphasic calcium phosphate nanoparticles for bone tissue engineering," *J. Biomater. Sci. Polym. Ed.*, vol. 30, no. 17, pp. 1636–1657, 2019. https://doi.org/10.1080/09205063.2019.1654210

[127] Q. Sun, L. Yu, Z. Zhang, C. Qian, H. Fang, J. Wang, P. Wu, X. Zhu, J. Zhang, L. Zhong, and R. He, "A novel gelatin/carboxymethyl chitosan/nano-hydroxyapatite/β-tricalcium phosphate biomimetic nanocomposite scaffold for bone tissue engineering applications," *Front. Chem.*, vol. 10, p. 958420, 2022.

[128] M. Rahmanian, A. Seyfoori, M. M. Dehghan, L. Eini, S. M. Naghib, H. Gholami, S. F. Mohajeri, K. R. Mamaghani, and K. Majidzadeh-A, "Multifunctional gelatin–tricalcium phosphate porous nanocomposite scaffolds for tissue engineering and local drug delivery: In vitro and in vivo studies," *J. Taiwan Inst. Chem. Eng.*, vol. 101, pp. 214–220, 2019.

[129] Z. Du, Z. Zhao, H. Liu, X. Liu, X. Zhang, Y. Huang, H. Leng, Q. Cai, and X. Yang, "Macroporous scaffolds developed from $CaSiO_3$ nanofibers regulating bone regeneration via controlled calcination," *Mater. Sci. Eng. C*, vol. 113, p. 111005, 2020.

[130] Ş. Duman and B. Bulut, "Effect of akermanite powders on mechanical properties and bioactivity of chitosan-based scaffolds produced by 3D-bioprinting," *Ceram. Int.*, vol. 47, no. 10, pp. 13912–13921, 2021.

[131] X.-Y. Peng, M. Hu, F. Liao, F. Yang, Q.-F. Ke, Y.-P. Guo, and Z.-H. Zhu, "La-doped mesoporous calcium silicate/chitosan scaffolds for bone tissue engineering," *Biomater. Sci.*, vol. 7, no. 4, pp. 1565–1573, 2019.

[132] M. Forni, C. Bernardini, F. Zamparini, A. Zannoni, R. Salaroli, D. Ventrella, G. Parchi, M. D. Esposti, A. Polimeni, P. Fabbri, F. Fava, C. Prati, and M. G. Gandolfi, "Vascular wall–mesenchymal stem cells differentiation on 3D biodegradable highly porous CaSi-DCPD doped Poly (α-hydroxy) acids scaffolds for bone regeneration," *Nanomaterials*, vol. 10, no. 2, p. 243, 2020.

[133] P. Srinath, P. Abdul Azeem, and K. Venugopal Reddy, "Review on calcium silicate-based bioceramics in bone tissue engineering," *Int. J. Appl. Ceram. Technol.*, vol. 17, no. 5, pp. 2450–2464, 2020.

[134] Z. Liu, X. He, S. Chen, and H. Yu, "Advances in the use of calcium silicate-based materials in bone tissue engineering," *Ceram. Int.*, vol. 49, no. 11, pp. 19355–19363, 2023.

[135] H. Ismail and H. Mohamad, "Bioactivity and biocompatibility properties of sustainable wollastonite bioceramics from rice husk ash/rice straw ash: A review," *Materials (Basel).*, vol. 14, no. 18, p. 5193, 2021.

[136] T. C. Schumacher, E. Volkmann, R. Yilmaz, A. Wolf, L. Treccani, and K. Rezwan, "Mechanical evaluation of calcium-zirconium-silicate (baghdadite) obtained by a direct solid-state synthesis route," *J. Mech. Behav. Biomed. Mater.*, vol. 34, pp. 294–301, 2014.

[137] H. Gheisari, "In vitro behavior of a novel nanostructure hardystonite/biphasic calcium phosphate scaffolds (HT/BCPS); evaluation and investigation," *J. Nanoanal.*, vol. 8, no. 2, pp. 86–100, 2021.

[138] S. Shemshad, S. Kamali, A. Khavandi, and S. Azari, "Synthesis, characterization and in-vitro behavior of natural chitosan-hydroxyapatite-diopside nanocomposite scaffold for bone tissue engineering," *Int. J. Polym. Mater. Polym. Biomater.*, vol. 68, no. 9, pp. 516–526, 2019.

[139] N. Rafiee, S. Karbasi, A. A. Nourbakhsh, and K. Amini, "Natural hydroxyapatite/diopside nanocomposite scaffold for bone tissue engineering applications: Physical, mechanical, bioactivity and biodegradation evaluation," *Mater. Technol.*, vol. 37, no. 1, pp. 36–48, 2022.

[140] M. Arastouei, M. Khodaei, S. M. Atyabi, and M. J. Nodoushan, "The in-vitro biological properties of 3D printed poly lactic acid/akermanite composite porous scaffold for bone tissue engineering," *Mater. Today Commun.*, vol. 27, p. 102176, 2021.

[141] S. Saber-Samandari, M. Mohammadi-Aghdam, and S. Saber-Samandari, "A novel magnetic bifunctional nanocomposite scaffold for photothermal therapy and tissue engineering," *Int. J. Biol. Macromol.*, vol. 138, pp. 810–818, 2019.

[142] M. Sayed, E. M. Mahmoud, F. Bondioli, and S. M. Naga, "Developing porous diopside/hydroxyapatite bio-composite scaffolds via a combination of freeze-drying and coating process," *Ceram. Int.*, vol. 45, no. 7, pp. 9025–9031, 2019.

[143] S. Sadeghzade and R. Emadi, "Improving the mechanical and bioactivity of hydroxyapatite porous scaffold ceramic with diopside/forstrite ceramic coating," *Nanomed. J.*, vol. 6, no. 1, 2019.

[144] M. Hamvar, H. R. Bakhsheshi-Rad, M. Omidi, A. F. Ismail, M. Aziz, F. Berto, and X. Chen, "Biocompatibility and bioactivity of hardystonite-based nanocomposite scaffold for tissue engineering applications," *Biomed. Phys. Eng. Express*, vol. 6, no. 3, p. 35011, 2020.

[145] Y. Hosseini, R. Emadi, M. Kharaziha, and A. Doostmohammadi, "Reinforcement of electrospun poly (ε-caprolactone) scaffold using diopside nanopowder to promote biological and physical properties," *J. Appl. Polym. Sci.*, vol. 134, no. 6, 2017.

[146] Z. Ba, Z. Chen, Y. Huang, D. Feng, Q. Zhao, J. Zhu, and D. Wu, "Nanoporous diopside modulates biocompatibility, degradability and osteogenesis of bioactive scaffolds of gliadin-based composites for new bone formation," *Int. J. Nanomed.*, pp. 3883–3896, 2018.

[147] F. Shamoradi, R. Emadi, and H. Ghomi, "Fabrication of monticellite-akermanite nanocomposite powder for tissue engineering applications," *J. Alloys Compd.*, vol. 693, pp. 601–605, 2017.

[148] E. Askari, M. Khoshghadam-Pireyousefan, S. M. Naghib, H. Akbari, B. Khosravani, A. Zali, Z. Salehi, Y. Zare, and K. Y. Rhee, "A hybrid approach for in-situ synthesis of bioceramic nanocomposites to adjust the physicochemical and biological characteristics," *J. Mater. Res. Technol.*, vol. 14, pp. 464–474, 2021.

[149] B. Bulut and Ş. Duman, "Evaluation of mechanical behavior, bioactivity, and cytotoxicity of chitosan/akermanite-TiO_2 3D-printed scaffolds for bone tissue applications," *Ceram. Int.*, vol. 48, no. 15, pp. 21378–21388, 2022.

[150] M. Arastouei, M. Khodaei, S. M. Atyabi, and M. J. Nodoushan, "Poly lactic acid-akermanite composite scaffolds prepared by fused filament fabrication for bone tissue engineering," *J. Mater. Res. Technol.*, vol. 9, no. 6, pp. 14540–14548, 2020.

[151] M. Arastouei, M. Khodaei, S. M. Atyabi, and M. Jafari Nodoushan, "Improving the properties of the porous polylactic acid scaffold by akermanite nanoparticles for bone tissue engineering," *J. Adv. Mater. Process.*, vol. 8, no. 2, pp. 11–19, 2020.

[152] E. Askari, S. M. Naghib, A. Seyfoori, M. A. Javidi, and A. M. Ansari, "Highly bioactive Akermanite-Monticellite nanocomposites for bone tissue engineering: A tunable three-dimensional biological study," *J. Mater. Res. Technol.*, vol. 20, pp. 4066–4076, 2022.

[153] P. Dehghanpour, R. Emadi, and H. Salimijazi, "Influence of mechanochemically fabricated nano-hardystonite reinforcement in polycaprolactone scaffold for potential use in bone tissue engineering: Synthesis and characterization," *J. Mech. Behav. Biomed. Mater.*, vol. 146, p. 106100, 2023.

[154] Z. Hadisi, H. R. Bakhsheshi-Rad, T. Walsh, M. M. Dehghan, S. Farzad-Mohajeri, H. Gholami, A. Diyanoush, E. Pagan, and M. Akbari, "In vitro and in vivo evaluation of silk fibroin-hardystonite-gentamicin nanofibrous scaffold for tissue engineering applications," *Polym. Test.*, vol. 91, p. 106698, 2020.

[155] M. M. Salmani, M. Hashemian, H. J. Yekta, M. G. Nejad, S. Saber-Samandari, and A. Khandan, "Synergic effects of magnetic nanoparticles on hyperthermia-based therapy and controlled drug delivery for bone substitute application," *J. Supercond. Nov. Magn.*, vol. 33, pp. 2809–2820, 2020.

[156] S. Foroutan, M. Hashemian, and A. S. Khandan, "A novel porous graphene scaffold prepared using freeze-drying technique for orthopedic approaches: Fabrication and buckling simulation using GDQ method.," *Iran. J. Mater. Sci. Eng.*, vol. 17, no. 4, 2020.

[157] S. Sahmani, M. Shahali, M. Ghadiri Nejad, A. Khandan, M. M. Aghdam, and S. Saber-Samandari, "Effect of copper oxide nanoparticles on electrical conductivity and cell viability of calcium phosphate scaffolds with improved mechanical strength for bone tissue engineering," *Eur. Phys. J. Plus*, vol. 134, no. 1, 2019.

[158] X. Dong, A. Heidari, A. Mansouri, W. S. Hao, M. Dehghani, S. Saber-Samandari, D. Toghraie, and A. Khandan, "Investigation of the mechanical properties of a bony scaffold for comminuted distal radial fractures: Addition of akermanite nanoparticles and using a freeze-drying technique," *J. Mech. Behav. Biomed. Mater.*, vol. 121, p. 104643, 2021.

[159] S. Sadeghzade, R. Emadi, F. Tavangarian, and A. Doostmohammadi, "The influence of polycaporolacton fumarate coating on mechanical properties and in vitro behavior of porous diopside-hardystonite nanocomposite scaffold," *J. Mech. Behav. Biomed. Mater.*, vol. 101, p. 103445, 2020.

[160] M. Razavi, M. Fathi, O. Savabi, L. Tayebi, and D. Vashaee, "Biodegradable magnesium bone implants coated with a novel bioceramic nanocomposite," *Materials (Basel)*, vol. 13, no. 6, p. 1315, 2020.

[161] E. Abdollahi and H. Bakhsheshi-Rad, "Evaluation of mechanical properties and apatite formation of synthesized fluorapatite-hardystonite nanocomposite scaffolds," *Adv. Ceram. Prog.*, vol. 4, no. 3–4, pp. 8–15, 2018.

[162] P. N. Christy, S. K. Basha, and V. S. Kumari, "Nano zinc oxide and nano bioactive glass reinforced chitosan/poly (vinyl alcohol) scaffolds for bone tissue engineering application," *Mater. Today Commun.*, vol. 31, p. 103429, 2022.

[163] L. L. Hench, R. J. Splinter, W. C. Allen, and T. K. Greenlee, "Bonding mechanisms at the interface of ceramic prosthetic materials," *J. Biomed. Mater. Res.*, vol. 5, no. 6, pp. 117–141, 1971.

[164] M. Shaltooki, G. Dini, and M. Mehdikhani, "Fabrication of chitosan-coated porous polycaprolactone/strontium-substituted bioactive glass nanocomposite scaffold for bone tissue engineering," *Mater. Sci. Eng. C*, vol. 105, p. 110138, 2019.

[165] M. N. Rahaman, D. E. Day, B. S. Bal, Q. Fu, S. B. Jung, L. F. Bonewald, and A. P. Tomsia, "Bioactive glass in tissue engineering," *Acta Biomater.*, vol. 7, no. 6, pp. 2355–2373, 2011.

[166] M. Kazemi, M. M. Dehghan, and M. Azami, "Biological evaluation of porous nanocomposite scaffolds based on strontium substituted β-TCP and bioactive glass: An in vitro and in vivo study," *Mater. Sci. Eng. C*, vol. 105, p. 110071, 2019.

[167] S. Manafi, F. Mirjalili, and R. Reshadi, "Synthesis and evaluation of the bioactivity of fluorapatite–45S5 bioactive glass nanocomposite," *Prog. Biomater.*, vol. 8, no. 2, pp. 77–89, 2019.

[168] R. Iron, M. Mehdikhani, E. Naghashzargar, S. Karbasi, and D. Semnani, "Effects of nano-bioactive glass on structural, mechanical and bioactivity properties of Poly (3-hydroxybutyrate) electrospun scaffold for bone tissue engineering applications," *Mater. Technol.*, vol. 34, no. 9, pp. 540–548, 2019.

[169] A. M. Deliormanlı and R. Konyalı, "Bioactive glass/hydroxyapatite-containing electrospun poly (ε-Caprolactone) composite nanofibers for bone tissue engineering," *J. Aust. Ceram. Soc.*, vol. 55, no. 1, pp. 247–256, 2019.

[170] C. D. F. Moreira, S. M. Carvalho, R. M. Florentino, A. França, B. S. Okano, C. M. F. Rezende, H. S. Mansur, and M. M. Pereira, "Injectable chitosan/gelatin/bioactive glass nanocomposite hydrogels for potential bone regeneration: In vitro and in vivo analyses," *Int. J. Biol. Macromol.*, vol. 132, pp. 811–821, 2019.

[171] A. Akturk, M. Erol Taygun, and G. Goller, "Optimization of the electrospinning process variables for gelatin/silver nanoparticles/bioactive glass nanocomposites for bone tissue engineering," *Polym. Compos.*, vol. 41, no. 6, pp. 2411–2425, 2020.

[172] H. Zhu, M. Monavari, K. Zheng, T. Distler, L. Ouyang, S. Heid, Z. Jin, J. He, D. Li, and A. R. Boccaccini, "3D bioprinting of multifunctional dynamic nanocomposite bioinks incorporating Cu-doped mesoporous bioactive glass nanoparticles for bone tissue engineering," *Small*, vol. 18, no. 12, p. 2104996, 2022.

[173] P. Nikpour, H. Salimi-Kenari, F. Fahimipour, S. M. Rabiee, M. Imani, E. Dashtimoghadam, and L. Tayebi, "Dextran hydrogels incorporated with bioactive glass-ceramic: Nanocomposite scaffolds for bone tissue engineering," *Carbohydr. Polym.*, vol. 190, pp. 281–294, 2018.

[174] M. H. Monfared, F. E. Ranjbar, M. Torbati, S. A. Poursamar, N. Lotfibakkhshaiesh, J. Ai, and S. Ebrahimi-Barough, "Preparation and characterization of 3D nanocomposite scaffold from bioactive glass/β-tricalcium phosphate via robocasting method for bone tissue engineering," *J. Non. Cryst. Solids*, vol. 593, p. 121769, 2022.

[175] A. Kumar and S. S. Han, "Enhanced mechanical, biomineralization, and cellular response of nanocomposite hydrogels by bioactive glass and halloysite nanotubes for bone tissue regeneration," *Mater. Sci. Eng. C*, vol. 128, p. 112236, 2021.

[176] S. Seyedmajidi, R. Rajabnia, and M. Seyedmajidi, "Evaluation of antibacterial properties of hydroxyapatite/bioactive glass and fluorapatite/bioactive glass nanocomposite foams as a cellular scaffold of bone tissue," *J. Lab. Physicians*, vol. 10, no. 03, pp. 265–270, 2018.

[177] C. D. F. Moreira, S. M. Carvalho, R. G. Sousa, H. S. Mansur, and M. M. Pereira, "Nanostructured chitosan/gelatin/bioactive glass in situ forming hydrogel composites as a potential injectable matrix for bone tissue engineering," *Mater. Chem. Phys.*, vol. 218, pp. 304–316, 2018.

[178] D. A. Canales, F. Reyes, M. Saavedra, L. Peponi, A. Leonés, H. Palza, A. R. Boccaccini, A. Grünewald, and P. A. Zapata, "Electrospun fibers of poly (lactic acid) containing bioactive glass and magnesium oxide nanoparticles for bone tissue regeneration," *Int. J. Biol. Macromol.*, vol. 210, pp. 324–336, 2022.

[179] S. Mondal, G. Hoang, P. Manivasagan, M. S. Moorthy, T. P. Nguyen, T. T. V. Phan, H. H. Kim, M. H. Kim, S. Y. Nam, and J. Oh, "Nano-hydroxyapatite bioactive glass composite scaffold with enhanced mechanical and biological performance for tissue engineering application," *Ceram. Int.*, vol. 44, no. 13, pp. 15735–15746, 2018.

[180] W. Wu, J. Fang, W. Liu, Y. Zhao, T. Huang, Y. Zhao, X. Li, J. Cui, Y. Yang, and Z. Zhou, "Preparation and properties of BMPLGA/NBAG-β-TCP composite scaffold materials," *Int. J. Polym. Anal. Charact.*, vol. 23, no. 8, pp. 710–720, 2018.

[181] S. Seyedmajidi, M. Seyedmajidi, E. Zabihi, and K. Hajian-Tilaki, "A comparative study on cytotoxicity and genotoxicity of the hydroxyapatite-bioactive glass and fluorapatite-bioactive glass nanocomposite foams as tissue scaffold for bone repair," *J. Biomed. Mater. Res. Part A*, vol. 106, no. 10, pp. 2605–2612, 2018.

[182] K. Glenske, P. Donkiewicz, A. Köwitsch, N. Milosevic-Oljaca, P. Rider, S. Rofall, J. Franke, O. Jung, R. Smeets, and R. Schnettler, "Applications of metals for bone regeneration," *Int. J. Mol. Sci.*, vol. 19, pp. 826, 2018.

[183] S. K. Jaganathan and M. P. Mani, "Enriched mechanical, thermal, and blood compatibility of single stage electrospun polyurethane nickel oxide nanocomposite for cardiac tissue engineering," *Polym. Compos.*, vol. 40, pp. 2381–2390, 2019.

[184] J. E. Kim, J. Lee, M. Jang, M. H. Kwak, J. Go, E. K. Kho, S. H. Song, J. E. Sung, J. Lee, and D. Y. Hwang, "Accelerated healing of cutaneous wounds using phytochemically stabilized gold nanoparticle deposited hydrocolloid membranes," *Biomater. Sci.*, vol. 3, pp. 509–519, 2015.

[185] R. Eivazzadeh-Keihan, E. B. Noruzi, K. K. Chenab, A. Jafari, F. Radinekiyan, S. M. Hashemi, F. Ahmadpour, A. Behboudi, J. Mosafer, A. Mokhtarzadeh, A. Maleki, and M. R. Hamblin, "Metal-based nanoparticles for bone tissue engineering," *J. Tissue Eng. Regen. Med.*, vol. 14, no. 12, pp. 1687–1714, 2020.

[186] E. Okoampah, Y. Mao, S. Yang, S. Sun, and C. Zhou, "Gold nanoparticles–biomembrane interactions: From fundamental to simulation," *Colloids Surf. B Biointerfaces*, vol. 196, p. 111312, 2020.

[187] Y. C. Wang, E. Rheaume, F. Lesage, and A. Kakkar, "Synthetic methodologies to gold nanoshells: An overview, "*Molecules*, vol. 23, no. 11, p. 2815, 2018.

[188] S. Liu and M. Lammerhofer, "Functionalized gold nanoparticles for sample preparation: A review," *Electrophoresis*, vol. 40, no. 18–19, pp. 2438–2461, 2019.

[189] X. Bai, Y. Wang, Z. Song, Y. Feng, Y. Chen, D. Zhang, and L. Feng, "The basic properties of gold nanoparticles and their applications in tumor diagnosis and treatment," *Int. J. Mol. Sci.*, vol. 21, no. 7, pp. 2480, 2020.

[190] D. Pooja, S. Panyaram, H. Kulhari, S. S. Rachamalla, and R. Sistla, " Xanthan gum stabilized gold nanoparticles: Characterization, biocompatibility, stability and cytotoxicity," *Carbohydr. Polym.*, vol. 110, pp. 1–9, 2014.

[191] N. Yang and W. H. Li, " Preparation of gold nanoparticles using chitosan oligosaccharide as a reducing and capping reagent and their in vitro cytotoxic effect on human fibroblasts cells," *Mater. Lett.*., vol. 138, pp. 154–157, 2015.

[192] S. Vieira, S. Vial, F. R. Maia, M. Carvalho, R. L. Reis, P. L. Granja, and J. M. Oliveira, "Gellan gum-coated gold nanorods: An intracellular nanosystem for bone tissue engineering," *RSC Advances*, vol. 5, pp. 77996–78005, 2015.

[193] P. Varvarà, L. Tranchina, G. Cavallaro, and M. Licciardi, "Preparation and characterization of gold nanorods coated with gellan gum and lipoic acid," *Appl. Sci.*, vol. 10, no. 23, 2020. https://doi.org/10.3390/app10238322

[194] P. R. More, S. Pandit, A. De Filippis, G. Franci, and M. Galdiero, "Preparation and silver nanoparticles: Bactericidal and mechanistic approach against drug resistant pathogens," *Microorganisms*, vol. 11, no. 2, pp. 369, 2023.

[195] E. Mikhailova, "Silver nanoparticles: Mechanism of action and probable bio-application," *J. Funct. Biomater.*, vol. 11, no. 4, pp. 84, 2020.

[196] S. Wahab, A. Salman, Z. Khan, S. Khan, C. Krishnaraj and S. II Yun, "Metallic nanoparticles: A promising arsenal against antimicrobial resistance – Unraveling mechanisms and enhancing medication efficacy," *Int. J. Mol. Sci.*, vol. 24, no. 9, p. 14897, 2023.

[197] G. Jin, H. Qin, H. Cao, S. Qian, Y. Zhao, X. Peng, X. Zhang, X. Liu, and P. K. Chu, "Synergistic effects of dual Zn/Ag ion implantation in osteogenic activity and antibacterial ability of titanium," *Biomaterials*, vol. 35, pp. 7699–7713, 2014.

[198] Y. Yan, X. Zhang, Y. Huang, Q. Ding, and X. Pang, "Antibacterial and bioactivity of silver substituted hydroxyapatite/TiO2 nanotube composite coatings on titanium," *Appl. Surf. Sci.*, vol. 314, pp. 348–357, 2014.

[199] Y. Chen, S. I. Roohani-Esfahani, Z. Lu, H. Zreiqat, and C. R. Dunstan, "Zirconium ions up-regulate the BMP/SMAD signaling pathway and promote the proliferation and differentiation of human osteoblasts," *PLoS One*, vol. 10, p. e0113426, 2015.

[200] Y. Oshima, F. Iwasa, K. Tachi, and K. Baba, " Effect of nanofeatured topography on ceria-stabilized zirconia/alumina nanocomposite on osteogenesis and osseointegration," *Int. J. Oral Maxillofac. Implants*, vol. 32, pp. 81–91, 2017.

[201] A. Smieszek, J. Szydlarska, A. Mucha, M. Chrapiec, and K. Marycz, "Enhanced cytocompatibility and osteoinductive properties of sol gel-derived silica/zirconium dioxide coatings by metformin functionalization," *J. Biomater. Appl.*, vol. 32, pp. 570–586, 2017.

[202] M. A. Maghsoudlou, E. Nassireslami, S. Saber-Samandari, and A. Khandan, "Bone regeneration using bio-nanocomposite tissue reinforced with bioactive nanoparticles for femoral defect applications in medicine," *Avicenna J. Med. Biotechnol.*, vol. 12, pp. 68–76, 2020.

[203] Y. Qu and L. Liu, "Zirconia materials for dental implants: A literature review," *Front. Dent. Med.*, vol. 2, p. 687983, 2023.

[204] P. Altuna, E. Lucas-Taulé, J. Gargallo-Albiol, O. Figueras-Álvarez, F. Hernández-Alfaro, and J. Nart, "Clinical evidence on titanium zirconium dental implants: A systematic review and meta-analysis," *Int J Oral Maxillofac Surg*, vol. 45, pp. 842–850, 2016.

[205] A. Doostmohammadi, Z. Karimzadeh Esfahani, A. Ardeshirylajimi, and Z. Rahmati Dehkordi, "Zirconium modified calcium silicate based nanoceramics: An in vivo evaluation in a rabbit tibial defect model," *Int. J. Appl. Ceram. Technol.*, vol. 16, pp. 431–437, 2019.

[206] A. Bhowmick, N. Pramanik, P. Jana, T. Mitra, A. Gnanamani, M. Das, and P. P. Kundu, "Development of bone-like zirconium oxide nanoceramic modified chitosan based porous nanocomposites for biomedical application," *Int. J. Biol. Macromol.*, vol. 95, pp. 348–356, 2017.

[207] M. Alam, E. Manivannan, S. Saha, G. Gopan, M. Mani, and K. Sanjeevi, "Design, fabrication, mechanical, and in vitro evaluation of 3D printed ZrO_2 reinforced polylactide scaffolds through fused deposition modeling," *Mater. Chem. Front.*, vol. 7, pp. 464–475, 2023.

[208] K. Sakthiabirami, V. Soundharrajan, J.-H. Kang, Y. P. Yang, and S.-W. Park, "Three-dimensional zirconia-based scaffolds for load-bearing bone-regeneration applications: Prospects and challenges," *Materials (Basel)*, vol. 14, no. 12, pp. 3207, 2021.

[209] S. Pattnaik, S. Nethala, A. Tripathi, S. Saravanan, A. Moorthi, and N. Selvamurugan, " Chitosan scaffolds containing silicon dioxide and zirconia nano particles for bone tissue engineering," *Int. J. Biol. Macromol.*, vol. 49, pp. 1167–1172, 2011.

[210] K. Hoffman, D. Skrtic, J. Sun, and W. Tutak, "Airbrushed composite polymer Zr-ACP nanofiber scaffolds with improved cell penetration for bone tissue regeneration," *Tissue Eng. Part C Methods*, vol. 21, pp. 284–291, 2014.

[211] Q. Shen, Y. Qi, Y. Kong, H. Bao, Y. Wang, A. Dong, H. Wu, and Y. Xu, "Advances in copper-based biomaterials with antibacterial and osteogenic properties for bone tissue engineering," *Front Bioeng Biotechnol.*, vol. 9, p. 795425, 2021.

[212] S. K. Sehmi, S. Noimark, J. Weiner, E. Allan, A. J. MacRobert, and I. P. Parkin, "Potent antibacterial activity of copper embedded into silicone and polyurethane," *ACS Appl. Mater. Inter.*, vol. 7, pp. 22807–22813, 2015.

[213] S. Dhivya, J. Ajita, and N. Selvamurugan, "Metallic nanomaterials for bone tissue engineering," *J. Biomed. Nanotech.*, vol. 11, pp. 1675–1700, 2015.

[214] E. Tomaszewska, S. Muszynski, K. Ognik, P. Dobrowolski, M. Kwiecien, J. Juskiewicz, D. Chocyk, M. Swietlicki, T. Blicharski, and B. Gladyszewska, " Comparison of the effect of dietary copper nanoparticles with copper (II) salt on bone geometric and structural parameters as well as material characteristics in a rat model," *J. Trace Elem. Med. Biol.*, vol. 42, pp. 103–110, 2017.

[215] J. Forero, E. Roa, J. Reyes, C. Acevedo, and N. Osses, " Development of useful biomaterial for bone tissue engineering by incorporating nano-copper-zinc alloy (nCuZn) in chitosan/gelatin/nano-hydroxyapatite (Ch/G/nHAp) scaffold," *Materials*, vol. 10, pp. 1177, 2017.

[216] D. Solairaj, P. Rameshthangam, and G. Arunachalam, " Anticancer activity of silver and copper embedded chitin nanocomposites against human breast cancer (MCF-7) cells," *Int. J. Biol. Macromol.*, vol. 105, pp. 608–619, 2017.

[217] Y. Yang, Q. Yan, Q. Liu, Y. Li, H. Liu, P. Wang, L. Chen, D. Zhang, Y. Li, and Y. Dong, "An ultrasensitive sandwich-type electrochemical immunosensor based on the signal amplification strategy of echinoidea-shaped Au@Ag-Cu_2O nanoparticles for prostate specific antigen detection," *Biosens Bioelectron.*, vol. 99, pp. 450–457, 2018.

[218] B. E. Noruzi, M. Kheirkhahi, B. Shaabani, S. Geremia, N. Hickey, F. Asaro, P. Nitti, and H. S. Kafil, " Design of a thiosemicarbazide functionalized calix[4]arene ligand and related transition metal complexes: Synthesis, characterization and biological studies," *Front. Chem.*, vol. 7, pp. 663, 2019.

[219] B. E. Noruzi, B. Shaabani, S. Geremia, N. Hickey, P. Nitti, and H. S. Kafil, "Synthesis, crystal structure, and biological activity of a multidentate calix[4]arene ligand doubly functionalized by 2-hydroxybenzeledene-thiosemicarbazone," *Molecules*, vol. 25, p. 370, 2020.

[220] M. P. Sutunkova, Y. V. Ryabova, I. A. Minigalieva, T. V. Bushueva, R. R. Sakhautdinova, I. A. Bereza, D. R. Shaikhova, A. M. Amromina, A. I. Chemezov, I. G. Shelomencev, L. A. Amromin, I. E. Valamina, and L. V. Toropova, "Features of the response to subchronic low-dose exposure to copper oxide nanoparticles in rats," *Sci. Rep.*, vol. 13, p. 11890, 2023.

[221] I. C. Lee, J. W. Ko, S. H. Park, J. O. Lim, I. S. Shin, C. Moon, S. H. Kim, J. D. Heo, and J. C. Kim, "Comparative toxicity and biodistribution of copper nanoparticles and cupric ions in rats," *Int. J. Nanomed.*, vol. 11, pp. 2883–2900, 2016.

[222] Q. Chen and G. A. Thouas, " Metallic implant biomaterials," *Mater. Sci. Eng. R Rep.*, vol. 87, pp. 1–57, 2015.

[223] J. He, F. L. He, D. W. Li, Y. L. Liu, and D. C. Yin, " A novel porous Fe/Fe-W alloy scaffold with a double-layer structured skeleton: Preparation, in vitro degradability and biocompatibility," *Colloids Surf. B Biointerfaces*, vol. 142, pp. 325–333, 2016.

[224] G. Karunakaran, R. Suriyaprabha, V. Rajendran, and N. Kannan, " Effect of contact angle, zeta potential and particles size on the in vitro studies of Al_2O_3 and SiO_2 nanoparticles," *Colloids Surf. B Biointerfaces*, vol. 142, pp. 325–333, 2016.

[225] H. R. A. Hasanjani and K. Zarei, "Electrochemical sensor for ultrasensitive determination of ceftazidime using hollow platinum nanoparticles/reduced graphene oxide/pencil graphite electrode," *Chem. Pap.*, vol. 72, no. 8, pp. 1935–1944, 2018.

[226] S. Kianfar, A. N. Golikand, and B. ZareNezhad, "An investigation on the structure properties of platinum nanoparticle deposition on graphene sheets by gamma-ray irradiation: A study of methanol electro-oxidation by synthesis catalyst," *Chem. Pap.*, vol. 75, no. 4, pp. 1701–1714, 2021.

[227] H. Hasnain, R. Gul, A. Andleeb, S. Ullah, M. Shah, M. Khanum, I. Ullah, C. Hano, and B. H. Abbasi, "A detailed review on biosynthesis of platinum nanoparticles (PtNPs), their potential antimicrobial and biomedical applications," *J. Saudi Chem. Soc.*, vol. 25, p. 101297, 2021.

[228] S. Li, E. Porcel, H. Remita, S. Marco, M. Refregiers, M. Dutertre, F. Confalonieri, and S. Lacombe, "Platinum nanoparticles: An exquisite tool to overcome radioresistance," *Cancer Nanotechnol.*, vol. 8, no. 1, p. 4, 2017.

[229] A. Ali, H. Zafar, M. Zia, I. UlHaq, A. R. Phull, J. S. Ali, and A. Hussain, "Synthesis, characterization, applications, and challenges of iron oxide nanoparticles," *Nanotechnol. Sci. Appl.*, vol. 9, pp. 49–67, 2016.

[230] N. V. S. Vallabani and S. Singh, " Recent advances and future prospects of iron oxide nanoparticles in biomedicine and diagnostics," *Biotechnology*, vol. 8, no. 6, p. 279, 2018.

[231] Y. Zhang, T. R. Nayak, H. Hong, and W. Cai, "Biomedical applications of zinc oxide nanomaterials," *Curr. Mol. Med.*, vol. 13, no. 10, pp. 1633–1645, 2013.

[232] J. Jiang, J. Pi, and J. Cai, "The advancing of zinc oxide nanoparticles for biomedical applications," *Bioinorg. Chem. Appl.*, vol. 2018, p. 1062562, 2018.

4 Bionanocomposites in Cancer Targeted Drug Delivery

Iqra Arooj, Hamna Shahid, Saadia Ijaz, Sehrish Fiaz and Atif Amin Baig

4.1 INTRODUCTION

4.1.1 CANCER

Cancer is a group of disorders characterized by malignant aberrant tissue growth (neoplasm), which results in cells with abnormal appearance and/or activity [1, 2]. These abnormal cells can evade the immune system, multiply, accomplish angiogenesis, and occasionally invade other body areas, ultimately resulting in life-threatening disease, as illustrated in Figure 4.1 [3]. Cancer can arise from many factors, most commonly heritable genetic deficiencies, such as BRCA1 and BRCA2 gene mutations, infection, external variables like air pollution, and inadequate lifestyle choices, such as excessive smoking or alcohol consumption. Signs of cancer include tiredness, decreased appetite, changes in the skin, abnormal bleeding, chronic coughing, fever, lumps, and tissue masses [1, 4]. The global incidence of cancer has been growing to the point where it has recently placed second to heart disease as a significant cause of death [5]. Generally, females are affected mainly by breast, cervical, lung, thyroid, and colorectal cancers (CRCs), whereas males are more frequently experiencing lung, prostate, colorectal, liver, and stomach cancers [6].

The schematic illustration shows that the aberrant growth of normal cells driven by mutations converts them into tumor cells, ultimately forming a giant tumor, which is still benign. When these cells turn on the angiogenic switch and govern vessel synthesis, individual tumor cells can access the larger blood vessels and move to distant locations through circulation. Ultimately, it precipitates in the form of tumor development at the secondary site, termed metastasis.

4.1.2 TRADITIONAL TREATMENTS OF CANCER

Surgery, immunotherapy, hormone therapy, radiotherapy, chemotherapy, and intravenous administration of multiple RNA molecules have all been used to treat cancer. However, chemotherapy is still a highly effective treatment option for cancer [7]. Drugs used in chemotherapy kill cancerous cells through several different processes, such as (1) triggering internal and external apoptosis pathways; (2) triggering cell cycle arrest; (3) enhancing the autophagy pathway; (4) inhibiting DNA or RNA synthesis; (5) alkylating DNA; (6) interfering with microtubules production; (7) damaging DNA directly or indirectly by producing reactive oxygen species (ROS); and (8) inhibiting topoisomerases. In general, most of these pathways result in oxidative stress and the activation of the ATM/ATR repair response, followed by activation of p53 and its subsidiary p21 protein, which ultimately cause a cell cycle halt or hasten aging [8–10].

4.1.3 SIDE EFFECTS OF CHEMOTHERAPY

Many chemotherapy drugs have emerged, and these drugs are presently employed in diverse combinations with different treatment regimens depending on cancer type, risk classification group, and

DOI: 10.1201/9781003650812-4

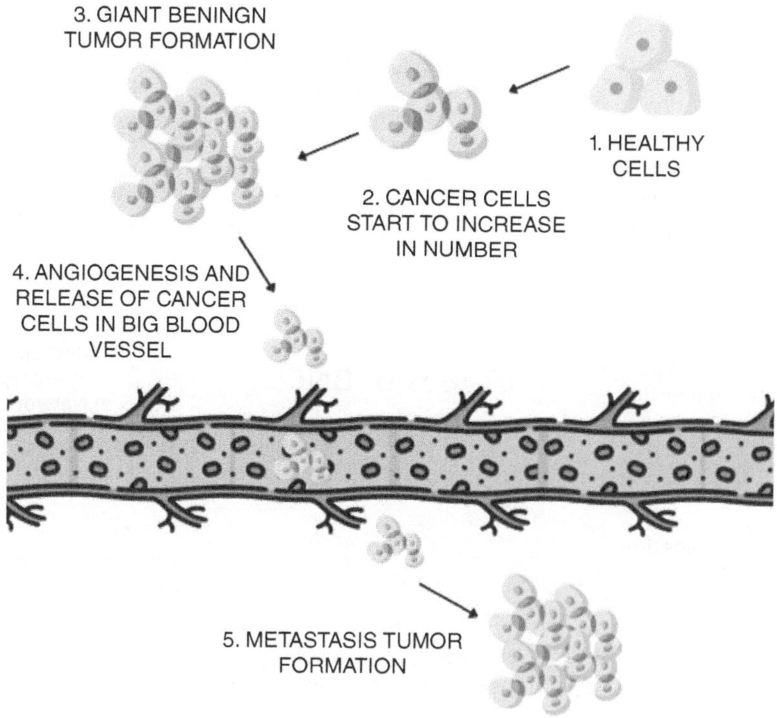

FIGURE 4.1 Tumorigenic transformation of normal cells and metastasis.

genomic background [11]. Treatment procedures are constantly being changed to improve rates of survival. Furthermore, the emphasis on therapeutic management has turned to reducing chemotherapy-related toxicity in patients. Secondary carcinomas, nephrotoxicity, cardiotoxicity, neurotoxicity, and hepatotoxicity are chemotherapy's most frequent side effects. Any chemotherapy drug cannot differentiate between cancer cells and normal dividing cells, for example, hair follicles. Thus, this also causes DNA damage in healthy cells, causing toxicities and rapid aging in cells [12–15].

4.2 BIONANOCOMPOSITES (BNCs): MEDIATED DRUG DELIVERY FOR CANCER

Bionanocomposites (BNCs) contain components of green nature, such as biological polymers and particulates, with a minimum of one dimension in the range of 1–100 nm [16]. The term "bionanocomposite (BNC)," also known as "nanobiocomposites (NBCs)," "green composites (GCs)," or "biohybrids (BHs)," was used for the first time in 2004 [17]. Combining a biodegradable polymer and a suitable nanofiller can make up a BNC. Incorporating a nanofiller improves the interactions between polymer matrix and filler because nanofillers have high surface-to-volume ratios, ultimately improving performance [18]. Additionally, nanofillers can enhance biopolymers' heating and permeability properties [19]. Various categories of BNCs have been depicted in Figure 4.2. BNCs have outstanding biodegradability and biocompatibility [20].

Any pharmaceutical ingredient can be transported inside the human body employing different technologies, compositions, innovations, and protocols to supply the desired therapeutic benefit, a process called drug delivery. Recent developments in drug delivery systems are directing focus toward the administration of drugs by providing the highest level of efficacy and safety at the appropriate time, location, and dose. In recent years, innovative drug delivery systems have attracted considerable attention. The development of prolonged or regulated drug delivery systems has

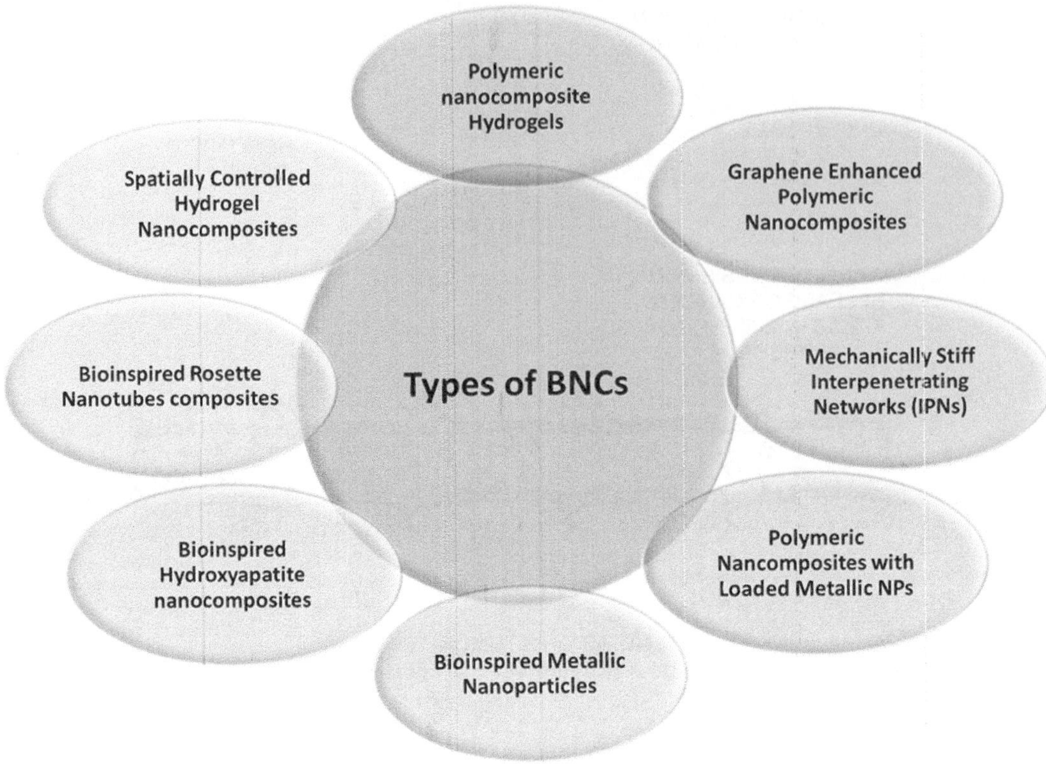

FIGURE 4.2 Different types of bionanocomposites (BNCs) can be incorporated into various drug delivery systems.

received consideration during the last few decades by aiming at maintained drug release, decreased dose frequency, and improved therapeutic efficacy compared to conventional administration [21–23].

Another potential improvement made possible by nanotechnology-based drug delivery systems is targeted delivery to tumors. The regulated release of pharmaceuticals made possible by nanoparticle (NP)-based drug delivery provides the prospect for more effective therapeutic action and allows drugs to react more quickly to some stimuli like enzymes, pH, heat, and light. Targeted drug delivery systems combine various disciplines of science (involving polymer science, pharmacology, bioconjugate chemistry, and molecular biology) for delivering the drug to particular sites in the body instead of the whole body or organ. Targeted drug delivery intends to direct and control the drug's pharmacodynamics, pharmacokinetics, toxicity, and immunogenicity. Besides that, another ultimate goal is exact drug efficiency combined with minimal adverse effects and molecular interactions between the drug and biopolymer. The levels of drug and biopolymer must be high at the tumor site while being nearly undetectable in healthy tissues [24].

BNCs can increase the effectiveness of nanomedicine because they have great targeting capabilities and can hold higher concentrations of a single drug [25]. Formulations should ideally be biofunctionalized to be effective in treating cancer. Biofunctionalization can be done by combining basic characteristics (surface charge and size) and other multifunctional characteristics (mixing various biopolymers). Additionally, different formulations should satisfy the following requirements:

1. Improve pharmacodynamic and pharmacokinetic characteristics of targeted drugs.
2. Eliminate tumor cells with precision while sparing normal cells.
3. Extend and manage the release of targeted drugs' active forms.

4. Enhance the cellular absorption of targeted drugs.
5. Reduce dose-limit toxicity [26, 27].

4.3 BIOPOLYMERS FOR CANCER THERAPY

The use of synthetic and natural biodegradable polymers as drug delivery systems has considerably risen in the past decade [28]. From polysaccharides to proteins, the full range of natural polymers demonstrates excellent properties and various capabilities that are used to create cutting-edge hybrid materials and nanocomposites (Figure 4.3). Important natural polysaccharides (such as alginate, fucoidan, cellulose, hyaluronic acid, and chitosan) and natural proteins (such as gelatin, silk, and collagen) can be used to create sustainable BNCs for cancer therapy [29]. Some important synthetic biopolymers, including PLA (poly-lactic acid), PCL (poly-caprolactone), PLGA (poly lactic-co-glycolic acid), PLLA (poly-l-lactic acid), and PEG (polyethylene glycol), have been frequently employed as substrates for the creation of BNCs [30, 31].

The choice of solvent is particularly crucial for developing BNCs as drug delivery systems; it must have sufficient solubility for both the drug and biopolymer. The consequent structure of the BNC is significantly influenced by the compatibility of the biopolymeric components and their physicochemical characteristics (such as surface tension, conductivity, and viscosity) [19, 32]. The release of drug kinetics is significantly influenced by the states of both components (biopolymer and nanofiller), their crystalline structure, and their distribution within the designed BNC. Additionally, the inclusion of amphiphilic molecules into designed BNCs can facilitate the release of hydrophobic drugs into the aqueous environment [33, 34]. Different chemotherapeutic drugs and metal or metal

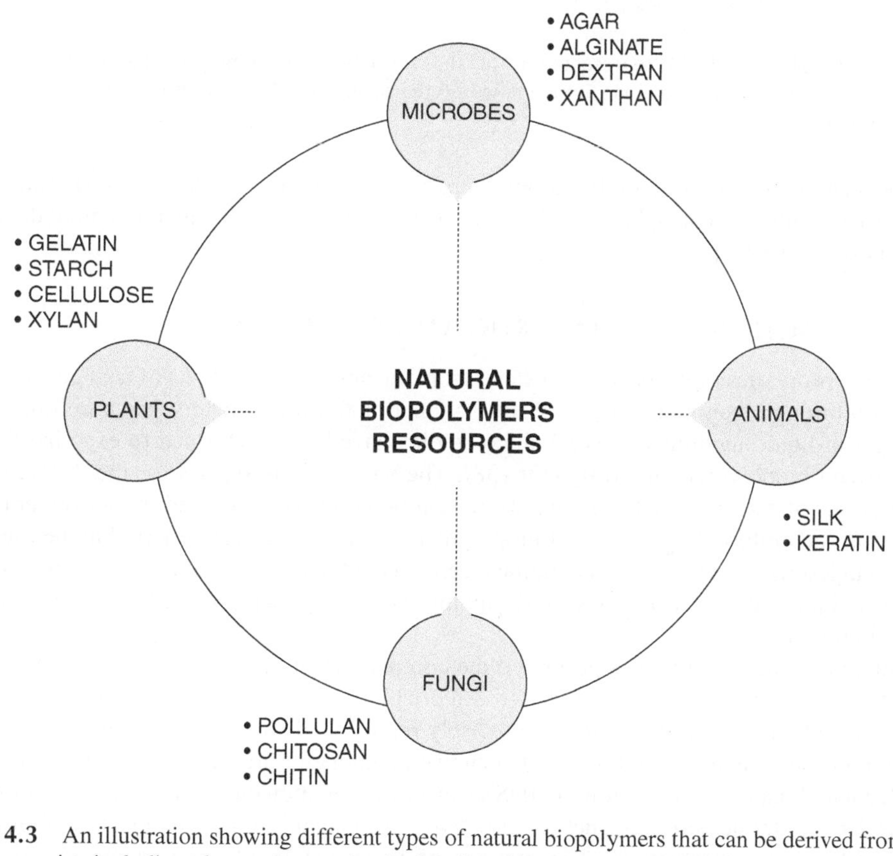

FIGURE 4.3 An illustration showing different types of natural biopolymers that can be derived from various natural reservoirs, including plants, algae, animals, fungi, and bacteria.

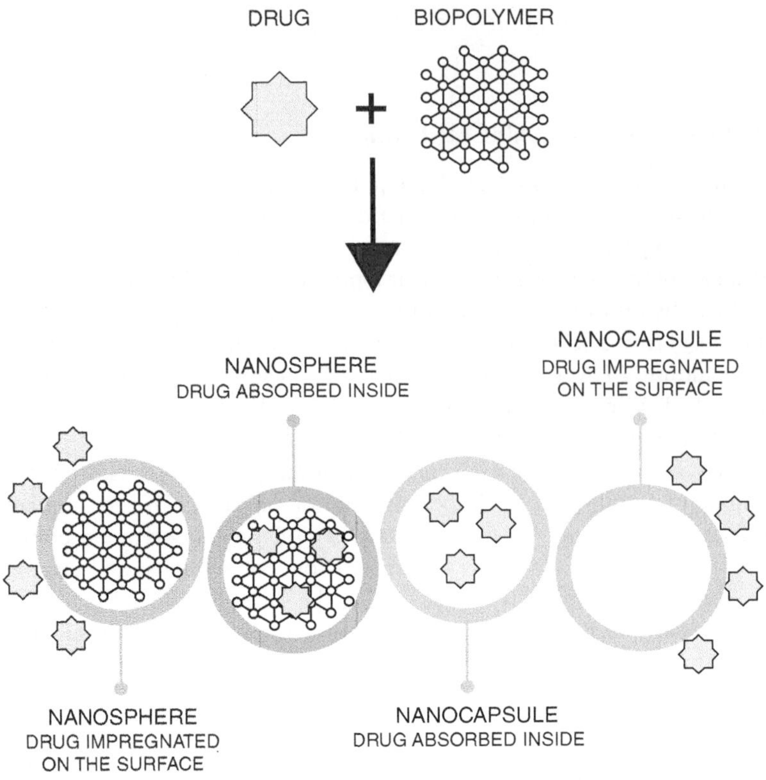

FIGURE 4.4 The graphical representation of the formation of biopolymer-based nanocapsules and nanospheres in which drugs are either impregnated on the surface or absorbed in the internal matrix for drug delivery systems.

oxide NPs can be incorporated into biopolymers by impregnation or absorption (Figure 4.4). As a result, nanocapsules or nanospheres of different sizes and shapes can be manufactured depending on the synthesis approach [35].

4.4 INTERACTION BETWEEN DRUG AND BIOPOLYMER

The specific properties of biopolymers extend from the angstrom level (Å) of a single atom-to-atom connection through nanometers (nm) of the polymer chain, micrometers (μm), millimeters (mm), and bigger in liquid mediums. Several silico studies have been performed to examine the interactions between biopolymers and drugs [36–38]. The various time frames for the different physical characteristics of each material can range from femtosecond (fs) to second (s) or even hour. Several instances of the multiscale character of biopolymer systems have been reported in the literature. As a result, numerous computational techniques were created to deal with these problems. These innovative techniques open new avenues for designing, perfecting, and predicting biopolymer architectures and properties.

Additionally, these techniques permitted the comparison of different biopolymers to each other. One of the primary techniques used today to explore biopolymer-drug interactions is atomistic modeling (AM). AM, in which every atom is precisely represented and handled as an individual sphere, and different chemical bonds or forces between two components are extensively studied [26, 36–38].

Molecular dynamics simulations (MDS) can represent molecular operations encompassing a wider variety of atomic particles, such as carbohydrates, nucleic acids, proteins, biopolymers, drugs, and other bioactive compounds. The number of hydrogen bonds, root mean square deviation

(RMSD), interaction energy, and solvent accessible surface area (SASA) variables are frequently used in MDS studies for analyzing interactions between biopolymers and drugs [26].

With these investigations, it is possible to examine how the biopolymer behaves both with and without the drug. These investigations also confirm drug exposure to and interaction with the solvent, drug attraction for the biopolymer, and the number of interactions between these two substances. Understanding the events is necessary to research relationships between biopolymers and drugs. Studying these relationships at the atomic scale is made possible by computational techniques, specifically MDS. This method can verify several key aspects of the relationship between biopolymers and drugs, resolving issues that experimental research cannot address [26, 36–38].

4.5 DIFFERENT FORMULATIONS OF BNCs FOR CANCER THERAPY

Both top-down (breakdown of bulk solids or liquids into smaller particles) and bottom-up (self-assembly of monomers into polymers due to certain changes in the environment) methods can be used to create BNCs. The synthesis method substantially manipulates the size and polydispersity index of BNCs. The desired properties of the polymeric NPs are considered when choosing an acceptable production method [39].

4.5.1 Top-Down Approaches for BNCs' Formulation

Electrospinning and emulsification are commonly used top-down approaches for BNC formulations (Table 4.1). These methods often rely on compression, impact, and shear as destructive forces to break up the bulk materials. These methods are frequently employed to produce BNCs, although they have significant drawbacks, including high equipment, maintenance, and operating expenses

TABLE 4.1
Top-Down Approaches for the Formulation of BNCs

Top-Down Approaches	Description	Examples	References
Homogenization method	Combine two immiscible liquids to create an emulsion using a mechanical tool. After emulsion formation, the internal mixture is gelled by adding gelling chemicals or by a specific temperature treatment. Several multivalent cations, such as Ca^{2+}, Cu^{2+}, Mg^{2+}, and Zn^{2+} can be used as gelling agents. Based on electrostatic screening, monovalent cations have also been employed to cause gelation.	Gelatin Hydrogels Alginate-based BNCs Dextran-based BNCs	[40]
Electrospinning method	In this method, the apparatus is made up of a collector plate, a needle tip, a high-voltage power source, a pump, and a syringe containing biopolymeric solution. When a high voltage is given, it changes the solution drop at the needle's edge into a Taylor cone. It further causes fibrous material to be blasted into the collector plate. This method allows for the control of the diameter and rate of drug release by selecting the proper compositional characteristics of the solution, such as the polymer concentration, the distance between the collector plate and needle, conductivity, elasticity, and viscosity.	Various core-shell NFs. Such as: Core: iron oxide NPs + The shell of collagen NF Core: cobalt ferrite and titanium oxide NPs + Shell: DOX-loaded chitosan NF	[41, 42]

and challenges in producing NPs with clearly specified structural features. Furthermore, they require significant volumes of bulk material and can degrade substances due to mechanical stress and grinding, which is typically inappropriate for some fragile and precious bioactive components [40].

4.5.2 Bottom-Up Approaches for BNCs' Formulation

With superior control over particle attributes (such as size, shape, and physical state), bottom-up techniques often enable the production of tiny particles. Additionally, compared to top-down solutions, the final product's contamination risk is frequently diminished. As outlined in Table 4.2, commonly used bottom-up approaches for BNC formulations are desolvation, coacervation, spray deposition, and microfluidics [40].

TABLE 4.2
Bottom-Up Approaches for the Formulation of BNCs

Bottom-Up Approaches	Description	Examples	References
Desolvation	Desolvation, sometimes called anti-solvent precipitation, is a common technique used to create BNCs from proteins and polysaccharides. When the quantity of the solvent used to dissolve the biopolymer is decreased, precipitation of the solute is promoted. The size of the nanoparticles can be optimized by adjusting variables like pH, the concentration of the cross-linking agent, and ionic strength. Water or any organic solvent is example of a solvent. The imbalance in the interactions between the solute, solvent, and anti-solvent propels the production of BNCs. This approach is highly recommended because it uses inexpensive and low-tech equipment.	Lactalbumin, ovalbumin, BSA, human serum albumin in desolvating agents like acetone, ethanol, and methanol	[43]
Coacervation	The approach separates the phases with high and low polymer content, just like the phase separation technique. When biopolymers with opposing charges interact, a rich biopolymer phase (coacervates) is created, which can help encapsulate the desired drug. The typical solvents used are acetone or ethanol. Typically, cross-linking chemicals like glutaraldehyde are used to stabilize the synthesized BNCs. The molecular weight and amount of the biopolymers are two variables that must be taken into consideration to manage the particle size.	Solid-lipid nanoparticle loaded (Arabic gum, sodium stearate) BSA-chitosan-based nano compositions	[39, 43]
Electrohydrodynamic atomization	The electrohydrodynamic atomization technique uses an electrical field to create charged droplets as a byproduct of the atomization process. The BNCs are firmly adhered to the substrate. The technique doesn't call for a specific surfactant or template. Variations in the charge, voltage supply, flow rate, and the separation between the substrate and the needle all affect the size of BNCs. Since there is no modification to the biological characteristics, this approach is highly recommended for synthesizing desired drug nanocrystals.	Very small-sized synthetic (PLGA) and natural (cellulose, alginate, zein, wool keratin, and gelatin) biopolymer-based nano compositions	[43, 44]

4.6 TARGETING MECHANISMS FOR BNCS

4.6.1 Cancer Cell Targeting

4.6.1.1 Transferrin-Conjugated BNCs (TC-BNCs)

The overexpression of a serum glycoprotein receptor called transferrin receptor occurs in certain cancer cells. TC-BNCs can be utilized as an active targeting technique because they have demonstrated improved intracellular drug deliveries and greater cellular uptake efficiencies. Furthermore, research suggests that TC-BNCs are essential in overcoming chemotherapeutic drug resistance [45–48].

4.6.1.2 Folate-Conjugated BNCs (FC-BNCs)

Folate receptors (FR-α and FR-ß) are responsible for folic acid uptake into the cells overexpressed in cancer cells compared to normal cells. Recently, novel FC-BNCs have been successfully employed to target the folate receptor for the treatment of cancer [48–50].

4.6.1.3 Lectins-Conjugated BNCs (LC-BNCs)

In certain cancer cells, lectin is overexpressed. Lectins are non-immunological glycoproteins that bind to specific carbohydrates to perform their function. Hence, to target these cancer cells, BNCs can be designed by using direct or indirect approaches. The direct approach involves the synthesis of LC-BNCs to target the carbohydrates, whereas the indirect approach involves using specific carbohydrates integrated into a nanocomposite matrix to target lectins [48, 51].

4.6.1.4 EGFR-BNCs

The overexpressed gene *EGFR* (epidermal growth factor receptor), which plays a role in several tumor development and progression pathways, is currently being explored as an avenue for drug delivery. For instance, human epidermal receptor-2 (HER-2)-positive breast cancer commonly responds to therapies targeting HER-2. EGFR-BNCs created to comprise enhanced ligands that adhere only to over-expressing *EGFR* gene cancer cells are a viable targeted drug delivery technique. Another approach is designing a single BNC with two EGFR-specific ligands [48, 52, 53].

4.6.2 Endothelium Targeting

Some BNCs stop the angiogenesis process rather than directly targeting specific cancer cells. Developing new blood vessels depends on the interaction of vascular endothelial growth factor (VEGF) and its receptors. Furthermore, it has been demonstrated that simultaneous targeting of the two main VEGFR-2 and VEGFR-3 receptors can increase the therapeutic efficacy of the drug [51, 54].

The neovascular endothelial cancer cells exhibit high levels of the αvß3 integrins that promote endothelial cell migration. Previous in vivo studies have described designing cationic BNCs combined with an αvß3 integrin-targeting ligand. Furthermore, blocking of αvß3 integrins may increase the efficiency of drug therapy because αvß3 integrin is linked to VEGFR-2 signaling pathways. Vascular Cell Adhesion Molecule-1 (VCAM-1), found at the surface of tumor cells, plays an important role in angiogenesis. Previous studies on multiple malignancies have shown them to overexpress VCAM-1, suggesting that BNCs can target this glycoprotein for drug delivery [48].

4.6.3 Passive Targeting

Passive targeting uses the compromised vasculature and lymphatic outflow in the typical tumor cellular microenvironment under conditions like inflammation/hypoxia [55]. It takes a lot of nutrients and oxygen for a tumor to develop, and in the interim, tumor-induced angiogenesis produces a lot of premature vasculatures that inhibit lymphatic outflow [56]. A nanocarrier-based DDS can penetrate the malignant site through these leaky blood vessels, traversing the interstitial space and entering the capillary endothelium through enhanced permeability and retention (EPR) [57]. Thus, nanocarrier extravasation from the tumor microvasculature triggers drug release, which causes a buildup of therapeutic agents in the tumor interstitium [58].

This distinctive characteristic, nonetheless, is not pertinent to small molecule drugs, as they possess a nearly brief circulation time and quick washout from tumors. Hence, utilizing nanosized drug carriers for packaging small-molecule drugs improves their pharmacokinetics (extended systemic circulation), presents tumor discernment, and reduces side effects. Passive targeting depends upon attributes of the carrier (size and circulation time) as well as the biology of the tumor (vascularity and leakiness, for instance), although there is no involvement of ligands for binding to particular tissue or organ [59]. A schematic representation of passive targeting-induced NP aggregation within a tumor is shown in Figure 4.5a.

4.6.4 Active Targeting

Active targeting of nanoscale drug delivery systems to cells can be accomplished by modifying aptamers or high-affinity ligands, which can specifically target cancer cells to deliver anticancer

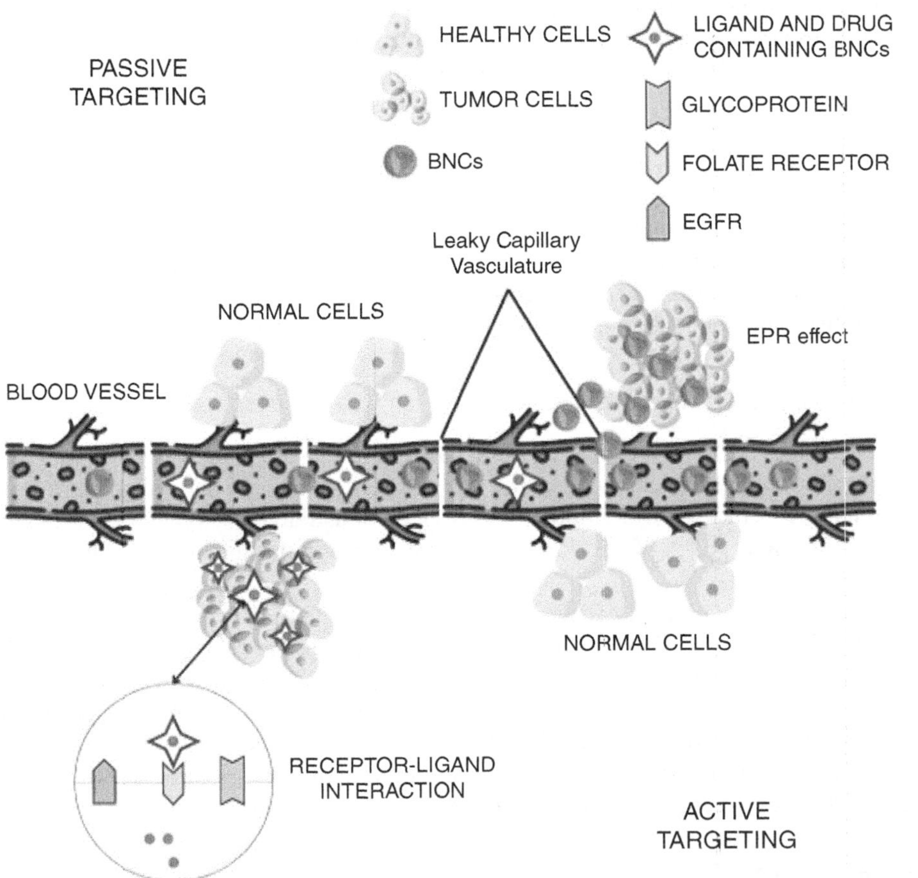

FIGURE 4.5 A schematic representation of passive and active targeting-induced aggregation of BNCs within tumors. (a) Passive targeting depicting extravasation of BNCs through leaky tumor vasculature circulates in the bloodstream and accumulates in tumor tissue. (b) Active targeting exploits ligand-modified BNCs, which bind to highly expressed receptors on the tumor cell, internalizing through receptor-mediated endocytosis.

drugs [60]. Overexpression of surface receptors is manifested by the cancer cells, and these receptors represent the capability for targeted intervention [61]. Additionally, every cancer cell demonstrates a distinctive feature that may be efficiently employed to recognize the cell successfully [62]. Examples of active targeting ligands for cancer therapy comprise aptamers, folate, and transferrin, as well as short RNA or DNA oligonucleotides, which may be folded in different configurations for engagement in the binding of ligands, antibodies, and peptides, for instance [63]. Receptor-mediated endocytosis can deliver medicine payload inside the cancerous tissue [64]. An advantage of active targeting is that it is less toxic for normal tissue because overexpression of targeting ligands is manifested by tumor tissue specifically, enabling its widespread use in cancer treatment. Active targeting may not forever indicate successful delivery to the entire tumor. Consequently, both passive and active targeting methodologies are utilized in concert to harness the maximum capability of nano-designed "magic bullets" [65]. Figure 4.5b depicts a schematic mechanism of active targeting.

4.6.5 Triggered-Release Targeting

The triggered release of drugs is dependent upon various stimuli, which may be physical or biological. It can be employed for modulation of payload release inside the tumor macro-environment. Diverse physical as well as chemical (for instance, temperature and pH) characteristics possessed by the nanocomposites enable modulation of the active and passive delivery of therapeutic medications and promotion of their buildup inside the tumor site [66]. pH inside the majority of the sites in the body is consistent and neutral. Nevertheless, in certain body sites, the pH is naturally acidic. Therefore, the nanoformulations can exploit and get an edge and release the medicine only if they encounter a specific pH [67].

An additional peculiar trigger mechanism depends upon the redox potential: the redox potential at the site adjacent to tumor tissue differs from other sites because hypoxia, a side effect of the tumor, modifies the redox potential [68]. Vesicles containing drugs may selectively target various tumors by manipulating the redox potential for triggering payload release. The drug-loaded nanocomposites gain an intensified benefit compared to conventional drugs because they can employ both passive and active targeting mechanisms. Such formulations are circulated across the body for an extended period until they are drawn toward their target successfully via magnetic positioning, cell-specific ligands, or pH-responsive materials [69].

4.7 OVERCOMING MULTIDRUG RESISTANCE (MDR) IN CANCER CELLS

The failure of diverse cancer treatments because of multidrug resistance has resulted in accelerated disease progression and poor prognosis. The processes underlying drug resistance inside the tumor mass encompass cellular and physiological elements; for instance, overexpression of ABC transporters, an acidic tumor microenvironment (TME), and faulty apoptotic machinery [70].

4.7.1 Targeting of ABC Transporters

Members of the ABC transporter family include efflux transporters, which are crucial in the appearance of resistance to drugs inside various tumors. These transporters lower the concentration of drugs across cells by pumping them out of the cells. P-glycoprotein (P-gp) is among the most extensively studied transporters. Among various tumors, including breast and ovarian tumors, elevated P-gp expression has been correlated with inadequate responses to therapy. Numerous studies have shown that drugs loaded with NPs can escape these overexpressing efflux transporters as the NPs gain entrance to the cell predominantly via endocytosis instead of diffusion to achieve drug release at the target site. The control of drug release can be altered by NP-based drug delivery technology. For instance, redox and low pH levels have been used in numerous studies as triggers to release the drug from NPs. Specific polymers can also be utilized as MDR modulators [48, 71–73].

Another method to combat resistance to treatment is combination therapy. It involves combining chemotherapeutic agents inside any individual nanocarrier. The combination approach depending on NPs has manifested considerable success when used to fight drug resistance and improve the effectiveness of cancer treatment. Additionally, inhibition of the expression and function of the efflux transporters by these nanocarriers is another good approach. It involves either lowering the quantity of ATP given to efflux pumps or manufacturing NPs which encompass chemotherapeutics as well as inhibitors of efflux pumps. A selective COX-2 inhibitor may reduce P-gp overexpression because COX-2 has been shown to contribute to the P-gp-mediated MDR inside the tumors. A recent study showed that doxorubicin and COX-2 inhibitors delivered via NPs reduced resistance in breast cancer cells (BCCs). Additionally, multiple studies have shown inhibition of ABC transporters' expression by similar combination approaches in treating MDR malignancies [48, 74–76].

4.7.2 Targeting of Apoptosis

Another main reason for MDR in cancer cells is their impaired apoptosis machinery, which does not allow cancer cells to undergo apoptosis. The nuclear factor kappa B (NF-B) and Bcl-2 pathways are frequently dysregulated, and Bcl-2 is an extensively studied antiapoptotic protein in multiple cancer cells. Thus, the Bcl-2 protein can be sought after as an attractive target to combat MDR. An NP-based combination approach can be employed to target these two antiapoptotic proteins. For example, NP-based combination therapy has employed NF-B inhibitors like curcumin. Another approach is combining a pro-apoptotic substance, ceramide, with the PTX (paclitaxel), and it can improve therapeutic efficiency in various tumor simulations with drug resistance [48].

A new study revealed that ceramide may be used to control alternative pre-mRNA splicing and re-establish synthesis of the normal form of essential tumor suppressor p53 protein. Regarding this, NPs provide an increasingly efficient platform to transfer ceramide to tumor cells. Restoring the function of p53 is a possible strategy to combat MDR because p53 performs a crucial function in apoptotic program. Consequently, extensive research has been done on the gene therapy of p53 by employing an NP-based approach for drug delivery. It has been documented that PLGA BNCs can restore the p53 gene in both lung and BCCs [48, 77].

Similarly, another study showed the management of MDR in prostate cancer cells. Researchers designed novel folic acid-conjugated NPs encapsulated with docetaxel drug. The results showed suppression of ABC transporters and less expression of antiapoptotic genes [78].

Furthermore, novel BNCs can be designed to target mitochondria. The efflux transporters need ATP to function; hence, targeting mitochondria can decrease ATP production in cancer cells. Recently, a novel hyaluronic acid nano micelle-PTX was designed to target mitochondrial outer membrane permeabilization by enabling the release of cytochrome C and activation of caspase-3 and caspase-9, causing MDR lung cancer cells to undergo apoptosis [76].

4.7.3 Targeting of Hypoxia

Another element contributing to MDR is hypoxia (high oxygen concentrations), which can happen in various circumstances. For instance, slow-replicating cells in hypoxic sites normally escape destruction by cytotoxic response. Hypoxia also creates oxygen gradients within the cancer cells, automatically boosting heterogeneity and encouraging violent phenotypes. Moreover, the research has exhibited that the upregulation of several proteins that usually take part in drug efflux is mediated by hypoxia. HIF-1 (hypoxia-inducible factor 1) is a crucial target and has been overexpressed in multiple malignancies [79–81].

The advantage of BNCs has been considerably reviewed in the therapy for hypoxia. One such approach is to silence the HIF-1 gene, and numerous studies have demonstrated the potency of HIF-1 siRNA-containing NPs in efficiently combating MDR in cancer cells [82, 83]. Besides that, NP-based combination therapy (PEGylated, PLGA-PEG, and non-PEGylated liposomes) may also present superior modalities with significant results. Furthermore, the transcriptional activity of HIF-1 is dependent upon HSP90. It has been revealed that the treatment of bladder cancer can be principally improved by utilizing HSP90 inhibitors inside the 17AAG-loaded nanocomposites [48, 84].

4.8 BNCs USED FOR TARGETED DELIVERY OF ANTICANCER DRUGS

4.8.1 Protein-Based BNCs

4.8.1.1 Albumin-Based BNCs

One of the protein polymers that occur naturally is albumin, the most prevalent in the bloodstream and involved in the binding and transportation of water, minerals, fatty acids, hormones, toxins, metals, and drug molecules in the body [85]. There are three types of albumin: bovine serum albumin, ovalbumin, and human serum albumin. These albumins are extensively exploited in cancer DDS because of their biocompatibility, high ligand interactions, accessibility, low cost, ability to form emulsions, rapid response toward pH and temperature changes, and biodegradable and inert properties [86].

Albumin-based BNCs are a versatile option against many types of tumors since they can offer targeting through passive and active routes, drug release in a controlled manner, evading drug resistance strategies of cancer cells, and inhibition of apoptosis [87]. The albumin-based DDS's ability to augment tumor targeting and subsequent accumulation accounts for its effectiveness. The increased tumor accumulation is caused by passive uptake through the EPR effect [88]. By this uptake process, the albumin-based BNCs bypass the tumor cell's drug efflux mechanism [89]. Furthermore, albumin can improve the binding and incorporation of BNCs by interacting with unique receptors overexpressed on cancer cells, such as glycoprotein-60kDa (gp60) receptor and secreted protein acidic and rich in cysteine (SPARC) receptor [90]. When compared to Cremophor EL-paclitaxel, it was found that nab-paclitaxel's endothelium binding increased 9.9-fold, and paclitaxel was delivered more efficiently by 4.2-fold [91]. Additionally, albumin possesses amino and carboxylic functional groups, which are amenable to the functionalization of albumin BNCs with therapeutically effective ligands [92].

4.8.1.2 Collagen-Based BNCs

One of the most prevalent structural proteins in the living body is collagen, a naturally occurring polymer that serves as the main constituent of the extracellular matrix (ECM) and is an integral part of connective tissues in the cartilage, tendons, and bones [93]. Collagen is a commonly used biomaterial for developing BNC DDS due to its biocompatibility, versatility, non-inflammatory properties, low antigenicity, and low cytotoxic responses [65]. According to a previous study, collagen-based NPs can aid in administering anticancer drugs by infiltrating tumors since collagen has the benefit of resembling the milieu of a tumor. This study used HCT116, 95-D, and U87 cell lines to create and refine collagen-based tumor spheroids to investigate antitumor and delivery efficacies through cytotoxicity and uptake studies on the drug-conjugated NPs. Based on their findings, the conjugated NPs penetrated the gel matrix to access the tumor cells [94].

4.8.1.3 Gelatin-Based BNCs

Another biodegradable, multifunctional polymer that occurs naturally is gelatin. It is made of proteins and peptides that are derived from partially hydrolyzed collagen [95]. Gelatin is a considerable reservoir of the amino acids hydroxyproline, proline, and glycine due to the enormous amounts of these amino acids present in its polymeric chain [96]. Gelatin possesses properties like hydrophilic nature, amphoteric behavior, sol-gel transition, and ease of cross-linking, making them excellent DDS for cancer therapy [56]. Due to its ability to swell, gelatin has been used in various DDS to create hydrogels. [97] made PLA/gelatin BNCs with two antitumor compounds (doxorubicin and dasatinib) for targeted DDS in cancer therapy.

4.8.2 Polysaccharide-Based BNCs

Natural polysaccharides, which are composed of monosaccharides linked together by glycosidic linkages, can be used to create BNCs and can be obtained from several sources, including animals (chitosan and chondroitin), plants (e.g., cellulose), seaweed (carrageenan (CR)), and microbes (alginate and pullulan) [98]. Polysaccharides can be used to create functionalized materials for cancer DDS since they differ chemically in chain length, charge, the configuration of the monosaccharides, and stereochemistry [99]. Polysaccharides can reduce and stabilize metal salts to create metallic nanoparticles (MNPs) [100]. Moreover, because they have hydrophilic functional groups (such as -OH, -COOH, and -NH_2), they can generate bio-adhesive polymers that can increase the effectiveness of many drugs by forming non-covalent interactions with biological cells [101]. Polysaccharides are also beneficial against cancer cells because they have selectivity to multiple sites and play a significant role in cell-to-cell recognition [102].

4.8.2.1 Chitosan-Based BNCs

Natural polysaccharide chitosan is created by partially deacetylating chitin, a biopolymer derived from marine sources that frequently makes up a sizeable portion of the fungal cell wall and crustacean exoskeleton [103]. Chitosan is composed of N-acetylglucosamine and possesses a cationic charge. Their distinctive designs, greater sustainability, simplicity, safety, cost-effective synthesis, biodegradability, biocompatibility, and non-immunogenic properties have made them an exemplary choice in drug delivery applications [104].

The successful development of its nanocomposites as anticancer drug carriers in recent years has demonstrated efficient and targeted drug delivery through active and passive mechanisms in tumor therapy [105]. The chitosan-based BNCs can stabilize and safeguard anticancer agents quite well and efficiently. Recently, chitosan-magnetic nanoparticle (CS-MNP)-based DDS has been developed for cancer treatments involving drug carrier systems such as doxorubicin-CS-MNP, significantly showing a stronger repressive influence on the growing tumor cells [106].

Abdel-Bary et al. (2020) investigated the cisplatin loading capability of chitosan functionalized with silicon dioxide (S), magnetite (M), and graphene oxide (GO) inorganic NPs [111]. For this reason, BNCs with formulations CS/M/S/GO; CS/M/S; CS/S; and CS/M were developed. The results revealed the highest efficacy of CS/M (87%) and CS/M/S/GO (84%) BNCs. At the same time, CS/M BNC showed the highest (91%) releasing potentiality compared with the others.

In another study, stimuli-responsive hydrogel BNC was fabricated using chitosan to co-polymerize acrylic acid and N-isopropyl acrylamide, after which the Fe_3O_4 magnetic NPs were synthesized *in situ*. To obtain regulated and modulated release of the antitumor drug doxorubicin, hydrogel BNC was used as a DDS, which showed drug-loading capacity of up to 89%. Furthermore, the BNC showed responsiveness to both pH and temperature, and within 48 hours, 82% of the drug doxorubicin was released from the hydrogel [107].

In a different study, using spherical particles of N, N, N-trimethyl chitosan chloride (TMC) with a diameter ranging from 11 to 17.5 nm, silver BNCs were produced. Lung cancer cell line A-549 showed decreased viability when treated with TMC/Ag BNCs with an IC_{50} value of 12.3 g/ml, whereas an IC_{50} value of 357.2 µg/ml was recorded with normal lung cells WI 38 [108].

4.8.2.2 Alginate-Based BNCs

Alginate is an anionic linear natural polysaccharide consisting of 1,4-linked β-d-mannuronic acid and α-l-guluronic acid monomers [109]. One interesting property of sodium alginate in aqueous conditions is that it undergoes ionic gelation when exposed to metal cations such as Ca^{2+}, Zn^{2+}, Ba^{2+}, and Al^{3+} [110].

Alginates have been extensively used as BNC DDS over the past few decades. Recently, a study done by Taşkın Çakıcı in 2023 developed TiO_2-doped sodium alginate/hydroxypropyl methylcellulose (NaAlg/HPMC/TiO2) BNC membrane for controlled release of 5-fluorouracil, which is an anticancer drug [111].

In another study by Sheng et al. (2021), researchers showed co-entrapment of methotrexate-loaded $CaCO_3$ ($CaCO_3$/MTX) and aspirin in hydrogels made from alginate and sodium carboxymethyl cellulose by crosslinking with Ca^{2+} for chemotherapy and simultaneous relief of pain in patients who have CRC. According to the findings, the BNC DDS shielded the anticancer therapeutic agent from absorbing in the stomach and small intestine and ensured effectiveness at the target location inside the colorectum. [112].

4.8.2.3 Cellulose-Based BNCs

Cellulose, a structural protein found in plants and eukaryotic algae, is formed via β (1 → 4)-glycosidic bonds among D-glucose units. The characteristics which make cellulose a resource for fabricating BNC DDS contribute to its non-toxic nature, renewability, biodegradability, chemical stability, mechanical robustness, biocompatibility, hydrogen bonding interactions, mechanical robustness, high molecular weight, and enzymatic resistance [113].

Sun et al. (2019) engineered hydrogel beads containing the anticancer drug 5-fluorouracil, which ZnO-carboxymethylcellulose-chitosan encapsulated to treat colon cancer. The results indicated that the cellulose-based BNCs delivered 5-fluorouracil in a pH-responsive manner [114].

In another study, Javanbakht et al. (2018) developed a CMC/MOF-5/graphene oxide carrier encapsulating doxorubicin, significantly enhancing its anticancer properties. When exposed to the acidic tumor microenvironment with a pH of 5, higher than the physiological pH of 7.4, doxorubicin was released at a considerably higher rate. The findings of the cytotoxicity test showed that doxorubicin-encapsulated CMC/MOF-5/GO BNCs significantly reduced the viability of K562 tumor cells [115].

4.8.2.4 Starch-Based BNCs

Plant-derived starches are biodegradable polymers with excellent biocompatibility. In one study, hydrogel beads using zinc oxide BNCs, carboxymethyl cellulose, and starch were developed [116]. By doing this, doxorubicin was designed to be released under controlled conditions. The *in vitro* testing showed that the quantities of carboxymethyl cellulose, the physiological pH, and the intervention of ZnO BNCs all impacted the hydrogel's swelling and therapeutic drug release capacity.

Another study by Gholamali et al. (2021) used oxidized starch/polyvinyl alcohol/CuO BNC hydrogels loaded with doxorubicin against human colon cancer cell line SW480. The findings revealed that the percentage of doxorubicin loading increased as the CuO NP content increased [117].

4.8.2.5 Xanthan Gum-Based BNCs

A biopolymer, xanthan gum, is created when extracellular polysaccharides are fermented with the help of the bacterium *Xanthomonas campestris* in the presence of sugars [118]. D-glucose (1-4) linkage and a linear structure without branches are both characteristics of xanthan gum. It exhibits excellent water solubility as well as good biocompatibility [119]. Xanthan gum is more effective at various pH levels, ionic concentrations, and temperature ranges [120]. Recent advancements have been made in the delivery of anticancer medications using xanthan gum-based BNCs.

El-Sawy et al. (2020), in one study, showed the development of BNC where xanthan gum (Xan), acrylic acid (AA), and magnesium oxide (MgO) were combined to form hydrogels that serve as drug carriers. Furthermore, methotrexate (MTX) was utilized as an anticancer drug model. The findings demonstrated that adding MgO to Xan-AAc hydrogel increased the drug loading effectiveness and boosted the release of MTX to the maximum at a neutral pH of 7. Additionally, the drug release property of hydrogel concurred well with its swelling capacity, making Xan-AAc)/MgO BNC hydrogels a potential therapeutic DDS [121].

4.8.2.6 Guar Gum-Based BNCs

Galactomannan polysaccharide, also known as guar gum or guaran, is obtained from guar beans and is an exopolysaccharide made up of galactose as well as mannose with a backbone of linearly linked β-1,4-mannose residues [122]. It exhibits advantageous characteristics such as biodegradability, biocompatibility, mechanical strength, physicochemical stability, and bioavailability [123]. It is a good candidate for delivering the drug due to its effective gelling characteristics and enzymes' degradation inside the colonic fluids [124]. Several guar gum-based BNCs DDS have been developed for targeted cancer therapy. Bhatt et al. (2021) developed chitosan (CS)/guar gum (GG)/gum ghatti (GGh)/AgNPs BNCs [125]. In another study, Muthaiah and Ramachandran also showed guar gum nanospheres containing the anticancer drug gemcitabine as DDS for targeted drug delivery [126].

4.8.2.7 Pectin-Based BNCs

Pectin is a complex biopolymer that occurs naturally in plant cell walls and is water-soluble, starch-free, and non-toxic [127]. Its linear polymer structure is primarily made up of D-galacturonic acid residues joined together using α-(1-4) glycosidic bonds, along with L-rhamnopyranose, which also exists via α-(1-2) linkages connecting methoxy groups, which esterify the pectin [128]. When added to an acidic environment, a sizable amount of sucrose (>50%) has been found to improve the gelling ability of high methoxy pectins. In divalent cations like Ca^{2+} and Zn^{2+}, low methoxy pectin can develop gelatinous structures through ionotropic gelation (Abitbol et al., 2021). [129]. These cations can be potential vehicles in DDS. Recently, several pectin-based BNC DDS have been developed for anticancer drug delivery.

To specifically target the colon when administering 5-fluorouracil orally, Wang et al. (2020) have developed a strategy by utilizing 3-Amino propyl tri-ethoxy silane modified-pectin-Ca^{2+}-nanocarbon sphere-based BNC gel films, which improved the pectin-based DDS's ability to release the therapeutic drug under control. This oral BNC film-based colon-specific DDS exhibited efficient encapsulation. The total release rates of simulated gastric, colonic, and small intestinal fluid were 22.77%, 32.17%, and 63.89%, respectively, showing favorable release performance of the BNCs [130].

4.8.2.8 Hyaluronic Acid-Based BNCs

A polyanionic natural polymer, hyaluronic acid, is widely distributed inside the extracellular environment of connective tissues in the human body. It is made up of repeating glucuronic acid and N-acetylglucosamine units connected by β-1,4 linkage [131]. It is an intriguing biopolymer due to its remarkable viscoelasticity, water solubility, biocompatibility, and lack of immunogenicity, making it an appealing candidate for creating BNCs for cancer DDS [132].

Using hyaluronic acid along with fluorochrome indocyanine green, doxorubicin, and carboxyl terminated dendrimer, Wu et al. (2019), in an intriguing study, created a hyaluronic-based BNC known as high-penetrating cationic liposomes (HPCID). The HPCID formulation showed improved therapeutic effects and efficient targeting of metastatic cancer cells. Subsequently, the hyaluronidase in 4T1 cells broke down the HA shell, causing a drug release that immediately responded to enzymatic activity. Furthermore, by using ultrasound radiation and chemotherapy to produce large amounts of ROS, the HPCID significantly increased cellular apoptosis. Additionally, in mice with 4T1 xenografts receiving HPCID along with ultrasonic radiation, without any systemic side effects, a significant decrease was observed in tumor growth and pulmonary metastasis. [133].

4.9 APPLICATIONS OF BNCs IN VARIOUS CANCERS

According to reports in 2005, cancer was the cause of 13% of all fatalities worldwide. Although many cancers require an early diagnosis to be effectively treated, the sensitivity limitations of existing diagnostic techniques limit their efficacy. Using nanoscale materials as agents for cancer imaging and therapy has been demonstrated to be successful in cancer treatment and diagnosis. The method used to generate responsive and multifunctional composite systems is functionalizing inorganic nanomaterials with biocompatible polymers, either naturally existing or synthetic molecules. Nanocomposite materials have demonstrated potential and effectiveness in cancer detection and treatment, even though only a few such advancements have been evaluated in humans [134].

4.9.1 Breast Cancer

Breast cancer (BC) affects more women than any other type of cancer, resulting in 25% of cancer incidents worldwide. In women, breast cancer is supposed to be responsible for 15% of all cancer-related deaths. Primary breast cancer treatment usually involves surgery, followed by adjuvant radio/chemotherapy. Radiotherapy reduces and eliminates tumor cells in around 50% of BC patients [135]. Despite recent advances in radiation, tumor radiotherapy resistance persists. It may lead to tumor recurrence and treatment failure, presenting a significant problem [136]. In this scenario, BNCs proved to be the most effective strategy to combat breast cancer. The minimum side effects of these nanomaterials make them a suitable choice over traditional treatment options.

4.9.1.1 ZnO/Chitosan (Ppy/C/Z)

The creation of a BNC matrix involving ZnO/chitosan grafted with polypyrrole (Ppy/C/Z) has been achieved by in-situ polymerization of pyrrole and different weight sections of ZnO. Adding ZnO NPs to polypyrrole improves the composite's photocatalytic, antibacterial, and cytotoxic characteristics: X-ray diffraction (XRD) and thermal analysis (TGA and DTA). FTIR, thermal analysis, and other techniques have been used to analyze the produced product. Particle size and surface morphology were evaluated using SEM and TEM. Using EDX and SEM together, the sample's elemental makeup was examined. Electrochemical double-layer capacitance (EDLC) data were used to calculate the electrochemical surface area. To evaluate the photocatalytic activity, dyes methylene blue (MB), reactive orange-16 (RO-16), and coomassie brilliant blue R-250 (CBB-R-250) were reduced with the availability of UV light.

For the photocatalytic process, the reactive species involved were discovered using a variety of scavengers. Recyclability tests were also carried out to confirm the photocatalyst's stability. The BNC, namely Ppy/C/Z, also demonstrated antibacterial and anticancer effects on cancer cell lines of humans, such as MCF-7 (the cell line for breast cancer). These effects were shown against Gram-negative as well as Gram-positive pathogenic bacteria. Experimental results show that Ppy/C/Z BNC outperforms pure polypyrrole combined with chitosan formulation (Ppy/C). Research has demonstrated these bio nanocomposites' efficacy in breast cancer therapeutics [137].

4.9.1.2 Chitosan-Based BNCs

As a natural biopolymer, chitosan has several uses owing to its biodegradability, antibacterial capabilities, non-toxicity, and other biological features. Due to their functional groups, they are coupled with different nanofillers for diverse biological applications. Chitosan does have anticancer properties; however, bio nanocomposites, which incorporate chitosan with nanofillers, outperform conventional cancer treatments. Nanocomposites based on chitosan are being investigated for photodynamic therapy, medication delivery, necrosis and/or apoptosis induction, and tumor imaging. Because of these exceptional properties, chitosan-based BNCs are effectively employed in treating breast cancer [137].

4.9.1.3 Silver Nanoparticles

Metal NPs are crucial elements with a wide range of astounding advantages in antibacterial, engineering, chemical, electronics, catalysis, etc., because of their small size, large surface area, distribution, and morphology. They are also inexpensive, highly efficient, and have high active performance. Physical, chemical, and biological processes are all used for the creation of AgNPs. The small size and vast surface area of AgNPs significantly contribute to their antimicrobial and anticancer effects. Because it requires minimal effort and is inexpensive, BNC reduction is often employed to create AgNPs without interparticle aggregation. In forming AgNPs, reducing agents perform an important part [138].

Naturally existing biological substances with reducing properties, significant water solubility, and anticancer properties are gallic acid (GA). Due to their distinctive features, BNCs have recently received increased interest in the disciplines of biological science, nanotechnology, engineering, and pharmaceuticals. These are a new class of nanomaterials with better structural and functional characteristics than traditional nanocomposites used in various applications because they are made of naturally occurring biopolymers from plants, microorganisms, and inorganic solids on the nanometer scale. Natural polymers' unique qualities, such as biocompatibility and biodegradability, provide these materials with novel possibilities in nanoscience [138].

Because smaller particles have a more substantial antimicrobial and anticancer impact, stabilizers are crucial in regulating AgNP particle size during synthesis. Because they are so good at avoiding particle collection and precipitation, biodegradable polymers are employed as stabilizers to provide particles with a great distribution. Nowadays, clay matrix interlayer space is extensively used due to its distinctive intercalation, swelling, and ion exchange capabilities, with a marked increase in mechanical qualities. Due to its distinct properties, bentonite is mainly utilized to create polymeric nanocomposites. Artificial neural networks (ANNs) would allow for the optimization and assessment of AgNPs while saving time and money, allowing for the creation of the best-fit optimized model. These bio nanocomposites' remarkable qualities make them a potent breast cancer treatment [138].

4.9.1.4 ZnO-NPs and CS-ZnO BNCs for BCCs in MCTSs

According to studies, 3D multicellular tumor spheroids (MCTSs) may realistically replicate the treatment responses of in vivo tumor cells. Using the 3D-MCTSs model, the ability of pure NPs synthesized from zinc oxide (ZnO-NPs) and chitosan-ZnO BNCs (CS-ZnO BNCs) to induce radiosensitization of BCCs (MDA-MB-231) was examined. ZnO-NPs and CS-ZnO BNCs were created using the standard co-precipitation technique. The homogenous, spherical ZnONPs were efficiently disseminated across chitosan. MDA-MB-231 MCTSs exhibited functional hallmarks of an in vivo mass of cancer cells in a culture plate. Importance of this approach for culturing over the commonly utilized 2D monolayer (or parental) cell culture strategy is because it mimics the tumor microenvironment [138].

To assess the toxicity of pure ZnO-NPs and CS-ZnO BNCs against MDA-M 231 BCCs, an MTT colorimetric test was performed. CS-ZnO BNCs were shown to be more biocompatible than pure ZnO-NPs (even at excessive concentrations of 100 g/mL). MCTSs were more radioresistant than parental cells, according to research that looked at the survival proportion of cells that had been treated with clinical X-ray radiation (6 MV). Furthermore, the clonogenic potential of irradiated MCTSs was reduced considerably when CS-ZnO BNCs were added, the way it was in monolayer cells. The sensitivity enhancement ratios (SER) of MCTSs and monolayer cells were 1.5 and 1.63, respectively. CS-ZnO BNCs were discovered to not only increase the amount of radiation-induced complex DNA breaks as well as mortality in MCTSs but to suspend DNA repair pathways additionally. A non-toxic amount of CS-ZnO BNCs was shown to boost radiosensitivity among resistant MCTSs, serving as an improved *in vitro* cancer model. As a result, CS-ZnO BNCs could become a viable strategy to reduce radiation resistance in BCC [138].

It should be highlighted that the development and validation of novel and effective anticancer therapies can be greatly helped by using precise and applicable cell-based assays in screening chemotherapy medications. Two-dimensional (2D) culture (monolayer) has frequently been employed for cell-based testing as a practical platform [136]. However, since there are no appropriate microenvironmental settings, for example, cell-extracellular matrix and cell-cell interactions, 2D culture cannot adequately mimic the complex cellular activity in tissues, resulting in incorrect cancer response prediction to novel therapies. This difference is a major factor in drug development's high failure rate at all stages of clinical testing. The 3D culture model is gaining popularity because it involves imitation of *the in vivo model, which can* overcome affirmational constraints and give more exact data on anticancer therapeutic effectiveness [139].

4.9.2 Lung Cancer

Accounting for around 29% of cancer deaths (particularly in males) and 26% of cancer deaths in females, lung cancer is the predominant reason for mortality globally. Lung cancer is the most prevalent type of malignant tumor globally. Chemotherapy is restricted by cancer cells developing drug resistance and using hazardous substances, which causes undesirable side effects. Nanobiotechnology is now gaining popularity in the field of biomedical applications. Due to its extensive medicinal and therapeutic applications, including its anticancer, antioxidant, and antibacterial properties, copper oxide NPs (CuO NPs) have captured greater interest than other metal or metal oxide NPs, particularly bio-synthesized CuO NPs. Recent studies have concentrated on manufacturing metal oxide NPs incorporated with chitosan, which has been demonstrated to have good biocompatibility. (1,4)-linked D-glucosamine and N-acetyl-D-glucosamine are randomly distributed throughout the polysaccharide known as chitosan. Because of its unique qualities, including biocompatibility, biodegradability, antibacterial properties, and drug delivery capabilities, chitosan has gained appeal. As a result, researchers have been working on biopolymer metal oxide nanocomposites [140].

4.9.2.1 Chitosan/Copper Oxide Nanocomposite

UV-visible spectroscopy, TEM, FE-SEM, XRD, FTIR, and EDS examined the bio-synthesized nanocomposite of CS-CuO. The synthesized nanocomposite's TEM scans and FE-SEM scans revealed an average size of 10 to 30 nm. EDS analysis was used to validate the component constituents of the CS-CuO nanocomposite. The CS-CuO nanocomposite had a monoclinic structure, according to XRD analysis. In A549 (human lung cancer cell line), the anti-growth action of the nanocomposite was examined. Having depicted the IC_{50} value of 20.50 g/mL, the CS-CuO nanocomposite suppressed the growth of A549 cancer cells. The resulting nanocomposites were shown to induce apoptosis in A549 cells (that were previously treated). Finally, the CS-CuO nanocomposite produced with rutin can be used as an anticancer medication in the biomedical and medical industries [140].

4.9.2.2 Polymeric BNCs

Polymeric BNC demonstrated substantial cytotoxicity against human lung cancer cell lines. A versatile antifouling hydrophilic polymer with multiple applications in both biomedicine and industry is polyethylene glycol (PEG). The surface coating of PEG on various substrates gives unique characteristics that improve host material biocompatibility. It is well known that PEG-coated surfaces have antifouling properties that reduce cell adherence, microbial attachment, and protein adsorption. Additionally, the antifouling capabilities of PEG and PEG-conjugated proteins may delay blood clotting, improve proteolytic stability, and increase mechanical and thermal stability. Many typical polymer nanofillers, such as talc, fumed silica, calcium carbonate, noble metals, and carbon nanotubes, increase the performance of polymers made from renewable resources. The resulting bio nanocomposite shows a broad range of practical applications in biomedical and industrial domains, combining the advantages of the high surface area of NPs with low-dimensional layers [141].

4.9.2.3 BNCs Combined with *P. cylindraceus* Oil

Using the prior described approach, *P. cylindraceus* oil and polymeric bio nanocomposite were assessed for cytotoxicity in human lung cancer (A549) cell lines. The A549 cancer cells were cultured in DMEM medium supplemented by 10% FBS, 100 mg mL1 streptomycin, 2 mM glutamine, and 100 IU mL1. Cell cultures were maintained at 37°C in humidified incubator that continuously supplied 5% CO_2. In 96-well plates, A549 cell culture was seeded with a density of 1*104 cells in each well. Polymeric BNC and *P. cylindraceus* oil in varying concentrations (0 to 200 g mL1) cultivated the cells for one day. After 24 hours, the cells were fed 100 L of MTT (3-(4,5-dimethylthiazol-2-yl)-2,5-diphenyltetrazolium bromide). Cells were later kept at 37°C for another 4 hours. The addition of purple formazan solution in 100 L of dimethyl sulfoxide after 4 hours of incubation. OD at 570 nm was recorded after 30 minutes with the help of an ELISA multiwell plate reader to calculate the IC50 value. The performance of the lactate dehydrogenase (LDH) leakage experiment was done in order to evaluate the cell membrane impairment and loss of membrane integrity. The consequences of modifying BNC on mitochondrial membrane potential (m) were studied using the rhodamine 123 staining technique. To avoid mistakes, all tests were carried out in triplicate. It was revealed by this research that the designed bio nanocomposites were highly effective in combating lung cancer [142].

4.9.3 Colorectal Cancer

It has been reported that CRC can be held responsible for 10% of global cancer occurrences and 9.4% of cancer mortalities in 2020, just below lung cancer, which can be attributed to 18% of casualties. In accordance with estimations of population expansion, aging, and human progress, the worldwide number of new CRC cases is expected to rise to 3.2 million in 2040. The heightened occurrence of CRC is largely because of greater susceptibility to environmental hazards due to a change in lifestyle and nutrition in the direction of Westernization. Advances in understanding the pathophysiology of CRC have resulted in more therapy alternatives. These medicines have effectively slowed cancer progression and increased overall survival. Population-based screening for CRC, including endoscopy, improves overall survival and quality of life [143].

4.9.3.1 5-Fluorouracil-Loaded Magnetic Cellulose BNCs

Natural multifunctionality and a wide range of physiochemical characteristics make magnetic polymer nanocomposites promising for application as novel drug nanocarriers. In a published study, 5-fluorouracil, often known as MC/5-FU, was supported on rice straw cellulose as a carrier for Fe_3O_4 NPs as a potential treatment for CRC. Several investigations revealed that MC/5-FU BNCs had multifunctional characteristics. Fe_3O_4 nanofillers covered the matrix with the help of transmission and scanning electron microscopy. While evaluating the release of drug from MC/5-FU at different temperatures and pH levels, pH 7.4 at 44.2°C produced the highest level of release. MC/5-FU indicated improved discernment and antitumor activity against CRC cells in 2D monolayer and 3D tumor spheroid models while employing an *in vitro* antitumor assay. This readily prepared MC/5-FU showed promise as an inexpensive drug formulation for treating CRC [144].

4.10 CONCLUSION

Today, the core component of cancer treatment is chemotherapy, an agonizing and time-consuming method. Toxic antimetabolites, antitumor antibiotics, topoisomerase inhibitors, alkylating agents, and mitotic inhibitors are a few of the traditional chemotherapy drugs that are frequently used. BNC-based drug delivery systems are novel techniques and exhibit remarkable qualities relevant to the successful treatment of cancer, including enhanced targeting efficacy and diminished adverse effects. Natural polymeric BNCs have been found to be more advantageous in cost, biocompatibility, sustainability, inherently low immunogenicity, and biodegradability. Various *in vivo* and *in vitro* investigations have been conducted on the successful synthesis of natural polymeric BNCs and their underlying mechanisms to deliver chemotherapeutic drugs at targeted sites. In the near future, researchers, regulatory authorities, and pharmaceutical companies must collaborate to ensure that these novel drug delivery systems reach from benchtop to bedside with enhanced safety and efficacy.

REFERENCES

[1] A. Ali, M. F. Manzoor, N. Ahmad, R. M. Aadil, H. Qin, R. Siddique, S. Riaz, A. Ahmad, S. A. Korma, and W. Khalid, "The burden of cancer, government strategic policies, and challenges in Pakistan: A comprehensive review," *Frontiers in Nutrition*, vol. 9, pp. 1553, 2022.

[2] C. Kaur, and U. Garg, "Artificial intelligence techniques for cancer detection in medical image processing: A review," *Materials Today: Proceedings*, vol. 81, pp. 806–809, 2021.
[3] M. Arifin, A. Parikesit, and D. Agustriawan, "Molecular simulation oF MDM2 and E6AP proteins as P53 regulator in cervical cancer," *Biointerface Research in Applied Chemistry*, vol. 10, pp. 5875–5879, 2020.
[4] W. You, and M. Henneberg, "Cancer incidence increasing globally: The role of relaxed natural selection," *Evolutionary Applications*, vol. 11, p. 140–152, 2018.
[5] F. Bray, J. Ferlay, I. Soerjomataram, R. L. Siegel, L. A. Torre, and A. Jemal, "Global cancer statistics 2018: GLOBOCAN estimates of incidence and mortality worldwide for 36 cancers in 185 countries," *CA: A Cancer Journal for Clinicians*, vol. 68, no. 6, pp. 394–424, 2018.
[6] K. Bukowski, M. Kciuk, and R. Kontek, "Mechanisms of multidrug resistance in cancer chemotherapy," *International Journal of Molecular Sciences*, vol. 21, no. 9, pp. 3233, 2020.
[7] C. Chakraborty, A. R. Sharma, G. Sharma, B. K. Sarkar, and S.-S. Lee, "The novel strategies for next-generation cancer treatment: miRNA combined with chemotherapeutic agents for the treatment of cancer," *Oncotarget*, vol. 9, no. 11, p. 10164, 2018.
[8] N. Behranvand, F. Nasri, R. Zolfaghari Emameh, P. Khani, A. Hosseini, J. Garssen, and R. Falak, "Chemotherapy: A double-edged sword in cancer treatment," *Cancer Immunology, Immunotherapy*, vol. 71, no. 3, pp. 507–526, 2022.
[9] M. Demaria, M. N. O'Leary, J. Chang, L. Shao, S. Liu, F. Alimirah, K. Koenig, C. Le, N. Mitin, and A. M. Deal, "Cellular senescence promotes adverse effects of chemotherapy and cancer relapsecellular senescence and chemotherapy," *Cancer Discovery*, vol. 7, no. 2, pp. 165–176, 2017.
[10] M. Xiao, J. Cai, L. Cai, J. Jia, L. Xie, Y. Zhu, B. Huang, D. Jin, and Z. Wang, "Let-7e sensitizes epithelial ovarian cancer to cisplatin through repressing DNA double strand break repair," *Journal of Ovarian Research*, vol. 10, no. 1, pp. 1–13, 2017.
[11] W. M. van den Boogaard, D. S. Komninos, and W. P. Vermeij, "Chemotherapy side-effects: Not all DNA damage is equal," *Cancers*, vol. 14, no. 3, pp. 627, 2022.
[12] S. H. Armenian, C. J. Gibson, R. C. Rockne, and K. K. Ness, "Premature aging in young cancer survivors," *JNCI: Journal of the National Cancer Institute*, vol. 111, no. 3, pp. 226–232, 2019.
[13] J. L. Guida, T. A. Ahles, D. Belsky, J. Campisi, H. J. Cohen, J. DeGregori, R. Fuldner, L. Ferrucci, L. Gallicchio, and L. Gavrilov, "Measuring aging and identifying aging phenotypes in cancer survivors," *JNCI: Journal of the National Cancer Institute*, vol. 111, no. 12, pp. 1245–1254, 2019.
[14] V. Schirrmacher, "From chemotherapy to biological therapy: A review of novel concepts to reduce the side effects of systemic cancer treatment," *International Journal of Oncology*, vol. 54, no. 2, pp. 407–419, 2019.
[15] S. Wang, A. Prizment, B. Thyagarajan, and A. Blaes, "Cancer treatment-induced accelerated aging in cancer survivors: Biology and assessment," *Cancers*, vol. 13, no. 3, pp. 427, 2021.
[16] B. Arora, R. Bhatia, and P. Attri, "Bionanocomposites: Green materials for a sustainable future," *New Polymer Nanocomposites for Environmental Remediation*, pp. 699–712: Elsevier, 2018.
[17] A. Kalsoom Khan, A. U. Saba, S. Nawazish, F. Akhtar, R. Rashid, S. Mir, B. Nasir, F. Iqbal, S. Afzal, and F. Pervaiz, "Carrageenan based bionanocomposites as drug delivery tool with special emphasis on the influence of ferromagnetic nanoparticles," *Oxidative Medicine and Cellular Longevity*, vol. 2017, p. 8158315, 2017.
[18] B. Joseph, S. Krishnan, V. Sagarika, A. Tharayil, N. Kalarikkal, and S. Thomas, "Bionanocomposites as industrial materials, current and future perspectives: A review," *Emergent Materials*, vol. 3, pp. 711–725, 2020.
[19] R. Sharma, S. M. Jafari, and S. Sharma, "Antimicrobial bio-nanocomposites and their potential applications in food packaging," *Food Control*, vol. 112, p. 107086, 2020.
[20] M. U. Akbar, Z.-E. Huma, M. Salman, R. Hussain, A. F. Zahoor, A. Mansha, S. Asim, and M. Zuber, "Synthetic materials to bionanocomposites: An overview," *Bionanocomposites*, pp. 1–20, 2020.
[21] M. Akhtar, M. Jamshaid, M. Zaman, and A. Z. Mirza, "Bilayer tablets: A developing novel drug delivery system," *Journal of Drug Delivery Science and Technology*, vol. 60, p. 102079, 2020.
[22] Z. Mohammad, A. Zeeshan, S. Faisal, A. Suhail, I. Sahar, S. Mohd, and K. Nazma, "Vesicular drug delivery system used for liver diseases," *World Journal of Pharmaceutical Sciences*, vol. 5, no. 4, pp. 28–35, 2017.
[23] A. Thakur, A. Roy, S. Chatterjee, P. Chakraborty, K. Bhattacharya, and P. P. Mahata, *Recent Trends in Targeted Drug Delivery*, SMGroup, 2015.

[24] A. Tewabe, A. Abate, M. Tamrie, A. Seyfu, and E. Abdela Siraj, "Targeted drug delivery—From magic bullet to nanomedicine: Principles, challenges, and future perspectives," *Journal of Multidisciplinary Healthcare*, vol. 14, pp. 1711–1724, 2021.

[25] S. Mumtaz, S. Khattak, F. U. Rehman, P. Muhammad, and S. Hanif, "Bionanocomposites as a new platform for drug delivery systems," *Novel Platforms for Drug Delivery Applications*, pp. 289–315, Elsevier, 2023.

[26] L. S. Reinhardt, P. R. Arantes, J. G. Henn, and D. J. Moura, "Bionanocomposites for in situ drug delivery in cancer therapy: Early and late evaluations," *Biomedical Composites: Perspectives and Applications*, pp. 145–165, Springer, 2021.

[27] P. Yingchoncharoen, D. S. Kalinowski, and D. R. Richardson, "Lipid-based drug delivery systems in cancer therapy: What is available and what is yet to come," *Pharmacological Reviews*, vol. 68, no. 3, pp. 701–787, 2016.

[28] R. Sahoo, S. Sahoo, P. Nayak, S. Sahoo, and P. Nayak, "Controlled release of the drug cefadroxil from polycaprolactone-polylactic acid nanocomposites," *European Journal of Scientific Research*, vol. 53, no. 2, pp. 154–162, 2011.

[29] A. Silvestre, C. Freire, and C. Vilela, "Special issue: Advanced biopolymer-based nanocomposites and hybrid materials," *Materials*, vol. 14, p. 493, 2021.

[30] A. Lau, F. Hussain, and K. Lafdi, "Biopolymeric nanofibers for tissue engineering," *Nano-and Biocomposites*, pp. 157–192, CRC Press, 2010.

[31] R. Nanda, A. Sasmal, and P. Nayak, "Preparation and characterization of chitosan–polylactide composites blended with Cloisite 30B for control release of the anticancer drug paclitaxel," *Carbohydrate Polymers*, vol. 83, no. 2, pp. 988–994, 2011.

[32] J. Širc, R. Hobzova, N. Kostina, M. Munzarová, M. Juklíčková, M. Lhotka, Š. Kubinová, A. Zajícová, and J. Michálek, "Morphological characterization of nanofibers: Methods and application in practice," *Journal of Nanomaterials*, vol. 2012, pp. 1–14, 2012.

[33] N. Goonoo, A. Bhaw-Luximon, and D. Jhurry, "Drug loading and release from electrospun biodegradable nanofibers," *Journal of Biomedical Nanotechnology*, vol. 10, no. 9, pp. 2173–2199, 2014.

[34] J. Hrib, J. Sirc, R. Hobzova, Z. Hampejsova, Z. Bosakova, M. Munzarova, and J. Michalek, "Nanofibers for drug delivery – Incorporation and release of model molecules, influence of molecular weight and polymer structure," *Beilstein Journal of Nanotechnology*, vol. 6, no. 1, pp. 1939–1945, 2015.

[35] M. Sharma, "Transdermal and intravenous nano drug delivery systems: Present and future," *Applications of Targeted Nano Drugs and Delivery Systems*, pp. 499–550, Elsevier, 2019.

[36] M. Jafari, F. Doustdar, and F. Mehrnejad, "Molecular self-assembly strategy for encapsulation of an amphipathic α-helical antimicrobial peptide into the different polymeric and copolymeric nanoparticles," *Journal of Chemical Information and Modeling*, vol. 59, no. 1, pp. 550–563, 2018.

[37] A. Kyrychenko, D. A. Pasko, and O. N. Kalugin, "Poly (vinyl alcohol) as a water protecting agent for silver nanoparticles: The role of polymer size and structure," *Physical Chemistry Chemical Physics*, vol. 19, no. 13, pp. 8742–8756, 2017.

[38] L. Weng, S. L. Stott, and M. Toner, "Molecular dynamics at the interface between ice and poly (vinyl alcohol) and ice recrystallization inhibition," *Langmuir*, vol. 34, no. 17, pp. 5116–5123, 2017.

[39] R. Sreena, and A. J. Nathanael, "Biodegradable biopolymeric nanoparticles for biomedical applications-challenges and future outlook," *Materials*, vol. 16, no. 6, p. 2364, 2023.

[40] I. J. Joye, and D. J. McClements, "Biopolymer-based nanoparticles and microparticles: Fabrication, characterization, and application," *Current Opinion in Colloid & Interface Science*, vol. 19, no. 5, pp. 417–427, 2014.

[41] L. Patwekar, "Nanobiocomposite: A new approach to drug delivery system," *Asian Journal of Pharmaceutics (AJP)*, vol. 10, no. 4, pp. S646–S656, 2016.

[42] L. Tzounis, M. Doña, J. M. Lopez-Romero, A. Fery, and R. Contreras-Caceres, "Temperature-controlled catalysis by core–shell–satellite AuAg@ pNIPAM@ Ag hybrid microgels: A highly efficient catalytic thermoresponsive nanoreactor," *ACS Applied Materials & Interfaces*, vol. 11, no. 32, pp. 29360–29372, 2019.

[43] R. Indiarto, L. P. A. Indriana, R. Andoyo, E. Subroto, and B. Nurhadi, "Bottom–up nanoparticle synthesis: A review of techniques, polyphenol-based core materials, and their properties," *European Food Research and Technology*, vol. 248, no. 1, pp. 1–24, 2022.

[44] J. A. Tapia-Hernández, F. Rodríguez-Félix, and I. Katouzian, "Nanocapsule formation by electrospraying," *Nanoencapsulation Technologies for the Food and Nutraceutical Industries*, pp. 320–345, Elsevier, 2017.

[45] Y.-N. Cui, Q.-X. Xu, P. Davoodi, D.-P. Wang, and C.-H. Wang, "Enhanced intracellular delivery and controlled drug release of magnetic PLGA nanoparticles modified with transferrin," *Acta Pharmacologica Sinica*, vol. 38, pp. 943–953, 2017.

[46] M. Santi, G. Maccari, P. Mereghetti, V. Voliani, S. Rocchiccioli, N. Ucciferri, S. Luin, and G. Signore, "Rational design of a transferrin-binding peptide sequence tailored to targeted nanoparticle internalization," *Bioconjugate Chemistry*, vol. 28, pp. 471–480, 2017.

[47] Z. C. Soe, J. B. Kwon, R. K. Thapa, W. Ou, H. T. Nguyen, M. Gautam, K. T. Oh, H.-G. Choi, S. K. Ku, and C. S. Yong, "Transferrin-conjugated polymeric nanoparticle for receptor-mediated delivery of doxorubicin in doxorubicin-resistant breast cancer cells," *Pharmaceutics*, vol. 11, pp. 63, 2019.

[48] Y. Yao, et al., "Nanoparticle-based drug delivery in cancer therapy and its role in overcoming drug resistance," *Frontiers in Molecular Biosciences*, vol. **7**, p. 193, 2020.

[49] R. Muralidharan, A. Babu, N. Amreddy, K. Basalingappa, M. Mehta, A. Chen, Y. D. Zhao, U. B. Kompella, A. Munshi, and R. Ramesh, "Folate receptor-targeted nanoparticle delivery of HuR-RNAi suppresses lung cancer cell proliferation and migration," *Journal of Nanobiotechnology*, vol. 14, pp. 1–17, 2016.

[50] H. Samadian, S. Hosseini-Nami, S. K. Kamrava, H. Ghaznavi, and A. Shakeri-Zadeh, "Folate-conjugated gold nanoparticle as a new nanoplatform for targeted cancer therapy," *Journal of Cancer Research and Clinical Oncology*, vol. 142, pp. 2217–2229, 2016.

[51] G. Obaid, I. Chambrier, M. J. Cook, and D. A. Russell, "Cancer targeting with biomolecules: A comparative study of photodynamic therapy efficacy using antibody or lectin conjugated phthalocyanine-PEG gold nanoparticles," *Photochemical & Photobiological Sciences*, vol. 14, pp. 737–747, 2015.

[52] S. Balasubramanian, A. R. Girija, Y. Nagaoka, S. Iwai, M. Suzuki, V. Kizhikkilot, Y. Yoshida, T. Maekawa, and S. D. Nair, "Curcumin and 5-fluorouracil-loaded, folate-and transferrin-decorated polymeric magnetic nanoformulation: A synergistic cancer therapeutic approach, accelerated by magnetic hyperthermia," *International Journal of Nanomedicine*, vol. 9, pp. 437–459, 2014.

[53] S. Sigismund, D. Avanzato, and L. Lanzetti, "Emerging functions of the EGFR in cancer," *Molecular Oncology*, vol. 12, pp. 3–20, 2018.

[54] R. S. Apte, D. S. Chen, and N. Ferrara, "VEGF in signaling and disease: Beyond discovery and development," *Cell*, vol. 176, pp. 1248–1264, 2019.

[55] B. Wang, Q. Zhao, Y. Zhang, Z. Liu, Z. Zheng, S. Liu, and X. Jiang, "Targeting hypoxia in the tumor microenvironment: A potential strategy to improve cancer immunotherapy," *Journal of Experimental & Clinical Cancer Research*, vol. 40, pp. 1–16, 2021.

[56] X. Jiang, J. Wang, X. Deng, F. Xiong, S. Zhang, Z. Gong, and W. Xiong, "The role of microenvironment in tumor angiogenesis," *Journal of Experimental & Clinical Cancer Research*, vol. 39, pp. 1–19, 2020.

[57] X. Cheng, Q. Xie, and Y. Sun, "Advances in nanomaterial-based targeted drug delivery systems," *Frontiers in Bioengineering and Biotechnology*, vol. 11, p. 1177151, 2023.

[58] M. A. Subhan, S. S. K. Yalamarty, N. Filipczak, F. Parveen, and V. P. Torchilin, "Recent advances in tumor targeting via EPR effect for cancer treatment," *Journal of Personalized Medicine*, vol. 11, pp. 571, 2021.

[59] M. F. Attia, N. Anton, J. Wallyn, Z. Omran, and T. F. Vandamme, "An overview of active and passive targeting strategies to improve the nanocarriers efficiency to tumour sites," *Journal of Pharmacy and Pharmacology*, vol. 71, pp. 1185–1198, 2019.

[60] O. K. Nag, and J. B. Delehanty, "Active cellular and subcellular targeting of nanoparticles for drug delivery," *Pharmaceutics*, vol. 11, p. 543, 2019.

[61] M. Brisset, M. Grandin, A. Bernet, P. Mehlen, F. Hollande, "Dependence receptors: New targets for cancer therapy," *EMBO Molecular Medicine*, vol. 13, no. 11, p. e14495, 2021.

[62] W. Le, B. Chen, Z. Cui, Z. Liu, and D. Shi, "Detection of cancer cells based on glycolytic-regulated surface electrical charges," *Biophysics Reports*, vol. 5, pp. 10–18, 2019.

[63] S. D. Steichen, M. Caldorera-Moore, and N. A. Peppas, "A review of current nanoparticle and targeting moieties for the delivery of cancer therapeutics," *European Journal of Pharmaceutical Sciences*, vol. 48, pp. 416–427, 2013.

[64] T. Tashima, "Effective cancer therapy based on selective drug delivery into cells across their membrane using receptor-mediated endocytosis," *Bioorganic & Medicinal Chemistry Letters*, vol. 28, pp. 3015–3024, 2018.

[65] A. Mondal, A. K. Nayak, P. Chakraborty, S. Banerjee, and B. C. Nandy, "Natural polymeric nanobiocomposites for anti-cancer drug delivery therapeutics: A recent update," *Pharmaceutics*, vol. 15, p. 2064, 2023.
[66] M. N. Hafeez, C. Celia, and V. Petrikaite, "Challenges towards targeted drug delivery in cancer nanomedicines," *Processes*, vol. 9, p. 1527, 2021.
[67] S. Waheed, Z. Li, F. Zhang, A. Chiarini, U. Armato, and J. Wu, "Engineering nano-drug bio interface to overcome biological barriers toward precision drug delivery," *Journal of Nanobiotechnology*, vol. 20, p. 395, 2022.
[68] S. Peng, F. Xiao, M. Chen, and H. Gao, "Tumor-microenvironment-responsive nanomedicine for enhanced cancer immunotherapy," *Advanced Science*, vol. 9, 2103836, 2022.
[69] E. V. Balaji and A. Selvan, "Nanopharmacology: A novel approach in therapeutics," *Asian Journal of Research in Pharmaceutical Science*, vol. 9, pp. 9–16, 2019.
[70] Z. Medarova, P. Pantazopoulos, and B. Yoo, "Screening of potential miRNA therapeutics for the prevention of multi-drug resistance in cancer cells," *Scientific Reports*, vol. 10, no. 1, pp. 1970, 2020.
[71] M. Kundu, P. Sadhukhan, N. Ghosh, S. Chatterjee, P. Manna, J. Das, and P. C. Sil, "pH-responsive and targeted delivery of curcumin via phenylboronic acid-functionalized ZnO nanoparticles for breast cancer therapy," *Journal of Advanced Research*, vol. 18, pp. 161–172, 2019.
[72] M. Murakami, H. Cabral, Y. Matsumoto, S. Wu, M. R. Kano, T. Yamori, N. Nishiyama, and K. Kataoka, "Improving drug potency and efficacy by nanocarrier-mediated subcellular targeting," *Science Translational Medicine*, vol. 3, p. 64ra2, 2011.
[73] L. Qin, L. Wu, S. Jiang, D. Yang, H. He, F. Zhang, and P. Zhang, "Multifunctional micelle delivery system for overcoming multidrug resistance of doxorubicin," *Journal of Drug Targeting*, vol. 26, pp. 289–295, 2018.
[74] B. Yu, N. Song, H. Hu, G. Chen, Y. Shen, and H. Cong, "A degradable triple temperature-, pH-, and redox-responsive drug system for cancer chemotherapy," *Journal of Biomedical Materials Research Part A*, vol. 106, pp. 3203–3210, 2018.
[75] J. He, C. Gong, J. Qin, M. Li, and S. Huang, "Cancer cell membrane decorated silica nanoparticle loaded with miR495 and doxorubicin to overcome drug resistance for effective lung cancer therapy," *Nanoscale Research Letters*, vol. 14, pp. 1–10, 2019.
[76] H. Wang, F. Zhang, H. Wen, W. Shi, Q. Huang, Y. Huang, J. Xie, P. Li, J. Chen, and L. Qin, "Tumor-and mitochondria-targeted nanoparticles eradicate drug resistant lung cancer through mitochondrial pathway of apoptosis," *Journal of Nanobiotechnology*, vol. 18, pp. 1–21, 2020.
[77] S. K. Khiste, Z. Liu, K. R. Roy, M. B. Uddin, S. B. Hosain, X. Gu, S. Nazzal, R. A. Hill, and Y.-Y. Liu, "Ceramide–rubusoside nanomicelles, a potential therapeutic approach to target cancers carrying p53 missense mutations," *Molecular Cancer Therapeutics*, vol. 19, pp. 564–574, 2020.
[78] S. K. Singh, J. W. Lillard Jr, and R. Singh, "Reversal of drug resistance by planetary ball milled (PBM) nanoparticle loaded with resveratrol and docetaxel in prostate cancer," *Cancer Letters*, vol. 427, pp. 49–62, 2018.
[79] X. Jing, F. Yang, C. Shao, K. Wei, M. Xie, H. Shen, and Y. Shu, "Role of hypoxia in cancer therapy by regulating the tumor microenvironment," *Molecular Cancer*, vol. 18, pp. 1–15, 2019.
[80] R. Vadde, et al., Role of hypoxia-inducible factors (HIF) in the maintenance of stemness and malignancy of colorectal cancer. *Critical Reviews in Oncology/Hematology*, vol. 113, pp. 22–27, 2017.
[81] S. Xia, S. Yu, X. Yuan, and S. Xu, "Effects of hypoxia on expression of P-glycoprotein and multidrug resistance protein in human lung adenocarcinoma A549 cell line," *Zhonghua yi xue za zhi*, vol. 84, no. 8, pp. 663–666, 2004.
[82] F. Hajizadeh, S. M. Ardebili, M. B. Moornani, A. Masjedi, F. Atyabi, M. Kiani, A. Namdar, V. Karpisheh, S. Izadi, and B. Baradaran, "Silencing of HIF-1α/CD73 axis by siRNA-loaded TAT-chitosan-spion nanoparticles robustly blocks cancer cell progression," *European Journal of Pharmacology*, vol. 882, p. 173235, 2020.
[83] X. Luan, Y. Y. Guan, H. J. Liu, Q. Lu, M. Zhao, D. Sun, J. F. Lovell, P. Sun, H. Z. Chen, and C. Fang, "A tumor vascular-targeted interlocking trimodal nanosystem that induces and exploits hypoxia," *Advanced Science*, vol. 5, no. 8, pp. 1800034, 2018.
[84] Q. Long, T.-Y. Lin, Y. Huang, X. Li, A.-H. Ma, H. Zhang, R. Carney, S. Airhart, K. S. Lam, and R. W. D. White, "Image-guided photo-therapeutic nanoporphyrin synergized HSP90 inhibitor in patient-derived xenograft bladder cancer model," *Nanomedicine: Nanotechnology, Biology and Medicine*, vol. 14, no. 3, pp. 789–799, 2018.

[85] E. Kianfar, "Protein nanoparticles in drug delivery: Animal protein, plant proteins and protein cages, albumin nanoparticles," *Journal of Nanobiotechnology*, vol. 19, pp. 159, 2021.
[86] F. F. Visentini, A. A. Perez, L. G. Santiago, "Bioactive compounds: Application of albumin nanocarriers as delivery systems," *Critical Reviews in Food Science and Nutrition*, vol. 63, pp. 1–31, 2022.
[87] S. Paranthaman, M. Goravinahalli Shivananjegowda, M. Mahadev, A. Moin, S. Hagalavadi Nanjappa, N. D. Nanjaiyah, D. V. Gowda, "Nanodelivery systems targeting epidermal growth factor receptors for glioma management," *Pharmaceutics*, vol. 12, p. 1198, 2020.
[88] M. Izci, C. Maksoudian, B. B. Manshian, S. J. Soenen, "The use of alternative strategies for enhanced nanoparticle delivery to solid tumors.," *Chemical Reviews*, vol. 121, pp. 1746–1803, 2021.
[89] Y. Almoshari, H. Iqbal, A. Razzaq, K. Ali Ahmad, M. K. Khan, S. Saeed Alqahtani, and B. Ali Khan, "Development of nanocubosomes co-loaded with dual anticancer agents curcumin and temozolomide for effective colon cancer therapy," *Drug Delivery*, vol. 29, pp. 2633–2643, 2022.
[90] P. Famta, S. Shah, N. Jain, D. A. Srinivasarao, A. Murthy, T. Ahmed, and S. Srivastava, "Albumin-hitchhiking: Fostering the pharmacokinetics and anticancer therapeutics," *Journal of Controlled Release*, 353, pp. 166–185, 2023.
[91] N. Gupta, H. Hatoum, G. K. Dy, "First line treatment of advanced non- small-cell lung cancer–specific focus on albumin bound paclitaxel," *International Journal of Nanomedicine*, vol. 9, pp. 209–221, 2014.
[92] V. Hornok, "Serum albumin nanoparticles: Problems and prospects," *Polymers*, vol. 13, p. 3759, 2021.
[93] M. R. Alam, M. A. Shahid, S. Alimuzzaman, and A. N. Khan, "Sources, extractions and applications of bio-maker collagen – A review," *Biomedical Engineering Advances*, vol. 4, p. 100064, 2022.
[94] A. Berthold, K. Cremer, and J. Kreuter, "Collagen microparticles: Carriers for glucocorticosteroids," *European Journal of Pharmaceutics and Biopharmaceutics*, vol. 45, pp. 23–29, 1998.
[95] Z. Fu, L. Ouyang, R. Xu, Y. Yang, and W. Sun, "Responsive biomaterials for 3D bioprinting: A review," *Materials Today*, vol. 52, pp. 112–132, 2022.
[96] W. Z. Siburian, E. Rochima, Y. Andriani, and D. Praseptiangga, "Fish gelatin (definition, manufacture, analysis of quality characteristics, and application): A review," *International Journal of Fisheries and Aquatic Studies*, vol. 8, pp. 90–95, 2020.
[97] C. Moya-Lopez, A. Juan, M. Donizeti, J. Valcarcel, J. A. Vazquez, E. Solano, and D. Hermida-Merino, "Multifunctional PLA/gelatin bionanocomposites for tailored drug delivery systems," *Pharmaceutics*, vol. 14, p. 1138, 2022.
[98] Y. Meng, C. Qiu, X. Li, D. J. McClements, S. Sang, A. Jiao, and Z. Jin, "Polysaccharide-based nano-delivery systems for encapsulation, delivery, and pH- responsive release of bioactive ingredients," *Critical Reviews in Food Science and Nutrition*, vol. 64, pp. 1–15, 2022.
[99] D. Raikwar, K. Van Aelst, T. Vangeel, S. Corderi, J. Van Aelst, S. Van den Bosch, and B. F. Sels, "Elucidating the effect of the physicochemical properties of organosolv lignins on its solubility and reductive catalytic depolymerization," *Chemical Engineering Journal*, vol. 461, p. 141999, 2023.
[100] M. Fernandes, J. Padrão, A. I. Ribeiro, R. D. Fernandes, L. Melro, T. Nicolau, and A. Zille, "Polysaccharides and metal nanoparticles for functional textiles: A review," *Nanomaterials*, vol. 12, p. 1006, 2022.
[101] D. Nishimoto-Sauceda, L. E. Romero-Robles, and M. Antunes-Ricardo, "Biopolymer nanoparticles: A strategy to enhance stability, bioavailability, and biological effects of phenolic compounds as functional ingredients," *Journal of the Science of Food and Agriculture*, vol. 102, pp. 41–52, 2022.
[102] A. M. Elbagory, R. M. Marima, and Z. Dlamini, "Role and merits of green based nanocarriers in cancer treatment," *Cancers*, vol. 13(22), p. 5686, 2021.
[103] S. Roy, T. Chakraborty, J. Begum, M. S. Hasnain, and A. K. Nayak, "Chitosan: A versatile biopolymer," *Chitosan in Biomedical Applications*, pp. 1–11, Academic Press, 2022.
[104] A. R. Bilia, V. Piazzini, L. Risaliti, G. Vanti, M. Casamonti, M. Wang, and M. C. Bergonzi, "Nanocarriers: A successful tool to increase solubility, stability and optimise bioefficacy of natural constituents," *Current Medicinal Chemistry*, vol. 26, pp. 4631–4656, 2019.
[105] A. Kumar, and A. Kumar, "Chitosan-based drug conjugated nanocomposites: Advances and innovation in cancer therapy," *Regenerative Engineering and Translational Medicine*, 10, pp. 1–8, 2023.
[106] A. S. Abdel-Bary, D. A. Tolan, M. Y. Nassar, T. Taketsugu, and A. M. El-Nahas, "Chitosan, magnetite, silicon dioxide, and graphene oxide nanocomposites: Synthesis, characterization, efficiency as cisplatin drug delivery, and DFT calculations," *International Journal of Biological Macromolecules*, vol. 154, pp. 621–633, 2020.

[107] S. Hosseinzadeh, H. Hosseinzadeh, S. Pashaei, and Z. Khodaparast, "Synthesis of stimuli-responsive chitosan nanocomposites via RAFT copolymerization for doxorubicin delivery," *International Journal of Biological Macromolecules*, vol. 121, pp. 677–685, 2019.
[108] M. M. Abdel-Aziz, M. H. A. Elella, and R. R. Mohamed, "Green synthesis of quaternized chitosan/silver nanocomposites for targeting mycobacterium tuberculosis and lung carcinoma cells (A-549)," *International Journal of Biological Macromolecules*, vol. 142, pp. 244–253, 2020.
[109] D. Bi, X. Yang, L. Yao, Z. Hu, H. Li, X. Xu, and J. Lu, "Potential food and nutraceutical applications of alginate: A review," *Marine Drugs*, vol. 20, p. 564, 2022.
[110] A. Hurtado, A. A. Aljabali, V. Mishra, M. M. Tambuwala, and A. Serrano-Aroca, "Alginate: Enhancement strategies for advanced applications," *International Journal of Molecular Sciences*, vol. 23, p. 4486, 2022.
[111] G. Taşkın Çakıcı, "Nano TiO_2-doped sodium alginate/hydroxypropyl methylcellulose synthesis of bionanocomposite membrane and its use in controlled release of anti-cancer drug 5-fluorouracil," *Polymer Bulletin*, vol. 80, pp. 1–22, 2023.
[112] Y. Sheng, J. Gao, Z. Z. Yin, J. Kang, and Y. Kong, "Dual-drug delivery system based on the hydrogels of alginate and sodium carboxymethyl cellulose for colorectal cancer treatment," *Carbohydrate Polymers*, vol. 269, p. 118325, 2021.
[113] E. Piorkowska, "Overview of biobased polymers", *Thermal Properties of Bio-based Polymers*, pp. 1–35, 2019. https://doi.org/10.1007/12_2019_52
[114] X. Sun, C. Liu, A. M. Omer, W. Lu, S. Zhang, X. Jiang, ... and X. K. Ouyang, "pH-sensitive ZnO/carboxymethyl cellulose/chitosan bio-nanocomposite beads for colon-specific release of 5-fluorouracil," *International Journal of Biological Macromolecules*, vol. 128, pp. 468–479, (2019).
[115] S. Javanbakht, and H. Namazi, "Doxorubicin loaded carboxymethyl cellulose/graphene quantum dot nanocomposite hydrogel films as a potential anticancer drug delivery system," *Materials Science and Engineering: C*, vol. 87, pp. 50–59, 2018.
[116] I. Gholamali, and M. Yadollahi, "Doxorubicin-loaded carboxymethyl cellulose/starch/ZnO nanocomposite hydrogel beads as an anticancer drug carrier agent," *International Journal of Biological Macromolecules*, vol. 160, pp. 724–735, 2020.
[117] I. Gholamali, S. N. Hosseini, and E. Alipour, "Doxorubicin-loaded oxidized starch/poly (vinyl alcohol)/CuO bio-nanocomposite hydrogels as an anticancer drug carrier agent," *International Journal of Polymeric Materials and Polymeric Biomaterials*, vol. 70, pp. 967–980, 2021.
[118] A. R. Rashidi, N. I. W. Azelee, D. N. A. Zaidel, L. F. Chuah, A. Bokhari, H. A. El-Enshasy, and D. J. Dailin, "Unleashing the potential of xanthan: A comprehensive exploration of biosynthesis, production, and diverse applications," *Bioprocess and Biosystems Engineering*, vol. 46, pp. 1–17, 2023.
[119] P. B. S. Albuquerque, W. F. de Oliveira, P. M. dos Santos Silva, M. T. dos Santos Correia, J. F. Kennedy, and L. C. B. B. Coelho, "Epiphanies of well-known and newly discovered macromolecular carbohydrates – A review," *International Journal of Biological Macromolecules*, vol. 156, pp. 51–66, 2020.
[120] A. Dzionek, D. Wojcieszyńska, and U. Guzik, "Use of xanthan gum for whole cell immobilization and its impact in bioremediation – A review," *Bioresource Technology*, vol. 351, p. 126918, 2022.
[121] N. M. El-Sawy, A. I. Raafat, N. A. Badawy, and A. M. Mohamed, "Radiation development of pH-responsive (xanthan-acrylic acid)/MgO nanocomposite hydrogels for controlled delivery of methotrexate anticancer drug," *International Journal of Biological Macromolecules*, vol. 142, pp. 254–264, 2020.
[122] M. D. Soltani, H. Meftahizadeh, M. Barani, A. Rahdar, S. M. Hosseinikhah, M. Hatami, and M. Ghorbanpour, "Guar (Cyamopsis tetragonoloba L.) plant gum: From biological applications to advanced nanomedicine," *International Journal of Biological Macromolecules*, vol. 193, pp. 1972–1985, 2021.
[123] P. Nezhad-Mokhtari, M. Ghorbani, and N. Abdyazdani, "Reinforcement of hydrogel scaffold using oxidized-guar gum incorporated with curcumin-loaded zein nanoparticles to improve biological performance," *International Journal of Biological Macromolecules*, vol. 167, pp. 59–65, (2021).
[124] D. Verma, and S. K. Sharma, "Recent advances in guar gum based drug delivery systems and their administrative routes," *International Journal of Biological Macromolecules*, vol. 181, pp. 653–671, 2021.
[125] V. G. Bhat, S. P. Masti, S. S. Narasagoudr, R. B. Chougale, S. K. Praveen Kumar, and A. B. Vantamuri, "Development and characterization of chitosan/guar gum/gum ghatti bionanocomposites with in situ silver nanoparticles," *Chemical Data Collections*, vol. 44, p. 101009, 2023.

[126] G. Muthaiah, and D. Ramachandran, "Preparation of cross-linked gum nano spheres containing Gemcitabine by single step emulsion in place compound cross-linking technique and its tested with different analytical techniques," *International Journal of ChemTech Research*, vol. 12, pp. 240–250, 2019.
[127] M. Khotimchenko, "Pectin polymers for colon-targeted antitumor drug delivery," *International Journal of Biological Macromolecules*, vol. 158, pp. 1110–1124, 2020.
[128] S. T. Minzanova, V. F. Mironov, D. M. Arkhipova, A. V. Khabibullina, L. G. Mironova, Y. M. Zakirova, and V. A. Milyukov, "Biological activity and pharmacological application of pectic polysaccharides: A review," *Polymers*, vol. 10, p. 1407, 2018.
[129] T. Abitbol, A. Mijlkovic, L. Malafronte, J. S. Stevanic, P. T. Larsson, and P. Lopez-Sanchez, "Cellulose nanocrystal/low methoxyl pectin gels produced by internal ionotropic gelation," *Carbohydrate Polymers*, vol. 260, p. 117345, 2021.
[130] S. Y. Wang, Y. J. Meng, J. Li, J. P. Liu, Z. Q. Liu, and D. Q. Li, "A novel and simple oral colon-specific drug delivery system based on the pectin/modified nano-carbon sphere nanocomposite gel films," *International Journal of Biological Macromolecules*, vol. 157, pp. 170–176, 2020.
[131] T. Kobayashi, T. Chanmee, and N. Itano, "Hyaluronan: Metabolism and function," *Biomolecules*, vol. 10, p. 1525, 2020.
[132] J. Zhu, X. Tang, Y. Jia, C. T. Ho, and Q. Huang, "Applications and delivery mechanisms of hyaluronic acid used for topical/transdermal delivery – A review," *International Journal of Pharmaceutics*, vol. 578, p. 119127, 2020.
[133] P. Wu, Y. Sun, W. Dong, H. Zhou, S. Guo, L. Zhang, and Y. Zong, "Enhanced anti-tumor efficacy of hyaluronic acid modified nanocomposites combined with sonochemotherapy against subcutaneous and metastatic breast tumors," *Nanoscale*, vol. 11, pp. 11470–11483, 2019.
[134] C. Minelli, S. B. Lowe, and M. M. Stevens, "Engineering nanocomposite materials for cancer therapy," *Small*, vol. 6, pp. 2336–2357, 2010.
[135] K. J. Ray, N. R. Sibson, and A. E. Kiltie, "Treatment of breast and prostate cancer by hypofractionated radiotherapy: Potential risks and benefits," *Clinical Oncology*, vol. 27, pp. 420–426, 2015.
[136] Z. Arab-Bafrani, E. Zabihi, S. M. Jafari, A. Khoshbin-Khoshnazar, E. Mousavi, M. Khalili, and A. Babaei, "Enhanced radiotherapy efficacy of breast cancer multi cellular tumor spheroids through in-situ fabricated chitosan-zinc oxide bio-nanocomposites as radio-sensitizing agents," *International Journal of Pharmaceutics*, vol. 605, pp. 120828, 2021.
[137] N. Ahmad, S. Sultana, S. M. Faisal, A. Ahmed, S. Sabir, and M. Z. Khan, "Zinc oxide-decorated polypyrrole/Chitosan bionanocomposites with enhanced photocatalytic, antibacterial and anticancer performance," *RSC Advances*, vol. 9, pp. 41135–41150, 2019.
[138] A. Jayakumar, V. P. Kumar, S. Radoor, I. C. Nair, S. Siengchin, J. Parameswaranpillai, and E. K. Radhakrishnan, "Chitosan-based bionanocomposites for cancer therapy," *Bionanocomposites in Tissue Engineering and Regenerative Medicine*, pp. 277–292, 2021.
[139] A. Doctor, V. Seifert, M. Ullrich, S. Hauser, and J. Pietzsch, "Three-dimensional cell culture systems in radiopharmaceutical cancer research," *Cancers*, vol. 12, p. 2765, 2020.
[140] R. Edmondson, J. J. Broglie, A. F. Adcock, and L. Yang, "Three-dimensional cell culture systems and their applications in drug discovery and cell-based biosensors," *ASSAY and Drug Development Technologies*, vol. 12, pp. 207–218, 2014.
[141] D. Bharathi, R. Ranjithkumar, B. Chandarshekar, and V. Bhuvaneshwari, "Bio-inspired synthesis of chitosan/copper oxide nanocomposite using rutin and their anti-proliferative activity in human lung cancer cells," *International Journal of Biological Macromolecules*, vol. 141, pp. 476–483, 2019.
[142] M. Amina, N. M. Al Musayeib, N. A. Alarfaj, M. F. El-Tohamy, and G. A. Al-Hamoud, "Antibacterial and anti cancer potentials of presynthesized photosensitive plectranthus cylindraceus oil/TiO_2/polyethylene glycol polymeric bionanocomposite," *Bioinorganic Chemistry and Applications*, vol. 2021, pp. 1–20, 2021.
[143] Y. Xi, and P. Xu, "Global colorectal cancer burden in 2020 and projections to 2040," *Translational Oncology*, vol. 14, p. 101174, 2021.
[144] M. Yusefi, M. S. Lee-Kiun, K. Shameli, S.-Y. Teow, R. R. Ali, K.-K. Siew, H.-Y. Chan, M. M.-T. Wong, W.-L. Lim, and K. Kuča, "5-fluorouracil loaded magnetic cellulose bionanocomposites for potential colorectal cancer treatment," *Carbohydrate Polymers*, vol. 273, p. 118523, 2021.

5 Bionanocomposites in Nasal Drug Delivery

RajaSekhar Reddy Alavala, S. N. Koteswara Rao Gudhanti, Sree Harsha Nagaraja, Diya Karbhari, Roja Rani Budha and Khushwant S. Yadav

5.1 INTRODUCTION TO NANOCOMPOSITES

Nanocomposites, in general, are materials that have been nanoengineered and have structures that are modified in the nanosizing scales [1, 2]. In general, a "composite" is defined as a material that does not exist naturally and is made up of a combination of two or more physicochemically distinct materials arranged so that the new character of the composite material is entirely different from the individual compounds used for production. This definition is applicable to both general material scientists and biomedical engineers. In general, the larger surface-to-volume ratio for the reinforcing phase, increased ductility without a decrease in the material strength profile, and scratch resistance are what set nanocomposites apart from conventional composites [3]. A composite typically consists of a reinforcement and a matrix phase. In contrast to the reinforcement, which has a high load capacity and favorable physical and mechanical properties, the bulk phase, or matrix, typically has a lower Young's modulus and more flexibility [4].

In biomedical engineering, an inorganic bioactive material is often taken into consideration for reinforcement, while a biopolymer often serves as the composite's matrix. Many different types of bionanocomposites were prepared using various methods and have been studied for biomedical applications during the last few decades. Natural, semi-synthetic, and synthetic polymers; metals and their oxides; ceramics; structured carbons; and other inorganic materials make up the majority of these nanocomposites [5, 6]. To improve the biological, mechanical, and physicochemical characteristics of the nanocomposite matrix, different materials are often reinforced. Polymeric nanoparticles (NPs), inorganic nanomaterials (such as nanostructured carbons, metallic NPs, metal oxide NPs, and nanoceramics), nanofibers (such as electrospun fibers), nanotubes (such as carbon nanotubes), nanosheets (such as exfoliated clay stacks), etc. are among the materials reinforced for the syntheses of nanocomposites [7–9]. On the basis of composition and matrix reinforcement, different types of nanocomposites can be categorized: (i) organic-inorganic (e.g., polymeric nanocomposites), (ii) organic–organic (e.g., polymeric-ceramic and polymeric metallic), and (iii) inorganic–inorganic (e.g., metallic nanocomposites, ceramic nanocomposites, metallic–ceramic, carbon nanotube–ceramic, metallic–ceramic, and carbon nanotube-metallic) [10].

Many types of nanocomposites are being synthesized using a variety of synthetic techniques. Physical mixing, film casting, dip coating, in situ preparation, co-precipitation, ionic gelation, covalent coupling, electrospinning, colloidal assembly, layer-by-layer assembly, etc., are some of the widely utilized nanocomposite synthesis techniques [6, 9]. The benefits of hydrogen bonding, electrostatic interactions, coulombic interactions, ionic interactions, covalent bonding, hydrophobic effects, assembly formation, etc. are made possible by these synthesis approaches [6].

Controlling synthesis procedures, ensuring compatibility with component materials, and producing a product with both distinctive and desirable material qualities are the problems in the synthesis of various nanocomposites [7, 9]. Applications of nanocomposites have steered a number of novel

 DOI: 10.1201/9781003650812-5

technologies in recent years, along with elegant and useful perspectives for many sectors, including the biomedical area [4–8].

5.2 BIONANOCOMPOSITES APPLICATION IN DRUG DELIVERY

"Biocomposites" is the name given to these composites, which have particular uses in biomedical engineering [4, 11]. The continuous bulk phase, or matrix, in composites enhances the mechanical and physical characteristics required for a certain biological application while supporting the reinforced material. Additionally, it has been noted that the matrix enhances the biocomposites' properties and processing parameters [4]. Polymers, ceramics, and metals that independently or collectively have a specific biological activity or should sometimes be bio-inert but always biocompatible can be found in biocomposites. Biofunctionality, bioinertness, bioactivity, and biodegradability are all included in the phrase biocompatibility. These days, selecting materials that will function as biomaterials requires careful thought. Prevent biofouling, one of the greatest risks to human health that can lead to infections that require immediate medical attention, is biofouling of biomaterials [12].

Drug administration, gene delivery, antibacterial, tissue regeneration, wound healing, dentistry, bioimaging, biosensors, and other uses are among the most significant applications of biomedical nanocomposites [6–9, 13]. The field of drug delivery applications necessitates the creation of effective dosage forms that can administer diverse medications to the body for the management and treatment of a range of illnesses and conditions [14]. Drug delivery has long been acknowledged as a crucial area of healthcare, where the administration of dosage forms to deliver diverse pharmaceuticals is necessary to achieve the best possible therapy to treat a range of illnesses and disorders [15, 16]. To create drug delivery systems, a variety of biomaterials are used, including metal and metal oxides, bioceramics, natural, synthetic, and semi-synthetic biopolymers, and more [15, 17]. The numerous dosage forms that are being developed for a range of drugs and used for the treatment or management of numerous diseases include hydrogels, tablets, capsules, in situ gels, topical gels, beads, microparticles, NPs or nanocapsules, dental pastes, buccal patches, emulsions, and implants [18]. Because of its superior mechanical, biological, physicochemical, and physical properties, nanocomposite has emerged as a promising drug delivery carrier system in the recent past. Furthermore, high drug stocking capacity and reinforcement at the nanoscale have opened up new directions in the drug delivery industry.

5.3 SYNTHESIS OF BIONANOCOMPOSITES

Various standard techniques are available for the preparation of nanocomposites, including melt intercalation, solution intercalation, freeze-drying, drop casting, in situ intercalative polymerization, and electrospinning. Inorganic/organic polymer-based bio-nanocomposites can be made in different ways, including colloidal suspension, molecular beam epitaxy, chemical vapor deposition, microwave synthesis, chemical vapor deposition, and the solvothermal approach. Every process could have drawbacks, particularly in large quantities. Thus, it is imperative to introduce a practical process for producing high-quality graphene on a big scale.

For example, a durable biopolymer-graphene/graphene oxide (GO) bionanocomposite requires a correct material distribution in polymeric matrices, which can affect the bionanocomposites' mechanical, thermal, electrical, water vapor permeability, and gas-barrier properties [19]. To create graphene/GO bionanocomposites with starch, chitosan, PLA, cellulose, alginate, gelatin, and poly(hydroxyalkanoates), several researchers have used the solution intercalation approach [19]. However, the most significant problem in this area is the restacking, partial exfoliation, and aggregation of graphene or GO particles when they are added to biopolymers [20]. In actuality, a poor dispersion may jeopardize the properties of the nanocomposites. Since GO can be exfoliated in water, it offers additional processing advantages. As a result, water-soluble polymers like poly(vinyl alcohol) [21] and poly(ethylene oxide) [22] or water-based latex technology [23] can be used to readily construct nanocomposites from GO.

Out of all the production methods, solution intercalation is the most widely used. It involves shear mixing or stirring the colloidal suspensions with the appropriate polymers, followed by solvent evaporation. This causes the adsorbed polymer to congregate and produce a sandwich among the polymers, resulting in the creation of bionanocomposites. The process involves slightly altering the polymeric matrix's chemical structure in the bionanocomposite with increased biopolymer quantity. This indicates that while there could be a mild chemical reaction between the biopolymers, the main interactions that will take place are physical ones, such as hydrogen bonding. In the following sections, some of the widely used synthetic techniques with suitable examples are mentioned.

5.3.1 Intercalation of the Solution

By using the intercalation method, the ability of a guar gum/bentonite bionanocomposite to sequester lead (Pb) and crystal violet dye in an aqueous solution was assessed. Temperature, pH, dosage, and length of contact all had an impact on the adsorption of Pb (II) and crystal violet [24]. Thermodynamic analyses demonstrated that the adsorption at the solid-solution interface was endothermic, spontaneous, and more unpredictable. Using 0.1 N HCl, Pb, and crystal violet was desirable, and the process had good regeneration power up to the fifth cycle. Additionally, the bionanocomposite shows great practical utility in the treatment of wastewater from various sources [25].

Sustainable bionanocomposites of carboxymethyl cellulose, polyvinyl alcohol, and copper oxide (CuO). Using compositions of 0.3, 0.6, and 0.9% (w/v) of CuO, copper oxide NPs (CuO-NPs) were synthesized and introduced to a mixed solution of carboxymethyl cellulose (CMC)/polyvinyl alcohol (PVA) [26]. The solution casting technique was utilized to create the CMC/PVA/CuO bionanocomposites, which were then coated over processed cheese. The produced film's gas transmission rate (GTR) and water vapor transmission rate (WVTR) were both reduced by the addition of CuO-NPs. Furthermore, the bionanocomposite suspensions showed strong but erratic inhibitory effects against a number of harmful fungi and bacteria. During six months of cold storage, the effects of covering processed cheese surfaces with the made bionanocomposite films on the microbiological, physicochemical, textural, and sensory qualities of the processed cheese were evaluated. Applying a layer containing CuO-NPs to cheese prevented the growth of mold on its surface and markedly ($P < 0.05$) reduced the overall number of bacteria present in the cheese. Moreover, cheese coating reduced moisture loss and postponed the hardening of the cheese during storage [27].

5.3.2 Reduction of Chemicals

Numerous methods have been presented to produce silver nanocomposites, comprising chemical, photochemical, sonochemical, microwave, and radiochemical reduction methods. By using the reduction method, silver NPs (AgNPs) of small size were prepared by using the montmorillonite (MMT), and chitosan (Ct) formed the bionanocomposite $AgNO_3$/MMT/Cts by UV irradiation [28, 29]. Large AgNPs are concurrently reduced and fragmented under UV irradiation. Without using the chemical reducing agents or any heat treatment, the interaction of tiny amounts of AgNPs into the lamellar space of MMT/Cts was achieved by using the reduction method with UV irradiation. AgNP production in the MMT/Cts suspension was indicated by the prepared samples' color gradually changing from colorless for $AgNO_3$/MMT/Cts to light grey, grey, and finally dark grey at varying UV irradiation periods [30].

There has been an increase in the synthesis of AgNPs using various other techniques also [31–35]. Using a chemical reducing agent, AgNPs were created in suspensions of chitosan (Cts), and gelatin. Cts and gelatin were employed as natural stabilizers and firm support, whereas the silver precursor was $AgNO_3$. As the reducing agent, sodium borohydride ($NaBH_4$) was employed. Stabilizers are one type of agent that should be used in the synthesis of AgNPs since they are crucial in regulating both the NPs' formation and their dispersion stability. Because polymers are good at avoiding particle agglomeration and precipitation, they are frequently utilized as particle stabilizers. When creating NPs with uniform distributions, this is crucial [35].

5.3.3 Alternative Techniques

The enzyme lysozyme causes titania and amorphous silica to precipitate quickly at room temperature. These materials then serve as good support matrices for other enzymes that are added to the reaction. With a notable retention of antimicrobial activity, this type of one-pot process of lysozyme-mediated precipitation also encapsulates the lysozyme within the titania or silica. The lysozyme provides protection against microbial degradation, and the inorganic mediums shield the immobilized biomolecules from physical degradation that happens with the free form of the enzymes in the solution. This appealing approach to biomineralization and bioencapsulation offers a simple and cost-effective way to create a variety of useful bionanocomposites that contain biomacromolecules encased in silica or titania nanostructures [36, 37].

The NPs of silver-loaded ZnO were produced by means of the sol–gel technique with a template of gelatin. The bionanocomposite films were created by green chemistry methodology, employing a solution casting process. Mechanical property testing indicated that the toughness and strength are due to the addition of NPs to the composite. The composites' elasticity and durability increased dramatically [38].

A variety of chitosan (CS) and MMT clay-based polyurethane bionanocomposites were manufactured by step-growth polymerization, reacting hydroxyl-terminated polybutadiene (HTPB) with toluene diisocyanate (TDI) to improve thermal and antibacterial properties of polyurethane (PU) [39]. Functionalization of synthetic polymers by adding natural polymers like chitin or chitosan is a suitable technique for biomaterial creation [40]. Chitosan-based PUs are attractive scaffolds as they exhibit amazing mechanical plasticity and biostability and can be employed for a wide variety of biomedical purposes. Many researchers described the production of functionalized, biocompatible, and biodegradable PUs by chemical alteration of their structure by incorporating chitin, chitosan, or starch [41]. Chitosan was utilized as an extender of the chain in the PU synthesis, which has exhibited better thermo-mechanical and structural properties. Xu and his coworker manufactured PUs by employing chitosan as a chain extender and used this polymer for blood compatibility as an anticoagulant agent [42]. The biocompatibility of chitosan-PU films was tested for pharmaceutical applications, and it was discovered that films with greater chitosan contents had increased adhesive power and biocompatibility that could be used in bandages [43]. Yang et al. created a hydrogel based on chitosan and poly(vinyl alcohol) and covered the synthetic PUs in a thin layer. They discovered that because of their increased hydrophilicity and slippery, slimy surface, these chitosan-coated PUs have high antibacterial action and also reduce protein absorption [44].

5.4 BIONANOCOMPOSITES TO NASAL DELIVERY

5.4.1 The Nasal Route—The Alternate to Deliver Drugs to the CNS

Nasal route is one of the alternate routes to transport drugs to the CNS, including the brain, for treating various neurological diseases. Many limitations exist; for example, blood–brain barrier (BBB) penetration prevents many therapeutic agents from having the intended pharmacological impact. Therefore, for the effective treatment of NDs, it is imperative to guarantee the safe and efficient delivery of active moieties in the brain [45]. Several benefits come with administering drugs intranasally, including escaping the liver's first-pass metabolism, avoiding the intestine, and minimizing overall negative effects. It also bypasses the BBB, giving it immediate entree to the brain through the trigeminal and olfactory nerve pathways. Although several APIs now have the chance to enter the brain by nasal administration, doing so is quite difficult. Due to reduced nasal absorption, factors such as mucociliary clearance, which reduces the medication's residence time at the administration site, may jeopardize nasal drug delivery [46, 47]. Micro- and nanotechnological techniques were extensively employed to get beyond these restrictions and improve the bioavailability of medications in the cerebral tissue. Natural or artificial materials make up micro- and nanoparticulate carriers, which interact molecularly with biological structures to change the way NDs are treated. By causing interaction between the target areas, they could reduce the negative consequences [47].

Without a doubt, the brain is the one crucial organ in the human that is most shielded from the introduction of outside elements like poisons and drug compounds. At three interfaces—the BBB, the blood–cerebrospinal fluid barrier (BSB), and the arachnoid barrier—different cells provide this protection [48]. Drug molecules must fulfill specific requirements in order to enter the brain: they must be lipophilic, non-ionized, have a molecular weight of less than 400 Da, and be able to establish fewer than eight hydrogen bonds [49]. The majority of medications used to treat neurodegenerative diseases don't meet the specified criteria for efficient brain delivery. This has prompted researchers to look for ways to administer drugs to get over the BBB and maximize their therapeutic effects. Intracerebral, intraparenchymal, and intracerebroventricular injections and infusions are possible routes of administration of therapeutics directly to the central nervous system (CNS); however, these methods are invasive and unsuitable for long-term drug administration [50, 51].

The last one or two decades have witnessed an increase in curiosity about the nasal route due to its non-invasiveness, ease of self-administration, quick absorption, and ability to prevent primary liver metabolism of medications. An increasing quantity of approvals of intranasal formulations is available for the treatment of dementia linked to Alzheimer's disease, such as an intranasal spray of rivastigmine (Rivamist®). Nasal formulations have the advantage of strong patient compliance and self-medication potential. The human nasal cavity is 12 to 14 cm long, extending after the nostrils toward the nasopharynx. It is lined with squamous, respiratory, transitional, and olfactory epithelia, which are located beneath the mucosa [52, 53]. Drugs delivered by nasal route deposit in the olfactory or respiratory epithelium [52]. Drugs can enter the blood circulation from the respiratory epithelium and reach the CNS if they can enter through the BBB. The trigeminal nerve, which connects both the olfactory and respiratory mucosa and the olfactory mucosa itself, is of particular relevance with regard to nasal delivery.

The medicine is delivered straight to the brain via the nasal route, which offers two routes for this purpose: extracellular and intracellular [54]. The intracellular route entails exocytosis into the olfactory bulb by neurons projecting to different parts of the brain, endocytosis by sensory olfactory cells, and axonal transport to their synaptic clefts [55]. Drug molecules are immediately transported by the extracellular pathway into the cerebrospinal fluid (CSF), which travels via the nasal epithelium's paracellular space, the perineural space, and finally the brain's subarachnoid space [55]. Both mechanisms assist in the transportation of drug molecules, notwithstanding the intracellular channel's extreme sluggishness and inability to demonstrate that intranasal markers are transported to all brain regions far beyond the olfactory bulb projections. The extracellular pathway seems to be the major component of drug transport and should be the main focus despite the lack of strong kinetic evidence supporting this [55]. Given the drug's physicochemical characteristics, formulation features, and the kind of drug-delivery device, it makes sense that an amalgamation of these paths might take place. The olfactory epithelium in the upper nose is the target area for nose-to-brain transfer. The nasal mucosa often functions as an efficient absorption site for medicinal medicines because of its extensive vascularization. On the other hand, the nose-to-brain (nose-to-CNS) connection to the olfactory area is direct because of its close proximity to the CSF [56].

The development of devices for nasal brain delivery has drawn more consideration in the recent past. PAMAM dendrimers attracted the attention of drug carriers to supply medications through the nasal route. The nasal route transports pharmaceuticals straight to the CNS by biological paths without any targeted alteration, in contrast to targeted drug delivery systems that pass into the cerebral tissue through the BBB. Furthermore, nasal brain transport will be very convenient for the clinical application of medications as a non-invasive mode of delivery [57]. Fluorescence-tagged small interfering RNA (fluorescence-tagged siRNA) was discovered in the cytoplasm and processes of neurons and glial cells in a variety of brain areas, including the striatum, cerebral cortex, amygdala, and hypothalamus, after nasal delivery of PAMAM-loaded siRNA [58, 59].

PAMAM-loaded haloperidol improved brain targeting after nasal administration, with 6.7 times lower doses of the dendrimer-haloperidol formulation administered via the intranasal route producing behavioral responses that were comparable to those induced by haloperidol formulations administered via an intraperitoneal injection [60]. The primary restriction on nasal delivery is the quick drug removal by the cilia and nasal mucosa, which shortens the period that the preparation adheres to the nasal mucosa [60]. A novel kind of ecologically sensitive gel for nasal delivery is called in situ gel; it responds to ionic changes, temperature variations, or pH changes in the nasal cavity to undergo a transition from a solution phase to a gel state. Prior to the gel phase transition, the solution state is suitable for dose control and medication administration because it keeps the preparation's viscosity at a consistently low level and allows for good fluidity. After phase change, a gel state with a higher viscosity level is created, which can stick to the nasal mucosa's surface and inhibit the nasal cavity's clearance to lengthen the contact time and absorb more material [61]. It's been proven that in situ gels are efficient polymer carriers for nasal brain transfer. In order to target the brain, Youssef Naha produced unique nasal almotriptan-loaded solid lipid NPs in mucoadhesive in situ gel formulation [62]. A liposomal mucoadhesive, thermosensitive in situ gel was created by Mura for the prolonged nasal delivery of opiorphin [63]. The gel phase transition matrix was chosen to be the ionotropic substance deacetylated gellan gum, which responds to K^+, Na^+, and Ca^{2+} in the nasal mucosa. As a bio-adhesive material, HMPC was employed. Because the hydroxyl groups in HPMC molecules interacted with the water molecules in the nasal mucosa by H-bonds, the adhesion strength between the mucosa and gel was strengthened, so the gel's clearance time was extended. Vitamin E was added as an antioxidant, chlorine acetate was added as a preservative, and mannitol was used as an isotonic agent.

5.4.2 APIs Suitable for Nasal Drug Delivery

The nasal cavity of humans has a total volume of approximately 15 to 20 mL and a surface area of approximately 150 cm^2 [64, 65]. Mucous secretions and hairs line the inside of the nose, contributing significantly to its ability to trap pathogens and inhaled particles. Mucin, a crucial mucus protein, has an affinity for foreign solutes, which restricts the solute's ability to diffuse [65]. Consequently, the old layer of mucus is rapidly replaced, and fresh mucus is continuously secreted. As a result, the particles that are stuck in the mucus barrier are transferred along with it, eventually leaving the nasal space [66]. The term mucociliary clearance refers to this essential defense mechanism. Drugs with poor absorption can overcome the nasal mucosal barrier by being encapsulated into the appropriate delivery systems, such as liposomes, microspheres, and NPs, or coadministered with other absorption enhancers [67]. By extending the intranasal residence time and overcoming the mucociliary clearance barrier, an ideal nasal carrier system should be able to address bioavailability issues and produce a tolerable therapeutic effect.

Dosage forms with targeted nose-to-brain delivery include mainly drugs that do not reach therapeutic concentrations in the brain tissue when otherwise administered, for example, orally; drugs with a pronounced first-pass effect; and drugs with many peripheral side effects [68]. The main properties that affect the rate and extent to which drug molecules will be transported from the nasal cavity to the brain tissue are molecular weight, lipophilicity, and the degree of dissociation [54].

Since dopamine cannot penetrate the BBB, it cannot be used to treat Parkinson's disease on its own. Dopamine levels in the blood and CSF were examined in an animal investigation to determine whether the medication was transported to the CNS *via* the olfactory pathway after nasal delivery. The drug was administered either nasally or intravenously. Compared to intravenous administration, higher brain dopamine levels were observed thirty minutes after nasal treatment. These results indicate that unchanged dopamine is transferred into the olfactory bulb via the olfactory pathway in rats [69]. Human studies have indicated that following intranasal delivery, peptides that have been found to impact brain processes, such as learning, memory, and cognition, such as insulin, vasopressin, and melanocortin, concentrate in the brain tissue. Intranasal insulin was found to improve cognitive functions in patients with Alzheimer's disease with no increase in peripheral blood levels [70].

5.4.3 Desired Properties of Bionanocomposites for Productive Nasal Delivery

Numerous dosage forms, such as suspensions, solutions, microemulsions, and gels, have been prepared for nasal delivery to reach the brain. Conventional forms usually do not provide a controlled release of drug molecules and are not capable of targeted delivery [71–73]. Soon after delivery, the active molecules are often released and absorbed quickly, resulting in a sudden rise in plasma concentration that may have harmful properties. After a very short length of time, this concentration decreases below therapeutic levels, and this may lead to more frequent usage of the dose form [47]. Nano-formulations can provide benefits over regular forms, for instance, better stability, accessibility, and an extended residence period in the nasal cavity. Another key point to consider when looking at nose-to-brain drug administration is to guarantee that the formulation is deposited in the olfactory region, which can be achieved with the use of appropriate devices for both liquid and solid systems [47]. Furthermore, the nasal dose form should be developed to give an extended residence duration and maintain a high local concentration for drug diffusion [74]. Another important consideration while developing the best delivery strategy for nose-to-brain is particle size. For example, because the tight connections of the nasal epithelium are less than 15 nm, NPs can pass through phospholipid membranes more readily than microparticles because of their reduced size. Bigger particles discharge the drug into the mucosal tissue, which is often absorbed by passive diffusion because they cannot break through the epithelium. Extending the duration of contact between the carrier and the mucosa is largely dependent on the carrier's surface charge. Because mucin has a net-negative charge, positively charged microparticles may adhere to the mucosa.

5.5 BIOMATERIALS FOR FORMULATIONS

5.5.1 Polymers Produced from Animal Sources

Chitosan is generated from chitin, the second most prevalent carbohydrate. Chitin includes β-(1–4)-poly-N-acetyl-D-glucosamine (Figure 5.1) and can be detected in a wide range of creatures, mostly in the exoskeletons of animals (e.g., insects, shrimp, lobsters, and crabs) [75]. The largest chitosan source is generated by the removal of the acetyl group largely from chitin. Because of its cationic properties, particularly when it comes to nucleic acid and negatively charged DNA because of the electrostatic interaction that results in polyplexes, chitosan is an excellent immunomodifier for drug delivery. Many studies have been done on chitosan as a possible biopolymer for use in biomedical applications; however, chitosan has certain disadvantages, including low solubility in physiological environments (pKa value of 6.3–6.4), the possibility of toxicity based on chitosan type and molecular weight, and intrinsic properties that can be impacted by crosslinking with other materials [75, 76].

Gelatin is a soluble protein that is produced from collagen, an insoluble fibrous protein that serves as the primary building block of the extracellular matrix in animal tissues like skin, cartilage, and bone [77]. Gelatin (both type A and type B) was produced by pre-treating collagen with acid and alkaline solutions, respectively. This biopolymer, hydrophilic biodegradable polypeptide polymer with a range of accessible functional groups, has been effectively applied to a wide range of vaccine delivery systems and offers a promising window into the encapsulated high payload of antigens [78]. In addition, gelatin is a well-known drug delivery vehicle since it can be manipulated to couple with numerous cross-linkers and has low antigenicity.

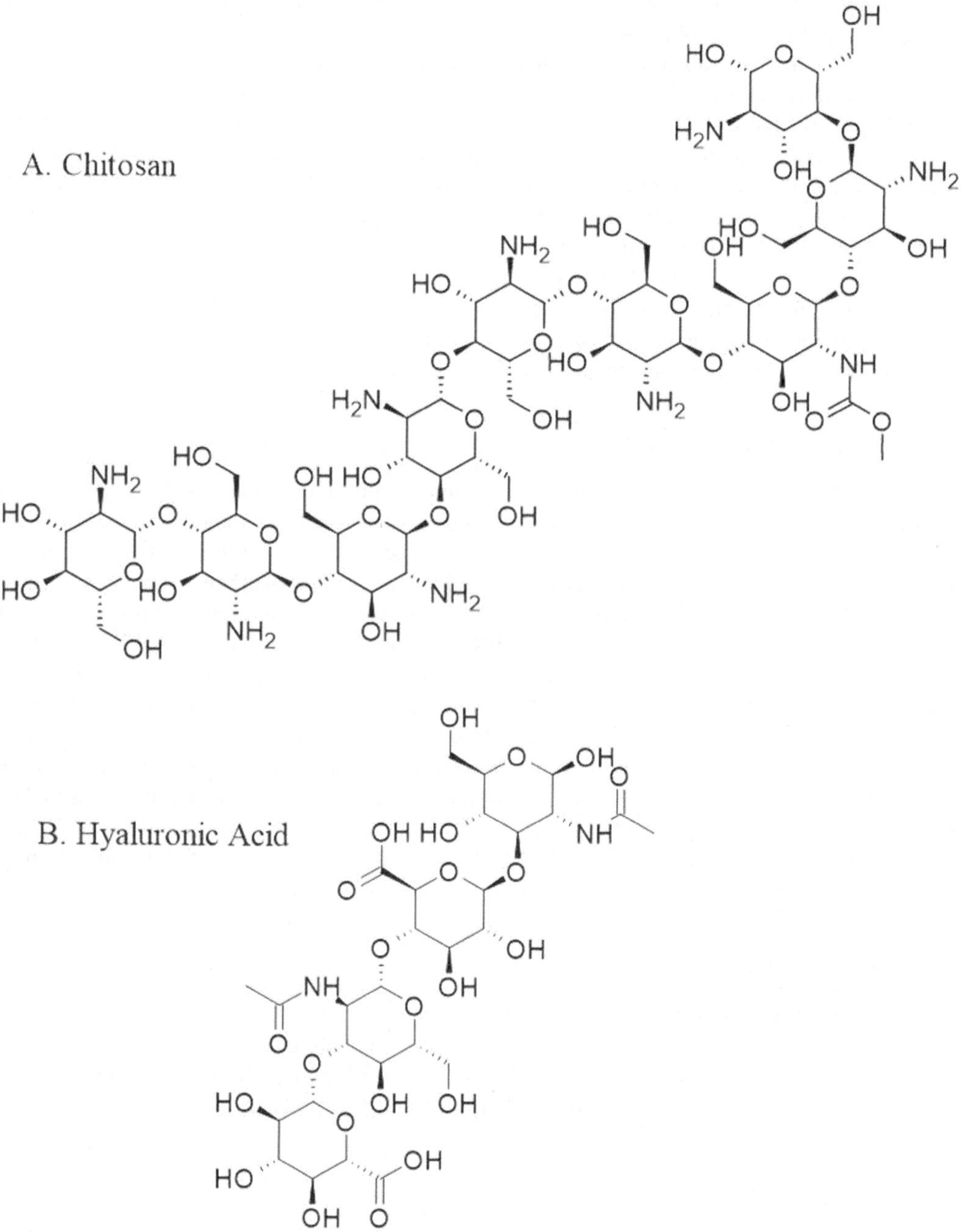

FIGURE 5.1 Chemical structures of (A) chitosan and (B) hyaluronic acid.

Albumin is the most abundant serum protein in the blood, making up 80 to 90% of the total protein content. Because albumin has an exceptionally long serum half-life—19 to 21 days in humans—it has been identified as a potential polymeric biomaterial with serum stability and longevity [64]. Albumin attacks the Fc receptor (FcRn), which has a wide distribution in various cell types, including DCs, endothelial, and epithelial cells. Through FcRn-mediated transport, "albumin trafficking" facilitates lymph node drainage and active endosomal escape to trigger different immune signaling events. Because of this mechanism, many therapeutic agents being developed can use the immunomodulatory capabilities of albumin [79, 80].

Hyaluronic acid (HA), a naturally occurring mucopolysaccharide, is a lengthy polymer of sugar units that is widely distributed throughout the body, including in joint fluid and mucus (Figure 5.1). This polymer is defined as an anionic consisting of N-acetyl-D-glucosamine (NADA) and D-glucuronic acid disaccharides combined by β (1 to 4) and β (1 to 3) glycosidic connections. Certain cancer cells have membrane-bound proteins on their cell surfaces that are bound to CD44 receptors, which HA specifically targets [80]. In order to generate different gene translations, such as cell endurance, which is essential in vaccine cancer therapy, CD44 must be integrated with cellular microenvironment signals. A therapeutic window for life-threatening cancer is demonstrated by a cancer vaccine that targets CD44 biomarkers by using HA, which plays a crucial role in self-restoration, tumor induction, metastasis, and chemoradioresistance [81]. Targeting CD44 was the goal of several investigations on cancer vaccines filled in HA.

5.5.2 Polymers Made from Plants

Most plant cell walls are made of cellulose, a symmetric polymer made of surplus glucose (Figure 5.2). Because of its rigidity, limited solubility, and tendency to form long particles, it is naturally unaffected by biological degradation. Because it is inexpensive, safe for use in pharmaceuticals, and resistant to chemical reactions, it performs well as an immunosorbent or transport medium. According to the literature, a range of cellulose derivatives, including ethyl cellulose (EC), methylcellulose (MC), hydroxypropyl cellulose (HPC), hydroxypropyl cellulose (HPMC), and ethyl hydroxy ethylcellulose (EHEC), have been employed in vaccine administration applications [82, 83].

Alginate is formed of (1–4) linkages of D-mannuronic acid and L-guluronic acid and is available in the brown sea algae cell walls (Figure 5.2). Due to its potential to increase immunogenicity and extend antigen release beyond that of conventional vaccines, alginate has been used extensively in vaccine administration. Furthermore, because of its mucoadhesive properties, it may lessen degradation during nasal and oral delivery in an acidic environment. Yu et al. examined the application of layered double hydroxide NPs (ALG-CHT-LDH) covered with alginate and chitosan polymers as a pH-sensitive and mucoadhesive polymer for oral vaccine administration [84].

5.5.3 Polymers Produced by Microorganisms

Dextran is a microbe-based natural polymer mainly obtained from Gram-positive bacteria such as facultatively anaerobic cocci from strains Leuconostoc and Streptococcus [85]. Dextran's neutral complex amylopectin-chain glucan, which consists of α-1,6-glycosidic connections between glucose monomers (Figure 5.3), contributes to its high water solubility [86]. Dextran's high solubility

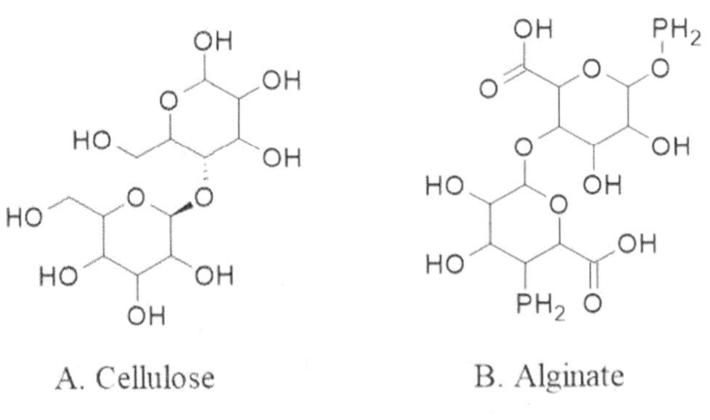

FIGURE 5.2 Chemical structures of (A) cellulose and (B) alginate.

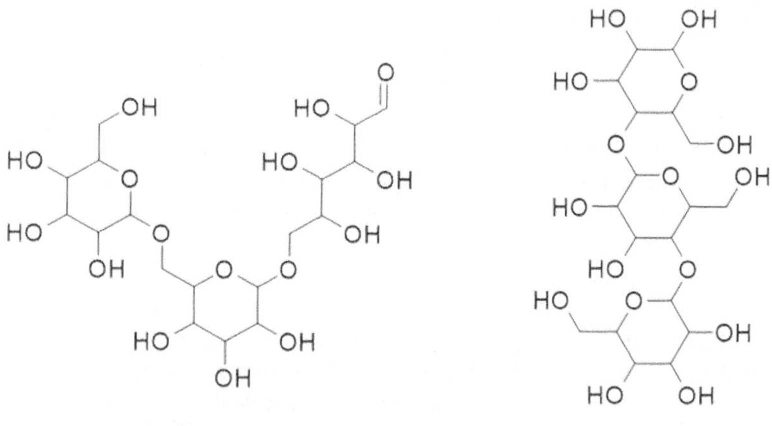

A. Dextran β-Glucan

FIGURE 5.3 Chemical structures of (A) dextran and (B) β-glucan.

makes it undesirable for use in the manufacturing of MP. In order to create an insoluble modified biopolymer, dextran was first converted into acetylated form (dextran-Ace-DEX) using 2-methoxy-propene in a single-stage acetyl synthesis process.

In the yeast and fungi cell walls, like *Saccharomyces cerevisiae*, the most abundant glucose polymer is called β-glucan (Figure 5.3). Depending on the carbon bonds in the D-glucose units (1-3), (1-4), and (1-6), there are many different types of β-glucan [87]. β-glucan has a significant deal of potential as a vaccine adjuvant due to its immunomodulatory activities, which are known to be induced by trained immunity. Tissue-resident memory (TRM) and epigenetic reprogramming of transcriptional pathways are examples of adaptive immune responses that elicit trained immunity, which is a de facto innate immunological memory [88]. The therapeutic effectiveness of the vaccines administered in combination with β-glucan is enhanced by taking advantage of receptors of β-glucan on immune cells, such as CR3, Dectin-1, TLR lactosylceramide, and specific scavenger receptors. The fact that β-glucan typically exists in a triple-helix structure sets it apart from other polymers, such as LNT obtained from *Lentinus edodes*, SPG derived from *Schizophyllum commune*, CUR extracted from *Alcaligenes faecalis*, Sclg obtained from *Sclerotium glucanicum*, and many more. Triple-helix β-glucan can be unwound using chemical modification, high temperature or pH change, and dimethyl sulfoxide (DMSO) solution to produce single chains [89].

5.6 UTILIZING BIONANOCOMPOSITES FOR NASAL ADMINISTRATION

5.6.1 Nanocomposites Based on Chitosan and Its Derivatives

Because of its remarkable biological qualities, chitosan has become a crucial component in the creation of biomaterials and has been thoroughly investigated for use in the delivery of drugs. In addition, a few additional essential characteristics are fungistatic, anticholesteremic, bacteriostatic, hemostatic, and anticarcinogenic [90, 91].

The process of adding nanofillers, or particles smaller than 100 nm, to naturally occurring biopolymers, or "nano-biocomposite," such as chitosan, has produced materials that show great promise for improved biological characteristics, primarily for use in biomedical applications. The traditional disadvantages of biopolymers have been effectively addressed by the chitosan matrix's integration of nano-reinforcements. The food industries, healthcare, biotechnology, agriculture, cosmetics, textiles, environmental protection, and other fields could benefit from the use of chitosan-based nanocomposites [92, 93]. Even at very low levels of nanofillers (5–10 wt %), chitosan-based nanocomposites exhibit or demonstrate notable enhancement in characteristics when compared to conventional composites that contain 40–50% classical fillers. Typically, a high chitosan content is maintained in the nanocomposites, producing goods with good biological activity and compatibility. Improved mechanical and barrier qualities, thermal stability, increased transparency, and other characteristics are among the additional attributes [94]. Innovative methods of drug delivery have endeavored to minimize the systemic dispersion of chemotherapeutic drugs while concentrating their amount at the particular location of effect (targeted delivery).

Chitosan nanocomposites, which offer a stable, non-toxic, target-specific, biocompatible, and biodegradable delivery mechanism, have been significant in these sectors. Similar to this, nanocomposites are gaining a lot of attention for target-specific diagnostic applications because of how simple it is to formulate them by adding imaging and therapeutic chemicals, which is recognized as a significant global public health issue [95]. Due to their distinct electrical, optical, and magnetic characteristics, several nanomaterials have attracted a great deal of consideration, especially in the fields of cancer imaging, diagnostics, and treatment. Targeted therapy is becoming a crucial process in cancer treatment primarily because it helps to enhance anticancer therapies that are based on imaging and treatment.

Various chitosan nanocomposites with distinct characteristics and uses have been studied as drug delivery systems. With its high drug association efficiencies and sustained release profiles, as well as its ability to resolve a serious side effect that continues to be a major obstacle to its application in cancer therapy, Venkatesan et al. demonstrated the effectiveness and potential of using hydroxyapatite-chitosan (Hap-Cs) nanocomposite loaded with celecoxib for colon cancer therapy [96]. In vitro experiments on colon cancer cells confirmed notable anti-proliferation and apoptosis, and showed cytoplasmic absorption of celecoxib-loaded Hap-Cs NPs based on time. Additionally, in vivo research using xenografted human colon tumors in naked mice showed a noticeably higher level of tumor development inhibition.

Chemical modification is a crucial first step to increase chitosan's solubility, hydrophobicity, biological activity, biocompatibility, and other qualities and to expand its uses. Without changing its intrinsic properties, chitosan can be derived in ways that improve its solubility in water in an alkaline environment by adding additional functional groups, such as carboxymethyl or alkyl [97]. The most popular techniques for modifying the chitosan backbone are graft copolymerization and quaternization [98]. Using X-ray irradiation polymerization, Yu Li et al. created the nanocomposite based on poly(butyl acrylate)-modified chitosan. The resulting nanocomposite showed enhanced water absorption resistance, thermal stability, and mechanical properties [99]. Using a layer-by-layer assembly method, a novel folate-linked carboxymethyl chitosan-ferroferric oxide doped with cadmium telluride quantum dot NPs (CFLMNPs) was created for targeted drug administration and cell imaging [100]. At room temperature, the resulting composite system demonstrated a robust superparamagnetic outcome and photoluminescence character. An anti-cancer medication, Adriamycin, has been examined for its target efficacy and release studies. Its loading efficiency is roughly 36.6 wt%. Adriamycin's release profile was pH-dependent, and the folate receptor controlled it.

A different study created a hybrid polysaccharide-based nanocarrier system grafted on a magnetic NP (Fe_3O_4) to carry the hydrophobic anticancer drug 5-fluorouracil [101]. It consisted of chitosan (polyvalent cation) cross-linked with a polyvalent anion like carboxymethyl-cyclodextrin. The composites show an increase in the capacity of the insoluble drug to bind to the hydrophobic cavity of cyclodextrin through a host-guest interaction. The composite exhibits good filling capacity and great saturation magnetization (43.8 emu/g). The release behavior was type-controlled by diffusion, pH-dependent, and swollen. Higher release rates at low pH have been ascribed to the bulge effect and electrostatic repulsion brought on by the protonation of the amino group.

Spray-drying was employed in a study by Gavini et al. to generate mucoadhesive microspheres filled with cyclodextrin (CD), which were then used as a nasal delivery system for brain targeting [102]. The capability of cyclodextrins to obstruct the production of b-amyloid fibrils in vitro was investigated, using alginate and chitosan as structure-making polymers. None of the examined CDs in this study—hydroxypropyl-cyclodextrin and cyclodextrin—exhibited toxicity at the cellular level; instead, they both showed a capacity to shield cells against the b-peptide. It was discovered that the kind of polymer, CD, and the proportion between the two have the greatest effects on the characteristics of microparticles. Compared to spherical particles, alginate microspheres possess a surface with numerous invaginations, which results in a greater explicit surface and improved aerodynamic performance. Furthermore, there could be a reaction between the Ca^{2+} ions in the extracellular fluid and alginate, which would improve adherence. The authors come to the conclusion that their microparticulate formulation represents a viable nasal medication delivery technology with the potential to target the brain [47].

Spray-drying produced spherical methyl-cyclodextrin and chitosan chloride microparticles filled with DFO at great fabrication yields, surpassing 50%. Both the API content and the encapsulation efficiency were within theoretical bounds, ranging from 93% to 98%. The authors of the study examined the qualities of powders that had been spray-dried and freeze-dried in terms of how well-suited they were for nasal delivery. The findings showed that, since spray-drying enables the manufacture of NPs with a slim size distribution, it is the method of choice for creating nasal formulations. Furthermore, it seems that methyl-cyclodextrin (MCD)-based microparticles are quite effective at promoting medication absorption through the olfactory mucosa's neuronal component. Given the low systemic bioavailability achieved through nasal delivery of the microparticles, the MCD method seems to hold the potential for a non-invasive therapeutic use of DFO as a neuroactive medication in a range of brain disorders [103]. Varshosaz et al. showed how chitosan microparticles may be used to deliver insulin through the nasal route [104]. They showed that, in comparison to intravenous insulin, insulin-loaded microspheres showed a 67% reduction in blood glucose levels.

5.6.2 Alginate-Based Bionanocomposites

Another study by Hussein et al. shows how to use the spray-drying method to prepare alginate microparticles coated with ropinirole hydrochloride [105]. Patients with moderate-to-advanced Parkinson's disease can benefit from the use of ropinirole, a dopamine receptor agonist, to treat their motor abnormalities [106]. However, because of its significant first-pass metabolism in the liver, ropinirole has a relatively poor oral bioavailability. Furthermore, ropinirole used orally can produce gastrointestinal issues [106]. The medication was more stable and non-toxic to an excised sheep nasal mucosa when incorporated into alginate microspheres, suggesting that it was effectively delivered to the brain and CSF fluid.

Alginate is an unbranched anionic biopolymer made up of glucuronic and mannuronic acid units. Due to its mucoadhesive, biodegradable, non-antigenic, gelation, and biocompatibility qualities, alginate has been widely suggested for use in the progress of innovative drug delivery systems. Furthermore, alginate's anionic nature gives it a high degree of interaction potential with cationic substances. As a result, it can be utilized to set up delivery systems for the addition of cationic medicinal compounds. Because of their adjuvant properties, alginate NPs can both boost immune responses and extend the release of antigens as compared to traditional vaccines. Alginate NPs have been created more recently to carry the medication venlafaxine (VLF) from the nasal route. Related to the VLF solution, the produced NPs had a mean particle size of 173.7 nm and showed an extraordinary potential for VLF transport to the brain by quick extra- or intracellular distribution alongside the olfactory neurons, avoiding blood circulation. Nonetheless, the documented information verified that medication concentration in the nasal cavity olfactory region has vanished through nasal breathing, and a portion of the NPs can cross the nasal barrier and reach the lungs.

5.6.3 Poloxamer-Based Liposomes

Several strategies have been proposed to enable nose-to-brain drug administration, including drug delivery nanosystems and gelling formulations that block mucociliary clearance [107]. An attempt was made to integrate the two approaches by creating a composite nanosystem for nasal drug delivery of APIs directly into the cerebral tissue. Liposomes make up this formulation, which is a thermogelling system [108].

First off, these carriers might give the medication advantageous properties like improved stability, mucoadhesion, and absorption. Second, employing gels improves absorption by lengthening the drug's residence duration in the nasal cavity. For the purpose of treating AD, several APIs that were loaded onto NPs and delivered intravenously were investigated [109]. For instance, compared to the commonly used products, the intranasal injection of a liposome containing donepezil greatly enhanced drug transport to the brain [110]. In a similar vein, rivastigmine-loaded liposomes administered intranasally increased rivastigmine concentrations in the brain in comparison to the free medication [111]. These outcomes supported earlier research using liposomal rivastigmine formulations [112], suggesting that this strategy is appropriate for treating AD.

The drug biopharmaceutics classification system (BCS) classifies our API as a class III medication due to its restricted permeability and high water solubility (> 10 mg/mL). The nasal mucosa is not an appropriate route of absorption for hydrophilic APIs. Therefore, this barrier is removed and drug transfer across mucosa is facilitated by putting the drug into a flexible liposome [113]. Both hydrophobic and hydrophilic medications can be encapsulated in liposomes. Hydrophobic medicines attach themselves to the phospholipid bilayer, whereas hydrophilic medicines become stuck in the aqueous cavity.

Liposomes are safe, non-immunogenic, fully biodegradable, and biocompatible [114]. Therefore, encapsulation within their aqueous core seems to be a viable method for the delivery of hydrophilic API through the intranasal route to the brain. To create an in situ gel, one has to decide on a polymer solution that gels in reaction to exterior stimuli, in this case, temperature, in order to maximize API remanence. Due to its thermoresponsive nature, the formulation is designed to function as a solution at room temperature to facilitate administration and transform into a gel in the nasal cavity at 34°C.

Poloxamer is a non-ionic triblock copolymer that dissolves in water. It is composed of two hydrophilic polyoxyethylene (POE) blocks and a hydrophobic polyoxypropylene (POP) center block. Poloxamers vary widely in terms of their molecular weight (MW) and the proportion of POP to POE components they contain. Poloxamers 407 and 188 are two of the most commonly found poloxamers. Poloxamer-based hydrogels become intriguing possibilities for drug carriers because of their reversible thermal properties. As a result, a lot of research has been done to create mucoadhesive formulations using these thermoreversible and non-irritating gels [115]. It is intriguing to utilize P188 in conjunction with P407 to adjust the Tsol-gel and gel's characteristics. In fact, P188 enhanced the Tsol-gel and mucoadhesive force of in situ thermosensitive gels for the vaginal delivery of sildenafil, as demonstrated by Soliman et al. [116].

In situ hydrogels for the treatment of neurological diseases, such as Alzheimer's disease, have recently been prepared using poloxamer 407 alone or in combination with mucoadhesive polymer [117]. Improved drug permeability, prolonged and regulated distribution, and mucoadhesion are all made possible by the liposome-containing in situ gel system [57]. It could be beneficial to employ mucoadhesive formulations, which include additional polymers in the gel formulation, to maximize the gel's persistence in the intranasal cavity. Therefore, the mucoadhesive qualities of the created formulation would be enhanced by the inclusion of well-known mucoadhesive polymers such as HPMC or chitosan.

Because intranasal delivery is a painless, non-invasive approach that can be used for mobile treatment, it has been given preference [118]. Therefore, this work aims to create and describe a novel composite formulation that combines the hydrogel and liposome techniques and is appropriate for intranasal delivery. We made sure that this formulation met the isotonic (280–20 mOsmol) and stabilized pH (6–3) requirements of the European Pharmacopoeia for nasal preparations in order to prevent negatively affecting the functions of the nasal mucosa and its cilia [108].

An attempt to create the poloxamer 407® (P407) erodible in situ gel-forming systems was made as a potentially useful platform, such as poly(lactic-co-glycolic acid) (PLGA) NPs, that could extend the release of rivastigmine hydrogen tartrate (RHT). Following their formulation and characterization, PLGA NPs containing RHT were implanted in a P407 gel-making matrix. Sol-gel temperature (Tsol-gel) was found to have a linear dependence on P407 concentration; an 18% P407 content was chosen. It was discovered that the loading efficiencies of the formulations ranged from 100.22% to 104.31%. On A549 cells, the RHT-filled NPs demonstrated appropriate cytocompatibility and a time-dependent rise in cellular uptake. Furthermore, compared to ordinary drug gel, nanocomposites demonstrated greater drug penetration through the nasal mucosa of sheep [119, 120].

5.6.4 Pullulan-Based Bionanocomposites

Several polymers have been used to create particulate systems that serve as vaccine carriers, but biodegradable polyesters like PLA, PLGA, and polycaprolactone have received much attention [121–123]. Regretfully, using organic solvents during the creation of these particulate systems has the primary disadvantage of potentially damaging proteomic structures [124]. The biopolymer chitosan and its products have also been extensively studied in relation to vaccine delivery. There was a trial to create a nanocomposite with chitosan derivatives for use as vaccine transporters by selecting carboxymethyl pullulan (CMP), a pullulan derivative, as a polyanion for the first time. A fungal strain known as Aureobasidium pullulan is the source of pullulan, which is frequently defined as a (1–6)-linked maltotriose [125]. Pullulan is a biodegradable exopolysaccharide that is not derivatized. It has been utilized as a vaccine adjuvant, where it was conjugated to different toxoids and demonstrated immunogenic results that were better than those of alum [126].

Pullulan becomes more soluble in cold water when carboxymethylation is added. Additionally, the carboxylate groups give the polymer's backbone structure a negative charge, which allows the polymer to rejoin with polycations through polyion complexation to generate nanocomposites. Additionally, compared to other organs, it was shown that CMP had a stronger affinity for the spleen and lymph nodes [127, 128]. The polyion complexation approach was utilized to manufacture nanocomposites loaded with diphtheria toxoid by employing polycationic chitosan derivatives (CG, TMC, and CCl) and polyanionic pullulan, CMP. According to the study's findings, CS derivatives and polyanion CMP can combine to form nanocomposites through the polycondensation method. These NPs are non-toxic and can potentially be highly effective new nasal vaccine delivery systems that can elicit strong cellular responses and strong and long-lasting systemic humoral responses [129].

The nanocomposite surface charge could be adjusted by varying the mass quotient of polycation to polyanion. All nanocomposite formulations displayed positive zeta potential values ranging from +14 to +33 mV. When chitosan derivatives and polyanionic pullulan derivatives (CMP) were complexed to produce NPs, the cytotoxicity to respiratory cells (Calu-3 cells) was much lower than when polycation polymers (TMC, CG, and CCl) were used alone. Macrophages effectively incorporated all of the NP formulations that were produced (J774A.1), indicating the potential utility of these innovative nanoparticulate carriers for nasal immunization [130].

5.6.5 Other Bionanocomposites Based on Polymers

Pectin has been researched and utilized in oral, ophthalmic, and nasal therapies for particular delivery needs. Pectin's mucoadhesive properties make it a promising treatment for localized diseases such as allergies, nasal congestion, and infections [131]. As a result, this specific polymer is suggested as a vehicle to attain a controlled release of drugs by hydrating and diffusing the mucosal tissue. Pectin's low esterification degree may have the ability to bind mucin through hydrogen bonding with mucin in an aqueous media, as well as through pectin's adsorption mechanism on the mucin molecule. When a quick medication release is required to treat cancer pain, pectin has been shown to enhance the analgesic onset, treatment efficacy, and acceptance [132, 133].

An increasing number of effectively developed brain-targeted drug delivery systems have been built using polyamidoamine (PAMAM) dendrimers through modifications at different points in the structure. PAMAM dendrimers, whose starting nucleus is ethylenediamine, are resulting in extremely branching nanocomposites. Dendrimers' surface contains a multitude of surface groups that can be utilized to modify their functional properties. Effective methods of drug loading by dendrimers include the physical trapping of large hydrophobic voids inside the cell and surface electrostatic adsorption or bonding. It was established that the brain-targeting primers transferrin (Tf) and serine-arginine-leucine (SRL) may successfully alter PAMAM dendrimers [59, 134, 135].

But in vivo, the dendrimer's brain-targeted delivery mechanism was altered by target proteins and proven unstable. The stability of the nanocomposites was challenged by complex enzymatic, ionic, and pH conditions [136]. The development of nasal delivery devices has drawn more attention in the recent past. Furthermore, nasal brain transport will be very convenient for the clinical application of medications as a non-invasive mode of delivery [57]. Fluorescence-tagged small interfering RNA (fluorescence-tagged siRNA) was discovered in the cytoplasm and processes of neurons and glial cells in a variety of brain areas, including the striatum, cerebral cortex, amygdala, and hypothalamus, after nasal delivery of PAMAM-loaded siRNA [58].

After nasal administration, PAMAM-loaded haloperidol improved brain targeting; behavioral responses induced by haloperidol formulations administered intraperitoneally were comparable to those induced by 6.7 times lower doses of the dendrimer-haloperidol formulation administered via the intranasal route [60]. The primary restriction on nasal delivery is the quick drug removal by the cilia and nasal mucosa, which shortens the period that the preparation adheres to the nasal mucosa [60]. In situ gel is a novel kind of ecologically sensitive gel for nasal delivery. Prior to the gel phase transition, the solution state is suitable for dose control and medication administration because it keeps the preparation's viscosity at a consistently low level and allows for good fluidity. After phase change, a gel state with a higher viscosity level is created, which can stick to the nasal mucosa's surface and inhibit the nasal cavity's clearance to lengthen the contact time and absorb more material [61]. It has been established that in situ gels are efficient polymer carriers for nasal brain transfer. In order to target the brain, Youssef Naha [62] produced unique nasal almotriptan-loaded solid lipid NPs in mucoadhesive in situ gel formulation. A liposomal mucoadhesive, thermosensitive in situ gel was created by Mura [63] for the prolonged nasal delivery of opiorphin.

Paeonol was enclosed in cavities by PAMAM dendrimers that had undergone functional modification. It is possible to successfully manufacture ionic responsive gel of nanocomposites in situ by employing gellan gum. It has been demonstrated that in situ gel is a non-Newtonian fluid with yield stress, shear thinning, and thixotropy. Following nasal delivery, the gel solution underwent a transition of phase that resulted in a gel state and enhanced bioadhesion. In situ gel improved mucosal absorption and extended the release period. The nasal absorption level of PAMAM nanocomposite solution is poor, and the nasal transport competence of nanocomposites can be greatly enhanced by in situ gel. A possible nasal brain medication delivery device is the PAMAM dendrimer nanocomposite/DGG delivery system [59, 63].

5.7 FUTURE PERSPECTIVES

Because of their enhanced physicochemical characteristics, nanocomposites—which have been more popular in the recent past—have drawn a lot of attention from the biomedical community. When medications are delivered using targeted nanocomposites, the negative effects of highly specific drugs are avoided and a controlled release rate is ensured at the intended site. Combining two or more components to create a single material with special qualities, including high loading capacity, increased mechanical capabilities, reduced toxicity, improved biocompatibility and biodegradability, and the ability to image guidance.

Because bionanocomposites are less likely to cause adverse effects and are stable in biological fluids, they represent a novel approach to improving drug delivery for the treatment of cancer. They are made up of two components: matrix and filler, which can be combined in different ways to create them. Drug delivery uses synthetic biopolymers such as polylactic acid (PLA) and polyglycolic acid

(PLGA); however, their mechanical stiffness, transparency, and thermal stability are all compromised. Nanocomposites are a more effective in situ drug delivery strategy since they have demonstrated superior impacts on drug stability as well as prolonged and controlled release. They can be made using polysaccharides like methylcellulose and hyaluronan, and they are employed as carriers for medications that treat cardiovascular issues, inflammation, antimicrobial issues, and cancer. The distribution of drugs to appropriate organs and tissues has garnered interest due to advancements in drug delivery development. Silver, gold, ZnO, TiO_2, silica and clay NPs, carbon nanotubes, carbon quantum dots, graphene, hydroxyapatite, and bioglass are among the most widely used nanomaterials. In summary, pullulan, a polysaccharide polymer derived from the fermentation of starch, exhibits superior film formability and antibacterial properties. Composites using biopolymers such as gelatin, chitosan, and others are being investigated to improve their film-forming properties. Moxifloxacin-loaded chitosan-pullulan-silver nanocomposites exhibit significant antibacterial efficacy, showcasing the potential for treating infections associated with cancer therapy. Magnetic NP technology is highlighted as a promising approach for targeted drug therapy in cancer. These composites show potential for applications in drug delivery, especially in the context of cancer treatment. Collagenous tissues yield gelatin, which is used to create 5-aminopyrazole-conjugated gelatin hydrogel, which is used to administer the anticancer medication 5-fluorouracil rectally. The hydrogel exhibits cytotoxicity toward human colon adenocarcinoma cells, implying a possible therapeutic approach for rectal cancer. The production of silver NPs with a focus on their anti-liver cancer and antioxidant qualities, employing gelatin as a stabilizing agent. Moreover, g-C3N4 nanosheets integrated into PVA/gelatin films demonstrate improved thermal stability and tensile strength, as well as possible drug delivery properties. Tissue engineering is used to describe hydrogels, especially those based on hyaluronic acid. Adipose-derived stem cell proliferation is supported by injectable hyaluronic acid-based hydrogels that incorporate cellulose nanocrystals, exhibiting enhanced structural characteristics and indicating potential for use in biomedical applications. Examined is the function of hyaluronic acid in cancer therapy, with a focus on how it interacts with cell surface receptors such as CD44. Possible options for cancer treatment are reviewed, including modification of HA and its effect on CD44-HA interactions. In order to increase stability and postprint fixing, double crosslinking of HA-based bioinks for 3D bioprinting combines noncovalent bonding with ionic crosslinking caused by sodium alginate. Finally, the conversation moves on to bionanocomposites, where drug delivery methods involving layered double hydroxides (LDH) coupled with biopolymers such as zein and alginate are being investigated. Additionally covered are bionanocomposites based on carrageenan, emphasizing how adaptable and customizable they are for a range of uses. The potential of biopolymers, hydrogels, and nanocomposites to improve cancer therapy and healthcare is demonstrated by their many uses in tissue engineering, drug delivery, and biomedical research.

It has been found that particle carriers work well for delivering drugs through various administration routes. Numerous studies in the literature demonstrate the great potential that nasal delivery offers for specifically directing to cerebral tissue in the treatment of various CNS illnesses. Drug transport via the trigeminal and olfactory nerve routes avoids the BBB and side effects associated with other routes, such as liver first-pass metabolism and enzyme degradation. As a result, there is a significant reduction in systemic exposure, systemic side effects, and brain bioavailability. The limits of the nasal route of administration have been extensively studied through the use of novel techniques, such as the use of micro- and nanosized drug carriers. These delivery systems shield the drug from the environment, which also lengthens the drug's residence period, improves drug permeability via the nasal mucosa, raises drug bioavailability, and boosts therapeutic efficacy.

The number of possible biomolecules, including RNA, proteins, peptides, and monoclonal antibodies, for the therapy of neurodegenerative diseases is continually rising. Nevertheless, a number of restrictions connected to important physicochemical and pharmacokinetic properties limit their therapeutic potential. It looks like a workable strategy to carry complex macromolecules directly from the nasal cavity to the brain is nose-to-brain delivery. In this field of study, optimizing the drug carriers' physicochemical characteristics would be crucial. An alternative viewpoint involves enhancing the carriers' effectiveness by adding ligands that target cells or peptides that penetrate cells. Future studies would likely center on the application of tailored, multi-targeted techniques in order to guarantee a customized therapeutic approach. More innovative delivery systems should be able to move from the experimental stage of development into the clinical setting thanks to new technologies that leverage the nose-to-brain pathway.

5.8 CONCLUSION

To put it simply, intranasal medicine delivery is an additional means of delivering bioactive molecules to the brain, systemic circulation, and local tissues to produce the intended therapeutic outcome. Following intranasal administration, medication dosage forms are quickly removed from the nasal canal, which lowers drug absorption. To extend the duration of medication formulation's residency at the nasal mucus site over several hours or days, a variety of mucoadhesive nanosystems might be employed. Hydrogel NPs and nanocomposites, out of all the nanosystems that are currently on the market, are the most stimuli-responsive and multifunctional due to their easy design, low cost, ability to include a wide range of drugs, and ability to attain the perfect model of a controlled discharge of drugs. These attributes make these materials perfect for nasal drug and vaccine delivery. Future studies will need to address this important issue because the toxicity, transport, and uptake by the NALT cells of nanogels and NPs trapped in the hydrogel network in the nasal cavity or central nervous system have not been extensively studied. Additionally, the medicinal market for hydrogel nanosystems is being driven by advances in CNS delivery and BBB crossing, particularly in the treatment of CNS tumors.

Growing interest has been seen in creating diverse nanomaterials for various biomedical uses in recent years. For use in biomedical applications, various nanocomposites, including organic-inorganic, inorganic-inorganic, and organic-organic nanocomposites, are being created from these nanomaterials. We can infer from this chapter that these biomedical nanocomposites have a variety of special qualities, including mechanical, physicochemical, biological, and drug delivery capabilities. These properties are useful for a wide range of applications, including dentistry, bioimaging, drug delivery, gene delivery, antimicrobials, tissue regeneration, wound healing, and wound healing.

REFERENCES

[1] Jian, Wei, David Hui, and Denvid Lau. "Nanoengineering in biomedicine: Current development and future perspectives." *Nanotechnology Reviews* 9, no. 1 (2020): 700–715.

[2] Nepal, Dhriti, Saewon Kang, Katarina M. Adstedt, Krishan Kanhaiya, Michael R. Bockstaller, L. Catherine Brinson, Markus J. Buehler et al. "Hierarchically structured bioinspired nanocomposites." *Nature Materials* 22, no. 1 (2023): 18–35.

[3] Kumar, Sanat K., and Ramanan Krishnamoorti. "Nanocomposites: Structure, phase behavior, and properties." *Annual Review of Chemical and Biomolecular Engineering* 1 (2010): 37–58.

[4] Kumar, Ashwini, and Awanish Kumar. "Biomedical applications of nanosilicate composites." In *Biomedical Composites: Perspectives and Applications*, pp. 1–18. Springer, 2021.

[5] Hasnain, M. S., S. A. Ahmad, N. Chaudhary, M. N. Hoda, and A. K. Nayak. "Biodegradable polymer matrix nanocomposites for bone tissue engineering." In Inamuddin, Asiri, A. M., and Mohammad, A. (eds.), *Applications of Nanocomposite Materials in Orthopaedics*. Woodhead Publishing Series in Biomaterials, pp 1–37. Elsevier Inc., 2019.

[6] Hasnain, M. S. and A. K. Nayak. "Nanocomposites for improved orthopedic and bone tissue engineering applications." In Inamuddin, Asiri, A. M., and Mohammad, A. (eds.), *Applications of Nanocomposite Materials in Orthopaedics*. Woodhead Publishing Series in Biomaterials, pp 145–177. Elsevier Inc., 2019.

[7] Camargo, Pedro Henrique Cury, Kestur Gundappa Satyanarayana, and Fernando Wypych. "Nanocomposites: Synthesis, structure, properties and new application opportunities." *Materials Research* 12 (2009): 1–39.

[8] Zheng, Yingying, Jonathan Monty, and Robert J. Linhardt. "Polysaccharide-based nanocomposites and their applications." *Carbohydrate Research* 405 (2015): 23–32.

[9] Hu, Weili, Shiyan Chen, Jingxuan Yang, Zhe Li, and Huaping Wang. "Functionalized bacterial cellulose derivatives and nanocomposites." *Carbohydrate Polymers* 101 (2014): 1043–1060.

[10] Parida, Santosh K. "Recent advances on polymer-based nanocomposite: A brief review." *Micro and Nanosystems* 14, no. 2 (2022): 121–132.

[11] Verma, Deepak, Vaishally Dogra, Arun Kumar Chaudhary, and Ravikant Mordia. "Advanced biopolymer-based composites: Construction and structural applications." In *Sustainable Biopolymer Composites*, pp. 113–128. Woodhead Publishing, 2022.

[12] Wang, Min, and Qilong Zhao. "Biomedical composites." In *Reference Module in Biomedical Sciences: Encyclopedia of Biomedical Engineering*. Elsevier, 2019.

[13] Das, Saumya, Dharmajit Pattanayak, Amit Kumar Nayak, Dong Kee Yi, Sitansu Sekhar Nanda, Mohammed Tahir Ansari, and Md Saquib Hasnain. "Alginate–montmorillonite composite systems as sustained drug delivery carriers." In *Alginates in Drug Delivery*, pp. 187–201. Academic Press, 2020.

[14] Holban, Alina Maria, and Alexandru Grumezescu, eds. *Materials for Biomedical Engineering: Nanomaterials-based Drug Delivery*. Elsevier, 2019.

[15] Hasnain, Md Saquib, Syed Anees Ahmed, Saad Alkahtani, Milan Milivojevic, Chandi Charan Kandar, Amal Kumar Dhara, and Amit Kumar Nayak. "Biopolymers for drug delivery." In *Advanced Biopolymeric Systems for Drug Delivery*, pp. 1–29. Springer, 2020.

[16] Nayak, Amit Kumar, Md Saquib Hasnain, Amit Kumar Nayak, and Md Saquib Hasnain. "Background: Multiple units in oral drug delivery." *Plant Polysaccharides-based Multiple-unit Systems for Oral Drug Delivery*, pp. 1–17. Springer, 2019.

[17] Nayak, Amit Kumar, and Md Saquib Hasnain, eds. *Advanced Biopolymeric Systems for Drug Delivery*. Springer, 2020.

[18] Nayak, Amit Kumar, Saad Alkahtani, and Md Saquib Hasnain. "Biomedical nanocomposites." In *Biomedical Composites: Perspectives and Applications*, pp. 35–69. Springer, 2021.

[19] Azizi-Lalabadi, Maryam, and Seid Mahdi Jafari. "Bio-nanocomposites of graphene with biopolymers; fabrication, properties, and applications." *Advances in Colloid and Interface Science* 292 (2021): 102416.

[20] Sarode, H., D. Barai, B. Bhanvase, R. Ugwekar, and V. Saharan. "Investigation on preparation of graphene oxide-CuO nanocomposite based nanofluids with the aid of ultrasound assisted method for intensified heat transfer properties." *Materials Chemistry and Physics* 251 (2020): 123102.

[21] Cobos, Mónica, Iker De-La-Pinta, Guillermo Quindós, M. Jesús Fernández, and M. Dolores Fernández. "One-step eco-friendly synthesized silver-graphene oxide/poly(vinyl alcohol) antibacterial nanocomposites." *Carbon* 150 (2019): 101–116.

[22] Zeng, Qianqian, Ziran Du, Chenyuan Qin, Yaming Wang, Chuntai Liu, and Changyu Shen. "Enhanced thermal, mechanical and electromagnetic interference shielding properties of graphene nanoplatelets-reinforced poly (lactic acid)/poly (ethylene oxide) nanocomposites." *Materials Today Communications* 25 (2020): 101632.

[23] Tkalya, Evgeniy, Marcos Ghislandi, Alexander Alekseev, Cor Koning, and Joachim Loos. "Latex-based concept for the preparation of graphene-based polymer nanocomposites." *Journal of Materials Chemistry* 20, no. 15 (2010): 3035–3039.

[24] Ahmad, Rais, and Anam Mirza. "Synthesis of Guar gum/bentonite a novel bionanocomposite: Isotherms, kinetics and thermodynamic studies for the removal of Pb (II) and crystal violet dye." *Journal of Molecular Liquids* 249 (2018): 805–814.

[25] Wang, Huiyan, Gaoke Zhang, Huihu Gan, and Yuanyuan Gao. "Synthesis and characterization of ibuprofen-rectorite composites by solution intercalation method." *Journal of Wuhan University of Technology-Materials Science Edition* 24, no. 4 (2009): 654–657.

[26] Youssef, Ahmed M., Fayza M. Assem, Hoda S. El-Sayed, Samah M. El-Sayed, Mostafa Elaaser, and Mohamed H. Abd El-Salam. "Synthesis and evaluation of eco-friendly carboxymethyl cellulose/polyvinyl alcohol/CuO bionanocomposites and their use in coating processed cheese." *RSC Advances* 10, no. 62 (2020): 37857–37870.

[27] Ebrahimi, Yadollah, Seyed Jamaleddin Peighambardoust, Seyed Hadi Peighambardoust, and Sirous Zahed Karkaj. "Development of antibacterial carboxymethyl cellulose-based nanobiocomposite films containing various metallic nanoparticles for food packaging applications." *Journal of Food Science* 84, no. 9 (2019): 2537–2548.

[28] Shameli, Kamyar, Mansor Bin Ahmad, Mohsen Zargar, Wan Md Zin Wan Yunus, Nor Azowa Ibrahim, Parvaneh Shabanzadeh, and Mansour Ghaffari Moghaddam. "Synthesis and characterization of silver/montmorillonite/chitosan bionanocomposites by chemical reduction method and their antibacterial activity." *International Journal of Nanomedicine* 6 (2011): 271–284.

[29] Shameli, Kamyar, Mansor Bin Ahmad, Wan Md Zin Wan Yunus, Abdolhossein Rustaiyan, Nor Azowa Ibrahim, Mohsen Zargar, and Yadollah Abdollahi. "Green synthesis of silver/montmorillonite/chitosan bionanocomposites using the UV irradiation method and evaluation of antibacterial activity." *International Journal of Nanomedicine* 5 (2010): 875–887.

[30] Ahmad, Mansor B., Kamyar Shameli, Majid Darroudi, Wan MZW Yunus, and Nor A. Ibrahim. "Synthesis and characterization of silver/clay/chitosan bionanocomposites by UV-irradiation method." *American Journal of Applied Sciences* 6, no. 12 (2009): 2030.

[31] Ahmad, Mansor B., Kamyar Shameli, Majid Darroudi, Wan M. Z. W. Yunus, and Nor A. Ibrahim. "Synthesis and characterization of silver/clay nanocomposites by chemical reduction method." *American Journal of Applied Sciences* 6, no. 11 (2009): 1909.

[32] Gonzalez, Carlos Miguel, Yun Liu, and J. C. Scaiano. "Photochemical strategies for the facile synthesis of gold–silver alloy and core–shell bimetallic nanoparticles." *The Journal of Physical Chemistry C* 113, no. 27 (2009): 11861–11867.

[33] Darroudi, Majid, Mansor Bin Ahmad, Kamyar Shameli, Abdul Halim Abdullah, and Nor Azowa Ibrahim. "Synthesis and characterization of UV-irradiated silver/montmorillonite nanocomposites." *Solid State Sciences* 11, no. 9 (2009): 1621–1624.

[34] Salkar, R. A., S. T. Pethaiyan Jeevanandam, Yuri Koltypin Aruna, and A. Gedanken. "The sonochemical preparation of amorphous silver nanoparticles." *Journal of Materials Chemistry* 9, no. 6 (1999): 1333–1335.

[35] Bin Ahmad, Mansor, Jenn Jye Lim, Kamyar Shameli, Nor Azowa Ibrahim, and Mei Yen Tay. "Synthesis of silver nanoparticles in chitosan, gelatin and chitosan/gelatin bionanocomposites by a chemical reducing agent and their characterization." *Molecules* 16, no. 9 (2011): 7237–7248.

[36] Luckarift, Heather R., Matthew B. Dickerson, Kenneth H. Sandhage, and Jim C. Spain. "Rapid, room-temperature synthesis of antibacterial bionanocomposites of lysozyme with amorphous silica or titania." *Small* 2, no. 5 (2006): 640–643.

[37] Luckarift, Heather R., Jim C. Spain, Rajesh R. Naik, and Morley O. Stone. "Enzyme immobilization in a biomimetic silica support." *Nature Biotechnology* 22, no. 2 (2004): 211–213.

[38] Murali, Srinath, Santosh Kumar, Joonseok Koh, Sahadevan Seena, Poonam Singh, Amílcar Ramalho, and Abilio JFN Sobral. "Bio-based chitosan/gelatin/Ag@ZnO bionanocomposites: Synthesis and mechanical and antibacterial properties." *Cellulose* 26 (2019): 5347–5361.

[39] Javaid, Muhammad Asif, Rasheed Ahmad Khera, Khalid Mahmood Zia, Kei Saito, Ijaz Ahmad Bhatti, and Muhammad Asghar. "Synthesis and characterization of chitosan modified polyurethane bio-nanocomposites with biomedical potential." *International Journal of Biological Macromolecules* 115 (2018): 375–384.

[40] Yang, Jen Ming, Shu Jyuan Yang, Hao Tzu Lin, Te-Hsing Wu, and Haw-Jan Chen. "Chitosan containing PU/Poly (NIPAAm) thermosensitive membrane for wound dressing." *Materials Science and Engineering: C* 28, no. 1 (2008): 150–156.

[41] Kumar, P. T. Sudheesh, S. Abhilash, K. Manzoor, S. V. Nair, H. Tamura, and R. Jayakumar. "Preparation and characterization of novel β-chitin/nanosilver composite scaffolds for wound dressing applications." *Carbohydrate Polymers* 80, no. 3 (2010): 761–767.

[42] Xu, Dan, Zhen Meng, Ming Han, Kai Xi, Xudong Jia, Xuehai Yu, and Qingmin Chen. "Novel blood-compatible waterborne polyurethane using chitosan as an extender." *Journal of Applied Polymer Science* 109, no. 1 (2008): 240–246.

[43] Lin, Y. H., N. K. Chou, W. J. Wu, S. H. Hsu, S. W. Whu, G. H. Ho, C. L. Tsai, S. S. Wang, S. H. Chu, and K. H. Hsieh. "Physical properties of water-borne polyurethane blended with chitosan." *Journal of Applied Polymer Science* 104, no. 4 (2007): 2683–2689.

[44] Yang, Shu-Hua, Yu-Sheng J. Lee, Feng-Huei Lin, Jen-Ming Yang, and Ko-shau Chen. "Chitosan/poly (vinyl alcohol) blending hydrogel coating improves the surface characteristics of segmented polyurethane urethral catheters." *Journal of Biomedical Materials Research Part B: Applied Biomaterials* 83, no. 2 (2007): 304–313.

[45] Zecca, Luigi, Moussa BH Youdim, Peter Riederer, James R. Connor, and Robert R. Crichton. "Iron, brain ageing and neurodegenerative disorders." *Nature Reviews Neuroscience* 5, no. 11 (2004): 863–873.

[46] Lochhead, Jeffrey J., and Robert G. Thorne. "Intranasal delivery of biologics to the central nervous system." *Advanced Drug Delivery Reviews* 64, no. 7 (2012): 614–628.

[47] Boyuklieva, Radka, and Bissera Pilicheva. "Micro-and nanosized carriers for nose-to-brain drug delivery in neurodegenerative disorders." *Biomedicines* 10, no. 7 (2022): 1706.

[48] Liebner, Stefan, Rick M. Dijkhuizen, Yvonne Reiss, Karl H. Plate, Dritan Agalliu, and Gabriela Constantin. "Functional morphology of the blood–brain barrier in health and disease." *Acta Neuropathologica* 135 (2018): 311–336.

[49] Banks, William A. "Characteristics of compounds that cross the blood-brain barrier." *BMC Neurology* 9, no. 1 (2009): 1–5.

[50] Belur, Lalitha R., Megan Romero, Junggu Lee, Kelly M. Podetz-Pedersen, Zhenhong Nan, Maureen S. Riedl, Lucy Vulchanova et al. "Comparative effectiveness of intracerebroventricular, intrathecal, and intranasal routes of AAV9 vector administration for genetic therapy of neurologic disease in murine mucopolysaccharidosis type I." *Frontiers in Molecular Neuroscience* 14 (2021): 618360.

[51] Duskey, Jason T., Daniela Belletti, Francesca Pederzoli, Maria Angela Vandelli, Flavio Forni, Barbara Ruozi, and Giovanni Tosi. "Current strategies for the delivery of therapeutic proteins and enzymes to treat brain disorders." *International Review of Neurobiology* 137 (2017): 1–28.

[52] Wu, Hongbing, Kaili Hu, and Xinguo Jiang. "From nose to brain: Understanding transport capacity and transport rate of drugs." *Expert Opinion on Drug Delivery* 5, no. 10 (2008): 1159–1168.

[53] Vyas, Tushar K., Aliasgar Shahiwala, Sudhanva Marathe, and Ambikanandan Misra. "Intranasal drug delivery for brain targeting." *Current Drug Delivery* 2, no. 2 (2005): 165–175.

[54] Gänger, Stella, and Katharina Schindowski. "Tailoring formulations for intranasal nose-to-brain delivery: A review on architecture, physico-chemical characteristics and mucociliary clearance of the nasal olfactory mucosa." *Pharmaceutics* 10, no. 3 (2018): 116.

[55] Crowe, Tyler P., M. Heather West Greenlee, Anumantha G. Kanthasamy, and Walter H. Hsu. "Mechanism of intranasal drug delivery directly to the brain." *Life Sciences* 195 (2018): 44–52.

[56] Keller, Lea-Adriana, Olivia Merkel, and Andreas Popp. "Intranasal drug delivery: Opportunities and toxicologic challenges during drug development." *Drug Delivery and Translational Research* 12, no. 4 (2021): 1–23.

[57] Jain, Darshana S., Amrita N. Bajaj, Rajani B. Athawale, Shruti S. Shikhande, Abhijeet Pandey, Peeyush N. Goel, Rajiv P. Gude, Satish Patil, and Preeti Raut. "Thermosensitive PLA based nanodispersion for targeting brain tumor via intranasal route." *Materials Science and Engineering: C* 63 (2016): 411–421.

[58] Kim, Il-Doo, Joo-Hyun Shin, Seung-Woo Kim, Sunghyun Choi, Junseong Ahn, Pyung-Lim Han, Jong-Sang Park, and Ja-Kyeong Lee. "Intranasal delivery of HMGB1 siRNA confers target gene knockdown and robust neuroprotection in the postischemic brain." *Molecular Therapy* 20, no. 4 (2012): 829–839.

[59] Xie, Huichao, Lingjun Li, Yue Sun, Yuzhen Wang, Shuang Gao, Yuan Tian, Xuemei Ma, Chengcheng Guo, Fumin Bo, and Li Zhang. "An available strategy for nasal brain transport of nanocomposite based on PAMAM dendrimers via in situ gel." *Nanomaterials* 9, no. 2 (2019): 147.

[60] Katare, Yogesh K., Ritesh P. Daya, Christal Sookram Gray, Roger E. Luckham, Jayant Bhandari, Abhay S. Chauhan, and Ram K. Mishra. "Brain targeting of a water insoluble antipsychotic drug haloperidol via the intranasal route using PAMAM dendrimer." *Molecular Pharmaceutics* 12, no. 9 (2015): 3380–3388.

[61] Chu, Kedan, Lidian Chen, Wei Xu, Huang Li, Yuqin Zhang, Weirong Xie, and Jian Zheng. "Preparation of a paeonol-containing temperature-sensitive in situ gel and its preliminary efficacy on allergic rhinitis." *International Journal of Molecular Sciences* 14, no. 3 (2013): 6499–6515.

[62] Abou Youssef, Nancy Abdel Hamid, Abeer Ahmed Kassem, Ragwa Mohamed Farid, Fatma Ahmed Ismail, EL-Massik Magda Abd Elsamea, and Nabila Ahmed Boraie. "A novel nasal almotriptan loaded solid lipid nanoparticles in mucoadhesive in situ gel formulation for brain targeting: Preparation, characterization and in vivo evaluation." *International Journal of Pharmaceutics* 548, no. 1 (2018): 609–624.

[63] Mura, Paola, Natascia Mennini, Cristina Nativi, and Barbara Richichi. "In situ mucoadhesive-thermosensitive liposomal gel as a novel vehicle for nasal extended delivery of opiorphin." *European Journal of Pharmaceutics and Biopharmaceutics* 122 (2018): 54–61.

[64] Pires, Anaísa, Ana Fortuna, Gilberto Alves, and Amílcar Falcão. "Intranasal drug delivery: How, why and what for?." *Journal of Pharmacy & Pharmaceutical Sciences* 12, no. 3 (2009): 288–311.

[65] Salatin, Sara, Jaleh Barar, Mohammad Barzegar-Jalali, Khosro Adibkia, Mitra Alami Milani, and Mitra Jelvehgari. "Hydrogel nanoparticles and nanocomposites for nasal drug/vaccine delivery." *Archives of Pharmacal Research* 39 (2016): 1181–1192.

[66] Ugwoke, Michael Ikechukwu, Norbert Verbeke, and Renaat Kinget. "The biopharmaceutical aspects of nasal mucoadhesive drug delivery." *Journal of Pharmacy and Pharmacology* 53, no. 1 (2001): 3–22.

[67] Debache, Karim, Christian Kropf, C. A. Schütz, L. J. Harwood, P. Käuper, Thierry Monney, N. Rossi, C. Laue, K. C. McCullough, and Andrew Hemphill. "Vaccination of mice with chitosan nanogel-associated recombinant NcPDI against challenge infection with Neospora caninum tachyzoites." *Parasite Immunology* 33, no. 2 (2011): 81–94.

[68] Fortuna, Ana, Gilberto Alves, Ana Serralheiro, Joana Sousa, and Amílcar Falcão. "Intranasal delivery of systemic-acting drugs: Small-molecules and biomacromolecules." *European Journal of Pharmaceutics and Biopharmaceutics* 88, no. 1 (2014): 8–27.

[69] Dahlin, Maria, Björn Jansson, and Erik Björk. "Levels of dopamine in blood and brain following nasal administration to rats." *European Journal of Pharmaceutical Sciences* 14, no. 1 (2001): 75–80.

[70] Born, Jan, Tanja Lange, Werner Kern, Gerard P. McGregor, Ulrich Bickel, and Horst L. Fehm. "Sniffing neuropeptides: A transnasal approach to the human brain." *Nature Neuroscience* 5, no. 6 (2002): 514–516.

[71] Patel, Hetal P., Priyanka S. Chaudhari, Priyanshi A. Gandhi, Bhargavi V. Desai, Ditixa T. Desai, Praful P. Dedhiya, Bhavin A. Vyas, and Furqan A. Maulvi. "Nose to brain delivery of tailored clozapine nanosuspension stabilized using (+)-alpha-tocopherol polyethylene glycol 1000 succinate: Optimization and in vivo pharmacokinetic studies." *International Journal of Pharmaceutics* 600 (2021): 120474.

[72] Vyas, Tushar K., A. K. Babbar, R. K. Sharma, Shashi Singh, and Ambikanandan Misra. "Intranasal mucoadhesive microemulsions of clonazepam: Preliminary studies on brain targeting." *Journal of Pharmaceutical Sciences* 95, no. 3 (2006): 570–580.

[73] Jayachandra Babu, R. J., Pankaj Patrick Dayal, Kasturi Pawar, and Mandip Singh. "Nose-to-brain transport of melatonin from polymer gel suspensions: A microdialysis study in rats." *Journal of Drug Targeting* 19, no. 9 (2011): 731–740.

[74] Pardeshi, Chandrakantsing Vijaysing, and Veena Shailendra Belgamwar. "Direct nose to brain drug delivery via integrated nerve pathways bypassing the blood–brain barrier: An excellent platform for brain targeting." *Expert Opinion on Drug Delivery* 10, no. 7 (2013): 957–972.

[75] Ilyas, Rushdan Ahmad, Humaira Alias Aisyah, Abu Hassan Nordin, Norzita Ngadi, Mohamed Yusoff Mohd Zuhri, Muhammad Rizal Muhammad Asyraf, Salit Mohd Sapuan et al. "Natural-fiber-reinforced chitosan, chitosan blends and their nanocomposites for various advanced applications." *Polymers* 14, no. 5 (2022): 874.

[76] Tan, Rebecca Shu Ling, Pouya Hassandarvish, Chin Fei Chee, Lai Wah Chan, and Tin Wui Wong. "Chitosan and its derivatives as polymeric anti-viral therapeutics and potential anti-SARS-CoV-2 nanomedicine." *Carbohydrate Polymers* 290 (2022): 119500.

[77] Alipal, J., NAS Mohd Pu'Ad, T. C. Lee, N. H. M. Nayan, N. Sahari, H. Basri, M. I. Idris, and H. Z. Abdullah. "A review of gelatin: Properties, sources, process, applications, and commercialisation." *Materials Today: Proceedings* 42 (2021): 240–250.

[78] Ndlovu, Sindi P., Kwanele Ngece, Sibusiso Alven, and Blessing A. Aderibigbe. "Gelatin-based hybrid scaffolds: Promising wound dressings." *Polymers* 13, no. 17 (2021): 2959.

[79] Sand, Kine Marita Knudsen, Malin Bern, Jeannette Nilsen, Hanna Theodora Noordzij, Inger Sandlie, and Jan Terje Andersen. "Unraveling the interaction between FcRn and albumin: Opportunities for design of albumin-based therapeutics." *Frontiers in Immunology* 5 (2015): 682.

[80] Nordin, Abu Hassan, Siti Muhamad Nur Husna, Zuliahani Ahmad, Muhammad Luqman Nordin, Rushdan Ahmad Ilyas, Ahmad Khusairi Azemi, Noraznawati Ismail et al. "Natural polymeric composites derived from animals, plants, and microbes for vaccine delivery and adjuvant applications: A review." *Gels* 9, no. 3 (2023): 227.

[81] Parayath, Neha N., Avani Parikh, and Mansoor M. Amiji. "Repolarization of tumor-associated macrophages in a genetically engineered nonsmall cell lung cancer model by intraperitoneal administration of hyaluronic acid-based nanoparticles encapsulating microRNA-125b." *Nano Letters* 18, no. 6 (2018): 3571–3579.

[82] Onofrei, M., and A. Filimon. "Cellulose-based hydrogels: Designing concepts, properties, and perspectives for biomedical and environmental applications." *Polymer Science: Research Advances, Practical Applications and Educational Aspects*, pp. 108–120. Formatex Research Center, 2016.

[83] Singh, Bijay, Sushila Maharjan, Tao Jiang, Sang-Kee Kang, Yun-Jaie Choi, and Chong-Su Cho. "Attuning hydroxypropyl methylcellulose phthalate to oral delivery vehicle for effective and selective delivery of protein vaccine in ileum." *Biomaterials* 59 (2015): 144–159.

[84] Yu, Xinying, Tinggang Wen, Pei Cao, Liang Shan, and Li Li. "Alginate-chitosan coated layered double hydroxide nanocomposites for enhanced oral vaccine delivery." *Journal of Colloid and Interface Science* 556 (2019): 258–265.

[85] Huang, Gangliang, and Hualiang Huang. "Application of dextran as nanoscale drug carriers." *Nanomedicine* 13, no. 24 (2018): 3149–3158.

[86] Díaz-Montes, Elsa. "Dextran: Sources, structures, and properties." *Polysaccharides* 2, no. 3 (2021): 554–565.

[87] Geller, Anne, Rejeena Shrestha, and Jun Yan. "Yeast-derived β-glucan in cancer: Novel uses of a traditional therapeutic." *International Journal of Molecular Sciences* 20, no. 15 (2019): 3618.

[88] Ikewaki, Nobunao, Vidyasagar Devaprasad Dedeepiya, Masaru Iwasaki, and Samuel JK Abraham. "Commentary: Beyond "TRIM" benefits of β-glucan by blood glucose and lipid balancing potentials in its defense against COVID-19." *Frontiers in Immunology* 12 (2021): 620658.

[89] Meng, Yan, Fengzhi Lyu, Xiaojuan Xu, and Lina Zhang. "Recent advances in chain conformation and bioactivities of triple-helix polysaccharides." *Biomacromolecules* 21, no. 5 (2020): 1653–1677.

[90] Saikia, C., P. Gogoi, and T. K. Maji. "Chitosan: A promising biopolymer in drug delivery applications." *Journal of Molecular and Genetic Medicine* S4, no. 006 (2015): 899–910.

[91] Ali, Akbar, and Shakeel Ahmed. "A review on chitosan and its nanocomposites in drug delivery." *International Journal of Biological Macromolecules* 109 (2018): 273–286.

[92] Coradin, Thibaud, Joachim Allouche, Michel Boissière, and Jacques Livage. "Sol-gel biopolymer/silica nanocomposites in biotechnology." *Current Nanoscience* 2, no. 3 (2006): 219–230.

[93] Liu, Xiaowang, Qiyan Hu, Zhen Fang, Xiaojun Zhang, and Beibei Zhang. "Magnetic chitosan nanocomposites: A useful recyclable tool for heavy metal ion removal." *Langmuir* 25, no. 1 (2009): 3–8.

[94] Fernandes, Susana C. M., Carmen S. R. Freire, Armando J. D. Silvestre, Carlos Pascoal Neto, Alessandro Gandini, Lars A. Berglund, and Lennart Salmén. "Transparent chitosan films reinforced with a high content of nanofibrillated cellulose." *Carbohydrate Polymers* 81, no. 2 (2010): 394–401.

[95] Lim, Eun-Kyung, and Bong Hyun Chung. "Preparation of pyrenyl-based multifunctional nanocomposites for biomedical applications." *Nature Protocols* 11, no. 2 (2016): 236–251.

[96] Venkatesan, P., Nagaprasad Puvvada, Rupesh Dash, B. N. Prashanth Kumar, Devanand Sarkar, Belal Azab, Amita Pathak, Subhas C. Kundu, Paul B. Fisher, and Mahitosh Mandal. "The potential of celecoxib-loaded hydroxyapatite-chitosan nanocomposite for the treatment of colon cancer." *Biomaterials* 32, no. 15 (2011): 3794–3806.

[97] Thomas, Deepa, and Sabu Thomas. "Chemical modification of chitosan and its biomedical application." *Biopolymer Nanocomposites: Processing, Properties, and Applications* (2013): 33–51.

[98] Alves, Natalia M., and Joaifo Filipe Mano. "Chitosan derivatives obtained by chemical modifications for biomedical and environmental applications." *International Journal of Biological Macromolecules* 43, no. 5 (2008): 401–414.

[99] Yu, Li, Liu Li, Zhang Wei'an, and Fang Yue'e. "A new hybrid nanocomposite prepared by graft copolymerization of butyl acrylate onto chitosan in the presence of organophilic montmorillonite." *Radiation Physics and Chemistry* 69, no. 6 (2004): 467–471.

[100] Shen, Jian-Min, Wan-Jin Tang, Xiao-Li Zhang, Tong Chen, and Hai-Xia Zhang. "A novel carboxymethyl chitosan-based folate/Fe_3O_4/CdTe nanoparticle for targeted drug delivery and cell imaging." *Carbohydrate Polymers* 88, no. 1 (2012): 239–249.

[101] Ding, Yongling, Shirley Z. Shen, Huadong Sun, Kangning Sun, Futian Liu, Yushi Qi, and Jun Yan. "Design and construction of polymerized-chitosan coated Fe_3O_4 magnetic nanoparticles and its application for hydrophobic drug delivery." *Materials Science and Engineering: C* 48 (2015): 487–498.

[102] Gavini, Elisabetta, Giovanna Rassu, Tone Haukvik, Cristina Lanni, Marco Racchi, and Paolo Giunchedi. "Mucoadhesive microspheres for nasal administration of cyclodextrins." *Journal of Drug Targeting* 17, no. 2 (2009): 168–179.

[103] Rassu, Giovanna, Elena Soddu, Massimo Cossu, Antonio Brundu, Guido Cerri, Nicola Marchetti, Luca Ferraro et al. "Solid microparticles based on chitosan or methyl-β-cyclodextrin: A first formulative approach to increase the nose-to-brain transport of deferoxamine mesylate." *Journal of Controlled Release* 201 (2015): 68–77.

[104] Varshosaz, J., H. Sadrai, and R. Alinagari. "Nasal delivery of insulin using chitosan microspheres." *Journal of Microencapsulation* 21, no. 7 (2004): 761–774.

[105] Hussein, Nozad, Huner Omer, Ava Ismael, Mohamed Albed Alhnan, Abdelbary Elhissi, and Waqar Ahmed. "Spray-dried alginate microparticles for potential intranasal delivery of ropinirole hydrochloride: Development, characterization and histopathological evaluation." *Pharmaceutical Development and Technology* 25, no. 3 (2020): 290–299.

[106] Pahwa, Rajesh, Kelly E. Lyons, and Robert A. Hauser. "Ropinirole therapy for Parkinson's disease." *Expert Review of Neurotherapeutics* 4, no. 4 (2004): 581–588.

[107] Martins, Patricia P., Hugh DC Smyth, and Zhengrong Cui. "Strategies to facilitate or block nose-to-brain drug delivery." *International Journal of Pharmaceutics* 570 (2019): 118635.

[108] Adnet, Thomas, Anne-Claire Groo, Céline Picard, Audrey Davis, Sophie Corvaisier, Marc Since, Frédéric Bounoure et al. "Pharmacotechnical development of a nasal drug delivery composite nanosystem intended for Alzheimer's disease treatment." *Pharmaceutics* 12, no. 3 (2020): 251.

[109] Cunha, Sara, Ben Forbes, José Manuel Sousa Lobo, and Ana Catarina Silva. "Improving drug delivery for Alzheimer's disease through nose-to-brain delivery using nanoemulsions, nanostructured lipid carriers (NLC) and in situ hydrogels." *International Journal of Nanomedicine* 16 (2021): 4373–4390.

[110] Al Asmari, Abdulrahman K., Zabih Ullah, Mohammad Tariq, and Amal Fatani. "Preparation, characterization, and in vivo evaluation of intranasally administered liposomal formulation of donepezil." *Drug Design, Development and Therapy* 10 (2016): 205–215.

[111] Yang, Zhen-Zhen, Yan-Qing Zhang, Zhan-Zhang Wang, Kai Wu, Jin-Ning Lou, and Xian-Rong Qi. "Enhanced brain distribution and pharmacodynamics of rivastigmine by liposomes following intranasal administration." *International Journal of Pharmaceutics* 452, no. 1–2 (2013): 344–354.

[112] Arumugam, Karthik, Ganesa Subramanian, Surulivel Mallayasamy, Ranjith Averineni, Meka Reddy, and Nayanabhirama Udupa. "A study of rivastigmine liposomes for delivery into the brain through intranasal route." *Acta Pharmaceutica* 58, no. 3 (2008): 287–297.

[113] Agrawal, Mukta, Swarnlata Saraf, Shailendra Saraf, Sophia G. Antimisiaris, Mahavir Bhupal Chougule, Sunday A. Shoyele, and Amit Alexander. "Nose-to-brain drug delivery: An update on clinical challenges and progress towards approval of anti-Alzheimer drugs." *Journal of Controlled Release* 281 (2018): 139–177.

[114] Patel, Nishith, and Subhranshu Panda. "Liposome drug delivery system: A critic review." *Journal of Pharmaceutical Science and Bioscientific Research* 2, no. 4 (2012): 169–175.

[115] Dumortier, Gilles, Jean Louis Grossiord, Florence Agnely, and Jean Claude Chaumeil. "A review of poloxamer 407 pharmaceutical and pharmacological characteristics." *Pharmaceutical Research* 23 (2006): 2709–2728.

[116] Soliman, Ghareb M., Gihan Fetih, and Ahmed M. Abbas. "Thermosensitive bioadhesive gels for the vaginal delivery of sildenafil citrate: In vitro characterization and clinical evaluation in women using clomiphene citrate for induction of ovulation." *Drug Development and Industrial Pharmacy* 43, no. 3 (2017): 399–408.

[117] Agrawal, Mukta, Shailendra Saraf, Swarnlata Saraf, Sunil K. Dubey, Anu Puri, Umesh Gupta, Prashant Kesharwani et al. "Stimuli-responsive In situ gelling system for nose-to-brain drug delivery." *Journal of Controlled Release* 327 (2020): 235–265.

[118] Bitter, Christoph, Katja Suter-Zimmermann, and Christian Surber. "Nasal drug delivery in humans." *Topical Applications and the Mucosa* 40 (2011): 20–35.

[119] Salatin, S., J. Barar, M. Barzegar-Jalali, Kh Adibkia, and M. Jelvehgari. "Thermosensitive in situ nanocomposite as an intranasal delivery system of rivastigmine hydrogen tartrate: Development, characterization, ex vivo permeation and cellular studies." *Colloids and Surfaces B: Biointerfaces* 159 (2017): 629–638.

[120] Cunha, S., M. Swedrowska, Y. Bellahnid, Z. Xu, JM Sousa Lobo, Ben Forbes, and A. C. Silva. "Thermosensitive in situ hydrogels of rivastigmine-loaded lipid-based nanosystems for nose-to-brain delivery: Characterisation, biocompatibility, and drug deposition studies." *International Journal of Pharmaceutics* 620 (2022): 121720.

[121] Davis, Stanley S. "The use of soluble polymers and polymer microparticles to provide improved vaccine responses after parenteral and mucosal delivery." *Vaccine* 24 (2006): S7–S10.

[122] Tafaghodi, Mohsen, S. Abolghasem Sajadi Tabassi, and Mahmood Reza Jaafari. "Induction of systemic and mucosal immune responses by intranasal administration of alginate microspheres encapsulated with tetanus toxoid and CpG-ODN." *International Journal of Pharmaceutics* 319, no. 1–2 (2006): 37–43.

[123] Pandit, Sreenivas, Erdal Cevher, Mohammed Gulrez Zariwala, Satyanarayana Somavarapu, and H. Oya Alpar. "Enhancement of immune response of HBsAg loaded poly (L-lactic acid) microspheres against hepatitis B through incorporation of alum and chitosan." *Journal of Microencapsulation* 24, no. 6 (2007): 539–552.

[124] Freitas, Sergio, Hans P. Merkle, and Bruno Gander. "Microencapsulation by solvent extraction/evaporation: Reviewing the state of the art of microsphere preparation process technology." *Journal of Controlled Release* 102, no. 2 (2005): 313–332.

[125] Sugumaran, K. R., R. V. Sindhu, S. Sukanya, N. Aiswarya, and V. Ponnusami. "Statistical studies on high molecular weight pullulan production in solid state fermentation using jack fruit seed." *Carbohydrate Polymers* 98, no. 1 (2013): 854–860.

[126] Yamaya, Shun-ichi, Akio Yamamoto, Takako Komiya, Junichiro Mizuguchi, and Tyoku Matuhasi. "Preparation of a diphtheria toxin-pullulan conjugate that elicits good IgG antibody production with poor IgE synthesis." *Vaccine* 8, no. 1 (1990): 65–69.

[127] Horie, Kazutoshi, Masahiro Sakagami, Kazuyoshi Masuda, Mitsuru Notoya, Hiroshi Hamana, Takayoshi Yoshikawa, and Koichiro Hirano. "Sialyl Lewis X-carboxymethylpullulan conjugate: A novel homing device to spleen and lymph nodes." *Biological and Pharmaceutical Bulletin* 27, no. 8 (2004): 1275–1280.

[128] Scomparin, Anna, Stefano Salmaso, Sara Bersani, Ronit Satchi-Fainaro, and Paolo Caliceti. "Novel folated and non-folated pullulan bioconjugates for anticancer drug delivery." *European Journal of Pharmaceutical Sciences* 42, no. 5 (2011): 547–558.

[129] Cevher, Erdal, Stefan K. Salomon, Satyanarayana Somavarapu, Steve Brocchini, and H. Oya Alpar. "Development of chitosan–pullulan composite nanoparticles for nasal delivery of vaccines: In vivo studies." *Journal of Microencapsulation* 32, no. 8 (2015): 769–783.

[130] Cevher, Erdal, Stefan K. Salomon, Apostolos Makrakis, Xiong Wei Li, Steve Brocchini, and H. Oya Alpar. "Development of chitosan–pullulan composite nanoparticles for nasal delivery of vaccines: Optimisation and cellular studies." *Journal of Microencapsulation* 32, no. 8 (2015): 755–768.

[131] Sriamornsak, Pornsak, Nathaya Wattanakorn, and Hirofumi Takeuchi. "Study on the mucoadhesion mechanism of pectin by atomic force microscopy and mucin-particle method." *Carbohydrate Polymers* 79, no. 1 (2010): 54–59.

[132] Sriamornsak, Pornsak, Nathaya Wattanakorn, Jurairat Nunthanid, and Satit Puttipipatkhachorn. "Mucoadhesion of pectin as evidence by wettability and chain interpenetration." *Carbohydrate Polymers* 74, no. 3 (2008): 458–467.

[133] Joergensen, Lars, Beate Klösgen, Adam Cohen Simonsen, Jonas Borch, and Ellen Hagesaether. "New insights into the mucoadhesion of pectins by AFM roughness parameters in combination with SPR." *International Journal of Pharmaceutics* 411, no. 1–2 (2011): 162–168.

[134] Vidal, Felipe, Pilar Vásquez, Francisca R. Cayumán, Carola Díaz, Jorge Fuentealba, Luis G. Aguayo, Gonzalo E. Yévenes, Joel Alderete, and Leonardo Guzmán. "Prevention of synaptic alterations and neurotoxic effects of PAMAM dendrimers by surface functionalization." *Nanomaterials* 8, no. 1 (2017): 7.

[135] Zarebkohan, Amir, Farhood Najafi, Hamid Reza Moghimi, Mohammad Hemmati, Mohammad Reza Deevband, and Bahram Kazemi. "Synthesis and characterization of a PAMAM dendrimer nanocarrier functionalized by SRL peptide for targeted gene delivery to the brain." *European Journal of Pharmaceutical Sciences* 78 (2015): 19–30.

[136] Ayatollahi, Sara, Zahra Salmasi, Maryam Hashemi, Saeedeh Askarian, Reza Kazemi Oskuee, Khalil Abnous, and Mohammad Ramezani. "Aptamer-targeted delivery of Bcl-xL shRNA using alkyl modified PAMAM dendrimers into lung cancer cells." *The International Journal of Biochemistry & Cell Biology* 92 (2017): 210–217.

6 Bionanocomposites in Gene Delivery

Farwa Munir, Nida Islam, Muhammad Shahzaib, Emad Abdulrahman Alsaedi, Farrukh Jawad Alvi, Basma Ellahi, Tanzeela Mariam and Atif Amin Baig

6.1 INTRODUCTION

6.1.1 Overview of Gene Therapy

Around five centuries ago, pioneering scientists postulated the prospect of exogenous DNA-mediated gene editing as a potential solution for congenital disorders in humans. The "gene therapy" technique offered the possible advantage of a single therapy producing a long-lasting and possibly curative therapeutic impact. Despite the considerable time it takes from concept to practical implementation, gene therapy is expanding the range of viable treatments in various healthcare disciplines [1].

The injection of genetic information for treating an individual that alters how their cells work is known as gene therapy. Research into a treatment for a rare immunodeficiency condition started in 1990, with the first study in humans. The most crucial stage in gene therapy is effective gene transport to the desired tissues or cells, accomplished through vectors and vehicles for delivering genes [2, 3].

A family of viral-based medicines called virotherapy includes the long-established technique of using viruses as therapeutic agents during gene therapy [4]. Non-viral and viral vectors are the two types. In vivo, viral vector-based gene therapy aims to introduce the curative gene into the individual via vectors based on adeno-associated viruses (AAVs), adenoviruses (Ads), or retroviruses. A therapeutic transgene can also be introduced ex vivo, which involves removing cells from the ill person and growing them outside the body. Following the insertion of a therapeutic transgene, cells are genetically altered before being reintroduced into the recipient's body [5].

Gene replacement is the introduction of a functional gene to substitute a malfunctioning gene; gene silencing involves deactivating a mutation in a gene which is now harmful to tissues; gene addition consists of overexpressing a "foreign" or exogenous gene to affect the functioning of cells and gene editing, which involves permanently altering a gene in an individual's genome, are the four fundamental approaches to gene therapy [6].

By 2017, almost 3000 clinical trials had been completed, indicating substantial advancement in gene therapy. Unexpectedly, 64.6% of the trials are for the treatment of cancer. A total of 7.4% of attention is given to infectious disorders, 10.5% to cardiovascular diseases, and 7.4% to monogenic conditions. Viral vectors have been used in about 70% of the experiments. Viral vectors continue to be appealing despite recent advances in gene manipulation techniques like CRISPR and more effective means of distribution for non-viral vectors [7–9].

Even with caution, viral-based gene therapy has a promising future. Multiple medications have been approved for treating various illnesses using diverse viral vectors, offering considerable flexibility and alternate strategic possibilities. Viral vectors are now better positioned due to vector engineering and safety research developments.

DOI: 10.1201/9781003650812-6

6.1.2 Overview of Nanocomposites

Nanotechnology has applications in several industries, including agriculture, medicine, and warfare [10].

Nanotechnology plays a critical part in resolving issues with viruses and human health. However, a severe public health issue is the rapid development of medication resistance to subsequently developed treatments and the adverse effects of prolonged use. It is necessary to advance innovative therapeutic methods. The interactions of nanostructures with microbes, which have advantages in diagnostic and therapeutic domains, drive the rapid change in the biomedical industry [11, 12].

Nanotechnology has offered a powerful method for reducing infections by avoiding, diagnosing, and curing diseases. To provide preventive disinfectants and measures, quick and precise diagnostic tools, and vaccinations or therapeutic agents that contain antiviral components, these approaches include the development of nanomaterial-based methods. Since viruses and nanoparticles (NPs) share a similar size range, they can mimic viruses' functional and structural features, significantly impacting vaccine development and immune engineering [12–14].

The application of NPs in numerous fields of technology and science has been made possible by the advancement of nanotechnology. Materials with a minimum of one dimension of 100 nm or fewer are called NPs. The use of physical and chemical methods in conventional nano compound synthesis has a few limitations, including the need for poisonous toxic substances and costly processes in terms of energy and expense that make it challenging to be widely adopted. Scientists have searched for a simple, workable alternative strategy for producing nano compounds to overcome these constraints [15, 16].

When the NPs are formulated with the biomaterials such as biopolymers, they are defined as bionanocomposites, as illustrated in Figure 6.1. Researchers worldwide have expressed interest in using a substitute biogenic pathway for NP formation, employing the biological components of single-cell living creatures like bacteria, actinomycetes, and fungi [17].

Numerous NPs, including those made of gold, silver, zinc, carbon, graphene, polymeric compounds, and liposomes, have demonstrated promising antiviral activity and have been used to generate vaccines, treat illnesses, create nanosensors, and make diagnostic tools. For instance, silver's

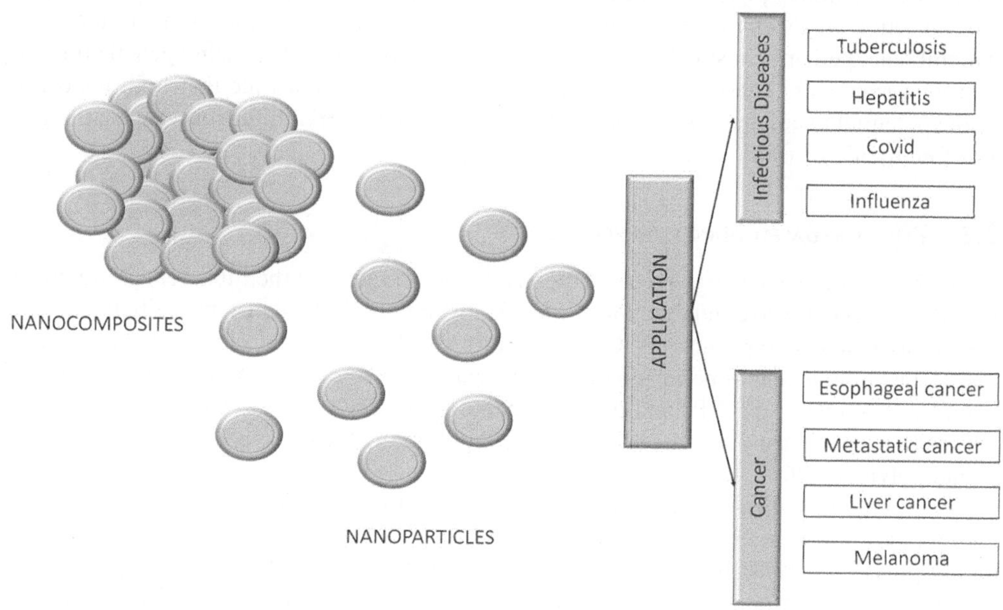

FIGURE 6.1 The difference between nanocomposites and bionanocomposites.

anti-angiogenesis, anti-inflammatory, antifungal, anticancer, antibacterial, and anti-platelet effects are well known [18].

Additionally, lipid-based NPs comprise lipid-lipid bilayer capsules employed for enclosing and transferring lipophilic and hydrophilic drugs because of their easy scaling, manageable biological behavior, minimal toxicology, high durability, reliability, and high stability [19].

6.2 TYPES OF NANOCOMPOSITES FOR GENE DELIVERY

6.2.1 Lipid-Based Nanocomposites

Lipid-based nanotechnology has become an essential delivery mechanism for medications for managing infections caused by bacteria. These approaches provide flexibility regarding the characteristics of the components used in formulation production, enabling enhanced interaction with microorganisms, precisely delivering drugs to the infection site, improving the solubility of antibacterial medications, and potentiating the effects of bioactive substances by improving the efficacy of therapies while reducing the unfavorable impact on healthy tissues [20].

Solid lipid NPs, liposomes, lipid nanocapsules, nanoemulsions, nanostructured lipid carriers, and microemulsions are notable examples of these systems that have shown possible effectiveness in reducing the number of resistant bacteria. Such lipid-based systems are up-and-coming for developing novel therapeutic approaches for managing bacterial infections [19]. Targeted drug delivery is made possible by the promising property of interaction with lipid membranes at the site of action in lipid-based nanosystems, which are arranged in nanometer-sized assemblies of ordered lipids. This capability offers a benefit for designing more effective interaction between particular types of cells [21].

These systems have several intrinsic qualities that make them an appealing choice for antibacterial therapies, including lower toxicity, smaller size, similarity to cell membranes, higher surface-to-volume ratio, capacity for penetrating cell membranes and walls, and ability to deliver concentrated doses of antibacterials or antibiotics to particular microbes. Lipid-based nanostructured systems have many prospects as an attractive option for antibacterial therapies [22, 23].

Lipid nanostructures have three significant effects on bacterial cells. The first two mechanisms of action both immediately affect the bacterial cell wall or membrane. In this case, the lipid nanostructures' pore formation or physical destabilization results in cellular content leakage. The third method entails an action on genetic material, specifically DNA. They instantly impact the bacterial cell wall and membrane, perhaps causing hereditary material instability and obstructing genetic transcription and protein synthesis. These three distinct modes of action demonstrate that lipid nanostructures have the potential to be a successful tool in the fight against bacterial infections, especially given the issue of antibiotic resistance. [24].

6.2.2 Polymer-Based Nanocomposites

Polymer-based composites have received much attention because of their inherent ability to be recycled and safe in their surroundings. More specifically, combining the benefits of both counterparts, polymer-based nanocomposites (PNCs) frequently exhibit improved chemical, mechanical, and physical capabilities and superior compatibility compared to single polymers [25]. The intricate interface zones among the NPs and polymer matrices are PNCs' most challenging feature. Those small scales produce many specific surface areas, highlighting the significance of interactions among NPs and polymers [26].

In addition to its numerous applications, PNCs have attracted academics from around the world during the past few years, and in-depth study has been done on these materials. PNCs exhibit outstanding physicochemical behavior that is impossible to achieve with single components and are becoming increasingly popular in various settings. PNCs, in particular, have drawn intense scientific interest in addressing energy and ecological issues [27, 28].

Additionally, PNCs offer additional benefits from cooperation because of the large interfacial area compared to the material volume and the NPs and polymeric supports on comparable length scales. The energy storage and dielectric properties of PNCs, which are prospective materials for candidates in the packaging of electronic technology, have received much attention recently. These nanocomposites (NCs) combine the outstanding mechanical properties of the NPs with the extensive pseudocapacitive nature of the conducting polymer (CP) via a double-layer capacitor. Additionally, environmentally friendly PNCs offer a way to maintain the ongoing development of commercially and ecologically advantageous technologies. As a result, environmentally friendly PNCs are attracting much attention along with their inherent qualities, including being toxic-free, biocompatible, and biodegradable and having improved morphological properties [28, 29].

6.2.3 Inorganic Nanoparticle-Based Nanocomposites

Because of inorganic NP-based NCs' distinctive physical and chemical characteristics, adaptable manufacturing techniques, ease of surface functionalization, and excellent biocompatibility, inorganic NPs have received extensive research attention as therapeutic agents for treating various diseases in healthcare sectors. The healthcare industry uses a variety of inorganic NP-based treatment medicines, such as mesoporous silica NPs, gold NPs, upconversion NPs, and magnetic NPs [30, 31].

Inorganic NP formulations have several benefits of easy manufacturing, a variety of surface conjugation chemistry, and excellent biocompatibility over other NP formulations. Inorganic NPs as carriers for drugs offer advantages over other organic drug delivery technologies. Systems for drug delivery that employ inorganic NPs typically offer more flexible surface modification techniques [32, 33].

First, the delivery capacity can be enhanced for some drugs with weak physiologic solubility. Second, the medicinal substances can be shielded from deterioration by the NPs. Third, by modifying the surface, NPs can lengthen the duration of the release of drugs and extend circulation time. To increase the circulation period, the feeling of inorganic NPs can be functionalized with molecules like polyethylene glycol (PEG) [34–36].

6.2.4 Types of Nanocomposites and Gene Therapy

Gene delivery is a pivotal aspect of modern biotechnology and medical research, offering the potential to treat genetic disorders, cancer, and other diseases by introducing therapeutic genetic material into target cells. In this context, inorganic NP-based nanocomposites, polymer-based NCs, and lipid NCs each play distinct roles, offering unique advantages in gene delivery [37, 38].

Inorganic NP-based NCs, such as those comprising gold or silica NPs, have garnered attention for their potential in gene delivery. These NPs can be functionalized with nucleic acids (such as DNA or RNA) and other targeting moieties to create nano complexes capable of efficiently delivering genes into cells. Their small size, high surface area, and tunable surface properties allow for effective cargo loading, protection of genetic material, and controlled release within target cells [39]. Additionally, their plasmonic properties can facilitate endosomal escape and enhance cellular uptake, crucial steps in successful gene delivery. The versatility of inorganic NPs permits the engineering of NCs with specific sizes, shapes, and surface chemistries to optimize transfection efficiency and minimize cytotoxicity.

Polymer-based NCs, frequently made from biodegradable polymers like poly(lactic-co-glycolic acid) (PLGA) or chitosan, provide a diverse platform for gene delivery. These NCs can encapsulate and protect genetic material, preventing enzymatic degradation and allowing for regulated release kinetics [40]. Incorporating inorganic NPs into polymer matrices can improve transfection efficiency by promoting endosomal escape or cellular absorption. Surface-modified NCs can be loaded with ligands or peptides for targeted distribution to specific cell types or regions. Furthermore, polymers allow for modifying NC features such as surface charge and hydrophobicity to improve cellular contacts and transfection efficacy. [41].

Meanwhile, lipid-based NCs, often referred to as lipid NPs or lipid-based carriers, offer an attractive solution for gene delivery due to their biocompatibility, ability to form stable complexes with nucleic acids, and low toxicity. Lipid NCs can encapsulate genetic material in lipid bilayers, creating structures like liposomes or lipid NPs. These lipid-based carriers can protect genetic material from degradation, facilitate cellular uptake through endocytosis, and promote endosomal escape for successful delivery [42]. Modifying the lipid composition allows for tailoring of NCs to optimize stability, release kinetics, and targeting capabilities.

In conclusion, inorganic NP-based NCs, polymer-based NCs, and lipid NCs contribute to advancing gene delivery technologies. Their unique properties and characteristics offer diverse tools for designing efficient and targeted gene delivery systems [43]. As researchers refine these NC platforms and explore their interactions with biological systems, the potential for safe and effective gene therapies becomes increasingly promising.

6.3 THERAPEUTIC IMPLICATIONS OF NANOCOMPOSITES

Gene therapy is a significant advancement in medical science. Gene therapy is a revolutionary way of treating genetic illnesses such as Parkinson's, cystic fibrosis, and various cancers. For efficient gene therapy, a gene vector that protects the desired gene from nuclease degradation and allows cellular DNA uptake with high transfection efficiency is required.

The most difficult challenge in the development of gene therapy is selecting an appropriate gene vector. Non-toxic nanocarriers utilized in successful gene therapy include graphene and graphene-covered substrates. Graphene-based nanosheets' sp2 hybridized orbitals can interact with pharmaceuticals and other substances, including nucleic acids like DNA and RNA. They can therefore be utilized for miRNA identification, gene delivery, or as carriers and guardians of probes. Polyethyleneimine (PEI) composite based on GO was created by Hyunwoo et al. and employed as an effective gene delivery vehicle in gene therapy [44]. Because of its potent binding to DNA and RNA and efficient cell uptake, polyethyleneimine (PEI) has traditionally been regarded as the "golden standard" cationic polymer in gene transfection. However, PEI polymers are only occasionally used in gene therapy due to their high cytotoxicity and low biocompatibility.

Nanotechnologies have improved nearly every branch of science, including engineering, material and biological science, and physical and chemical science. Many scientists have been interested in using nanotechnology to cure infectious diseases and cancer over the past ten years. Precise medications or genes must be delivered to exact places in the human body using NCs. Because of their innovative uses in the diagnosis and treatment of infectious disorders such as COVID-19, tuberculosis, hepatitis, and HIV infection, as well as cancer, NCs have drawn attention (Figure 6.2). The characteristics of NCs, such as their remarkable physicochemical behavior, superior antibacterial capacity, and anticancer and anti-inflammatory action, determine their broad and distinctive use. Various NPs were studied for possible antibacterial and anticancer properties. However, the most studied NPs are silver NPs (AgNPs).

6.3.1 Gene Therapy, Nanocomposites, and Cancer

Gene therapy is gaining popularity and is being used to treat various disorders, including cancer and other genetic issues. Exogenous, therapeutic genes are introduced into host cells, where a specific therapeutic protein can be translated to rectify or mediate the faulty intrinsic genes, resulting in the long-term eradication of numerous diseases at their source. Efficiently transporting fragile and relatively large therapeutic genes into cell nuclei without significant nuclease-mediated degradation is critical to gene therapy success. The delivery of nuclear-targeted genes was studied using NLS

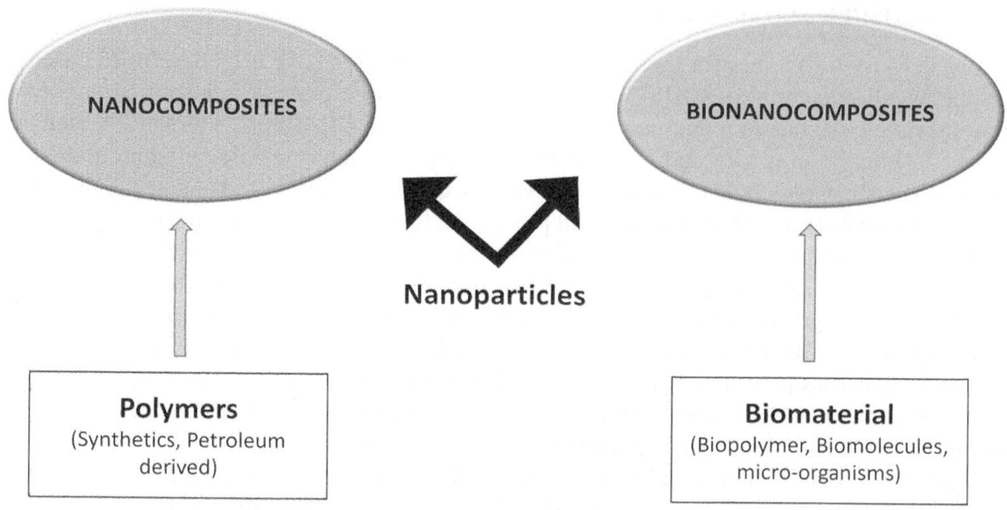

FIGURE 6.2 Therapeutic role of nanocomposites in cancer and infectious diseases.

peptide-linked liposomes as early as 1998. Despite the enormous work put into creating organic non-virus gene delivery systems, it has recently been shown that more reliable and controllable inorganic nanocarriers make better candidates for targeted gene delivery. Liang and colleagues have discussed the possibility of ultrasmall AuNPs for nuclear-targeted gene therapy. Due to their tiny size, AuNPs (2 nm) treated with a particular triplex-forming oligonucleotide could enter the nuclei of MCF-7 cancer cells. Because of the downregulated expression of the C-myc gene (a 50% decrease in word), such an NC might limit cell proliferation and cause 30% cell death at a concentration of 1 mM, providing a new way for manipulating gene expression via direct intra-nuclear delivery of genes. [45].

It is also better to encapsulate genes inside nanocapsules rather than conjugate or adsorb them on the surface to prevent genes from breaking down into nucleic acids.

A team of researchers developed biocompatible mesoporous organosilica NPs (MONs) with ultra-large mesopores for successful gene loading despite the genes' relatively large sizes (several nanometers). In the interim, the size of MONs was strictly adjusted to allow them to penetrate the cell nuclear membrane for intranuclear gene delivery. Uniform and monodispersed flower-like MONs with radial ultra-large 5–10 nm mesopore diameters were generated by assembling the micelle with the precursor. After conjugating the TAT peptide on the surface of the NCs, the transfection efficiency of plasmid DNA mediated by nuclear-targeting MONs was as high as 36.5%, substantially more significant than that produced by nonnuclear-targeting MONs (13.5%). Because of the higher transfection efficiency of nucleus-focused gene delivery, advanced gene therapy for successful cancer medicines is predicted to offer significant promise. With only a few FDA-approved gene therapy medications (Zolgensma, Kymriah, and Luxturna; however, none have been approved for BC yet) and many other promising therapies in the works, gene therapy has generated significant interest in both the research and therapeutic communities. Several genetic mutations and aberrations found in breast cancer are perfect triggers for gene therapy, in which cancer cells can be given a nucleic acid-based medication to either rectify the congenital abnormalities or eradicate the tumors. Nanomaterials are revolutionizing BC therapy and diagnostics objectives by removing present therapeutic barriers and reshaping the future treatment landscape. They do this by reducing the suffering connected to conventional chemotherapy. Nanodevices are a promising tool in the fight against cancer, despite worries about ethics and safety [46].

6.3.2 CRISPER and Nanocomposites

Various delivery techniques for therapeutic genetic modification have been developed based on the vast therapeutic potential of CRISPR/Cas systems. The cargo must be transported and protected from enzymatic degradation and metabolic clearance for the CRISPR/Cas tools to be delivered to the site of interest in a safe and targeted manner with sustained release (in some cases). Many attempts have been undertaken due to the convergence of biomaterials and nanotechnology to build multifunctional NP-based NCs for safe and practical CRISPR/Cas delivery. [47].

This section will review recent NP-based technologies for CRISPR/Cas tool delivery and therapeutic applications, including lipid NPs (LNPs), polymer-based NPs, and hybrid NPs. LNPs have recently garnered greater interest due to the enormous success of mRNA vaccine technology in combating the COVID-19 pandemic. LNPs are being developed and tested extensively for transporting genetic materials to establish their safety and usefulness as clinical delivery vehicles. Following electrostatic interaction with the car, the negatively charged genetic material payload is commonly carried utilizing the cationic carriers, DOTAP, DOPE, and cholesterol. [48].

Negatively charged nucleic acids are additionally transported by ionizable lipids. Traditional gears like cholesterol, phospholipid, and PEG derivatives are frequently combined with ionizable lipids in LNPs for particle, structural, and physiological stability. The liver has been chosen as the target organ for the NP-assisted delivery of CRISPR/Cas systems for in vivo genome editing due to NP accumulation upon systemic injection. Because of their excellent success rates and low toxicity, LNPs are extensively used for the targeted delivery of CRISPR/Cas systems to hepatocytes. Improvements in LNPs targeting liver cells for delivering CRISPR/Cas9 payloads have been successfully demonstrated in both in vitro and in vivo preclinical settings. [49].

LNP modification and the injection of different CRISPR systems have been tested to improve the efficacy of gene therapy. The clinical trial of NTLA-2001 for TTR gene editing in liver cells is an important step forward in this field. Systemic CRISPR/Cas administration to organs other than the liver had been problematic until the recent discovery of LNPs with such transport capacity. Sago and colleagues developed the high-throughput platform to detect LNPs. They discovered two LNPs, 7C2 and 7C3, capable of delivering mRNA to several endothelial cell types in vivo. Unlike LNPs, which target hepatocytes, 7C3 successfully delivered Cas9 RNA and its guide to splenic endothelial cells. [50].

Polymeric molecules, in combination with inorganic components, are used in a feasible CRISPR/Cas delivery strategy. Due to Cas9's affinity for crRNA, the Cas9 binding element is gold NPs linked with an SH-spacer-crRNA in the core region. The complex's surface was electrostatically pierced with donor ssDNA, which was then coated with PEI, downregulating HDR in hematopoietic stem and progenitor cells. Graphene oxide (GO) is also used to transport the Cas9 protein. The GO-PEG-PEI complex, formed by mixing PEG and PEI, enhanced and functionalized GO's biocompatibility and enabled rapid RNP delivery into human cells while preserving Cas9 activity, with a gene-editing efficacy of approximately 39%.

6.3.3 Drug Delivery Systems and Nanocomposites

As a result of the rapid development of advanced nanotechnology, various targeted drug delivery systems (DDSs) with unique advantages, such as improved drug encapsulation capacity, increased drug stability, controlled drug release, increased tumor accumulation by targeting modification, and so on, have been extensively developed and intensively investigated. Only a tiny percentage (0.7%) of the nanocarriers delivered were observed to reach and concentrate in solid cancer tissues eventually. Even worse, medications released into the cytoplasm from nanocarriers would travel a tortuous path and pass through several obstacles at the cellular and subcellular levels, such as endosomal trapping and lysosomal degradation, before they reach their molecular sites of action. Therefore, developing more sophisticated drug carriers and corresponding DDSs that can transport medications to specific subcellular locations more effectively will improve the therapeutic effectiveness and elucidate their pharmacological effect.

A nuclear envelope, a double-layered membrane containing many nuclear pore complexes (NPCs), separates the cell nucleus from the cytoplasm. NPCs comprise roughly 30 distinct types of proteins called nucleoporins and serve as the single route for all bidirectional exchanges between nucleoplasmic and cytoplasmic compartments [51].

Brownian motion through NPCs dominates passive intra-nuclear transport based on the diffusion process. Numerous studies have been conducted on the essential properties of NPs, such as size and shape, which can be controlled by the logical design and engineering of passive cancer cell nucleus-targeting nanotherapeutics, taking into account NPCs' proteinaceous nature and small size.

6.4 BARRIERS TO THE UTILIZATION OF NANOCOMPOSITES IN GENE THERAPY

Due to their capacity to encapsulate and distribute genetic material to target cells, NCs have demonstrated significant potential for application in gene therapy. For the successful and secure application of NCs in gene therapy, numerous obstacles must be overcome.

6.4.1 Biocompatibility, Toxicity, and Stability

The potential toxicity of NCs to cells and tissues is one of their key challenges. Some NPs could impair cell viability or provoke immunological reactions. NCs must be biocompatible to avoid unwanted side effects. NCs frequently contain NPs that must remain stable while being stored, transported, and used in physiological environments. Their aggregation or breakdown may hamper NPs' ability to transport genetic material properly [52].

6.4.2 Precision, Immune Reactions

Targeting particular cells or tissues can be challenging. NCs must be created to recognize and bind to the intended cells while preventing off-target effects. The immune system may recognize and attack NCs, which would reduce their efficiency and result in adverse side effects. It is crucial to develop methods for thwarting or controlling the immune response.

6.4.3 Effective Genetic Material Distribution

Effective genetic material distribution to the target cells is essential for the success of gene therapy. NCs should be able to shield genetic material from deterioration and make it easier for cells to absorb it.

6.4.4 Release of Cargo, Scale-Up, and Manufacturing

Once the NCs have made contact with the target cells, they must carefully release the genetic material. Uncontrolled or premature release could produce less-than-ideal therapeutic results. Switching from lab-scale synthesis to mass-produced NCs can be difficult. It's crucial to guarantee uniformity, quality control, and reproducibility on a broader scale.

6.4.5 Regulatory Approval and Ethical Implications

The regulatory environment for innovative treatments, such as NCs-based gene therapies, is complicated. It takes time and effort to meet regulatory criteria for safety and efficacy. The ethical implications of altering genetic material and passing those modifications on to future generations are the same as with any gene therapy. It might be costly to develop and produce NCs for gene therapy. An essential factor to consider is ensuring the treatment is still available and inexpensive for patients [53]. It is necessary to comprehend NCs' stability and long-term impacts on the cells they have been used to treat. Over time, NCs ought to hold up well and continue to function.

Researchers in nanotechnology and gene therapy are actively attempting to overcome these obstacles. Many of these obstacles might be overcome as technology develops and our knowledge of NCs grows, making gene therapies safer and more efficient.

6.5 CONCLUSION

A unique and promising platform for gene delivery applications has emerged in the form of NCs. These hybrid systems have several benefits in terms of biocompatibility, controlled release, target specificity, and decreased cytotoxicity by fusing the unique qualities of bio-derived materials with the adaptability of nanotechnology. Using NCs in gene delivery has great potential to get around the drawbacks of conventional delivery techniques like synthetic polymers and viral vectors. We have highlighted the various bio-based components that can be incorporated into NC structures to improve gene delivery efficacy, including proteins, polysaccharides, and nucleic acids. These materials' adaptable qualities enable the creation of NCs tailored to meet particular needs, including those for stability, cellular uptake, and intracellular release.

Recognizing the difficulties and complexity of creating and adapting bionanocomposites for gene delivery into therapeutic applications is crucial. Rigorous research is required to guarantee long-term safety, scalability, and reproducibility. Regulatory and ethical issues must also be considered as these technologies advance to clinical usage.

Enabling more effective and focused treatments for various genetic abnormalities and diseases, the confluence of bionanocomposites and gene delivery has the potential to revolutionize the field of therapeutics. As research develops, it will become increasingly important to close the gap between laboratory innovation and real-world application to fully unleash the transformative potential of bionanocomposites in gene delivery and enhance the lives of countless people worldwide.

REFERENCES

[1] C. E. Dunbar, K. A. High, J. Joung, D. B. Kohn, K. Ozawa, and M. Sadelain, "Gene therapy comes of age," *Science*, vol. 359, no. 6372, Jan. 2018, doi: 10.1126/science.aan4672

[2] R. Macarron et al., "Impact of high-throughput screening in biomedical research," *Nature Reviews Drug Discovery*, vol. 10, no. 3, pp. 188–195, Mar. 2011, doi: 10.1038/nrd3368

[3] H. G. Terheggen et al., "An unsuccessful gene substitution attempt in arginase deficiency," *Zeitschrift für Kinderheilkunde*, vol. 119, pp. 1–3, 1975.

[4] M. J. Cline, "Perspectives on gene therapy: Physical procedures and viral vectors for inserting new genetic information into mammalian cells by physical techniques and viral vectors," *Pharmacology & Therapeutics*, vol. 29, pp. 69–92, 1985.

[5] J. T. Bulcha, Y. Wang, H. Ma, P. W. Tai, and G. Gao, "Viral vector platforms within the gene therapy landscape," *Signal Transduction and Targeted Therapy*, vol. 6, no. 1, p. 53, 2021.

[6] B. N. Fields, D. M. Knipe, and P. M. Howley, *Fields' Virology*, Wolters Kluwer, 2007.

[7] M. Beitelshees, A. Hill, P. Rostami, C. H. Jones, and P. A. Pfefifer, "Pressing diseases that represent promising targets for gene therapy," *Discovery Medicine*, vol. 24, pp. 313–322, 2017.

[8] M. P. McCormack, and T. H. Rabbitts, "Activation of the T-cell oncogene LMO_2 after gene therapy for X-linked severe combined immunodeficiency," *The New England Journal of Medicine*, vol. 350, pp. 913–922, 2004.

[9] S. Hacein-Bey-Abina, A. Garrigue, G. P. Wang, J. Soulier, A. Lim, E. Morillon, E. Clappier, L. Caccavelli, E. Delabesse, K. Beldjord et al., "Insertional oncogenesis in 4 patients after retrovirus-mediated gene therapy of SCID-X1," *The Journal of Clinical Investigation*, vol. 118, pp. 3132–3142, 2008.

[10] D. S. Chauhan, R. Prasad, R. Srivastava, M. Jaggi, S. C. Chauhan, and M. M. Yallapu, "A comprehensive review of current interventions, diagnostics, and nanotechnology perspectives against SARS-CoV-2," *Bioconjugate Chemistry*, vol. 31, no. 9, pp. 2021–2045, 2020.

[11] H. Reza Rezaie, H. Beigi Rizi, M. M. Rezaei Khamseh, A. Öchsner, H. Reza Rezaie, H. Beigi Rizi, … and A. Öchsner, "Primary information about biomaterials," in *A Review on Dental Materials*, pp, 1–30, Springer, 2020.

[12] M. Radmansouri, E. Bahmani, E. Sarikhani, K. Rahmani, F. Sharifianjazi, and M. Irani, "Doxorubicin hydrochloride-loaded electrospun chitosan/cobalt ferrite/titanium oxide nanofibers for hyperthermic tumour cell treatment and controlled drug release," *International Journal of Biological Macromolecules*, vol. 116, pp. 378–384, 2018.

[13] D. Yang, "Application of nanotechnology in the COVID-19 pandemic," *International Journal of Nanomedicine*, vol. 16, pp. 623–649, 2021.

[14] A. H. Saleh, D. Kumar, I. Sirakov, P. Shafiee, and M. Arefian, "Application of nano compounds for preventing, diagnosing, and treating SARS-coronavirus: A review," *Journal of Composites and Compounds*, vol. 3, no. 9, pp. 230–246, 2021.

[15] N. Abdel-Raouf, N. M. Al-Enazi, and I. B. M. Ibraheem, "Green production of gold nanoparticles utilising Galaxaura elongate and their antibacterial properties," *Journal of Chemistry*, vol. 10, pp. S3029–S3039, 2013, doi: 10.1016/j.arabjc.2013.11.044

[16] M. Shah, D. Fawcett, S. Sharma, S. K. Tripathy, and G. E. J. Poinern, "Green synthesis of metallic nanoparticles via biological entities," *Materials*, vol. 8, no. 11, pp. 7278–7308, doi: 10.3390/ma8115377

[17] R. Singla, A. Guliani, A. Kumari, and S. K. Yadav, "Role of bacteria in nano compound formation and their application in medical," in *Microbial Applications Vol. 2: Biomedicine, Agriculture and Industry*, pp. 3–37, Springer, 2017.

[18] L. A. Dykman, "Gold nanoparticles for preparation of antibodies and vaccines against infectious diseases," *Expert Review of Vaccines*, vol. 19, no. 5, pp. 465–477, 2020.

[19] A. Pormohammad, N. K. Monych, and R. J. Turner, "Zinc and SARS-CoV-2: A molecular modelling study of Zn interactions with RNA-dependent RNA-polymerase and 3C-like proteinase enzymes," *International Journal of Molecular Medicine*, vol. 47, no. 1, pp. 326–334, 2021.

[20] K. Cerpnjak, A. Zvonar, M. Gašperlin, F. Vrečer, "Lipid-based systems as a promising approach for enhancing the bioavailability of poorly water-soluble drugs," *Acta Pharmaceutica*, vol. 63, pp. 427–445, 2013, doi: 10.2478/ACPH-2013-0040

[21] T. C. Lin, K. H. Hung, C. H. Peng, J. H. Liu, L. C. Woung, C. Y. Tsai, S. J. Chen, Y. T. Chen, and C. C. Hsu, "Nanotechnology-based drug delivery treatments and specific targeting therapy for age-related macular degeneration," *Journal of the Chinese Medical Association*, vol. 78, pp. 635–641, 2015, doi: 10.1016/J.JCMA.2015.07.008

[22] M. A. Dos Santos Ramos, P. B. Da Silva, L. Sposito, L. G. De Toledo, B. Vidal Bonifácio, C. F. Rodero, K. C. Dos Santos, M. Chorilli, and T. M. Bauab, "Nanotechnology-based drug delivery systems for control of microbial biofilms: A review," *International Journal of Nanomedicine*, vol. 13, pp. 1179–1213, 2018, doi: 10.2147/IJN.S146195

[23] M. Yousefi, A. Ehsani, and S. M. Jafari, "Lipid-based nano delivery of antimicrobials to control foodborne bacteria," *Advances in Colloid and Interface Science*, vol. 270, pp. 263–277, 2019, doi: 10.1016/J.CIS.2019.07.005

[24] M. A. dos Santos Ramos, L. G. de Toledo, L. Sposito, G. D. Marena, L. C. de Lima, G. C. Fortunato, V. H. S. Araújo, T. M. Bauab, and M. Chorilli, "Nanotechnology-based lipid systems applied to resistant bacterial control: A review of their use in the past two decades," *International Journal of Pharmaceutics*, vol. 603, p. 120706, 2021, doi: 10.1016/j.ijpharm.2021.120706

[25] A. C. Hatae, C. A. Roque-Borda, and F. R. Pavan, "Strategies for lipid-based nanocomposites with potential activity against Mycobacterium tuberculosis: Microbial resistance challenge and drug delivery trends," *OpenNano*, vol. 13, p. 100171, 2023.

[26] G. Zhao, X. Huang, Z. Tang, Q. Huang, F. Niu, and X. Wang, "Polymer-based nanocomposites for heavy metal ions removal from aqueous solution: A review," *Polymer Chemistry*, vol. 9, no. 26, pp. 3562–3582, 2018.

[27] S. H. Zaferani, "Introduction of polymer-based nanocomposites," in *Polymer-based Nanocomposites for Energy and Environmental Applications*, pp. 1–25, Woodhead Publishing, 2018.

[28] P. Arunachalam, "Polymer-based nanocomposites for energy and environmental applications," in *Polymer-based Nanocomposites for Energy and Environmental Applications*, pp. 185–203, Woodhead Publishing, 2018.
[29] N. Pandey, S. K. Shukla, and N. B. Singh, "Water purification by polymer nanocomposites: An overview," *Nanocomposites*, vol. 3, no. 2, pp. 47–66, 2017.
[30] N. Kaur, R. Kaur, and S. Rana, "Polymer and bionanomaterial-based electrochemical sensors for environmental applications," in *Handbook of Nanomaterials for Sensing Applications*, pp. 241–319, Elsevier, 2021.
[31] L. K. Bogart, G. Pourroy, C. J. Murphy, V. Puntes, T. Pellegrino, D. Rosenblum, D. Peer, and R. Lévy, "Nanoparticles for imaging, sensing, and therapeutic intervention," *ACS Nano*, vol. 8, pp. 3107–3122, 2014.
[32] G. Chen, I. Roy, C. Yang, and P. N. Prasad, "Nanochemistry and nanomedicine for nanoparticle-based diagnostics and therapy," *Chemical Review*, vol. 116, pp. 2826–2885, 2016.
[33] G. Bao, S. Mitragotri, and S. Tong, "Multifunctional nanoparticles for drug delivery and molecular imaging," *Annual Review of Biomedical Engineering*, vol. 15, pp. 253–282, 2013.
[34] D. K. Chatterjee, P. Diagaradjane, and S. Krishnan, "Nanoparticle-mediated hyperthermia in cancer therapy," *Therapeutic Delivery*, vol. 2, pp. 1001–1014, 2011.
[35] J. A. Hubbell, and A. Chilkoti, "Nanomaterials for drug delivery," *Science*, vol. 337, pp. 303–305, 2012.
[36] S. Mura, J. Nicolas, and P. Couvreur, "Stimuli-responsive nanocarriers for drug delivery," *Nature Materials*, vol. 12, pp. 991–1003, 2013.
[37] J. V. Jokerst, T. Lobovkina, R. N. Zare, and S. S. Gambhir, "Nanoparticle pegylation for imaging and therapy," *Nanomedicine*, vol. 6, pp. 715–728, 2011.
[38] J. D. Byrne, T. Betancourt, and L. Brannon-Peppas, "Active targeting schemes for nanoparticle systems in cancer therapeutics," *Advanced Drug Delivery Reviews*, vol. 60, pp. 1615–1626, 2008.
[39] Q. Erica, R. Serena, D. Luca, G. Francesca, S. Barbara, A. Heinz, T. Valentina, M. Laura, B. Roberto, C. Lishan, W. Junbiao, A. Augusto, M. Cristina, P. Daniela, and C. Giulio. "Microfluidic formulation of DNA-loaded multicomponent lipid nanoparticles for gene delivery," *Pharmaceutics*, vol. 13, no. 8, p. 1292, 2021, doi: 10.3390/PHARMACEUTICS13081292
[40] C. M. Bailey-Hytholt, P. Ghosh, J. Dugas, I. E. Zarraga, and A. Bandekar. "Formulating and characterizing lipid nanoparticles for gene delivery using a microfluidic mixing platform," *Journal of Visualized Experiments*, 2021, doi: 10.3791/62226
[41] X. Zhao, Z. Glass, J. Chen, L. Yang, D. L. Kaplan, and Q. Xu, "mRNA delivery using bioreducible lipidoid nanoparticles facilitates neural differentiation of human mesenchymal stem cells," *Advanced Healthcare Materials*, vol. 10, no. 4, p. e2000938, 2021, doi: 10.1002/ADHM.202000938
[42] M. Oves, M. A. Rauf, M. O. Ansari, M. K. Warsi, A. Hussain, I. M. Ismail, *Polysaccharide-based Nanocomposites for Gene Delivery and Tissue Engineering*, 2021, doi: 10.1016/B978-0-12-821230-1.00008-6
[43] A. Tariq, S. A. Bhawani, M. Nisar, M. R. Asaruddin, and K. M. Alotaibi, *Starch-based Nanocomposites for Gene Delivery*, 2021, doi: 10.1016/B978-0-12-821230-1.00007-4
[44] T. Mahmood, A. Ullah, and R. Ali, "Improved nanocomposite materials and their applications," in *Nanocomposite Materials for Biomedical and Energy Storage Applications*, IntechOpen, Nov. 02, 2022, doi: 10.5772/intechopen.102538
[45] L. Pan, J. Liu, and J. Shi, "Cancer cell nucleus-targeting nanocomposites for advanced tumour therapeutics," *Chemical Society Reviews*, vol. 47, no. 18, pp. 6930–6946, Jan. 2018, doi: 10.1039/c8cs00081f
[46] Z. Mirza, and S. Karim, "Nanoparticles-based drug delivery and gene therapy for breast cancer: Recent advancements and future challenges," *Seminars in Cancer Biology*, vol. 69, pp. 226–237, Feb. 2021, doi: 10.1016/j.semcancer.2019.10.020
[47] M. J. Mulligan et al., "Phase I/II study of COVID-19 RNA vaccine BNT162b1 in adults," *Nature*, vol. 586, no. 7830, pp. 589–593, Aug. 2020, doi 10.1038/s41586-020-2639-4
[48] D. Chatzikleanthous, D. T. O'Hagan, and R. Adamo, "Lipid-based nanoparticles for delivery of vaccine adjuvants and antigens: Toward multicomponent vaccines," *Molecular Pharmaceutics*, vol. 18, no. 8, pp. 2867–2888, Jul. 2021, doi: 10.1021/acs.molpharmaceut.1c00447
[49] Y. Granot, and D. Peer, "Delivering the right message: Challenges and opportunities in lipid nanoparticles-mediated modified mRNA therapeutics – An innate immune system standpoint," *Seminars in Immunology*, vol. 34, pp. 68–77, Dec. 2017, doi: 10.1016/j.smim.2017.08.015

[50] M. W. Ghani, A. Iqbal, H. Ghani, S. Bibi, Z. Wang, and R. Pei, "Recent advances in nanocomposite-based delivery systems for targeted CRISPR/Cas delivery and therapeutic genetic manipulation," *Journal of Materials Chemistry B*, vol. 11, no. 24, pp. 5251–5271, Jan. 2023, doi: 10.1039/d2tb02610d
[51] H. Yue, X. Zhou, M. Cheng, and D. Xing, "Graphene oxide-mediated Cas9/sgRNA delivery for efficient genome editing," *Nanoscale*, vol. 10, no. 3, pp. 1063–1071, Jan. 2018, doi: 10.1039/c7nr07999k
[52] S. A. Meenach, K. W. Anderson, and J. Z. Hilt, "Hydrogel nanocomposites: Biomedical applications, biocompatibility, and toxicity analysis," in *Nanostructure Science and Technology*, 2008, pp. 131–157, doi: 10.1007/978-0-387-78608-7_7
[53] M. Ebbesen, and T. G. Jensen, "Nanomedicine: Techniques, potentials, and ethical implications," *Journal of Biomedicine and Biotechnology*, vol. 2006, pp. 1–11, Jan. 2006, doi: 10.1155/job/2006/51516

7 Bionanocomposites in Peptide and Protein Delivery

Farwa Munir, Zainab Anis, Momina Maitla, Maryum Hamayoun, Farrukh Jawad Alvi, Basma Ellahi, Tanzeela Mariam and Atif Amin Baig

7.1 INTRODUCTION TO NANOCOMPOSITES IN PROTEIN AND PEPTIDE DELIVERY

7.1.1 A Brief Overview of the Importance of Protein and Peptide Therapeutics

Proteins and peptides have become increasingly essential biomolecules in medicine due to their potential to treat and prevent various human diseases [1]. Unlike traditional drugs, proteins can offer powerful medicinal effects. It implies that proteins are more specific in their actions, making them less likely to cause target-off effects.

However, delivering proteins and peptides into the targeted cells of our bodies remains a significant challenge due to their large size, complex structure, and interactions with water. All these properties make them incapable of penetrating the cell membrane [2].

This chapter comprehensively overviews nanocarrier-based approaches for delivering proteins and peptides inside cells and current discoveries, problems, and future research opportunities in this pharmacology topic.

7.1.2 Introduction to Nanotechnology and Its Applications in Drug Delivery

Nanotechnology has many possibilities in medication delivery; nanocomposites can also be functionalized with targeting ligands to improve their selectivity toward specific cells. In this approach, nanotechnology has significant promise for enhancing protein and peptide therapeutic delivery efficiency, stability, and intracellular activity, ultimately boosting human health and disease treatment. They have the advantage of being active and effective at even lower concentrations due to their characteristics of high substrate specificity, minimizing adverse effects, and off-target risks [3].

Furthermore, protein-based therapeutics have shown remarkable potential in targeting specific receptors and achieving the desired therapeutic effects.

Nanocomposites are produced and designed to interact with specific cellular pathways and processes to get precise and targeted treatments [4]. However, protein delivery inside mammalian cells remains a substantial barrier due to their vast size, complex structure, and hydrophilic nature, which results in poor cell membrane permeability [5].

As a result, designing practical and adaptable protein drug delivery techniques is critical for their safe and successful use. Nanosystems capable of inducing endocytosis and endosomal disruption and directly delivering proteins into the cytosol are required for successful therapeutic effects.

Furthermore, continuing research seeks to address the limitations and problems of protein and peptide treatments to promote human health and combat disease.

Using nanocomposites can improve the efficacy of novel and existing medications while allowing for selective diagnostics via disease indicators. This chapter also examines the opportunities and

 DOI: 10.1201/9781003650812-7

problems of nanomedicines in drug delivery and the field's current developments and perspectives. Nanomedicine and nano-delivery systems use nanoscale materials for diagnostic tools and precise drug delivery, offering benefits in treating chronic diseases. Recent advances in nanomedicines are reviewed, including the use of nanomaterials to improve drug efficacy and selective diagnosis, as well as information on trends and perspectives in the field.

7.1.3 The Rationale Behind Using Nanocomposites for Protein and Peptide Delivery

Nanocomposites have several benefits for delivering proteins and peptides because of their unique abilities. They can protect these molecules from breaking down, which helps them last longer in the body. Moreover, nanocomposites can make it easier for the body to absorb these molecules specially made to target cells or tissues.

Nanocomposites can even be set up to slowly release the proteins and peptides, which helps the treatment last longer. They are an excellent way to safely and effectively deliver proteins and peptides. They could change how we treat diseases in the future.

7.2 CHARACTERIZATION OF NANOCOMPOSITES

Nanocomposites combine nanoparticles with a matrix that enhances various applications' characteristics. Understanding these materials' performance and maximizing design depends heavily on their characterization. This paper focuses on three critical attributes of nanocomposites: particle size analysis techniques, surface characterization, encapsulation efficiency, and release kinetics.

7.2.1 Techniques for Particle Size Analysis

The particle size considerably impacts the properties and behavior of nanocomposites. An accurate particle size analysis can illuminate stability, agglomeration, and dispersion. Popular techniques include dynamic light scattering (DLS), scanning electron microscopy (SEM), and transmission electron microscopy (TEM). DLS, as opposed to SEM and TEM, which produce high-resolution images for direct size measurement, analyzes particle mobility in a liquid medium.

DLS, also known as photon-correlation spectroscopy, is a straightforward method for determining the quality of a protein in a sample solution, particularly in terms of stability and accumulation [6]. In real-time, particle size distributions can be ascertained using fluctuations in elastic laser light scattering brought on by the individual Brownian motion of the particles in a solvent. Visible light through a laser focused on a solution is typically utilized in DLS [7].

An easy, quick, and direct method for observing the process of protein-protein interaction and determining the binding affinity was provided by the nanoparticle tracking analysis (NTA). The strength of NTA has been demonstrated wonderfully in the direct and quantitative assessment of the protein-protein interaction by combining metal nanoparticle probes, particularly gold, as a read-out device with DLS as a light-scattering enhancer [8, 9]. It is essential to precisely measure the size and distribution of proteins at the nanoscale scale since the physicochemical properties of substances are dictated by their size and the material qualities of the materials that make them up [10].

7.2.2 Surface Characterization

Nanoparticles' chemical and physical characteristics that affect how they interact with the matrix and the environment are examined through surface characterization. Fourier-transform infrared spectroscopy (FTIR) and X-ray photoelectron spectroscopy (XPS) can determine surface functional groups and chemical compositions. Surface area analysis using Brunauer-Emmett-Teller (BET) adsorption isotherms is also performed to determine the potential active interaction areas. In research, atomic force microscopy (AFM) and SEM are robust characterization instruments that can show surface characteristics. The morphology of the sample surface, particle size, microorganism, and its fragments SEM is used to analyze by producing a high-resolution three-dimensional (3D) image [11]. Both technologies have benefits and drawbacks. AFM enables imaging while the samples are hydrated without sample pre-treatment. However, sample interactions on point might result in deterioration of the quality of the picture, such as distortion and minimum resolution power, as non-contact mode imaging has a maximum resolution of about 2 nm. SEM imaging provides a much greater solution because there are no source-sample interactions, but it also requires pre-treatment of the samples and is done in a high vacuum [12].

FTIR, or Fourier transform infrared spectroscopy, is a non-contact, non-destructive method that can characterize materials with excellent resolution and much light [13]. The advantages of FTIR over other processes are its fast scanning speed, high signal-to-noise ratio, high luminous flux, high measurement accuracy, and high resolution. However, it has disadvantages, like using spectral data for calibration [14].

7.2.3 Encapsulation Efficiency and Release Kinetics

Encapsulation efficiency measures how well nanoparticles are encapsulated and assesses the loading capacity of the particles within the matrix. This is crucial for drug delivery systems, controlled release applications, and other specific uses. The effectiveness of encapsulation can be assessed through methods like UV-Vis spectroscopy or high-performance liquid chromatography (HPLC), where the concentration of the encapsulated chemical is measured both before and after encapsulation.

A research study by Sang Hoon Lee evaluated the amount of protein loaded in nanocomposites, demonstrating 2.1–3.8-fold higher cellular uptake [15]. The pace and mechanism of nanoparticle release from the composite matrix are examined in release kinetics. For drug delivery systems and other time-sensitive applications, this is very crucial. Several mathematical models characterize the release profile and comprehend the underlying release process, including zero-order, first-order, Higuchi, and Korsmeyer-Peppas.

In conclusion, a thorough examination of particle size, surface characteristics, encapsulation effectiveness, and release kinetics is required to characterize nanocomposites. These methods help design, optimize, and grow nanocomposites' applications in various sectors by offering valuable insights into the behavior and performance of nanocomposites, as illustrated in Figure 7.1.

7.3 TYPES OF NANOCOMPOSITES IN GENE DELIVERY

Nanocomposites are materials that incorporate nanosized particles into a standard fabric, resulting in unique properties. They have various applications in various industries, including automobile, construction, electronics, information technology, food packaging, and biomedical applications. Despite the several carriers available, lipid nanoparticles (LNPs) are the most therapeutically advanced compared to other choices [16].

Nanocomposites utilized in gene delivery are amalgamations of nanoparticles with genetic material, such as DNA or RNA. Their primary purpose is to proficiently transport and convey the genetic payload into specific cells, thereby bolstering gene therapy and related endeavors.

Several classes of nanocomposites are commonly employed for gene delivery: LNPs, including liposomes and LNPs, are prevalent choices for gene delivery due to their compatibility with biological systems and adeptness at encapsulating genetic material. These nanoparticles safeguard the genetic payload from degradation and facilitate its ingress into target cells. Lipid-based nanocomposites can be customized to enhance stability and targeting precision.

Biomaterials such as polyethyleneimine (PEI), poly(lactic-co-glycolic acid) (PLGA), and polyethene glycol (PEG) are frequently mixed with nanoparticles to form gene delivery vehicles. These polymers condense the genetic material and provide a protective shield, aiding cellular uptake and controlled discharge of the genetic payload.

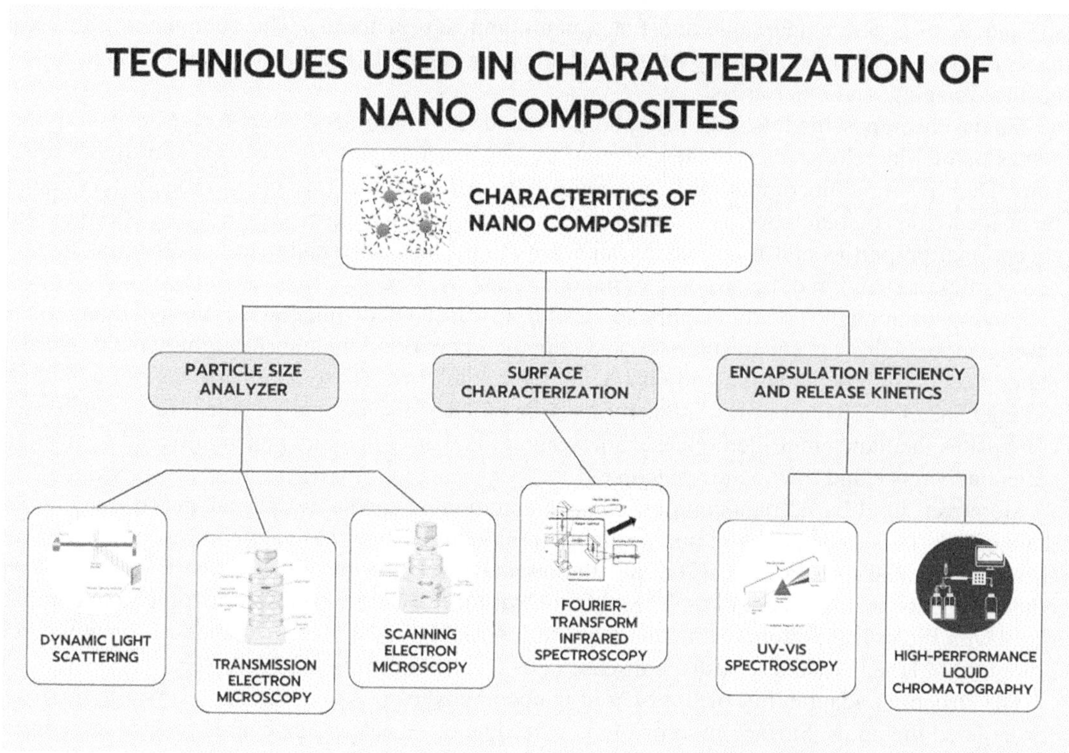

FIGURE 7.1 Techniques and methods that are typically used to characterize nanocomposites.

Inorganic nanoparticles like gold and silica can be tailored with molecules that interact with genetic material. These nanoparticles function as carriers with adjustable surface properties for improved stability, targeting, and liberation from endosomes.

7.3.1 Lipid Nanocomposites

These nanocomposite categories bring benefits and complexities, and ongoing research strives to optimize their properties for safe and efficient gene delivery applications. It's worth noting that the nanocomposites and gene delivery field is rapidly evolving, potentially yielding novel advancements and innovations. The advantages and limitations are summarized in Table 7.1.

Lipid-based nanocomposites are a captivating fusion of fields encompassing materials science, nanotechnology, and biomedical applications. This innovative domain leverages the distinctive attributes of lipids, fundamental molecules within biological systems, integrating them with nanoscale

TABLE 7.1
Advantages and Limitations of Lipid Nanocomposites

Advantages	Limitations
Biocompatibility	Limited stability in circulation
Versatile cargo loading	Low transfection efficiency
Controlled release	Challenges in large-scale production
Targeted delivery	Short circulation half-life

substances to generate adaptable and functional composite materials. The outcome is lipid-based nanocomposites, a domain gaining substantial attention due to their potential in drug delivery, diagnostics, imaging, and other areas.

Lipids, encompassing fats, oils, phospholipids, and cholesterol, constitute a diverse class of molecules pivotal in cellular membranes, serving as both barriers and organizers within living organisms. Their inherent biocompatibility and capacity to self-assemble into organized structures render them ideal for amalgamation with nanoscale materials. Researchers create hybrid designs with exceptional properties and functions by amalgamating lipids with nanoparticles, such as metallic nanoparticles, quantum dots, or polymer nanoparticles.

Foremost among the potential applications of lipid-based nanocomposites is drug delivery. Lipid-based nanoparticles can encapsulate drugs within their core or on their surface, thus shielding therapeutic agents from degradation and enhancing their solubility. These nanoparticles can be tailored to target specific cells or tissues, intensifying drug efficacy and mitigating side effects. Such nanocomposites facilitate controlled release, allowing gradual drug delivery and significantly enhancing patient adherence and therapeutic outcomes.

Moreover, lipid-based nanocomposites have emerged as candidates for advanced imaging and diagnostics. These composites improve imaging modalities such as magnetic resonance imaging (MRI), computed tomography (CT), and fluorescence imaging by infusing the lipid matrix with contrast agents or fluorescent dyes. Their biocompatibility ensures minimum toxicity and compatibility with biological systems, allowing them to be used in vivo. These advances in imaging technologies hold the potential to reshape disease detection, monitoring, and research.

The structural adaptability of lipid-based nanocomposites positions them as versatile platforms for targeted therapies. Surface modifications with ligands or antibodies enable precise targeting of specific cells or receptors, including cancer cells. Such a tailored approach intensifies treatment effectiveness by concentrating therapeutic intervention at particular locations and mitigating off-target effects.

External stimuli such as temperature, pH fluctuations, or light exposure can be built into lipid-based nanocomposites, allowing for triggered medication release or regulated reactions. Nonetheless, the development and application of lipid-based nanocomposites encounter challenges. Attaining consistent particle size, stability, and reproducibility proves intricate due to the complex nature of lipid self-assembly and interactions with other materials. Furthermore, comprehending the interactions between these nanocomposites and biological systems is essential to ensure their safety and efficacy.

The nanoparticles of lipids (LNPs), which include nucleic acids such as DNA and RNA, have emerged as promising carriers for gene delivery. LNPs have several advantages, including their tiny size, biocompatibility, and high encapsulation efficiency [17]. They can effectively encapsulate nucleic acids, protecting them from degradation and promoting cellular uptake [18].

In conclusion, lipid-based nanocomposites signify a captivating realm of innovation bridging materials science and biomedical research. Their potential to merge lipids' unique attributes with nanoparticles' functionalities holds immense promise for drug delivery, diagnostics, imaging, and targeted therapies. LNPs frequently comprise various lipid components, such as ionizable lipids, helper lipids, cholesterol, and PEG-conjugated lipids [19]. Effective encapsulation is possible because the ionizable lipid component can bind with negatively charged nucleic acids [20]. Moreover, as researchers deepen their understanding of these materials and their interplay with biological systems, the prospect of translating lipid-based nanocomposites into practical applications enhancing human health grows increasingly viable.

7.3.2 Polymer-Based Nanocomposite

Polymer-based nanocomposites emerge as a vibrant and rapidly advancing domain at the intersection of materials science, nanotechnology, and engineering. These novel materials amalgamate the

TABLE 7.2
Advantages and Limitations of Polymer-Based Nanocomposites

Advantages	Limitations
High payload capacity	Cytotoxicity
Tailorable surface	Challenges in endosomal escape
Enhanced stability	Variable transfection efficiency
Prolonged circulation	Immunogenicity

diverse characteristics of polymers with the exceptional properties of nanoscale fillers, resulting in a distinct class of materials boasting elevated mechanical, thermal, electrical, and functional traits. Integrating nanoparticles into polymer matrices holds promise across diverse sectors such as aerospace, automotive, electronics, and biomedical applications. The advantages and limitations are summarized in Table 7.2.

Polymer-based nanocomposites have shown promise in gene delivery applications. These nanocomposites, composed of polymers and nanomaterials, offer advantages such as biocompatibility, biodegradability, and targeted delivery. They've been used in various biomedical applications, including tissue engineering and gene therapy. Polysaccharide-based nanocomposites, such as starch and chitosan, have been widely researched for their potential in gene transfer [21, 22].

Polymers, consisting of long chains of repeating monomer units, have gained widespread use owing to their adaptability, low weight, and ease of processing. However, inherent limitations in terms of mechanical strength, thermal stability, and other properties have spurred exploration into polymer-based nanocomposites. Nanoparticles, commonly composed of inorganic materials like metals, metal oxides, clays, or carbon-based substances like carbon nanotubes or graphene, can be dispersed within polymer matrices to craft these nanocomposites.

A pivotal advantage of polymer-based nanocomposites lies in their heightened mechanical performance. Infusing nanoparticles into the polymer matrix imparts a reinforcement effect, enhancing stiffness, strength, and resilience. This development has engendered lightweight materials showcasing exceptional mechanical properties, rendering them apt for employment in structural components, sports gear, and automotive parts. Furthermore, these nanocomposites frequently exhibit augmented resistance to wear, fatigue, and impact, thereby extending the longevity of the materials.

Enhanced thermal properties also characterize polymer-based nanocomposites. These nanocomposites exhibit escalated thermal conductivity and improved resistance to temperature fluctuations. This renders them valuable in contexts where heat dissipation holds importance, such as electronics and heat-resistant coatings. The ability to customize the thermal attributes of polymer-based nanocomposites by manipulating the type and concentration of nanoparticles presents opportunities for tailored applications.

Notably, polymer-based nanocomposites have substantially influenced the sphere of electrical conductivity. While conventional polymers typically serve as insulators, the infusion of conductive nanoparticles can metamorphose them into functional conductive materials. This development has fueled applications in flexible electronics, sensors, and electromagnetic interference shielding. The capability to engineer polymers with specified electrical traits ushers in novel prospects for innovative technologies.

The biomedical arena has also experienced the ascendancy of polymer-based nanocomposites tailored for distinct properties. Nanoparticles laden with therapeutic agents can be incorporated into polymer matrices, enabling controlled release of drugs for targeted therapies. These nanocomposites can be engineered to react to specific stimuli like alterations in pH or temperature, heightening their potential for personalized medicine. Furthermore, polymer-based nanocomposites have been explored for applications in tissue engineering and regenerative medicine due to their biocompatibility and adjustable mechanical attributes.

However, the fusion of nanoparticles into polymer matrices presents challenges. Ensuring uniform dispersion of nanoparticles within the polymer matrix, sustaining adequate interfacial adhesion, and averting agglomeration are pivotal for achieving the desired characteristics. Furthermore, the scale of nanoparticle production and their potential toxicity necessitate careful consideration to ensure the safety and sustainability of these materials.

In summation, polymer-based nanocomposites represent a transformative category of materials that harness polymers' adaptability alongside nanoparticles' distinct properties. Their elevated mechanical, thermal, electrical, and functional characteristics bestow novel prospects across diverse industries and applications. As researchers continue to innovate in synthesizing, processing, and analyzing polymer-based nanocomposites, these materials are poised to mold the trajectory of materials engineering, contributing to advancements in science and technology.

7.3.3 Inorganic Nanoparticle-Based Nanocomposites

Inorganic nanoparticle-based nanocomposites are on the cutting edge of materials science, representing an amalgamation of nanotechnology and advanced materials engineering. These innovative composites merge the distinct attributes of inorganic nanoparticles with diverse matrices to produce versatile materials applicable across electronics, energy, medicine, and environmental remediation. This convergence of inorganic nanoparticles and different host materials has unlocked a spectrum of possibilities to tailor and amplify material properties for specific uses. The advantages and limitations are summarized in Table 7.3.

Inorganic nanoparticles, often on the nanometer scale, exhibit unique traits such as size-related optical, electronic, magnetic, and catalytic properties. These traits can be harnessed and integrated into nanocomposites by dispersing these nanoparticles within matrices made of metals, ceramics, polymers, or other nanoparticles. This fusion of components creates synergistic effects where each material's strengths combine, resulting in novel materials with properties unattainable by individual constituents alone. Inorganic nanoparticle-based nanocomposites have shown promise in gene delivery applications. These nanocomposites, composed of magnetic nanoparticles and a delivery platform, offer advantages such as excellent magnetic properties, stability, and biocompatibility [23].

Plus, they can be used to encapsulate genes and promote cell uptake, making them an effective and safe gene delivery system [24]. The use of magnetic nanocomposites in gene delivery has been reported in various studies, highlighting their potential for practical applications [25]. One noteworthy feature of inorganic nanoparticle-based nanocomposites is their adjustable optical properties. Nanoparticles like quantum dots or metallic nanoparticles can display distinct visual behaviors due to quantum confinement and plasmonic effects. By embedding these nanoparticles into appropriate matrices, nanocomposites can be tailored to emit specific colors, rendering them valuable in sensors, displays, and biomedical imaging. This customizability has paved the way for advancements in lighting technology, anti-counterfeiting strategies, and cutting-edge imaging methods.

TABLE 7.3
Advantages and Limitations of Inorganic Nanocomposites

Advantages	Limitations
Optical properties	Limited cargo capacity
Targeted delivery	Clearance by the reticuloendothelial system
Therapeutic potential	Complex surface chemistry
Imaging capabilities	Potential cytotoxicity

Additionally, integrating inorganic nanoparticles into nanocomposites can enhance mechanical and structural characteristics. For instance, fortifying polymers with nanoparticles bolsters their tensile strength, stiffness, and resistance to deformation. This finds use in lightweight structural materials, protective coatings, and even flexible electronics, where mechanical resilience is paramount.

In the energy sector, inorganic nanoparticle-based nanocomposites hold great potential. Infusing nanoparticles into electrode materials can significantly enhance the performance of energy storage devices like batteries and supercapacitors. These nanocomposites can boost energy density, charging rates, and long-term stability, addressing crucial challenges in energy storage technology. Similarly, in catalysis, nanoparticles' elevated surface area and distinctive surface properties can yield efficient catalysts for various chemical reactions.

Inorganic nanoparticle-based nanocomposites have changed diagnostic and therapeutic approaches in the medical field. Magnetic nanoparticles embedded in biocompatible matrices have been used in MRI and targeted medication delivery. Gold nanoparticles have been explored for their potential in cancer therapy and photothermal treatments, capitalizing on their ability to convert light into heat. These applications underscore nanocomposites' potential to revolutionize disease diagnosis, treatment, and monitoring.

Despite their immense promise, hurdles exist in the synthesis, scalability, and stability of inorganic nanoparticle-based nanocomposites. Achieving uniform nanoparticle dispersion within matrices, managing their interactions, and preserving their properties over time are areas necessitating ongoing research and development.

To conclude, inorganic nanoparticle-based nanocomposites are reshaping the forefront of modern materials science and technology. Their aptitude to merge the distinctive attributes of inorganic nanoparticles with versatile matrices yields materials with customized functionalities, with implications spanning diverse industries. As researchers refine synthesis methods, deepen the comprehension of underlying principles, and address challenges, these nanocomposites are poised to play an increasingly pivotal role in advancing technological boundaries and tackling intricate global predicaments.

7.4 ENHANCED BIOAVAILABILITY AND TARGETING

Drug delivery has undergone a revolution since the advancement in the field of nanotechnology, which has provided inventive solutions to problems with bioavailability and targeted therapy. Creating nanocomposites, which combine different nanoparticles with therapeutic substances to increase their efficacy, bioavailability, and targeting accuracy, is one of the significant elements in this field. Nanocomposites have the enormous potential to revolutionize the treatment of many diseases by combining active and passive targeted techniques.

7.4.1 Passive Targeting

Targeting is dependent on various biochemical and physicochemical interactions, many of which are heavily influenced by the physiochemical properties of nanocarriers and the specific characteristics of the biological environment [26]. The most well-known phenomenon in this regard is the enhanced permeability and retention (EPR) effect. Our tissues' vasculature is abnormal, with leaky blood vessels and poor lymphatic drainage. These anomalies cause an accumulation of nanoparticles within the cancer microenvironment due to the EPR effect. As a result, therapeutic agent-loaded nanocomposites can preferentially assemble in cancer tissues, increasing medicine concentrations while decreasing systemic toxicity [27].

Endosomal absorption prefers specifically shaped nanoparticles over other kinds. Similarly, the charge of the nanoparticle influences the immune response, with positively charged nanoparticles eliciting a more robust immunological response than negatively charged or neutral nanoparticles.

The ability of nanocarriers to preferentially target cancer cells, increasing therapeutic efficacy while preserving healthy cells from injury, is a critical component of their usage as drug delivery systems [28]. The siRNA molecules are transported for gene silencing in nanoparticle-based RNA interference (RNAi) treatment, which can potentially treat cancer [29].

7.4.2 Active Targeting

Nanocomposites are functionalized with ligands that precisely interact with receptors overexpressed on target cells as part of active targeting. This method minimizes off-target effects while enabling accurate administration of medicinal substances to the desired spot. The potential of nanocomposites is increased by incorporating ligand-receptor interactions, which provides a more individualized and focused approach to therapy [30].

It is possible to achieve even higher levels of bioavailability and specificity by combining passive and active targeting techniques in nanocomposites. While active targeting promotes selectivity by activating particular cell-surface receptors, passive targeting uses the EPR effect to collect nanoparticles at the disease location. Drug resistance is less likely due to this combination, which improves the accuracy of drug delivery. Hyaluronic acid, polyethene glycol, and 5-colanic acid were chemically combined to form tumor-targeted nanoparticles (P-HA-NPs). DOX and camptothecin, two anticancer medicines, were successfully encapsulated into the lipophilic inner core of these nanoparticles [31].

In an experiment by Jokerst et al. (2012), nanoparticles encapsulating both therapeutic payload and targeting ligands were created, dramatically illustrating this synergy [32]. This dual-targeting strategy demonstrated the potential of combining both techniques by increasing tumor accumulation and treatment efficacy.

7.5 CLINICAL APPLICATIONS AND FUTURE DIRECTIONS

Hyaluronic acid, polyethene glycol, and 5-colanic acid were chemically combined to form tumor-targeted nanoparticles (P-HA-NPs). DOX and camptothecin, two anticancer medicines, were successfully encapsulated into the lipophilic inner core of these nanoparticles. Moreover, nanocomposites with distinct surface qualities enable targeted distribution to specific cells or tissues. Nanocomposites ensure sustained release and prolonged therapeutic effects by protecting proteins and peptides from degradation. Additionally, they can improve the cellular uptake and intracellular delivery of proteins and peptides, leading to better therapeutic outcomes [33].

In the future, nanocomposites will likely be developed with improved biocompatibility, controlled release kinetics, and targeted delivery capabilities. However, more research is necessary to optimize nanocomposite design and formulation for specific protein and peptide therapeutics, considering factors like stability, toxicity, and immunogenicity [34]. Overall, nanocomposites are promising to advance protein and peptide drug delivery in clinical applications, providing improved treatment options for various diseases.

7.5.1 Overview of Ongoing Clinical Trials Involving Nanocomposite-Based Protein and Peptide Delivery Systems

Recent advances in nanomedicines and nano-based drug delivery systems have demonstrated the promising ability to deliver therapeutic substances to specific places within a patient's body in a targeted and regulated manner. Furthermore, nanotechnology provides several benefits in treating chronic human diseases by enabling the delivery of precise, site-specific, and target-oriented drugs. This chapter discusses these advancements [35].

Nanomedicines have been applied in treating various diseases, including chemotherapeutic, biological, and immunotherapeutic agents [36]. The development and use of nanomaterials have increased the efficacy of new and old medications, including natural products, and have enabled selective diagnostics using disease marker molecules [37]. Nanomedicines have also demonstrated the ability to improve drug solubility, absorption, bioavailability, and controlled release.

Ongoing research aims to develop advanced nano-based drug delivery systems to overcome obstacles and successfully deliver medications to their intended places [38].

The field of nanomedicine continues to evolve, with ongoing efforts to explore new technologies, trends, and perspectives in drug delivery and diagnosis. Nanocarrier-based delivery approaches involve encapsulating the antibody in a nanoparticle that can enter the cell through endocytosis and release the antibody into the cytosol.

Moreover, direct delivery into the cytosol can be achieved using techniques such as electroporation or microinjection. Despite the potential of these solutions, efficiency constraints and safety problems must be addressed. As a result, more effective and varied delivery mechanisms are required to safely and successfully use protein medicines, including antibodies.

7.5.2 Highlighting Successful Outcomes and Challenges

Achievements in protein and peptide drug delivery through bio nanocomposites encompass enhancements in drug stability, bioavailability, and therapeutic effectiveness. Bio-nanocomposites have paved the way for precise and extended release of protein- and peptide-based medications at specified anatomical sites, resulting in heightened therapeutic impacts.

However, delivering bio nanocomposites within protein and peptide drug delivery is challenging. Ensuring harmonious interaction and compatibility between these nanocomposites' biological and synthetic constituents poses a significant challenge.

Furthermore, it remains a noteworthy challenge to attain a meticulously controlled release mechanism for drugs encapsulated within nanocomposites and fine-tune their release kinetics. Creating bio nanocomposites capable of effectively crossing biological barriers, including the formidable blood-brain barrier, adds a layer of complexity to the landscape of protein and peptide drug delivery.

Continual research comprehensively addresses these challenges, primarily focusing on refining nanocomposites' blueprint and operational prowess to elevate drug delivery efficacy and therapeutic outcomes [39].

7.5.3 Emerging Trends in Nanocomposite Design for Optimized Protein and Peptide Delivery

Emerging trends in nanocomposite design aimed at optimizing protein and peptide delivery involve the advancement of nanocomposites with enhanced stability, precise release mechanisms, and the ability to target specific sites. Researchers are actively investigating inventive approaches to improve the interaction and compatibility between nanocomposites' biological and synthetic constituents, thus enhancing their efficiency in drug delivery [38].

The integration of bioresponsive elements within bionanocomposites holds the potential to enable tailored drug release in response to distinct physiological triggers. Moreover, the exploration of multifunctional nanocomposites that combine drug delivery with imaging or diagnostic capabilities is underway, particularly for applications in personalized medicine. The ongoing research tackles challenges like achieving well-regulated drug release from nanocomposites and refining their release kinetics.

The prospects on the horizon encompass progress in both nanotechnology and biotechnology, which are poised to steer the evolution of bionanocomposite systems for protein and peptide delivery. Such advancements promise to translate into improved therapeutic outcomes and elevated standards of patient care.

7.5.4 Potential Integration with Personalized Medicine and Combination Therapies

Bionanocomposites possess the potential to integrate with personalized medicine and combination therapies seamlessly. By amalgamating biological and synthetic components, these nanocomposites can be customized to cater to the specific requirements of individual patients, thereby facilitating personalized drug delivery.

The design of nanocomposites can be refined to facilitate the release of drugs in response to precise physiological cues, thereby achieving targeted and controlled therapeutic delivery. The inherent multifunctionality of bionanocomposites enables the amalgamation of drug delivery with imaging or diagnostic capabilities, thereby facilitating the adoption of personalized medicine approaches.

The efficacy of combination therapies, which involve the concurrent or sequential administration of multiple therapeutic agents, can be heightened by integrating various medicinal substances into bionanocomposites. This integration opens the door to synergistic effects and improved treatment outcomes.

Combining nanocomposites with personalized medicine and combination therapies presents a promising avenue for developing more effective and individualized treatment strategies [40].

7.6 CONCLUSION

Bionanocomposites have become a potential platform for transporting proteins and peptides in biomedicine. These materials mix biopolymers with nanoparticles to improve bioactive chemical stability, controlled release, and targeted distribution. Bio-nanocomposites increase the therapeutic effectiveness of proteins and peptides because they provide adjustable characteristics, biocompatibility, and protection from degradation. Bio-nanocomposites have the potential to revolutionize protein and peptide delivery through creative formulations and engineering, resolving issues with bioavailability, immunogenicity, and delivery effectiveness in numerous medical applications. With solutions for multiple biomedical applications, including medication administration and regenerative medicine, this groundbreaking method can potentially revolutionize the field of protein and peptide delivery.

REFERENCES

[1] S. Zhang, J. Shen, D. Li, and Y. Cheng, "Strategies in the delivery of Cas9 ribonucleoprotein for CRISPR/Cas9 genome editing," *Theranostics*, vol. 11, pp. 614–648, 2020. DOI: 10.7150/thno.47007

[2] R. Tang, C. S. Kim, D. J. Solfiell, S. Rana, R. Mout, E. M. Velázquez-Delgado, et al., "Direct delivery of functional proteins and enzymes to the cytosol using nanoparticle-stabilized nanocapsules," *ACS Nano*, vol. 7, pp. 6667–6673, 2013. DOI: 10.1021/nn402753y

[3] J. Xie, D. Gonzalez-Carter, T. A. Tockary, N. Nakamura, Y. Xue, M. Nakakido, et al., "Dual-sensitive nano micelles enhance the systemic delivery of therapeutically active antibodies, specifically into the brain," *ACS Nano*, vol. 14, pp. 6729–6742, 2020. DOI: 10.1021/acsnano.9b09991

[4] A. V. Ulasov, A. A. Rosenkranz, and A. S. Sobolev, "Transcription factors: Time to deliver," *Journal of Controlled Release*, vol. 269, pp. 24–35, 2018. DOI: 10.1016/j.jconrel.2017.11.004

[5] D. Lembo and R. Cavalli, "Nanoparticulate delivery systems for antiviral drugs," *Antiviral Chemistry & Chemotherapy*, vol. 21, no. 2, pp. 53–70, 2010. DOI: 10.3851/IMP1684

[6] T. O. C. Kwan, R. Reis, and I. Moraes, "In situ measurements of polypeptide samples by dynamic light scattering: Membrane proteins, a case study," in *Polypeptide Materials*, M. Ryadnov, Ed. Humana, 2021.

[7] S. Falke and C. Betzel, "Dynamic light scattering (DLS)," in *Radiation in Bioanalysis*, A. Pereira, P. Tavares, and P. Limão-Vieira, Eds. Springer, 2019.

[8] A. E. James and J. D. Driskell, "We are monitoring gold nanoparticle conjugation and analysis of biomolecular binding with nanoparticle tracking analysis (NTA) and dynamic light scattering (DLS)," *Analyst*, vol. 138, no. 4, pp. 1212–1218, 2013.

[9] W. L. Chong, K. Chupradit, S. P. Chin, M. M. Khoo, S. M. Khor, C. Tayapiwatana, P. Nimmanpipug, W. Thongkum, and V. S. Lee, "Protein-protein interactions: Insight from molecular dynamics simulations and nanoparticle tracking analysis," *Molecules*, vol. 26, no. 18, p. 5696, Sep. 20, 2021.

[10] A. Kim, W. B. Ng, W. Bernt, et al., "Validation of size estimation of nanoparticle tracking analysis on polydisperse macromolecule assembly," *Scientific Report*, vol. 9, p. 2639, 2019.

[11] J. Rydz, A. Šišková, and A. Eckstein, "Scanning electron and atomic force microscopy: Topographic and dynamical surface studies of blends, composites, and hybrid functional materials for sustainable future," *Advances in Materials Science and Engineering*, vol. 2019, no. 1, p. 6871785, 2019.

[12] J. Wang, J. Zhang, S. Li, D. Liu, A. Bhambhani, and H. Zeng, "Characterization of structures and molecular interactions of RNA and lipid carriers using atomic force microscopy," *Advances in Colloid and Interface Science*, vol. 313, p. 102855, 2023.

[13] H. H. Radamson, "Raman spectroscopy, Fourier transform infrared spectroscopy (FTIR) and X-ray photoelectron spectroscopy (XPS)," in *Analytical Methods and Instruments for Micro- and Nanomaterials*, Springer International Publishing, 2023, pp. 87–114.

[14] H. Wei, X. Y. Yang, H. C. Van der Mei, and H. J. Busscher, "X-ray photoelectron spectroscopy on microbial cell surfaces: A forgotten method for characterizing microorganisms encapsulated with surface-engineered shells," *Frontiers in Chemistry*, vol. 9, p. 666159, 2021.

[15] S. H. Lee, J. G. Song, and H. K. Han, "Development of pH-responsive organic-inorganic hybrid nanocomposites as an effective oral delivery system of protein drugs," *Journal of Controlled Release*, vol. 311, pp. 74–84, 2019.

[16] V. L. Demchenko, S. Kobylinskyi, M. Iurzhenko, S. V. Riabov, A. Vashchuk, N. Rybalchenko, S. Zahorodnia, K. Naumenko, O. Demchenko, G. Adamus, and M. Kowalczuk, "Nanocomposites based on polylactide and silver nanoparticles and their antimicrobial and antiviral applications," *Reactive & Functional Polymers*, vol. 170, p. 105096, 2022. DOI: 10.1016/J.REACTFUNCTPOLYM.2021.105096

[17] C. Li, T. Yang, Y. Weng, M. Zhang, D. Zhao, S. Guo, B. Hu, W. Shao, X. Wang, A. Hussain, X.-J. Liang, and Y. Huang, "Ionizable lipid-assisted efficient hepatic delivery of gene editing elements for monotherapy," *Bioactive Materials*, vol. 9, pp. 590–601, 2022. DOI: 10.1016/J.BIOACTMAT.2021.05.051

[18] E. Quagliarini, S. Renzi, L. Digiacomo, F. Giulimondi, B. Sartori, H. Amenitsch, V. Tassinari, L. Masuelli, R. Bei, L. Cui, J. Wang, A. Amici, C. Marchini, D. Pozzi, and G. Caracciolo, "Microfluidic formulation of DNA-loaded multicomponent lipid nanoparticles for gene delivery," *Pharmaceutics*, vol. 13, no. 8, p. 1292, 2021. DOI: 10.3390/PHARMACEUTICS13081292

[19] C. M. Bailey-Hytholt, P. Ghosh, J. Dugas, I. E. Zarraga, and A. Bandekar, "Formulating and characterizing lipid nanoparticles for gene delivery using a microfluidic mixing platform," *Journal of Visualized Experiments*, no. 168, p. e62226, 2021. DOI: 10.3791/62226

[20] X. Zhao, Z. Glass, J. Chen, L. Yang, D. L. Kaplan, and Q. Xu, "mRNA delivery using bioreducible lipidoid nanoparticles facilitates neural differentiation of human mesenchymal stem cells," *Advanced Healthcare Materials*, vol. 10, no. 4, p. 2000938, 2021. DOI: 10.1002/ADHM.202000938

[21] M. Oves, M. Ahmar Rauf, O. Ansari, W. M. Khan, A. Hussain, and M. I. Iqbal, "Polysaccharide-based nanocomposites for gene delivery and tissue engineering," in *Biodegradable and Biocompatible Polymer Composites: Processing, Properties and Applications*, N. G. Shimpi, Ed. Woodhead Publishing, 2017, pp. 3–32.

[22] A. Tariq, S. A. Bhawani, M. Nisar, R. A. Mohd, and K. M. Alotaibi, *Starch-based Nanocomposites for Gene Delivery*, 2021. DOI: 10.1016/B978-0-12-821230-1.00007-4

[23] S. Bhattacharya, *Nanostructures in Gene Delivery*, 2021. DOI: 10.1016/B978-0-12-814657-6.00007-0

[24] M. Singh, "Assessing nucleic acid: Cationic nanoparticle interaction for gene delivery," in *Methods of Molecular Biology*, 2021. DOI: 10.1007/978-1-0716-0943-9_4

[25] S. El-Andaloussi, T. Lehto, E. Smith, R. Sillard, and K. Ezzat, "*Nanoparticle-like delivery system*. U.S. Patent Application 17/777, 227, 2023.

[26] G. Onzi, S. S. Guterres, A. R. Pohlmann, and L. A. Frank, "Passive targeting and the enhanced permeability and retention (EPR) effect," in *The ADME Encyclopedia: A Comprehensive Guide on Biopharmacy and Pharmacokinetics*, Springer, 2021, pp. 1–13.

[27] M. Bamburowicz-Klimkowska, M. Poplawska, and I. P. Grudzinski, "Nanocomposites as biomolecule delivery agents in nanomedicine," *Journal of Nanobiotechnology*, vol. 17, p. 1–32, 2019.

[28] A. Kumar, "Chitosan-based drug conjugated nanocomposites: Advances and innovation in cancer therapy," *Regenerative Engineering and Translational Medicine*, vol. 10, pp. 1–8, 2023. DOI: 10.1007/s40883-023-00310-4

[29] D. Mundekkad and W. C. Cho, "Nanoparticles in clinical translation for cancer therapy," *International Journal of Molecular Sciences*, vol. 23, no. 3, p. 1685, 2022.

[30] X. Qin, H. Zhang, X. Xing, P. Wang, J. Yan, D. Liu, et al., "Robust strategies in nuclear-targeted cancer therapy based on functional nanomaterials," *Materials & Design*, vol. 221, p. 110999, 2022.

[31] S. Arpicco, P. Milla, B. Stella, and F. Dosio, "Hyaluronic acid conjugates as vectors for the active targeting of drugs, genes and nanocomposites in cancer treatment," *Molecules*, vol. 19, no. 3, pp. 3193–3230, Mar. 2014.

[32] J. V. Jokerst, T. Lobovkina, R. N. Zare, and S. S. Gambhir, "Nanoparticle PEGylation for imaging and therapy," *Nanomedicine*, vol. 6, no. 4, pp. 715–728, 2011.

[33] Y. Feng, Z. Guo, J. Chen, S. Zhang, J. Wu, H. Tian, et al., "Cationic polymer synergizing with a disulfide-containing enhancer achieved efficient nucleic acid and protein delivery," *Biomaterials Science*, vol. 10, pp. 6230–6243, 2022. DOI: 10.1039/d2bm01211a

[34] J. Lv, E. Tan, Y. Wang, Q. Fan, J. Yu, and Y. Cheng, "Tailoring guanidyl-rich polymers for efficient cytosolic protein delivery," *Journal of Controlled Release*, vol. 320, pp. 412–420, 2020. DOI: 10.1016/j.jconrel.2020.01.056

[35] S. Z. Razzacki, P. K. Thwar, M. Yang, V. M. Ugaz, and M. A. Burns, "Integrated microsystems for controlled drug delivery," *Advanced Drug Delivery Review*, vol. 56, pp. 185–198, 2004.

[36] Y. I. Golovin, S. L. Gribanovsky, D. Y. Golovin, N. L. Klyachko, A. G. Majouga, A. M. Master, M. Sokolsky, and A. V. Kabanov, "Towards nanomedicines of the future: Remote magneto-mechanical actuation of nanomedicines by alternating magnetic fields," *Journal of Controlled Release*, vol. 219, pp. 43–60, 2015.

[37] Y. Saadeh and D. Vyas, "Nanorobotic medical applications: Current proposals and designs," *American Journal of Robotic Surgery*, vol. 1, pp. 4–11, 2014.

[38] M. A. Obeid, M. M. Al Qaraghuli, M. Alsaadi, A. R. Alzahrani, K. Niwasabutra, and V. A. Ferro, "Delivering natural products and biotherapeutics to improve drug efficacy," *Therapeutic Delivery*, vol. 8, pp. 947–956, 2017.

[39] B. Pelaz, et al., "Diverse applications of nanomedicine," *ACS Nano*, vol. 11, pp. 2313–2381, 2017.

[40] A.B. Balaji, H. Pakalapati, M. Khalid, R. Walvekar, and H. Siddiqui, "Natural and synthetic biocompatible and biodegradable polymers," in *Biodegradable and Biocompatible Polymer Composites: Processing, Properties and Applications*, N. G. Shimpi, Ed. Woodhead Publishing Series in Composites Science and Engineering, Woodhead Publishing, 2017, pp. 3–32.

8 Polymer Nanocomposites in Gene and Drug Delivery

Mehmethan Yıldırım and Serap Yalcin

8.1 INTRODUCTION

Today, bionanocomposites (BNCs) are environmentally friendly materials designed to be used in various application areas and can replace traditional materials. They also have great potential in the biomedical field.

In particular, the production of BNCs from natural polymers makes them environmentally friendly and biocompatible. While these materials contribute to reducing environmental problems, they can also be used safely and effectively for human health [1].

Studies show that BNCs can be customized by combining different components and that these materials can be directed to different application areas. For example, BNCs for bone tissue engineering can promote bone tissue formation by increasing durability. At the same time, they provide antibacterial properties, allowing them to be used in hygienic conditions.

The use of BNCs in medical applications indicates great potential for the development of new treatment methods and materials. Since these materials have biocompatible and biodegradable properties, they can be used in fields such as medical devices, drug delivery systems, and tissue engineering [2].

As a result, we can say that BNCs are of great importance in terms of environmental sustainability, medical applications, and material science. Further research and development of these materials may contribute to reducing environmental problems and improving human health in the future [3].

The role of nanomaterials in drug delivery systems offers many advantages by enabling more effective targeting, transport, and release of drugs. Nanomaterials can increase the stability of drugs and solve solubility problems. When drugs are protected within nanomaterials, chemical degradation or solubility problems are minimized [4]. Nanoparticles can provide a controlled release of drugs. This allows the medication to be released slowly into the body over a long period of time, allowing for long-term treatments where medication doses do not need to be taken frequently. Nanomaterials can make it easier for the drug to reach specific target cells or tissues. This can help the medicine keep unwanted side effects to a minimum. Drugs can be used in nanomaterials at lower doses, which can reduce the toxicity of the drug. Nanomaterials can help enhance therapeutic effects by enabling better penetration of drugs into target cells [5].

The use of nanomaterials allows for safer and more effective use of drugs while also enabling better management and storage of drugs. Therefore, nanomaterials play an important role in the field of drug development.

In addition, new treatment methods such as gene therapy are promising in the treatment of diseases. Gene therapy aims to treat diseases at the genetic level, and research in this field continues. Both drug delivery systems and emerging fields such as gene therapy can lead to significant advances in medical practices and contribute to more effective treatment of various diseases [6]. In this section, the role of BNC materials, which are bionanomaterials, in gene transfer will be discussed.

DOI: 10.1201/9781003650812-8

8.1.1 What Are Bionanocomposites?

BNCs are materials in which nanoscale materials are integrated into natural or synthetic polymer matrices. These materials are used in many industrial sectors and have various applications, especially in the healthcare and food sectors. Here are some examples of the use of BNCs in these areas:

1. Food Packaging: BNCs are widely used in the food packaging industry. Nanoscale materials can increase the durability of packaging and preserve the freshness of foods. Additionally, BNCs can provide environmentally friendly packaging options by increasing the natural solubility of food packaging.
2. Food Supplements: The delivery of health-beneficial ingredients (e.g., probiotics or antioxidants) in BNCs can be used in the production of food supplements. This can ensure better absorption and preservation of the ingredients.
3. Drug Delivery: BNCs can be used in drug delivery and delivery systems. Nanoscale materials can help drugs reach targeted areas more effectively.
4. Dental Materials: In dental practices, BNCs are used for dental fillings and coatings. Nanoscale materials allow the development of durable materials that are compatible with teeth.
5. Wound Care Materials: In the healthcare sector, BNCs can be used as wound care materials. Nanoscale materials can be used to accelerate wound healing and reduce the risk of infection.
6. Food Processing and Storage: In food production, BNCs are used in processing, packaging, and storing foods. This can extend the shelf life of products and ensure food safety.
7. Cosmetic Products: In the cosmetic industry, BNCs can be used in the formulation of beauty products. Nanoscale materials can enable cosmetics to be better dispersed and effective [7].

These various applications of BNCs can provide many advantages to the industry, both by increasing the use of environmentally friendly materials and by improving the efficiency of food and healthcare products. However, the safety and regulation of these materials are also important and should therefore be examined carefully [8].

BNC coating films are versatile materials created by combining natural or synthetic biodegradable polymers with nanoscale materials. The properties and applications of these films may vary depending on the type, ratio, molecular arrangement, and bonding nature of the materials used. Below is more information about some of the properties and applications of BNC coating films:

Features:

1. Molecular Arrangement: The molecular arrangement of the natural or synthetic biodegradable polymers used can affect the mechanical strength, flexibility, and permeability of the coating film.
2. Active Functional Groups: Some biopolymers may have active functional groups to provide surface functionality. These groups can improve the surface properties and adhesion ability of the coating film.
3. Thermal Behavior: The thermal behavior of the coating film can be critical to application temperatures and conditions. Coating films resistant to high temperatures can be used in industrial processes.
4. Solubility: The solubility of the coating film plays an important role in the production process and final application. Its solubility in a particular solvent can affect the methods of forming the coating film [9].

8.1.1.1 Natural Polymers

8.1.1.1.1 Cellulose-Based Polymers

Cellulose is one of the essential components of plant cell walls and is considered a naturally occurring biopolymer. Cellulose nanocrystals (CNCs) are microscopic crystal structures of cellulose fibers and are generally obtained from wood and plant-derived materials. These CNCs play an important role in the production of nanocomposite materials for use in many industrial applications [10].

Cellulose and CNCs:

- Cellulose Molecular Arrangement: Cellulose is a biopolymer formed by arranging glucose molecules in long chains. These chains have a structure consisting of crystalline and amorphous regions. CNCs are microscopic crystalline fragments obtained from these crystalline regions of cellulose fibers.
- Production Methods: Different mechanical and chemical processes are used for the production of CNCs. These processes include methods such as acid hydrolysis, mechanical digestion, enzymatic methods, and cryo-crushing. These processes reduce cellulose fibers to microscopic sizes, enabling the formation of CNCs.
- Microcrystals and Nanofibers: CNCs are often referred to as microcrystals, microcrystallines, whiskers, nanofibers, or nanofibrils. These terms are used based on the sizes and shapes of CNCs. Dividing CNCs into smaller sizes, especially at the nanometer scale, offers opportunities for greater individualization and optimization in different applications.

Applications:

- Polymer-Based Nanocomposites: CNCs are used in the production of nanocomposite materials by integrating them into polymer matrices. These nanocomposites can improve the mechanical properties, thermal behavior, and barrier properties of polymers.
- Food Packaging: CNCs increase the barrier properties of food packaging, keeping foods fresher for longer.
- Biomedical Applications: CNCs are used in coatings of biomedical devices, drug delivery systems, and tissue engineering applications. This can increase biocompatibility and improve the performance of biomedical materials.
- Paint and Coating Materials: CNCs can increase the durability and adhesion abilities of paint and coating materials.
- Paper Industry: CNCs can be used in paper production to increase the durability and printing quality of paper.
- Environmentally Friendly Materials: CNCs can contribute to the development of environmentally friendly products by using them in the production of sustainability-oriented materials.

CNCs allow the development of environmentally friendly materials because they are obtained from cellulose, a natural and sustainable resource. These CNCs can be used in the production of new and advanced materials in many industrial sectors and may find more applications in the future [11].

8.1.1.1.2 Chitosan-Based Polymers

Chitosan is a biopolymer derived from chitin, a natural polysaccharide, and has many advantageous properties. These properties enable the use of chitosan in a number of industrial applications [12].

Chitosan Properties:

1. Active Primary Amine Groups: Active primary amine groups present in the molecular structure of chitosan serve as primary reagents suitable for chemical modifications and cross-linking reactions.
2. Hydroxyl Groups: Chitosan is open to surface modifications and various chemical reactions due to the presence of hydroxyl groups.
3. Polyelectrolyte Properties: Chitosan is a positively charged polyelectrolyte, so it can form electrostatic interactions with negatively charged anionic components.
4. Biocompatibility: Chitosan is biocompatible and suitable for use in medical applications.
5. Antibacterial Properties: Due to the antibacterial properties of chitosan, it can be used in wound care and hygiene products.

Scope of Application:

1. Medical and Drug Delivery: Chitosan is used in drug delivery systems and medical applications. It is especially effective in wound dressings and coating drug delivery nanoparticles.
2. Food Industry: Chitosan is used in coating food packaging and food preservation. It can prolong the freshness of foods and inhibit bacterial growth.
3. Agriculture: Chitosan can be used to control plant diseases and pests.
4. Environmentally Friendly Materials: Chitosan can be used in the production of environmentally friendly plastics and water purification processes.
5. Bioactive Coatings: Chitosan can improve the surface properties of materials by using it in the production of bioactive coatings.
6. Biopolyurethanes: Chitosan contributes to the production of biodegradable materials by integrating them into various polymer matrices such as biopolyurethanes.
7. Protein Separation and Identification: Chitosan is used for protein separation and identification in the fields of biochemistry and biotechnology.
8. Cosmetic Products: Chitosan can be used in the formulations of cosmetic products and hair care products.

The uses of chitosan are diverse, and this polymer can be modified to suit different application requirements. Therefore, chitosan has become an important component in the production of biopolymer-based materials and BNCs. By various chemical and physical modifications, the properties and application potential of chitosan can be further expanded [13].

8.1.1.1.3 Lignin-Based Polymers

Lignin is an important component of plant cell walls and is one of the most common organic polymers found in nature. Lignin, obtained from various sources of plant materials such as wood, straw, and mushrooms, is considered an important biopolymer. Lignin serves as a component that makes plant materials mechanically durable and waterproof and allows plants to stand upright. Additionally, lignin contributes to the resistance of plants to harmful microorganisms and insects [14].

The properties and composition of lignin may vary from plant to plant. Essentially, lignin has a complex structure consisting of aromatic rings and side chains. This structure contains ether and ester bonds, aliphatic and aromatic hydroxyl groups, methyl groups, and other functional groups. This diversity reflects differences in lignin from different plant species, components, and origins.

Lignin has traditionally been viewed as a waste product in the wood processing industry and has often been used as fuel for energy production. However, lignin is increasingly recognized as a valuable biopolymer that can be used not only in energy production but also in the production of industrial products.

The ability to use lignin in these applications contributes to both more efficient plant material processing and increased adoption of materials derived from renewable resources. Additionally, since lignin-based materials have low environmental impacts, they offer sustainable material options [12].

8.1.1.1.4 Pullulan-Based Polymers

Pullulan is a water-soluble polysaccharide produced by certain strains of a polymorphic fungus called Aureobasidium pullulans. This natural polymer is a commercially produced biopolymer used in many industrial applications [15].

1. Water Solubility: Pullulan is highly soluble in water, which allows it to be used in a variety of water-based applications.
2. Structural Flexibility: Pullulan has a high structural flexibility due to the α-(1→6) glycosidic bonds in its molecular structure. This allows the pullulan to form different shapes and structures.
3. Oxygen Impermeability: Pullulan-based films provide oxygen barrier properties and can be used to preserve the freshness of products in applications such as food packaging.
4. Adhesiveness: Pullulan has adhesive properties and can be used in many adhesive applications.
5. Colloidal Stability: Pullulan provides colloidal stability and can be used in the stabilization of emulsions, foams, and other colloidal systems.
6. Low Viscosity: The viscosity of pullulan is lower than some other polysaccharides, making it easier to use in a variety of applications.

Pullulan can also be given greater functionality through various chemical modifications. In particular, surface modifications can help adapt pullulan to specific applications.

Industrial applications include the pharmaceutical, chemical, power generation, agriculture, and food industries. Pullulan can be used in the production and packaging of various products in these sectors. For example, it is used in drug delivery systems, food packaging, cosmetics, foams, and many other applications.

It has also been stated that pullulan is also used in the production of nanocomposites by combining it with materials such as nanoparticles and inorganic tactoids. These nanocomposites can play an important role in providing oxygen barriers, especially for packaging materials and films [16].

8.1.1.1.5 Polyhydroxyalkanoate-Based Polymers

Polyhydroxyalkanoate (PHA) is a linear biopolymer synthesized by microorganisms and has potential as a bioplastic. PHA is considered an attractive material in many application areas because it has properties similar to synthetic thermoplastics with biodegradability and biocompatibility.

PHA exists in two main categories: short chain length (SCL-PHA) and medium chain length (MCL-PHA) based on hydroxyalkonoic acids. These two categories are distinguished based on carbon chain length [17].

Short Chain Length PHA (SCL-PHA):

- Poly(3-hydroxybutyrate) (PHB): This SCL-PHA is the most common and well-defined type of PHA. It is often used as the basic building block of biodegradable plastics.
- Poly(3-hydroxyvalerate) (PHV): PHV is used primarily in medical applications and is considered a biocompatible material.
- Poly(3-hydroxybutyrate-C-hydroxyvalerate) (PHBV): This is a copolymer of PHB and PHV and generally offers more customizable properties.

Medium Chain Length PHA (MCL-PHA):

- Poly(3-hydroxyoctanoate) (PHO): PHO is a type of MCL-PHA with longer carbon chains and is sometimes used in the production of bioplastics.
- Poly(3-hydroxynonate) (PHN): PHN, like other types of MCL-PHA, can be used in different applications.

PHA is considered an important material in various medical and biomedical applications such as medical implants, drug delivery systems, bio-implants, and tissue engineering due to its biodegradability and biocompatibility. It also has potential in the development of environmentally friendly bioplastics and may contribute to the reduction of plastic waste [18].

8.1.1.2 Synthetic Polymers

8.1.1.2.1 Polyglycolic Acid-Based Polymers

Poly(glycolic acid) (PGA) stands out as a biopolymer and is used especially in biomedical applications. PGA can be synthesized via ring-opening polymerization starting from various monomers. This polymer has a hydrophilic structure and is generally highly degradable. However, it is insoluble in most organic solvents; it is soluble only in certain solvents such as hexafluoroisopropanol [19].

PGA has very high mechanical properties and high hardness. However, the hardness of PGA can be reduced by its copolymerization with other monomers. PGA copolymers thus obtained may exhibit properties suitable for more specific applications.

A number of manufacturing techniques are used when producing PGA-based structures and forms for biomedical applications. These techniques include methods such as extrusion, injection molding, compression molding, particle leaching, and solvent casting. These methods enable PGA to be used in the creation of desired biomedical products or structures [7].

In particular, PGA's ability to rapidly form diacid products has led to its use in the production of surgical sutures. These types of stitches can eliminate the need for a second surgery by allowing the stitches to dissolve within the body and contribute to better tissue healing. Therefore, PGA-based surgical sutures have an important application in the biomedical field [20].

8.1.1.2.2 Polylactide-Based Polymers

Polylactide (PLA) is a prominent material among biopolymers and is used in a number of different applications. It is synthesized from a cyclic dimer called lactide and begins with the D or L isomers of lactic acid, which are two stereoisomers. L-lactide is a natural optical isomer, while DL-lactide is a synthetic mixture [21].

PLA can be produced by different synthesis methods. PLA can be synthesized via polycondensation, ring-opening polymerization method, or melt-solid polycondensation. During this production, D-lactic acid or L-lactic acid can be used as a difunctional monomer for polycondensation, while D-lactide or L-lactide contributes to the ring-opening polymerization of PLA.

PLA is a material that can be elastic or rigid and is aroma resistant. Additionally, PLA polymers have the property of being transparent [22]. However, it is important to remember that different isomers of PLA have different physical properties. For example, since L-lactide is a natural isomer, it exhibits 37% crystallinity and has a semi-crystalline structure. On the other hand, DL-lactide is an amorphous polymer.

PLA is considered an important material in the biomedical field. In particular, the high degradation rate of PLA makes it suitable for certain applications, such as drug delivery systems. Additionally, the hydrophobic structure of PLA is strengthened by the steric shielding effect of methyl groups.

To increase the storage ability of PLA, L-lactide is sometimes used by grafting it onto the surface of chitosan. Such studies aim to make PLA and similar biopolymers more suitable for various applications [23].

8.1.1.2.3 Polybutylene Succinate-Based Polymers

Polybutylene succinate (PBS) is a polymer produced through chemical synthesis and belongs to the family of poly(alkene) dicarboxylates. PBS is obtained by the condensation reaction of succinic acid or adipic acid with ethylene glycol or 1,4-butane diol. This polymer is a material with diverse properties and is used in various applications [24].

High Melting Temperature: PBS has a relatively high melting temperature (Tm ~ 90–113 °C) compared to other commonly used polymers, polyethylene and polypropylene. This feature provides durability at high temperatures.

1. Mechanical Properties: PBS is a polymer that exhibits mechanical strength and durability. Therefore, it is used in engineering plastics and similar applications.
2. Nanocomposites: Properties of PBS, such as its electrical properties and viscoelastic behavior, have been studied in the field of nanotechnology. For example, PBS nanocomposites have been found to have anti-static properties.
3. Processing Ability: PBS exhibits processing ability in the production of various products such as textiles and plastic injection molding. This allows it to be used in different industrial applications.
4. Biodegradability: PBS can be copolymerized with adipate to increase biodegradability. This is a feature that is environmentally friendly and can be used in biomedical applications.

In conclusion, PBS is a versatile polymer that can be used in a variety of industrial applications. Its properties, such as mechanical durability, processability, and biodegradability, enable various applications in different fields [7].

8.1.1.2.4 Polyurethane-Based Polymers

Polyurethanes (PUs) are versatile polymers used in a variety of industries. These polymers can have different properties and can be designed to suit different applications. Bio-based PUs are PUs produced through environmentally friendly production processes and have biodegradable properties.

The main components used in the production of PUs are polyols and isocyanates. Isocyanates are reactive groups that form the urethane bonds of PU. Polyol contains hydroxyl groups, the other component of PU, and reacts with isocyanates to form PU bonds [25].

PUs with different properties can be obtained by using different types of polyols. In particular, the type of polyol greatly affects the structure and properties of PU. There are two main types of polyols: polyether-based polyol and polyester-based polyol.

- Polyether-Based PUs: Polyether polyols are organic compounds with hydroxyl groups and are generally synthesized from petrochemical derivatives ethylene oxide and propylene oxide. Polyether-based PUs are flexible, elastic, and durable. These properties are particularly desirable in applications such as the production of elastomers and flexible foams.
- Polyester-Based PUs: Polyester polyols are formed by the reaction of alcohols with hydroxyl groups with diacids or dicarboxylic acids. Polyester-based PUs are used in the production of harder and harder plastics. Furthermore, the use of polyester polyols provides a way to obtain biodegradable PUs.

Bio-based PUs are of great importance, especially today when the demand for environmentally friendly materials is increasing. Such PUs are produced using polyester polyols and are biodegradable. Thanks to these properties, they can be used in environmentally friendly packaging materials, medical implants, and other applications [26].

In conclusion, PUs are versatile polymers and can have different properties depending on the polyol type. Bio-based PUs are considered an important step in the development and use of environmentally friendly materials.

8.2 GENE AND DRUG DELIVERY

Gene therapy is a medical approach used in the treatment of genetic diseases and some other diseases. This treatment is used to replace genetic material (DNA or RNA), repair or replace missing genes, or correct genetic mutations that cause disease. Gene therapy is done through gene delivery systems [27, 28].

Gene delivery systems are technologies that enable the transportation of genetic material to be used for treatment into target cells. These systems are critical for the effective delivery of gene therapy.

Here are some gene delivery systems and applications:

Viral Vectors: Viral vectors are frequently used tools for gene therapy. These vectors are modified versions of viruses that carry their genetic material. These modified viruses can carry the desired genetic material into target cells. Viral vectors such as adenoviruses (AdV) and lentiviruses (LV) have been used in clinical studies.

Non-viral Vectors: Non-viral gene delivery systems are used as an alternative to viral vectors. These systems can deliver genetic material to target cells using lipid-based carriers, polymers, or other non-viral tools. Non-viral vectors may increase the safety of gene therapy, but their efficiency may be lower.

Ex Vivo and In Vivo Applications: Gene therapy can be applied both ex vivo (outside the body) and in vivo (inside the body). For example, the patient's tissue or cells can be genetically corrected outside the body and then returned *(ex vivo)*. Gene therapy can also be administered directly within the patient's body *(in vivo)*.

Applications for Specific Diseases: Gene therapy may be a promising option, especially in the treatment of inherited genetic diseases. For example, gene therapy used to treat neuromuscular diseases such as spinal muscular atrophy (SMA) can slow the course of the disease.

Cancer Treatment: Gene therapy can also be used in cancer treatment. For example, studies are being carried out to deliver special genetic materials that target and kill cancer cells to cancer patients.

Gene therapy is a promising field in the treatment of many different diseases, but it is not yet a fully developed treatment method. Research and clinical studies continue to advance in this field and may help develop effective gene therapies that can be used to treat more diseases in the future [29].

Gene therapy is developing as a promising treatment method in the treatment of genetic diseases and some other diseases. Gene therapy is used to change or correct genetic material and involves different approaches. Here are some of these approaches:

1. Treatment with Healthy Gene Addition: This approach involves adding a healthy gene to replace a gene that is not working or missing in the patient's body. In this way, problems caused by genetic diseases are corrected. For example, if a person is deficient in a gene related to the immune system, the disease can be treated by inserting a healthy copy in place of that gene.
2. Treatment in Which the Diseased Gene is Inactivated: This approach is used in cases where a diseased gene disrupts its normal function. Various methods are used to stop or inhibit the functioning of the diseased gene.
3. Addition of Protective Genes: This approach involves adding protective genes to cells to prevent diseases. It can be used especially in the prevention of diseases that require genetic predisposition, such as cancer.

When applying gene therapy, genetic material must be transported to target cells safely and effectively. Therefore, gene delivery systems are of great importance. Gene delivery systems are tools that enable the delivery of genetic material to target cells. This goal can be achieved by using different methods, such as viral and non-viral gene delivery systems [30].

Viral gene delivery systems use viruses as carriers of genetic material. Non-viral gene delivery systems, on the other hand, use lipid-based carriers, polymers, or other chemicals to deliver genetic material to target cells. Both approaches have advantages and disadvantages, and more studies are needed in terms of safety, efficiency, and effectiveness.

Although gene therapy is not yet a fully developed treatment method, it is considered a promising field for many diseases. Research and clinical studies continue to enable gene therapy to be used effectively in more diseases [31].

8.2.1 Development of Gene Delivery Systems

Genetic material plays an important role in the solution and management of genetic diseases. Genetic information can help understand genetic predisposition and identify the causes of genetic diseases. Additionally, genetic information allows individuals to develop more effective treatment methods by providing personalized medical treatments [32].

Gene therapy is also an important field of research in ensuring that genetic variables do not change. Gene therapy, or genetic treatment, aims to change or correct genetic material. This treatment approach involves treating genetic diseases by intervening in their root causes [33]. However, gene therapy is still in its early stages and poses many challenges and ethical issues.

Genetic therapy requires the participation of not only biomedical scientists but also genetic counselors, ethicists, and other health professionals. Additionally, it is important to continue genetic research to eliminate and treat genetic diseases.

These advances are promising as new treatment methods emerge to reduce or eliminate genetic diseases. However, it is important to remember that these processes are time-consuming [34].

Gene therapy is considered one of the important advances in the field of treatment. In addition to this treatment method having the potential to treat genetic diseases, other important methods of genetic engineering are also promising.

Gene therapy applications include various information tools such as DNA plasmids, siRNA, miRNA, shRNA, antisense oligonucleotides (ASO), and CRISPR/Cas9 [32, 35]. These tools are used to directly correct or modify genetic material. This offers the potential for treatment by correcting or replacing abnormal genes that cause genetic changes.

However, there are also several challenges and limitations associated with gene therapy. One of these challenges is the difficulty of effectively delivering gene therapies to their target nutrients. This is exemplified by its various properties, such as the ability of gene therapy drugs to be degraded by serum enzymes, the ability to encounter immunological responses, and the ability to get caught in other biological filters. However, the development of nanotechnology and materials science may enable new vectors and results to demonstrate these barriers [36].

The increase in gene therapy drugs approved by the FDA demonstrates the extent of progress in this field toward clinical application. However, more research and improvements are needed before gene therapy can be applied safely and effectively.

Viral vectors and non-viral vectors are often used to effectively deliver gene therapy drugs to target sites. Both vector systems have advantages and disadvantages, so researchers carefully evaluate and maintain suitable carriers for gene therapy [32].

Viral vectors include viruses such as retroviruses, AdV, adenovirus-accessible viruses (AAV), and LV. The combination of viral vectors provides high ease of transfection and efficiency in gene transfer. However, the benefits of these vectors include high immunogenicity, safety concerns, and production difficulty [33].

Non-viral vectors generally include entities with biocompatible properties, such as cationic liposomes, micelles, polymers, and inorganic nanoparticles. The suite of these vectors includes large gene payload carrying capacity, low immunogenicity, and high safety for large diversity production.

With the advancement of research in the field of gene therapy, more advanced nanocarriers such as DNA nanoclews, metal-organic frameworks, and cell membranes have also been reported. These transporters may provide better performance, healing capacity, and gene therapy effects. They may also offer higher biosafety and higher targeting properties than viral vectors.

Therefore, it is important to maintain appropriate carriers to overcome the hallmarks of the gene therapy drug delivery process. These carriers are designed to target gene therapy drugs and deliver them to the target more effectively and safely. Advances in this field can be seen as opportunities for the development of more effective and safe treatment options in the field of gene therapy.

Viral Vector Gene Delivery Systems: Viral vector gene delivery systems generally have a structure that contains the information of viruses and takes advantage of their natural genetic material carrying capacity [37]. These systems include retroviruses, AdV, adenovirus-borne viruses (AAV), LV, and herpes simplex viruses. The combination of viral vectors is their high ease of transfection and efficiency in gene transfer. However, it also has problems such as high immunogenicity, safety concerns, and production options [38].

Viral vectors are generally divided into two categories: somatic gene delivery systems and germline gene delivery systems. Germline gene production systems are not generally used due to ethical issues. There are three types of somatic gene delivery systems: in vivo, ex vivo, and in situ delivery [39].

DNA-Based Viral Vectors: These vectors are generally longer lasting and can integrate into genomes. DNA-based viral vectors such as LV, smallpox virus, AdV, AAV, retrovirus, human foamy virus (HFV), and herpes virus are used. These vectors are designed to efficiently deliver genetic accommodation options and show promise in gene therapy [38].

RNA-Based Viral Vectors: RNA-based viral vectors have direct transcription capability for RNA transcripts. These systems are generally transient and are intended for the use of modified CD34(+) neutralization with lentiviral vectors in infectious diseases such as HIV [40].

Oncolytic Viral Vectors: Oncolytic viruses are a new option for the treatment of cancer. These viruses develop inside tumors, multiply, and kill. Oncolytic AdV vectors offer a promising strategy in cancer treatment [40].

Non-viral Vector Gene Delivery Systems: Non-viral gene delivery systems include physicochemical treatments. These systems use biocompatible materials and are generally less likely to trigger a metabolic reaction [41].

Non-viral vectors include liposomes and polymers. Liposome-based vectors enable gene delivery through the formation of lipoplexes. Polymer-based vectors, on the other hand, transfer genes, forming polyplexes [38].

These systems include methods such as physical delivery-mediated gene delivery, needle amplification, ballistic DNA assembly, sonoporation, photoporation, magnetofection, and hydroporation. Chemical modifications include synthetic vectors and non-viral vectors that use segments that facilitate gene transfer.

8.2.1.1 Gene Therapy Drugs

8.2.1.1.1 siRNA

Small interfering RNA (siRNA) is a technology that plays an important role in the field of gene therapy and can specifically inhibit gene expression.

Working Principle of siRNA:

1. siRNA Production: Endogenous or exogenous double-stranded RNA is processed into 21–23 nucleotide siRNA by the Dicer enzyme located in the cytoplasm registered in the cell.

2. RISC Complex: The antisense strand binds to a complex called RNA-induced complex (RISC).
3. mRNA Targeting: siRNA is used together with the formula that remains on the RISC complex to recognize and bind to the mRNA of the target gene.
4. Digestion and Gene Silencing: Under the guidance of siRNA, the RISC complex recognizes and digests the target mRNA. This process blocks protein synthesis of the target gene and ensures silencing of the gene [42].

Challenges of siRNA:

- Easy Degradability: siRNA can be easily degraded by enzymes.
- Kidney Filtration: It is filtered by the kidneys.
- Cell Engulfment: Engulfed by the host.

Nanocarriers and siRNA Gene Therapy:

- Nanocarriers Used: To overcome the challenges of siRNA, the aim is to use various nanocarriers to deliver it effectively. These include cationic lipid polymers, polypeptides, polyethyleneimine (PEI), and nucleic acid as self-dissolving associative carriers.
- Nucleic Acid Self-Associating Carriers: These carriers unravel the rigid structure of siRNA, increasing negative shifting and can significantly increase the gene silencing fraction.
- Example Application: Bujold and his team wrapped siRNA in a responsive gated DNA strand feature using a prismatic DNA nanocage to prevent nuclease degradation. With this approach, therapeutic genes used to control anti-apoptotic factors could be effectively released [43].

These advances allow the development of new and effective treatments in the field of siRNA-based gene therapy [44].

8.2.1.1.2 miRNA

MicroRNAs (miRNAs) are small RNA molecules that regulate gene expression and have a critical structure on biological properties such as cell development, proliferation, differentiation, and apoptosis.

Working Mechanism of miRNA:

1. Production: MiRNA is synthesized by eukaryotic developing genetic material.
2. Processing: These long miRNA precursors are made shorter and processable by the Dicer enzyme in the nucleus.
3. Activation: These short miRNAs are then activated through episodes of RNAi (RNA interference).
4. Targeting: miRNAs match the 3' untranslated regions of target mRNAs.
5. Translation Inhibition or mRNA Degradation: The communication between miRNA and target mRNA regulates gene expression by inhibiting the translation of the target mRNA or promoting the degradation of the mRNA [45].

The Role of miRNA in Genetic Diseases and Tumor Treatment:

- miR-451a in Hepatoma Carcinoma: Studies have examined miRNAs that play a role in the pathogenesis of hepatoma carcinoma. For example, miR-451a was found to be significantly downregulated in hepatoma carcinoma and exerts tumor suppressor effect [46].
- Kidney Damage and miRNA-218: Overexpression of miRNA-218 appeared to have a positive effect on damage and nephropathy of kidney disease. This miRNA reduces kidney damage by systemic regulation.

- miRNA in cardiovascular diseases: miRNAs play a potential role in the care used by regulating heart development, remodeling, regeneration, endothelial function, and angiogenesis.
- Vascular Inflammation and miRNA: miRNAs ensure E-selectin expression by regulating the implementation of the system.
- Depression and Clinical Biomarkers: Some miRNAs (miR-941 and miR-589) have been proposed to be used as clinical biomarkers to ensure major deposition.

These examples highlight the utility of miRNA as a tool with potential for gene therapy and disease treatment [47]. The ability of miRNA to target specific genes, its capacity to regulate gene expression, and its impact on various biological pathways offer significant potential in therapeutic applications.

8.2.1.1.3 Antisense Oligonucleotides

ASOs comply with the demanding guidelines for regulating gene expression. These oligonucleotides inhibit gene expression by specifically binding to target gene DNA or mRNA. The operating rates of ASO occur through complementary binding to a specific nucleotide sequence of the target mRNA [32].

Working Mechanism of ASO:

1. Binding: ASO specifically binds to a specific nucleotide sequence of the target gene.
2. Hybridization: The DNA sequence of ASO hybridizes with the target mRNA; that is, a DNA-RNA hybrid is formed.
3. RNase H Activation: Endogenous RNase H enzyme recognizes and attracts this DNA-RNA hybrid.
4. Cutting and Degradation: RNase H recognizes the DNA region of the hybrid and cuts and degrades the target mRNA.
5. Decrease in Gene Expression: Cutting and cleavage of the mRNA of the target gene leads to stabilization of gene expression [48].

FDA-Approved ASO Medicines:

1. Fomivirsen Sodium: Used for the treatment of cytomegalovirus retinitis of the eye.
2. Mipomersen Sodium: Used for the treatment of hypercholesterolemia.
3. Eteplilirsen: It is the first phosphoramidite morpholino oligonucleotide approved for the treatment of Duchenne muscular dystrophy (DMD).
4. Nusinersen Sodium: Used for the treatment of spinal muscular atrophy (SMA).

ASO and Nanotechnology:

- Biodegradable Lipid Nanoparticles: Biodegradable lipid nanoparticles are available for delivery of ASO to cultured and animal models. These nanoparticles provide a high economy of gene knockout and may contribute to the development of ASO-based therapy.
- Ethyl Cellulose Nanoemulsions: Positively charged ethyl cellulose nanoemulsions are successfully decomplexed with ASO. These complexes can be effective in in vitro transfection assays and in vivo gene therapy [21].

These studies demonstrate the emergence of comprehensive therapies such as nanotechnology and lipid nanoparticles for the development of ASO-based therapies.

8.2.1.1.4 CRISPR/Cas9

The CRISPR/Cas9 system is a revolutionary development in gene-editing technologies. This system involves targeted genetic edits using the Cas9 protein and single-stranded guide RNA (sgRNA).

CRISPR/Cas9 System Basis:

- Cas9 Protein and sgRNA: Cas9 protein is an enzyme that can bind to the targeted DNA sequence and cut and edit this sequence. Single-stranded director RNA (sgRNA) ensures the correct orientation of Cas9 to the targeted DNA. In this way, the Cas9 protein is targeted by specific sets of genetic edits in the targeted gene [49].

CRISPR/Cas9 Deployment Levels:

1. Plasmid-Based Delivery: Plasmids encoding Cas9 protein and sgRNA are a stable and convenient option.
2. RNA-Based Delivery: mRNA encoding the Cas9 protein has a lower rate of targeted knockdown, but multiple transfers can be made.
3. Protein-Based Delivery: Directly delivers Cas9 protein with low immunogenicity [32].

The Most Effective CRISPR/Cas9 Delivery Method:

- Cas9/sgRNA Ribonucleoprotein (RNP) Delivery: It is delivered directly as RNP, bypassing the plasmid or mRNA structure of Cas9 protein and sgRNA. Minimizing target disruptions is important at this stage.

Distribution Methods:

- Viral Vectors: Used for the CRISPR/Cas9 system. Viral vectors do not contain genetic materials.
- Electroporation: It is a method of combining genetic material by passing cell membranes using electric fields.
- Microinjection: It is the direct collection of genetic material using microscopic needles.
- High-Pressure Injection from the Tail Vein: Targeted insertion of genetic material is ensured by using the high pressures of the tail veins [50].

Application Example:

- Ghassemi and his team conducted a study of exon 2 and 3 regions of the Hbb-bs gene using plasmids encoding Cas9 protein and double sgRNA. These plasmids were delivered to fertilized eggs via microinjection. This resulted in fertilized eggs being implanted into pregnant mice, progeny screening, and genotyping and a β-thalassemia mouse model with Hbb-bs gene knockout [49].

Developments in nanotechnology play an important role in the effective use of the CRISPR/Cas9 system and its delivery to tissues.

Arginine Gold Nanoparticles (ArgNPs): Mout and his team used arginine gold nanoparticles (ArgNPs) to achieve co-delivery of Cas9 protein and sgRNA. These nanoparticles effectively transported RNP into the cytoplasm, achieving up to a 90% distribution change and a 30% gene regulatory upregulation.

Cationic Liposomes: Cho et al. designed cationic liposomes encapsulated sgRNA with the CRISPR/Cas9 system. This organic material is widely preferred due to its high gene amount and transfection capacity. Thus, the Dipeptidyl Peptidase-4 gene (DPP-4) sgRNA was encapsulated in lecithin cationic liposomes. It effectively knocked out the DPP-4 gene, which facilitates intravenous transformation into type 2 diabetic mice [51].

Cas9 and sgRNA Modifications: Modification of Cas9 protein and sgRNA can increase off-target results and stability. Ferdosi and his team demonstrated that SpCas9 protein refinement retained functionality and specificity while eliminating immunodominant epitopes. By shortening the length of the sgRNA from 20 nt to 17 nt, Hendel et al. made structural changes to the terminal sections, reducing off-target effects and increasing the genome regulation [52].

These studies emphasize the need to increase the combination of nanotechnological and genetic materials to use the CRISPR/Cas9 system more effectively.

8.2.1.1.5 Gene Therapy Programs

Gene therapy programs are a significant research policy that includes various strategies to treat or cure various genes and genetic diseases.

1. shRNA (Short Hairpin RNA):
    - shRNA consists of two short inverted repeats and a stem-loop sequence in the middle to form a hairpin structure.
    - It remains stable through virus-mediated transmission due to its high viral encoding.
    - Dicer enzyme triggers gene silencing in the cell after transduction.
    - Zhang et al. were able to induce mitochondrial apoptosis and treat pancreatic fibrosis in pancreatic stellate by delivering TLR4 shRNA using cationic liposomes [53].
2. Plasmid-Based Therapeutic Gene Drugs:
    - A therapeutic gene is inserted into a plasmid and delivered to the target cell.
    - Gene plasmid containing foreign antigen is introduced directly into animal products, which stimulates the host cell to respond and produce by expressing the antigen protein.
    - By Tian et al., the pCMFO/DMT complex was evaluated as a tuberculosis vaccine by causing an anti-Th1 response and an increase in the specific IL2 + T CM cell reaction [54].
3. Gene Editing Drugs:
    - Gene editing changes are used to change the components of genetic products or gene changes.
    - Depending on climatic conditions and temperature ranges, gene therapy applications, drug studies, and gene knockout effectiveness in various cell lines targeting various genes vary in durability.
    - The CRISPR/Cas9 system can target gene transfer by removing DNA molecules of the gene; the performance of other genes can only be intervened at the level of targets of mRNA molecules and RNA [55].
4. Distribution of Gene Therapy Drugs:
    - Most gene drugs are negatively charged, hindering the drug's efficacy, and distribution size is an important factor.
    - Nucleic acids consisting of small molecules such as siRNA, miRNA, shRNA, and ASO are suitable for drug delivery efficiency thanks to their small size [56].
    - However, the survival and distribution of large molecules such as the CRISPR/Cas9 system or pDNA are among the current problems [32].

These studies on gene therapy provide important information about increasing the potential of gene therapy and the methods used.

8.2.1.2 Use of Viral Delivery Systems in Gene Therapies

Developments in the field of gene therapy have significantly increased the use of viral vectors in recent years. Viral vectors are tools designed to carry genetic material to the target site and make genetic changes. These vectors are preferred in gene therapy applications for advantages such as high transfection rate and stable transgene expression.

8.2.1.2.1 Adeno-Associated Virus (AAV)

AAV is an important viral vector for gene therapy applications. As a non-enveloped, double-stranded DNA virus, it attracts attention with its biological properties, genetic stability and high gene transfer processes. However, since AAV's packaging limit is only 4.5 kilobases (kb), the amount of genetic material it can carry is limited. Additionally, the sequences of AAV vectors are among the limited factors due to the complexity of the production process.

Various strategies can be used to optimize AAV expression for gene therapy. The most common of these strategies is genetic modification. Genetic changes, for example, with the CRISPR/Cas9 system, are used to increase the targeting range of AAV vectors. Furthermore, targeted regulation at the transcriptional level and disruption, such as covalent linkage modification of the capsid protein, have been developed to optimize the targeting of AAV infection.

An example of the use of this method is the study by Yoon and colleagues [57]. They modified mouse embryos by targeting the Tyr locus through the CRISPR/Cas9 system, resulting in genetically modified mice. Similarly, gene editing to alter Duchenne muscle nutrition and neuromuscular delivery via AAV vectors has revealed promising results [58]. Moreover, AAV-mediated gene therapy is also available as a novel therapeutic intervention method used to overcome drug resistance in cardiac cancer [59, 60]. These strategies accompany promising developments to improve the success of gene therapy AAV vectors and minimize cytotoxicity.

8.2.1.2.2 Adenovirus (AdV)

AdV is a non-enveloped, double-stranded DNA virus with an icosahedral nucleocapsid structure. It has features such as a wide host range, easy scrutability, genetic stability, and large foreign gene loading capacity. Therefore, approximately 25% of viral vectors used in clinical gene therapy applications are AdV vectors.

Ehrke-Schulz and his team performed a study using high-capacity adenoviral vectors (HCAdV) to minimize immunogenicity so that any viral genes could be expressed [61]. This created the CRISPR/Cas9 promoter system for the human papillomavirus (HPV) oncogene E6, the DMD dystrophin gene, and the HIV co-receptor CC chemokine receptor type 5 (CCR5) gene. In the experiments, it was determined that the highest gene insertion-deletion rate reached 93%. However, this system on HCAdV borders has not yet been implemented as an in vivo application.

Tan and his team evaluated the specific theoretical reaction induced by these vectors on immunized transgenic mice and the antiviral abilities of transgenic mice to obtain a recombinant AdV vector containing hepatitis B cell antigen (HBcAg) and TPPII genes [62]. The results obtained show that Adv-HBcAg-TPPII can break immune tolerance, adapt to HBV-specific fragments of cytotoxic T lymphocytes, and is prone to cure therapeutic diseases with better outcomes obtained in transgenic mice. These studies make an important contribution to the investigation of the potential efficacy of AdV vectors in gene therapy applications.

8.2.1.2.3 Lentivirus (LV)

LV is a virus with a spherical structure made of single-stranded RNA with an encapsulation volume of approximately 8 kb and is widely used in gene therapy to provide gene delivery-based drug systems. The activation feature of the immune system is similar to AdVs. However, the use of LVs as a carrier for genetic systems poses a safety risk due to their ability to integrate into the host genome. LV coupling may lead to unnecessary off-target splicing changes. For this reason, most laboratories are unable to prepare non-genomic integrated lentiviral vectors. This makes LV used less frequently than vectors such as AdV and AAV and is generally preferred for the purpose of generating disease models.

Integration-deficient lentiviral vectors (IDLV) reduce integration-related errors while preserving the highly transductive systems of LVs. Ahmed and his team confirmed that IDLVs can effectively deliver spinal motor development, demonstrating that a new strategy for the treatment of inherited early childhood neurodegenerative diseases may be provided [63].

In addition, Zhao and others demonstrate that RNA interference mediated by lentiviral vectors controls the expression of CLDN1 in the appearance of breast cancer, enabling the tumor cell to hide internally [64]. This highlights the potential of LV in gene delivery targeting breast cancer.

Finally, Lu and his team developed an LV-like bionanoparticle (LVLP) vector that can encapsulate mRNA expressing SaCas9 protein [65]. This enabled novel transduction by minimizing off-target and was presented as a safer option in gene therapy applications.

8.2.1.2.4 Bacteriophages

Bacteriophages are known as phage vectors that can realize targeted gene performance in the field of gene therapy and vary in gene therapy target and multidrug resistance research. However, due to narrow host selection and lower gene capacity efficiency than animal viruses, they have been little used in research applications so far.

Suwan and his team synthesized a multifunctional mixed adeno-associated virus/phage (AAVP) vector by enabling viral capsid replacement of phage vectors [66]. This directed evolutionary genetic strategy has conferred traits that may increase the availability of next-generation AAVP. These properties include the ability to neutralize antibodies, escape lysosomal degradation, and avoid transduction barriers before and after internalization. These advanced features aim to increase the potential of phage vectors in gene transfer through gene therapy.

On the other hand, Przystal and his team inserted the human AAV single-stranded genome into the M13 phage single-stranded genome, creating an AAVP (adeno-associated virus/bacteriophage) containing a bacteriophage capsid [67]. This phage vector allows dual targeting of the therapeutic gene to glioma, opening new method development possibilities for the treatment of glioblastoma multiforme (GBM). This study shows that bacteriophages can play a unique and effective role in gene therapy applications.

8.2.1.3 Use of Non-Viral Drugs in Gene Therapy and Gene Transfer

Although viral vectors have the ability to effectively deliver gene therapy drugs via cell transduction, safety issues such as high immunogenicity and high risk in clinical applications limit the overall translation of these vectors. Ingenious design of non-viral vectors for transfection reduction offers a solution to increase the potential shortcomings of gene therapy drugs.

The ideal gene therapy drug carrier should have a variety of options. These properties should include the ability to protect nucleic acid drugs, extend half-life, improve targeting, enhance endosomal dissemination, and enable intracellular release. Non-viral vectors have the advantage of having this feature [68].

Non-viral vectors have the ability to adapt more easily and respond more effectively to the safety issues mentioned above, especially when compared to viral vectors. In addition, the fact that non-viral vectors have a wider application area provides various application opportunities in the field of gene therapy. Therefore, non-viral vectors play an important role in using and safely treating gene therapy drugs [32].

8.2.1.3.1 Cationic Polymer

Cationic polymers are among the polymeric structures used to modify and effectively deliver gene therapy drugs. These polymers are formed by polymerization of short-chain repeating units with a controllable structure and can be precisely designed according to the scanning responses they contain. In general, these polymers attract attention with their advantages, such as biocompatibility, biodegradability, and structural controllability.

However, there is a problem with the cytotoxicity of cationic polymers, which increases with their dense weight and positive charge. This problem, in particular, can cause damage to the genetic material contained in the polymer and damage the modified gene structure. If cytotoxicity progresses in a controlled manner, gene therapy applications may become permanent.

Commonly used cationic polymers include PEI, polyaminoamine, polyaminoesters, and natural biocompatible polymer properties. These polymers are used by combining nucleic acids with electrostatic effect to target gene therapy drugs. In this way, it is used as a more effective portable structure targeting gene therapy treatment.

For example, Wang et al. have developed a therapeutic gene carrier encoding human tumor necrosis factor-replicated apoptosis-inducing ligand (PPR/pTRAIL) using PEG-modified PEI for breast cancer metastasis treatment [69]. This carrier demonstrated that PEI-PEG-R6dGR/pTRAIL exhibited multiple anti-tumor capacities.

In addition to PEGylation to enhance transfection cleavage, cationic polymers constitute an important avenue of research for the functional design of carriers. Duan et al. report that BPAE-NB, a poly(β-amino ester) with a multivalent cationic group arrangement, has higher nucleic acid binding ability and performs better compared to commercial reagents [70].

Polyamidoamine (PAMAM) dendrimer is an example of a cationic synthetic dendrimer with high branching degree, low dispersion, and high functionality. Gu and his team designed graphene oxide functionalized PAMAM dendrimer (GO-PAMAM) to deliver doxorubicin (DOX) and MMP-9 shRNA plasmids together to treat breast cancer [71]. This study demonstrates that the delivery system can be used as a gene therapy carrier with the potential to provide high drug loading, gene supply efficiency, and biocompatibility.

8.2.1.3.2 Inorganic Carriers

Inorganic nanocarriers are remarkable ingredients with wide application possibilities in the functioning of gene therapy drugs. These nanocarriers offer features such as uncomplicated preparation, convenient storage, specific large surface area, good stability, and easy replacement. However, its biosafety is still controversial and needs to be analyzed long-term. Factors based on surface modification, increasing transfection cross sections and efficiency of nanocarriers are important [72]. Currently, inorganic nanocarriers such as gold nanoparticles (AuNPs), carbon nanotubes (CNTs), graphene, quantum dots (QDs), upconversion nanoparticles (UCNs), and silica nanoparticles (MSNs) are widely used in the functioning of gene therapy drugs [32].

AuNPs are classical inorganic nanomaterials with low toxicity, high drug capacity, tunable size and shape, good chemical stability, and biocompatibility. Kong and his team constructed arginine-glycine-aspartate (Arg-Gly-Asp, RGD) peptide-modified dendrimer-trapped gold nanoparticles (Au DENPs), a device that can efficiently transfect both green fluorescent protein and the luciferase reporter gene into humans. Gene carriers were developed [73]. This study allowed specific binding of the radical properties of the designed carrier, in which RGD and AuNPs were prepared together.

With developing nanomaterials, new types of nanomaterials that play an effective role in gene transfer are emerging. For example, Karim and his team reported that they effectively used strontium sulfate nanoparticles as pH-sensitive inorganic nanocarriers to detect siRNA in breast cancer [74]. This study demonstrated the siRNA delivery potential of nanoparticles.

Alsaiari and his team used these structural carriers by effectively encapsulating large amounts of Cas9 protein and sgRNA into CC-ZIF nanoparticles [75]. These transporters, which contain imidazole groups and ions, are regulated in the gene-environment by promoting escape from endosomes by protonation at pH and transporting them to the nucleus. These examples demonstrate that inorganic nanocarriers have significant potential for gene therapy applications.

8.2.1.3.3 Endogenous Transporters

Endogenous nanocarriers can be seen as a breakthrough in the application of gene therapy drugs due to their natural structure and biological stability. Compared with synthetic nanocarriers, endogenous nanocarriers have advantages such as low immunogenicity, high stability, and high efficiency in therapeutic treatment.

Exosomes: Exosomes are nanometer-sized vesicles (40–100 nm) secreted by cells, playing an important role in material transport and intercellular signal communication. Exosomes have properties similar to cell membranes. They have advantages such as their small size, being negatively charged, and preventing phagocytosis. Exosomes from different cell sources vary in their biodensity properties. György and his team created an exosome-AAV vector by fusing exosomes with AAV [76]. This vector had higher transduction rates than conventional AAV transductions. Exosomes also encapsulate gene drugs, providing a high encapsulation regime [77].

Ferritin: Ferritin is a protein found in animals and plants and contains mineral core and subunit shells. Ferritin has a structure suitable for drug addiction and can achieve active targeting by seeing transferrin receptors. Due to these properties, ferritin has become an ideal nanocarrier for the delivery of gene therapy drugs. The inner surface of a mineralized ferrite has been used to prevent lysosomal escape and gene silencing [78]. This study demonstrates that ferritin nanocage is a potential carrier for gene therapy services.

Red Blood Cell Membrane: Red blood cell membrane can be used as a carrier derived from red blood. This membrane covers the surface of the gene complex through electrostatic interaction, prolonging circulation time and increasing biocompatibility. Phagocytic effects of gene-derived results by camouflage of the RBC membrane provide a new method of gene delivery [79].

8.2.2 Drug Delivery

Treatment for chronic diseases over an extended period typically depends on a prescription. Many chronic conditions like diabetes, cancer, asthma, and Parkinson's necessitate frequent administration of drugs. Some treatment plans also involve maintaining a consistent level of medication in the bloodstream, requiring varied doses at regular intervals. Usually, these doses are delivered through oral pills or intravenous injections, which can be inconvenient for certain patients. Effectively managing the specific distribution of drugs within the human body is a significant challenge in the development of drug delivery systems [80–82].

Drug delivery systems encompass a range of devices, formulations, and technologies designed to release a consistent dosage of a drug over a specified duration and at a particular location within the human body, ensuring a safe and efficient therapeutic impact [83–85]. These systems may involve various components and polymers, preferably biocompatible, such as implantable biosensors [86], catheters, microfluidic devices, controlled-release microchips, molecularly imprinted polymers, and diverse carriers like microspheres, liposomes, nanoparticles, and polymers, preferably biocompatible [87–89]. An ideal system is expected to transport the drug intact to the target site and regulate its release both in terms of dosage and timing [90]. In general, polymers have gained recognition as highly promising candidates for the development of controlled-release devices for clinical applications [91]. The emergence of innovative responsive polymers is expected to broaden the scope for creating cost-effective systems with enhanced capabilities [90, 91].

Nanoscale drug delivery systems are employed to minimize the adverse effects of medications, ensure efficient delivery, enhance the efficacy of drugs, and improve overall treatment efficiency, among other purposes [92–94]. The objectives of entrapping drugs in nanoparticles include improving the delivery to target cells, increasing uptake by target cells, and reducing the toxicity of the free drug to non-target organs. Achieving either of these goals can lead to an expanded therapeutic index, representing the margin between doses that produce therapeutic efficacy (such as tumor cell death) and doses causing toxicity to other organ systems. To fulfill these objectives, the development of nanoparticles that are both long-lived and specific to the target is essential [95].

There are many studies based on various nanocomposites. The studies carried out in recent years are given in Table 8.1.

8.3 NANOCOMPOSITES IN GENE DELIVERY

Materials chemistry has not made significant advances in recent years and has focused primarily on advanced pharmaceutical synthetic production with biological, magnetic, and portable storage. An important development in this field is the use of iron oxide nanoparticles (FENPs). FENPs have been

TABLE 8.1
List of Various Nanocomposites-Based Delivery Systems

Nanocomposite	Drug	References
Natural polymer-based graphene oxide bionanocomposite hydrogel beads	Doxorubicin	[96]
Mn3O4@PAA@ZIF-8 nanocomposite	Methotrexate	[97]
PLA/TiO_2 nanocomposites	Norfloxacin	[98]
Complex polysaccharide-based nanocomposites	Insulin	[99]
Bio-ceramic-based nanocomposite hydrogels	Dexamethasone	[95]
Fe_3O_4 magnetic nanocomposites	Doxorubicin	[100]
Fabricating gum polysaccharides-based nano-composites	Meropenem	[101]
Polymer-encapsulated upconversion nanoparticle/iron oxide nanocomposites	Doxorubicin	[95]
Water-dispersible PEG-curcumin/amine-functionalized covalent organic framework nanocomposites	Doxorubicin	[102]
Chitosan-PEG-gelatin polymer nanocomposites	5-fluorouracil	[103]

widely used as cancer treatment therapeutic tools, especially since they have excellent properties such as superparamagnetism and low Curie temperature [104].

In order for these nanoparticles to be used effectively, they must be stabilized using appropriate polymers. In this direction, a number of studies on polysaccharide-based magnetic nanocomposites have been reported [105]. Polysaccharides play an effective role in stabilizing these nanoparticles, providing a suitable environmental cycle for drug-targeted release.

Nanocomposites of naturally occurring polymers combined with semiconductor nanomoieties are called BNCs. This class of materials contributes to an interdisciplinary field that combines materials science, biology, and nanotechnology, also known as "nanobiocomposites" (NCs). BNCs have improved mechanical, gas barrier, and optical structure because they contain nanometer-sized particles homogeneously dispersed in the polymer matrix. These properties provide advantages, especially in drug delivery systems and biomedical applications (Muthiah et al., 2012).

One of the important advances of BNCs is that they are fundamental physiologically in the synthesis of biopolymers (such as polysaccharides, proteins, DNA, and poly(hydroxyalkanoates)) [106]. These natural polymers show the biodegradability and biocompatibility properties of BNCs. Additionally, these polymer matrices contain nanosized additives and are partially differentiated from biocomposites made from biopolymers.

In this context, nanobiocomposites (NNCs) have a number of advantages, such as drug delivery, biomedical applications, gas barrier, and optical properties. These materials have the potential to play a more effective and safe role in future drug delivery systems, gene delivery, and biomedical applications.

8.3.1 Production of Bionanocomposites for Gene Transfer

BNCs are nanomaterials designed to effectively distribute, grow, and deliver genetic material to the target in the general therapeutic area. These materials often contain an intricate detail of biopolymer matrix and inorganic nanoparticles. The design process is focused on ensuring the safe and effective delivery of genetic material into the cell. These materials are coated onto the gene delivery package, enabling gene transfer. Additionally, the targeted homing capacity enables specific or tissue-specific delivery of genetic material. The controlled release block allows genetic material to be operated safely within the cell, ensuring biocompatibility during long-term gene replacement. These BNCs have the potential to provide potential therapeutic solutions in various biomedical applications, especially in the fields of gene therapy and gene editing. However, more research and development is needed before clinical applications can be cost-effective.

8.3.1.1 Microfluidic Structure/Self-Assembly

Microfluidics represents an interdisciplinary technology in which small volumes of liquids are processed and includes engineering, physics, chemistry, nanotechnology, and biotechnology. This technology has a wide range of applications, used in biological modeling without the separation of chemical structure [107].

Microfluidics has focused on nanoparticle synthesis in the field of pharmaceutical processing. This technology aims to provide a solution to the repeatability and large variation production problems of nanoparticle production. Microfluidic systems offer significant advantages, especially in the synthesis of nanoparticles used in nanomedicine applications [108]. However, the potential for this technological clinical evaluation, reproducibility, and whether it provides a full solution to current challenges related to large-scale production have not yet been fully established.

Microfluidic technology offers several advantages. For example, microfluidic devices enable rapid prototyping, which significantly speeds up the process of newly deposited testing. Applicability has been demonstrated in microfluidic systems, especially in the field of nanoparticle synthesis for pharmaceutical processing [109].

One of the prominent features of microfluidic systems is that they enable the dissolution and assembly of amphiphilic molecules and facilitate the formation of nanoparticles. This differs from the parameters used to change the polarity of the solvent, unlike traditional methods. Microfluidic systems enable more effective stabilization in a homogeneous solution of these amphiphilic molecules, allowing the properties of smaller and homogeneous nanoparticles [110, 111].

8.3.1.2 Layer by Layer/Self-Assembly (LbL)

Layer-by-layer (LbL) dissolution is a method used in the field of nanotechnology. This method involves an alternative and repeated adsorption of nuclei with bulky charges to form multilayered structures [112]. The LbL method can be used in a variety of applications and plays an especially important role in drug delivery systems.

Qiu and colleagues used the center of LbL in the production of ibuprofen microparticles in 2001 [113]. In this method, biocompatible polyelectrolytes such as chitosan, dextran sulfate, carboxymethyl cellulose, and alginate were adsorbed on the core materials and formed a multilayered shell. This shell enabled the formation of polyelectrolyte microcapsules with a size of 20–60 nm. Encapsulation is an important factor in distributing drug release.

LbL-based multilayer structures offer many advantages over other fabrication methods. First, it can be adjusted to control the change of particles on the wall. Second, the selection of polyelectrolytes used for coating can be specifically designed to ensure nanoparticle stability. Third, the position and order of the layers can be controlled to manipulate drug release kinetics [114].

The electrostatic interaction between oppositely charged polyelectrolytes enables LbL to be realized; however, other forces such as relative bonding, hydrophobic interactions, and van der Waals forces can also contribute to this process. These forces act on film coating stability, morphology, handling, drug accumulation, and permeability.

As a result, LbL-based multilayer structures stand out as a powerful technique that offers various advantages in fields such as nanotechnology and drug delivery systems. This method can be used to control important rates such as drug release and gene transfer and to incorporate nanostructures suitable for specific needs into applications [115].

8.3.1.3 Printing Lithography: PRINT (Particle Multiplication in Non-Wetting Templates) Technology

Printing lithography, especially PRINT (Particle Multiplication in Non-Wetting Templates) technology, is considered a promising method that allows the preparation of colloidal degradables with specific shapes and sizes [116].

This technology is based on storing a rigid program for casting an elastomeric mold. This elastomeric mold for replicating the original template offers high files, high accuracy, and low cost for a wide variety of production. PRINTING is a manufacturing method that can produce uniform micro- and nanoparticles by providing absolute control over size, shape, and composition. This technology is suitable for the properties of structures endowed with various chemical structures.

DeSimone and colleagues successfully produced bionanoparticles using light-curable perfluoropolyether (PFPE)-based materials using high-cost printing lithography in 2004 [117]. PFPE-based molds are chemically sound, durable, and resistant to solvents. At the same time, problems with polydimethylsiloxane-based soft lithography, which allows high accuracy and quality options of nanomaterials, have been solved.

An important feature of PRINT compared to traditional printing lithography is that PFPE-based molds can be processed by both inorganic and organic methods. It allows the identification of insulated nanoparticles with this feature. Single-particle parts can be produced with various technologies using PFPE-based molding, and even fragile biological particles (such as DNA or protein) can be incorporated into these parts [118].

PRINT technology has the potential to produce biological molecules containing uniform nano- and microparticles, such as insulin, albumin, and albumin mixtures, in protein-based therapeutics by Kelly et al. This may offer new possibilities for many potential applications, such as pharmaceutical problems [119].

The unique feature of print lithography-based manufacturing is the ability for individuals to control the methods, allowing for a variety of options. Reciprocally, self-assembled nanoparticles are often assembled in a specific way, resulting in better control of the shape. Therefore, by printing lithography, a variety of shapes such as cylinders, spheres, elongated ellipsoids, and toroidal processes can be produced [117].

This diversity is important for the distribution of rates of purchases, especially in applications such as pharmaceutical retailers. The cellular uptake regime often accommodates distributions from factors such as disorder, surface distribution, targeting ligands, and shape. Particle size, surface charge, and targeting ligands can be varied by adjusting the input of building blocks during imprint lithography. However, its shape can be controlled, especially with molding.

For example, studies with the HeLa system revealed that both cubic and cylindrical structures can be internalized, but the cylindrical structure is taken up more efficiently. Therefore, in the design of the package of drug carriers, the shape of the particle is an important factor.

In conclusion, printing lithography provides control over part acquisition processes through its ability to fabricate shapes of a variety of diseases and highlights the importance of shape in the design of drug carriers. This could be an important tool for developing advanced and effective solutions, especially in nanotechnology and drug delivery stages [107].

8.3.2 Use of Bionanocomposites for Gene Transfer

Implementation efforts are ongoing for the understanding of the effective delivery of nucleic acid-based therapeutics. Focusing on the understanding and development of ideal bionanoparticles, researchers have designed complex nanoparticle platforms that exhibit high efficiency and specificity. Advances in this field have led to the emergence of a change in material focus. However, as existing obstacles to gene transfer continued, it was realized that a single ingredient was not sufficient.

In this context, the use of various functional materials and their integration into a single nanoparticle has led to further development studies on BNCs with obstacles in gene transfer. This modular design approach offers an effective strategy to overcome a variety of solutions. These efforts have led to the development of composite nanoparticles, focusing on ensuring that critical barriers to gene transfer are maintained.

Major barriers to gene transfer include serum protein adsorption, clearance by the reticuloendothelial system, cytoplasmic membrane passage, endo/lysosome trapping, and nuclear envelope passage. BNC structures that need to be decomposed to overcome these obstacles attract attention with their ability to prevent the adsorption of serum protein, provide more effective passage into the cell, and reach the nucleus.

In conclusion, advances in this field show that significant progress has been made in the design of composite nanoparticles that can cope with inhibitions in gene transfer and enable more effective delivery of therapeutic genes to targets.

8.3.2.1 Use of Lipid-Coated Bionanocomposites

Lipid-coated BNCs are a common strategy used in gene delivery. Lipids are a type of material that can be easily formulated into other nanoformulations through electrostatic or hydrophobic communication. Lipid coating enables nanoparticles to gain liposomal properties, and liposome modification can be made on surfaces with simple and stable protocols. This makes it possible to control various properties of nanoparticles. For example, PEGylation of nanoparticles can be achieved by adding lipid-PEG conjugates. Additionally, targeting ligands or other functional motifs may also be incorporated [120].

The cores of lipid-coated composite nanoparticles can be diverse. Polyplex-based cores refer to nanosized complexes between negatively charged polyanions and positively charged polycations. These polyplexes have been used as gene promoters, but difficulties may be encountered, such as serum instability and nonspecific uptake by the reticuloendothelial system after systemic administration. Lipid coating of polyplexes is a common method to overcome this failure. Lipid coating of polyplexes can be achieved by mixing with liposomes or by rehydrating the dry lipid membrane with a polyplex solution. This method takes advantage of the low risk and immunogenicity of liposomes and their ability to PEGylate, allowing for prolonged circulation [121].

An important example of these lipid-coated composite nanoparticles was developed by Dr. Created in Leaf Huang's laboratory. Using poly(l-lysine) and protamine, negatively charged polyplexes were converted into lipid-protamine-DNA (LPD) nanoparticles, which were used by mixing with liposomes containing DC-Chol and DOPE for lipid coating [122]. This lipid coating, as opposed to lipoplexes, allowed nanoparticles to be obtained that are smaller in size and more resistant to nuclease degradation. LPD nanoparticles achieved more effective targeted delivery after systemic administration, ensuring serum protein adsorption and longer retention in circulation in in vivo applications. PEGylation further enhanced this process, and the binding access of siRNA was greatly increased [115].

These lipid-coated composite nanoparticles stand out as an important strategy to overcome challenges in gene transfer and achieve effective targeted delivery.

8.3.2.2 Mesoporous Silica Nanoparticle Cores

Mesoporous silica nanoparticles are one of the inorganic nanoparticles that stand out as an effective strategy for providing filter and contrast properties. These nanoparticles have large surface area and high storage volume, offering unique properties such as high drug loading capacity and tunable size [123]. The surfaces of MSNs can be subjected to various modifications. Specifically, to deliver nucleic acid agents, the silica surface of MSNs is transformed to carry positive charges for binding DNA or siRNA. This transformation can be achieved by grafting amine groups or coating them with polycations [124].

MSNs generally appear small in size, with nucleic acid therapeutics usually immobilized on the outside of MSNs. Broadly protected MSNs are designed to be open to developments in this situation. For example, MSNs with large cationic selves can be used as an effective carrier in gene therapy by retaining plasmid DNA in the cell and providing better protection against nuclease degradation.

The "protocells" developed by the Brinker laboratory are MSN-based composite nanoparticles produced by fusing liposomes on MSNs and simultaneously loading and separating the available birth cargos with the lipid membrane [125]. These protocols have higher drug loading capacity and stability compared to conventional liposomes. Chemodrugs can encapsulate various structures such as proteins, quantum dots, and siRNAs. Compartments of MSNs can be modified by targeting peptides and molecules such as lipidated endosomolytic peptides, facilitating recruitment and endosomal escape of structures into cells. These breaks enable MSNs to be used as effective carriers in gene therapy applications [126].

8.3.2.3 Use of Polymeric Nanoparticle-Based Cores (PNPs)

Polymeric nanoparticles (PNPs) represent an important class of nanomaterials for drug therapy by gene delivery using biodegradable and biocompatible polymers. PNPs with high integrity, stability, and persistence, such as controlled drug release, can be produced by various preparation methods through different synthetic or natural biopolymers [107].

Lipid-coated polymeric bionanoparticles have been developed to avoid the weak factors of PNPs, such as in vivo instability, nonspecific stability, and premature drug release. These nanoparticles are designed to target nucleic acid therapeutics, proteins, and peptides through entrapment, adsorption, or covalent conjugation. Essentially, lipid-coated PNPs have a threefold structure with specific solutions: (1) the polymeric core on which it is loaded; (2) a lipid membrane that imparts liposomal properties to the core and prevents the properties from leaking through the filter; and (3) a functionalized PEG layer for targeting, membrane penetration, or endosomal escape. Polymers such as PLGA (poly lactic-co-glycolic acid) and polycaprolactone are frequently used in such nanoparticles due to their high surface area and easy functionalization [127, 128].

One method used to process nucleic acids into PLGA nanoparticles is to use a polycation-based condensing agent to intensify the hydrophobicity of the packages so that they can be loaded into the hydrophobic core. This strategy effectively carries gene therapy applications by providing a slow release of the drug. Various formulations are available for the delivery of siRNA using lipid/polymer biocomposite nanoparticles. These formulations allow for a variety of loading methods, settings, and positive effects on targeted gene expression [129].

Those used by Gao et al. were designed as a composite bionanoparticle platform consisting of a dispersant-grafted poly(amidoamine) (rPAA-Chol) core and a lipid coating [130]. This amphiphilic polymer was dissolved into a nanoparticle in an aqueous solution by thin film hydration method, and then siRNA molecules were added. The anionic core was then coated with DOTAP-based cationic liposomes for lipid coating. Lipid-polymer nanoparticles were then subjected to PEGylation by subsequent uptake of a lipid-PEG conjugate. An endosomolytic peptide, T7 (HAIYPRH) or transferrin, is conjugated to the distal end of the PEG chain for the purpose of targeting or targeting endosomal escape. The size of lipid-rPAA-Chol composite nanoparticles is small (100 nm) compared to lipid-PLGA nanoparticles, and a significant tumor inhibition effect was demonstrated when delivering a tumor model containing anti-EGFR siRNA [130].

In a study by Hasan et al., the production of lipid-PLGA nanoparticles was carried out using PRINT technology to create a PLGA/siRNA with high siRNA loading [129]. siRNA and PLGA (85:15 lactic/glycolic acid) were prepared in dimethyl sulfoxide/dimethylformamide/water and molded with PRINT technology. The cores were designed as an 80 x 320 nm monodisperse needle for better uptake. The core was then subjected to cationic lipid coating and PEGylation. These nanoparticles were tested in multiple cell lines and appeared to knock out target genes. This study was an important milestone in the development of the composite bionanoparticle-based siRNA process. Nanoparticles have demonstrated great translational potential due to their high batch-to-batch reproducibility and easy scale-up production for clinical evaluation [129].

8.3.2.4 Use of Gold Nanoparticle-Based Cores

AuNPs are a class of nanomaterials that are of interest in many application areas, especially biomolecular sensing, computed tomography imaging, and photothermal therapy. They have also been investigated as effective nucleic acid generation systems due to their biocompatibility, versatility, and easy surface modification via gold-thiol linkages.

Chad Mirkin and his team studied citrate-stabilized AuNPs with thiolated siRNA [131]. In this method, siRNA duplexes were allowed to chemisorb through thio-gold bonds. This enabled extensive surface functionalization of nucleic acids, increasing the stability of the packaging to which siRNAs are attached while protecting their biological parts. However, it has been observed that negatively charged, nucleic acid-adsorbed AuNPs are in danger due to their poor uptake. To solve this problem, Rhim, Kim, and Nam coated nucleic acid-adsorbed AuNPs with cationic liposomes [132]. This used AuNPs of various sizes (15, 30, 50, and 80 nm) to attach pDNA for lipid coating. A double-ended lipid-gold nanoparticle was observed under cryo-TEM observation. In vitro transfection studies reveal significantly higher transfection processes of lipid-coated AuNPs compared to liposome-mediated or bare AuNPs-mediated DNA processing.

Additionally, Kong et al. used a different method for the production of lipid-coated AuNPs for the storage of siRNAs using 5 nm AuNPs [133]. This was dissolved in the content of AuNPs, DC-Chol, DOPE, and their chloroform, and then the system was emulsified. The resulting nanoparticles contain a cationic lipid membrane with a cluster of gold nanoparticle cores.

In an application supported by Alhasan et al. (2014), it was discovered that nucleic acid-adsorbed gold nanoparticles can naturally separate into exosomes during endocytosis [134]. Exosomes containing these nanoparticles can be isolated and enriched for miRNAs in vivo. With this approach, nanoparticle production represents engineered nanoparticles of biogenesis.

8.3.2.5 Use of Magnetic Nanoparticle-Based Cores

Magnetic nanoparticles (MNPs) have properties that can be dissolved, usually with cores consisting of large numbers of nanocrystals, can be directed to the target under an external magnetic field, and can respond to the energy used. These properties have been exploited to increase transfection fractions of non-viral gene transfer.

Lipid-coated magnetic nanocrystals called "LipoMag" created by Namiki et al. were designed to ensure effective storage of siRNA into tumor lesions under the influence of a magnetic field [38]. LipoMags were fabricated by dispersing oleic acid-coated magnetite nanocrystal cores with cationic lipids in chloroform and then removing the solvent. In this process, a single layer of cationic lipid was recoated onto the nanocrystal cores through hydrophobic interactions. In addition, siRNAs were able to adsorb LipoMag through electrostatic interaction. Under a magnetic field, siRNA delivered by LipoMag showed intense accumulation in tumor lesions and caused silencing of the target gene.

In another method by Jiang et al., iron oxide nanoparticles were coated with lipid or lipid-like methods [135]. Oleic acid-coated iron oxide nanoparticles and lipids were dispersed in chloroform, and N -methyl-2-pyrrolidone (NMP) solvent was added. Since NMP is a solvent that is miscible with both chloroform and water, the adhesive part between the surfaces of lipids and nanoparticles was undertaken by dialyzing the nanoparticles against water. This method prevented aggregation by promoting the organization and assembly of the outer leaflet lipid into a more complete layer. As a result, the produced magnetic nanoparticles were highly homogeneous and showed high efficiency in delivering pDNA and siRNA in vitro.

Yalcin (2019) formulated nanoparticles using dextran-coated iron oxide intended for delivering miR-29a to breast cancer cells and assessed its therapeutic effectiveness in a laboratory setting [136]. Findings revealed that the dextran-coated magnetic nanoparticles carrying miR-29a facilitated a more targeted delivery of the miRNA. Moreover, these nanoparticles led to the down-regulation of anti-apoptotic genes [136].

8.4 CONCLUSION AND FUTURE OUTLOOK

Recent advances in the synthesis, development, and applications of nanocomposites, especially polymer-based BNCs for gene and drug delivery, are summarized in this review. The structure and mechanisms of these nanocomposite systems are discussed. Nanocomposites have an important place in the studies carried out in the field of nanotechnology. Polymer-based nanocomposites have significant promise and are the subject of extensive research for applications in drug/gene delivery, but their widespread commercialization and large-scale production face challenges due to the associated costs and the difficulty of achieving consistent nanocomposite production. By way of designing nanocomposites, new formulations and drug/gene delivery systems continue to evolve; these technologies in the medical field will eventually lead to novel strategies, ease of production, and their use in clinical settings.

REFERENCES

[1] Armentano, I., Puglia, D., Luzi, F., Arciola, C. R., Morena, F., Martino, S., & Torre, L. (2018). Nanocomposites based on biodegradable polymers. *Materials (Basel, Switzerland)*, *11*(5), 795.

[2] Fortunati, E., Puglia, D., Armentano, I., Valdés, A., Ramos, M., Juárez, N., … & Kenny, J. M. (2017). Multifunctional antimicrobial nanocomposites for food packaging applications. In *Food Preservation* (pp. 265–303). Academic Press.

[3] Tripathy, D. K., & Sahoo, B. P. (2017). *Properties and Applications of Polymer Nanocomposites*. Berlin, Heidelberg: Springer.

[4] Yalcin, S., Yıldırım, M., Kamil, N. İ. K. (2023). Cytotoxicity and biocompatibility of biobased materials. In Mishra, A. K., & Hussain, C. M. (eds.), *Biobased Materials*. Singapore: Springer.

[5] Jahangirian, H., Lemraski, E. G., Webster, T. J., Rafiee-Moghaddam, R., & Abdollahi, Y. (2017). A review of drug delivery systems based on nanotechnology and green chemistry: Green nanomedicine. *International Journal of Nanomedicine*, *12*, 2957–2978. https://doi.org/10.2147/IJN.S127683

[6] Jacob, J., Haponiuk, J. T., Thomas, S., & Gopi, S. (2018). Biopolymer based nanomaterials in drug delivery systems: A review. *Materials Today Chemistry*, *9*, 43–55.

[7] Mhd Haniffa, M. A. C., Ching, Y. C., Abdullah, L. C., Poh, S. C., & Chuah, C. H. (2016). Review of bionanocomposite coating films and their applications. *Polymers*, 8(7), 246.

[8] Yıldırım, M., & Yalcin, S. (2022). 24 – Effect of bionanocomposites on human health. In *Woodhead Publishing Series in Composites Science and Engineering, Bionanocomposites for Food Packaging Applications*, Woodhead Publishing, pp.479–498.

[9] Darder, M., Aranda, P., & Ruiz-Hitzky, E. (2007). Bionanocomposites: A new concept of ecological, bioinspired, and functional hybrid materials. *Advanced Materials*, *19*(10), 1309–1319.

[10] Österberg, M., Peresin, M. S., Johansson, L. S., & Tammelin, T. (2013). Clean and reactive nanostructured cellulose surface. *Cellulose*, *20*, 983–990.

[11] Habibi, Y., Lucia, L. A., & Rojas, O. J. (2010). Cellulose nanocrystals: Chemistry, self-assembly, and applications. *Chemical Reviews*, *110*(6), 3479–3500.

[12] Saad, R., & Hawari, J. (2013). Grafting of lignin onto nanostructured silica SBA-15: Preparation and characterization. *Journal of Porous Materials*, *20*, 227–233.

[13] Gómez-Estaca, J., Gómez-Guillén, M. C., Fernández-Martín, F., & Montero, P. (2011). Effects of gelatin origin, bovine-hide and tuna-skin, on the properties of compound gelatin–chitosan films. *Food Hydrocolloids*, *25*(6), 1461–1469.

[14] Leple, J. C., Dauwe, R., Morreel, K., Storme, V., Lapierre, C., Pollet, B., … & Boerjan, W. (2007). Downregulation of cinnamoyl-coenzyme A reductase in poplar: Multiple-level phenotyping reveals effects on cell wall polymer metabolism and structure. *The Plant Cell*, *19*(11), 3669–3691.

[15] Trovatti, E., Fernandes, S. C., Rubatat, L., Freire, C. S., Silvestre, A. J., & Neto, C. P. (2012). Sustainable nanocomposite films based on bacterial cellulose and pullulan. *Cellulose*, *19*, 729–737.

[16] Fernandes, S. C., Sadocco, P., Causio, J., Silvestre, A. J., Mondragon, I., & Freire, C. S. (2014). Antimicrobial pullulan derivative prepared by grafting with 3-aminopropyltrimethoxysilane: Characterization and ability to form transparent films. *Food Hydrocolloids*, *35*, 247–252.

[17] Zhou, L., Chen, Z., Chi, W., Yang, X., Wang, W., & Zhang, B. (2012). Mono-methoxy-poly(3-hydroxybutyrate-co-4-hydroxybutyrate)-graft-hyper-branched polyethylenimine copolymers for siRNA delivery. *Biomaterials*, *33*(7), 2334–2344.

[18] Kai, D., & Loh, X. J. (2014). Polyhydroxyalkanoates: Chemical modifications toward biomedical applications. *ACS Sustainable Chemistry & Engineering*, *2*(2), 106–119.

[19] Oshiro, T., Wakamatsu, K., Nabekura, T., Moriyama, Y., & Kitahara, N. (2023). The potential of a polyglycolic acid sheet for preventing intrathoracic sleeve migration. *Minimally Invasive Therapy & Allied Technologies: MITAT: Official Journal of the Society for Minimally Invasive Therapy*, *32*(4), 199–206.

[20] Villanueva-Cabello, T. M., Gutiérrez-Valenzuela, L. D., Salinas-Marín, R., López-Guerrero, D. V., & Martínez-Duncker, I. (2022). Polysialic acid in the immune system. *Frontiers in Immunology*, *12*, 823637.

[21] Li, G., Zhao, M., Xu, F., Yang, B., Li, X., Meng, X., Teng, L., Sun, F., & Li, Y. (2020). Synthesis and biological application of polylactic acid. *Molecules (Basel, Switzerland)*, *25*(21), 5023.

[22] Ranakoti, L., Gangil, B., Mishra, S. K., Singh, T., Sharma, S., Ilyas, R. A., & El-Khatib, S. (2022). Critical review on polylactic acid: Properties, structure, processing, biocomposites, and nanocomposites. *Materials (Basel, Switzerland)*, *15*(12), 4312.

[23] Singhvi, M. S., Zinjarde, S. S., & Gokhale, D. V. (2019). Polylactic acid: Synthesis and biomedical applications. *Journal of Applied Microbiology*, *127*(6), 1612–1626.

[24] Steeves, D. M., Farrell, R., & Ratto, J. A. (2007). Investigation of polybutylene succinate-co-adipate (PBSA)/montmorillonite layered silicate (MLS) melt-processed nanocomposites. *Journal of Biobased Materials and Bioenergy*, *1*(1), 94–108.

[25] Nurman, S., Saiful, S., Ginting, B., Rahmi, R., Marlina, M., & Wibisono, Y. (2021). Synthesis of polyurethane membranes derived from red seaweed biomass for ammonia filtration. *Membranes*, *11*(9), 668.

[26] Marois, Y., & Guidoin, R. (2000–2013). Biocompatibility of polyurethanes. In *Madame Curie Bioscience Database [Internet]*. Austin (TX): Landes Bioscience.

[27] Sung, Y. K., & Kim, S. W. (2019). Recent advances in the development of gene delivery systems. *Biomaterials Research*, *23*, 8.

[28] Chen, C. K., Huang, P. K., Law, W. C., Chu, C. H., Chen, N. T., & Lo, L. W. (2020). Biodegradable polymers for gene-delivery applications. *International Journal of Nanomedicine*, 15, 2131–2150.

[29] Mali, S. (2013). Delivery systems for gene therapy. *Indian Journal of Human Genetics*, *19*(1), 3.

[30] Kamimura, K., Suda, T., Zhang, G., & Liu, D. (2011). Advances in gene delivery systems. *Pharmaceutical Medicine*, *25*, 293–306.

[31] Guo, X., & Huang, L. (2012). Recent advances in nonviral vectors for gene delivery. *Accounts of Chemical Research*, *45*(7), 971–979.

[32] Pan, X., Veroniaina, H., Su, N., Sha, K., Jiang, F., Wu, Z., & Qi, X. (2021). Applications and developments of gene therapy drug delivery systems for genetic diseases. *Asian Journal of Pharmaceutical Sciences*, *16*(6), 687–703.

[33] Liu, X., Liu, M., Wu, L., & Liang, D. (2018). Gene therapy for hemophilia and Duchenne muscular dystrophy in China. *Human Gene Therapy*, *29*(2), 146–150.

[34] Liras, A., Segovia, C., & Gabán, A. S. (2012). Advanced therapies for the treatment of hemophilia: Future perspectives. *Orphanet Journal of Rare Diseases*, *7*, 1–9.

[35] Bhattacharyya, N. P. (2008). Huntington's disease: A monogenic disorder with cellular and biochemical complexities. *The FEBS Journal*, *275*(17), 4251–4251.

[36] Cicalese, M. P., & Aiuti, A. (2020). New perspectives in gene therapy for inherited disorders. *Pediatric Allergy and Immunology*, *31*, 5–7.

[37] McDonough, P. G. (1997). The ethics of somatic and germline gene therapy. *Annals of the New York Academy of Sciences*, *816*, 378–382.

[38] Namiki, Y., Namiki, T., Yoshida, H., Ishii, Y., Tsubota, A., Koido, S., Nariai, K., Mitsunaga, M., Yanagisawa, S., Kashiwagi, H., Mabashi, Y., Yumoto, Y., Hoshina, S., Fujise, K., & Tada, N. (2009). A novel magnetic crystal-lipid nanostructure for magnetically guided in vivo gene delivery. *Nature Nanotechnology*, *4*(9), 598–606.

[39] Herrero, M. J., Sabater, L., Guenechea, G., Sendra, L., Montilla, A. I., Abargues, R., … & Aliño, S. F. (2012). DNA delivery to 'ex vivo' human liver segments. *Gene Therapy*, *19*(5), 504–512.

[40] Gonçalves, G. A. R., & Paiva, R. D. M. A. (2017). Gene therapy: Advances, challenges and perspectives. *Einstein (Sao Paulo)*, *15*, 369–375.

[41] Sung, Y. K., & Kim, S. W. (2018). The practical application of gene vectors in cancer therapy. *Integrative Cancer Science and Therapeutics*, *5*, 1–5.

[42] Chakraborty, C., Sharma, A. R., Sharma, G., Doss, C. G. P., & Lee, S. S. (2017). Therapeutic miRNA and siRNA: Moving from bench to clinic as next generation medicine. *Molecular Therapy-Nucleic Acids*, *8*, 132–143.

[43] Bujold, K. E., Hsu, J. C., & Sleiman, H. F. (2016). Optimized DNA "nanosuitcases" for encapsulation and conditional release of siRNA. *Journal of the American Chemical Society*, *138*(42), 14030–14038.

[44] Hu, B., Weng, Y., Xia, X. H., Liang, X. J., & Huang, Y. (2019). Clinical advances of siRNA therapeutics. *The Journal of Gene Medicine*, *21*(7), e3097.

[45] Zhao, S., Li, J., Zhang, G., Wang, Q., Wu, C., Zhang, Q., ... & Yang, S. (2019). Exosomal miR-451a functions as a tumor suppressor in hepatocellular carcinoma by targeting LPIN1. *Cellular Physiology and Biochemistry*, 53(1), 19–35.

[46] Samanta, S., Balasubramanian, S., Rajasingh, S., Patel, U., Dhanasekaran, A., Dawn, B., & Rajasingh, J. (2016). MicroRNA: A new therapeutic strategy for cardiovascular diseases. *Trends in Cardiovascular Medicine*, *26*(5), 407–419.

[47] McAnena, P., Lowery, A., & Kerin, M. J. (2018). Role of micro-RNAs in breast cancer surgery. *Journal of British Surgery*, *105*(2), e19–e30.

[48] Yang, L., Ma, F., Liu, F., Chen, J., Zhao, X., & Xu, Q. (2020). Efficient delivery of antisense oligonucleotides using bioreducible lipid nanoparticles in vitro and in vivo. *Molecular Therapy-Nucleic Acids*, *19*, 1357–1367.

[49] Ghassemi, B., Shamsara, M., Soleimani, M., Kiani, J., & Rassoulzadegan, M. (2019). Pipeline for the generation of gene knockout mice using dual sgRNA CRISPR/Cas9-mediated gene editing. *Analytical Biochemistry*, *568*, 31–40.

[50] Mout, R., Ray, M., Yesilbag Tonga, G., Lee, Y. W., Tay, T., Sasaki, K., & Rotello, V. M. (2017). Direct cytosolic delivery of CRISPR/Cas9-ribonucleoprotein for efficient gene editing. *ACS Nano*, *11*(3), 2452–2458.

[51] Cho, E. Y., Ryu, J. Y., Lee, H. A. R., Hong, S. H., Park, H. S., Hong, K. S., ... & Yoon, T. J. (2019). Lecithin nano-liposomal particle as a CRISPR/Cas9 complex delivery system for treating type 2 diabetes. *Journal of Nanobiotechnology*, *17*, 1–12.

[52] Ferdosi, S. R., Ewaisha, R., Moghadam, F., Krishna, S., Park, J. G., Ebrahimkhani, M. R., ... & Anderson, K. S. (2019). Multifunctional CRISPR-Cas9 with engineered immunosilenced human T cell epitopes. *Nature Communications*, *10*(1), 1842.

[53] Zhang, Y., Yue, D., Cheng, L., Huang, A., Tong, N., & Cheng, P. (2018). Vitamin A-coupled liposomes carrying TLR4-silencing shRNA induce apoptosis of pancreatic stellate cells and resolution of pancreatic fibrosis. *Journal of Molecular Medicine*, *96*, 445–458.

[54] Tian, M., Zhou, Z., Tan, S., Fan, X., Li, L., & Ullah, N. (2018). Formulation in DDA-MPLA-TDB liposome enhances the immunogenicity and protective efficacy of a DNA vaccine against Mycobacterium tuberculosis infection. *Frontiers in Immunology*, *9*, 310.

[55] Tan, S., Tao, Z., Loo, S., Su, L., Chen, X., & Ye, L. (2019). Non-viral vector based gene transfection with human induced pluripotent stem cells derived cardiomyocytes. *Scientific Reports*, *9*(1), 14404.

[56] Mirón-Barroso, S., Domènech, E. B., & Trigueros, S. (2021). Nanotechnology-based strategies to overcome current barriers in gene delivery. *International Journal of Molecular Sciences*, 22(16), 8537.

[57] Yoon, Y., Wang, D., Tai, P. W., Riley, J., Gao, G., & Rivera-Pérez, J. A. (2018). Streamlined ex vivo and in vivo genome editing in mouse embryos using recombinant adeno-associated viruses. *Nature Communications*, *9*(1), 1–12.

[58] Bengtsson, N. E., Hall, J. K., Odom, G. L., Phelps, M. P., Andrus, C. R., Hawkins, R. D., ... & Chamberlain, J. S. (2017). Corrigendum: Muscle-specific CRISPR/Cas9 dystrophin gene editing ameliorates pathophysiology in a mouse model for Duchenne muscular dystrophy. *Nature Communications*, *8*, 16007.

[59] Ma, S., Sun, J., Guo, Y., Zhang, P., Liu, Y., Zheng, D., & Shi, J. (2017). Combination of AAV-TRAIL with miR-221-Zip therapeutic strategy overcomes the resistance to TRAIL induced apoptosis in liver cancer. *Theranostics*, *7*(13), 3228.

[60] Naso, M. F., Tomkowicz, B., Perry III, W. L., & Strohl, W. R. (2017). Adeno-associated virus (AAV) as a vector for gene therapy. *Bio Drugs*, *31*(4), 317–334.

[61] Ehrke-Schulz, E., Schiwon, M., Leitner, T., Dávid, S., Bergmann, T., Liu, J., & Ehrhardt, A. (2017). CRISPR/Cas9 delivery with one single adenoviral vector devoid of all viral genes. *Scientific Reports*, *7*(1), 17113.

[62] Tan, Q., Ma, S., Hu, J., Chen, X., Yu, Y., Tang, Z., & Zang, G. (2017). Adenovirus vector harboring the HBcAg and tripeptidyl peptidase II genes induces potent cellular immune responses in vivo. *Cellular Physiology and Biochemistry*, *41*(2), 423–438.

[63] Ahmed, S. G., Waddington, S. N., Boza-Morán, M. G., & Yáñez-Muñoz, R. J. (2018). High-efficiency transduction of spinal cord motor neurons by intrauterine delivery of integration-deficient lentiviral vectors. *Journal of Controlled Release*, *273*, 99–107.

[64] Zhao, X., Zou, Y., Gu, Q., Zhao, G., Gray, H., Pfeffer, L. M., & Yue, J. (2015). Lentiviral vector mediated claudin1 silencing inhibits epithelial to mesenchymal transition in breast cancer cells. *Viruses*, *7*(6), 2965–2979.

[65] Lu, B., Javidi-Parsijani, P., Makani, V., Mehraein-Ghomi, F., Sarhan, W. M., Sun, D., ... & Atala, A. (2019). Delivering SaCas9 mRNA by lentivirus-like bionanoparticles for transient expression and efficient genome editing. *Nucleic Acids Research*, *47*(8), e44–e44.

[66] Suwan, K., Yata, T., Waramit, S., Przystal, J. M., Stoneham, C. A., Bentayebi, K., ... & Hajitou, A. (2019). Next-generation of targeted AAVP vectors for systemic transgene delivery against cancer. *Proceedings of the National Academy of Sciences*, *116*(37), 18571–18577.

[67] Przystal, J. M., Waramit, S., Pranjol, M. Z. I., Yan, W., Chu, G., Chongchai, A., ... & Hajitou, A. (2019). Efficacy of systemic temozolomide-activated phage-targeted gene therapy in human glioblastoma. *EMBO Molecular Medicine*, *11*(4), e8492.

[68] Li, Y., Bolinger, J., Yu, Y., Glass, Z., Shi, N., Yang, L., ... & Xu, Q. (2019). Intracellular delivery and biodistribution study of CRISPR/Cas9 ribonucleoprotein loaded bioreducible lipidoid nanoparticles. *Biomaterials Science*, *7*(2), 596–606.

[69] Wang, X., Yin, S., Li, M., Rao, J., Wan, D., Qiu, Y., ... & He, Q. (2020). Autophagy inhibition changes the disposition of non-viral gene carriers during blood-brain barrier penetration and enhances TRAIL-induced apoptosis in brain metastatic tumor. *Journal of Controlled Release*, *321*, 497–508.

[70] Duan, S., Cao, D., Li, X., Zhu, H., Lan, M., Tan, Z., ... & Chen, Y. (2020). Topology-assisted, photo-strengthened DNA/siRNA delivery mediated by branched poly (β-amino ester) s via synchronized intracellular kinetics. *Biomaterials Science*, *8*(1), 290–301.

[71] Gu, Y., Guo, Y., Wang, C., Xu, J., Wu, J., Kirk, T. B., ... & Xue, W. (2017). A polyamidoamne dendrimer functionalized graphene oxide for DOX and MMP-9 shRNA plasmid co-delivery. *Materials Science and Engineering: C*, *70*, 572–585.

[72] Caoduro, C., Hervouet, E., Girard-Thernier, C., Gharbi, T., Boulahdour, H., Delage-Mourroux, R., & Pudlo, M. (2017). Carbon nanotubes as gene carriers: Focus on internalization pathways related to functionalization and properties. *Acta Biomaterialia*, *49*, 36–44.

[73] Kong, L., Alves, C. S., Hou, W., Qiu, J., Möhwald, H., Tomás, H., & Shi, X. (2015). RGD peptide-modified dendrimer-entrapped gold nanoparticles enable highly efficient and specific gene delivery to stem cells. *ACS Applied Materials & Interfaces*, *7*(8), 4833–4843.

[74] Karim, M. E., Shetty, J., Islam, R. A., Kaiser, A., Bakhtiar, A., & Chowdhury, E. H. (2019). Strontium sulfite: A new pH-responsive inorganic nanocarrier to deliver therapeutic siRNAs to cancer cells. *Pharmaceutics*, *11*(2), 89.

[75] Alsaiari, S. K., Patil, S., Alyami, M., Alamoudi, K. O., Aleisa, F. A., Merzaban, J. S., ... & Khashab, N. M. (2018). Endosomal escape and delivery of CRISPR/Cas9 genome editing machinery enabled by nanoscale zeolitic imidazolate framework. *Journal of the American Chemical Society*, *140*(1), 143–146.

[76] György, B., Sage, C., Indzhykulian, A. A., Scheffer, D. I., Brisson, A. R., Tan, S., ... & Maguire, C. A. (2017). Rescue of hearing by gene delivery to inner-ear hair cells using exosome-associated AAV. *Molecular Therapy*, *25*(2), 379–391.

[77] Zhao, L., Gu, C., Gan, Y., Shao, L., Chen, H., & Zhu, H. (2020). Exosome-mediated siRNA delivery to suppress postoperative breast cancer metastasis. *Journal of Controlled Release*, *318*, 1–15.

[78] Huang, H., Sha, K., Veroniaina, H., Wu, Z., Wu, Z., & Qi, X. (2020). Ca 2+ participating self-assembly of an apoferritin nanostructure for nucleic acid drug delivery. *Nanoscale*, *12*(13), 7347–7357.

[79] Hao, X., Li, Q., Wang, H., Muhammad, K., Guo, J., Ren, X., ... & Feng, Y. (2018). Red-blood-cell-mimetic gene delivery systems for long circulation and high transfection efficiency in ECs. *Journal of Materials Chemistry B*, *6*(37), 5975–5985.

[80] Singh, A. P., Biswas, A., Shukla, A., & Maiti, P. (2019). Targeted therapy in chronic diseases using nanomaterial-based drug delivery vehicles. *Signal Transduction and Targeted Therapy*, *4*, 33.

[81] Lee, S. H., Piao, H., Cho, Y. C., Kim, S. N., Choi, G., Kim, C. R., Ji, H. B., Park, C. G., Lee, C., Shin, C. I., Koh, W. G., Choy, Y. B., & Choy, J. H. (2019). Implantable multireservoir device with stimulus-responsive membrane for on-demand and pulsatile delivery of growth hormone. *Proceedings of the National Academy of Sciences of the United States of America*, *116*(24), 11664–11672.

[82] Mallakpour, S., Azadi, E., & Hussain, C. M. (2021). Recent advancements in synthesis and drug delivery utilization of polysaccharides-based nanocomposites: The important role of nanoparticles and layered double hydroxides. *International Journal of Biological Macromolecules*, *193*(Pt A), 183–204.

[83] Jain, K. K. (2008). Drug delivery systems-An overview. *Methods in Molecular Biology*, *437*, 1–50.
[84] Liu, D., Yang, F., Xiong, F., & Gu, N. (2016). The smart drug delivery system and its clinical potential. *Theranostics*, *6*(9), 1306–1323.
[85] Yi, Y., Buttner, U., & Foulds, I. G. (2015). A cyclically actuated electrolytic drug delivery device. *Lab on a Chip*, *15*(17), 3540–3548.
[86] Yi, Y., Chiao, M., & Wang, B. (2021). An electrochemically actuated drug delivery device with in-situ dosage sensing. *Smart Materials and Structures*, *30*(5), 055003.
[87] Jackson, J., Chen, A., Zhang, H., Burt, H., & Chiao, M. (2018). Design and near-infrared actuation of a gold nanorod-polymer microelectromechanical device for on-demand drug delivery. *Micromachines*, *9*(1), 28.
[88] Liu, R., & Poma, A. (2021). Advances in molecularly imprinted polymers as drug delivery systems. *Molecules (Basel, Switzerland)*, *26*(12), 3589
[89] McCarthy, P. C., Zhang, Y., & Abebe, F. (2021). Recent applications of dual-stimuli responsive chitosan hydrogel nanocomposites as drug delivery tools. *Molecules (Basel, Switzerland)*, *26*(16), 4735.
[90] Mura, S., Nicolas, J., & Couvreur, P. (2013). Stimuli-responsive nanocarriers for drug delivery. *Nature Materials*, *12*(11), 991–1003.
[91] Liang, J., Peng, X., Zhou, X., Zou, J., & Cheng, L. (2020). Emerging applications of drug delivery systems in oral infectious diseases prevention and treatment. *Molecules (Basel, Switzerland)*, *25*(3), 516.
[92] Benoit, D. S., Overby, C. T., Sims Jr, K. R., & Ackun-Farmmer, M. A. (2020). Drug delivery systems. In *Biomaterials Science*. Academic Press, pp. 1237–1266.
[93] Khan, M. S., & Roberts, M. S. (2018). Challenges and innovations of drug delivery in older age. *Advanced Drug Delivery Reviews*, *135*, 3–38.
[94] Shirsath, N. R., & Goswami, A. K. (2019). Nanocarriers based novel drug delivery as effective drug delivery: A review. *Current Nanomaterials*, *4*(2), 71–83.
[95] De Jong, W. H., & Borm, P. J. (2008). Drug delivery and nanoparticles: Applications and hazards. *International Journal of Nanomedicine*, *3*(2), 133–149.
[96] Rehman, S., Madni, A., Jameel, Q. A., Usman, F., Raza, M. R., Ahmad, F., Shoukat, H., Aali, H., & Shafiq, A. (2022). Natural polymer-based graphene oxide bio-nanocomposite hydrogel beads: Superstructures with advanced potentials for drug delivery. *AAPS PharmSciTech*, *23*(8), 304.
[97] Samiei Foroushani, M., Zahmatkeshan, A., Arkaban, H., Karimi Shervedani, R., & Kefayat, A. (2021). A drug delivery system based on nanocomposites constructed from metal-organic frameworks and Mn_3O_4 nanoparticles: Preparation and physicochemical characterization for BT-474 and MCF-7 cancer cells. *Colloids and Surfaces. B, Biointerfaces*, *202*, 111712.
[98] Salahuddin, N., Abdelwahab, M., Gaber, M., & Elneanaey, S. (2020). Synthesis and design of norfloxacin drug delivery system based on PLA/TiO_2 nanocomposites: Antibacterial and antitumor activities. *Materials Science & Engineering. C, Materials for Biological Applications*, *108*, 110337.
[99] Collado-González, M., Ferreri, M. C., Freitas, A. R., Santos, A. C., Ferreira, N. R., Carissimi, G., Sequeira, J. A. D., Díaz Baños, F. G., Villora, G., Veiga, F., & Ribeiro, A. (2020). Complex polysaccharide-based nanocomposites for oral insulin delivery. *Marine Drugs*, *18*(1), 55.
[100] Davaran, S., Alimirzalu, S., Nejati-Koshki, K., Nasrabadi, H. T., Akbarzadeh, A., Khandaghi, A. A., Abbasian, M., & Alimohammadi, S. (2014). Physicochemical characteristics of Fe_3O_4 magnetic nanocomposites based on Poly(N-isopropylacrylamide) for anti-cancer drug delivery. *Asian Pacific Journal of Cancer Prevention: APJCP*, *15*(1), 49–54.
[101] Singh, B., Kumari, A., Sharma, D., Dhiman, A., & Kumar, S. (2023). Fabricating gum polysaccharides based nano-composites for drug delivery uses via sustainable green approach. *International Journal of Biological Macromolecules*, *235*, 123856.
[102] Zhang, G., Li, X., Liao, Q., Liu, Y., Xi, K., Huang, W., & Jia, X. (2018). Water-dispersible PEG-curcumin/amine-functionalized covalent organic framework nanocomposites as smart carriers for in vivo drug delivery. *Nature Communications*, *9*(1), 2785.
[103] Rajan, M., Raj, V., Al-Arfaj, A. A., & Murugan, A. M. (2013). Hyaluronidase enzyme core-5-fluorouracil-loaded chitosan-PEG-gelatin polymer nanocomposites as targeted and controlled drug delivery vehicles. *International Journal of Pharmaceutics*, *453*(2), 514–522.
[104] Kalsoom Khan, A., Saba, A. U., Nawazish, S., Akhtar, F., Rashid, R., Mir, S., Nasir, B., Iqbal, F., Afzal, S., Pervaiz, F., & Murtaza, G. (2017). Carrageenan based bionanocomposites as drug delivery tool with special emphasis on the influence of ferromagnetic nanoparticles. *Oxidative Medicine and Cellular Longevity*, *2017*, 8158315.

[105] Niemirowicz, K., Markiewicz, K. H., Wilczewska, A. Z., & Car, H. (2012). Magnetic nanoparticles as new diagnostic tools in medicine. *Advances in Medical Sciences*, *57*(2), 196–207.

[106] Muthiah, M., Park, I. K., & Cho, C. S. (2013). Surface modification of iron oxide nanoparticles by biocompatible polymers for tissue imaging and targeting. *Biotechnology Advances*, *31*(8), 1224–1236.

[107] Wang, Y., & Huang, L. (2014). Composite nanoparticles for gene delivery. *Advances in Genetics*, 88, 111–137.

[108] Valencia, P. M., Farokhzad, O. C., Karnik, R., & Langer, R. (2020). Microfluidic technologies for accelerating the clinical translation of nanoparticles. *Nano-Enabled Medical Applications*, pp. 93–112. https://doi.org/10.1201/9780429399039-3

[109] Liu, K., Wang, H., Chen, K. J., Guo, F., Lin, W. Y., Chen, Y. C., … & Shen, C. K. (2010). A digital microfluidic droplet generator produces self-assembled supramolecular nanoparticles for targeted cell imaging. *Nanotechnology*, *21*(44), 445603.

[110] Rhee, M., Valencia, P. M., Rodriguez, M. I., Langer, R., Farokhzad, O. C., & Karnik, R. (2011). Synthesis of size-tunable polymeric nanoparticles enabled by 3D hydrodynamic flow focusing in single-layer microchannels. *Advanced Materials*, *23*(12), H79–H83.

[111] Valencia, P. M., Basto, P. A., Zhang, L., Rhee, M., Langer, R., Farokhzad, O. C., & Karnik, R. (2010). Single-step assembly of homogenous lipid– polymeric and lipid– quantum dot nanoparticles enabled by microfluidic rapid mixing. *ACS Nano*, *4*(3), 1671–1679.

[112] Deshmukh, P. K., Ramani, K. P., Singh, S. S., Tekade, A. R., Chatap, V. K., Patil, G. B., & Bari, S. B. (2013). Stimuli-sensitive layer-by-layer (LbL) self-assembly systems: Targeting and biosensory applications. *Journal of Controlled Release*, *166*(3), 294–306.

[113] Qiu, X., Donath, E. and Möhwald, H. (2001), Permeability of ibuprofen in various polyelectrolyte multilayers. *Macromolecular Materials and Engineering*, *286*, 591–597.

[114] De Villiers, M. M., Otto, D. P., Strydom, S. J., & Lvov, Y. M. (2011). Introduction to nanocoatings produced by layer-by-layer (LbL) self-assembly. *Advanced Drug Delivery Reviews*, *63*(9), 701–715.

[115] Wang, Y., Zhang, L., Guo, S., Hatefi, A., & Huang, L. (2013). Incorporation of histone derived recombinant protein for enhanced disassembly of core-membrane structured liposomal nanoparticles for efficient siRNA delivery. *Journal of Controlled Release: Official Journal of the Controlled Release Society*, 172(1), 179–189.

[116] Merkel, T. J., Herlihy, K. P., Nunes, J., Orgel, R. M., Rolland, J. P., & DeSimone, J. M. (2010). Scalable, shape-specific, top-down fabrication methods for the synthesis of engineered colloidal particles. *Langmuir*, *26*(16), 13086–13096.

[117] Rolland, J. P., Van Dam, R. M., Schorzman, D. A., Quake, S. R., & DeSimone, J. M. (2004). Solvent-resistant photocurable "liquid teflon" for microfluidic device fabrication. *Journal of the American Chemical Society*, *126*(8), 2322–2323.

[118] Qin, D., Xia, Y., & Whitesides, G. M. (2010). Soft lithography for micro-and nanoscale patterning. *Nature Protocols*, *5*(3), 491.

[119] Kelly, J. Y., & DeSimone, J. M. (2008). Shape-specific, monodisperse nano-molding of protein particles. *Journal of the American Chemical Society*, *130*(16), 5438–5439.

[120] Li, S. D., & Huang, L. Y. (1997). In vivo gene transfer via intravenous administration of cationic lipid–protamine–DNA (LPD) complexes. *Gene Therapy*, *4*(9), 891–900.

[121] Gao, X., & Huang, L. (1996). Potentiation of cationic liposome-mediated gene delivery by polycations. *Biochemistry*, *35*(3), 1027–1036.

[122] Li, S. D., Chono, S., & Huang, L. (2008). Efficient gene silencing in metastatic tumor by siRNA formulated in surface-modified nanoparticles. *Journal of Controlled Release*, *126*(1), 77–84.

[123] Shen, J., Kim, H. C., Su, H., Wang, F., Wolfram, J., Kirui, D., Mai, J., Mu, C., Ji, L. N., Mao, Z. W., & Shen, H. (2014). Cyclodextrin and polyethylenimine functionalized mesoporous silica nanoparticles for delivery of siRNA cancer therapeutics. *Theranostics*, 4(5), 487–497.

[124] Kim, M. H., Na, H. K., Kim, Y. K., Ryoo, S. R., Cho, H. S., Lee, K. E., Jeon, H., Ryoo, R., & Min, D. H. (2011). Facile synthesis of monodispersed mesoporous silica nanoparticles with ultralarge pores and their application in gene delivery. *ACS Nano*, *5*(5), 3568–3576.

[125] Liu, J., Stace-Naughton, A., Jiang, X., & Brinker, C. J. (2009). Porous nanoparticle supported lipid bilayers (protocells) as delivery vehicles. *Journal of the American Chemical Society*, *131*(4), 1354–1355.

[126] Ashley, C. E., Carnes, E. C., Phillips, G. K., Padilla, D., Durfee, P. N., Brown, P. A., Hanna, T. N., Liu, J., Phillips, B., Carter, M. B., Carroll, N. J., Jiang, X., Dunphy, D. R., Willman, C. L., Petsev, D. N., Evans, D. G., Parikh, A. N., Chackerian, B., Wharton, W., Peabody, D. S., … Brinker, C. J. (2011). The targeted delivery of multicomponent cargos to cancer cells by nanoporous particle-supported lipid bilayers. *Nature Materials*, *10*(5), 389–397.

[127] Yang, X. Z., Dou, S., Wang, Y. C., Long, H. Y., Xiong, M. H., Mao, C. Q., Yao, Y. D., & Wang, J. (2012). Single-step assembly of cationic lipid-polymer hybrid nanoparticles for systemic delivery of siRNA. *ACS Nano*, *6*(6), 4955–4965.

[128] Shi, J., Xiao, Z., Votruba, A. R., Vilos, C., & Farokhzad, O. C. (2011). Differentially charged hollow core/shell lipid-polymer-lipid hybrid nanoparticles for small interfering RNA delivery. *Angewandte Chemie (International ed. in English)*, *50*(31), 7027–7031.

[129] Hasan, W., Chu, K., Gullapalli, A., Dunn, S. S., Enlow, E. M., Luft, J. C., Tian, S., Napier, M. E., Pohlhaus, P. D., Rolland, J. P., & DeSimone, J. M. (2012). Delivery of multiple siRNAs using lipid-coated PLGA nanoparticles for treatment of prostate cancer. *Nano Letters*, *12*(1), 287–292.

[130] Gao, L. Y., Liu, X. Y., Chen, C. J., Wang, J. C., Feng, Q., Yu, M. Z., Ma, X. F., Pei, X. W., Niu, Y. J., Qiu, C., Pang, W. H., & Zhang, Q. (2014). Core-shell type lipid/rPAA-Chol polymer hybrid nanoparticles for in vivo siRNA delivery. *Biomaterials*, *35*(6), 2066–2078.

[131] Choi, C. H., Hao, L., Narayan, S. P., Auyeung, E., & Mirkin, C. A. (2013). Mechanism for the endocytosis of spherical nucleic acid nanoparticle conjugates. *Proceedings of the National Academy of Sciences of the United States of America*, *110*(19), 7625–7630.

[132] Rhim, W. K., Kim, J. S., & Nam, J. M. (2008). Lipid-gold-nanoparticle hybrid-based gene delivery. *Small (Weinheim an der Bergstrasse, Germany)*, *4*(10), 1651–1655.

[133] Kong, W. H., Bae, K. H., Jo, S. D., Kim, J. S., & Park, T. G. (2012). Cationic lipid-coated gold nanoparticles as efficient and non-cytotoxic intracellular siRNA delivery vehicles. *Pharmaceutical Research*, *29*(2), 362–374.

[134] Alhasan, A. H., Patel, P. C., Choi, C. H., & Mirkin, C. A. (2014). Exosome encased spherical nucleic acid gold nanoparticle conjugates as potent microRNA regulation agents. *Small (Weinheim an der Bergstrasse, Germany)*, *10*(1), 186–192.

[135] Jiang, S., Eltoukhy, A. A., Love, K. T., Langer, R., & Anderson, D. G. (2013). Lipidoid-coated iron oxide nanoparticles for efficient DNA and siRNA delivery. *Nano Letters*, *13*(3), 1059–1064.

[136] Yalcin, S. (2019). Dextran-coated iron oxide nanoparticle for delivery of miR-29a to breast cancer cell line. *Pharmaceutical Development and Technology*, *24*(8), 1032–1037.

9 Bionanocomposites in Biomarkers

Tanzeela Mariam, Fatima Tul Zahra, Muniza Shehzad, Farwa Munir, Farrukh Jawad Alvi, Basma Ellahi, Sarfaraz Ahmad, Nimra Idrees and Atif Amin Baig

9.1 INTRODUCTION

Bionanocomposites are materials that stand out later because of their remarkable properties and potential applications in different fields. These materials are made of matrix material, like polymers or ceramics, and nanoscale fillers, such as nanoparticles or nanotubes [1]. The subsequent bionanocomposites have improved mechanical, electrical, and thermal properties compared with their pure matrix counterparts. Bionanocomposites can be grouped in light of their network material, for example, polymer-based, ceramic-based, or metal-based bionanocomposites [2].

Bionanocomposites represent a new elegance of nanostructured hybrid materials. They consist of a combination of natural polymers and inorganic solids at least one nanometer in size [3]. Combining metal, semiconductor, carbon, and leading polymers (CPs) nanomaterials into biomaterials shows special electronic, photonic, and catalytic properties [4]. Throughout recent years, bionanomaterials has turned into a general term to designate the nanocomposites by interfacing enzymes, antibodies (antigens), or DNA and biopolymers with inorganic species [5]. These nanocomposites exhibit elite, recognizable proof and catalytic characteristics, working with the plan of novel biosensor platforms [6]. The biomaterials and bionanocomposite materials offer the key future building blocks for bionanomaterial architectures with the following fundamental features [7].

Biomarkers, a rapidly developing field of research, offer promising avenues for fabricating and synthesizing bionanocomposites. They are quantifiable marks of biological processes in the body and can be utilized to identify diseases, monitor disease prognosis, and evaluate therapy reactions. Nonetheless, the performance of biomarkers can be restricted by sensitivity, specificity, and stability. Bionanocomposites combine biopolymers with nanomaterials to create bio-inspired materials with enhanced properties and functionalities [8].

Biomarkers play a crucial role in biomedicine, as they provide valuable information about the physiological state of an organism. With advancements in nanotechnology, the development of bionanocomposites has emerged as a promising tool for detecting and analyzing biomarkers [9]. Biomarkers are measurable substances or characteristics that can be objectively evaluated and are essential in determining the presence or severity of a particular disease or physiological change. Due to the diverse nature of biomarkers, they are classified into various groups according to their molecular composition, function, or application [10].

Biomarkers are measurable substances or indicators that reflect normal biological processes, pathogenic processes, or responses to therapeutic interventions. They can be detected in bodily fluids, such as blood, urine, and saliva [11]. They can be categorized into different types based on their nature and purpose. These include genetic, proteomic, metabolic, and imaging biomarkers. Each type has its own set of challenges and advantages when it comes to biomarker research [12].

Bionanocomposites have uncommon mechanical strength and bioactivity, which makes them an important candidate for different tissue engineering and drug delivery applications. The

 DOI: 10.1201/9781003650812-9

one-of-a-kind blend of hard and delicate parts in a designed bionanocomposite resembles the combination of various parts in natural tissues [13]. Probably the best test in planning bionanocomposites for tissue recovery and biomedical applications is high mechanical strength combined with biocompatibility, bioactivity, and hierarchical structure of natural tissue [14]. A few biopolymers have been joined with nanofillers in various classifications, for example, silicate-based materials, clays, silica nanoparticles, ceramics such as nanohydroxyapatite, inorganic nanoparticles, engineered layered twofold hydroxides, carbon-based nanomaterials such as like carbon nanotubes, and metal/metal oxides [15]. Due to the remarkable mechanical properties of bionanocomposites, much interest lies in mirroring the bone structure, like dental implants and other orthopedic applications, as they consider staggered coordination of underlying material—organic properties comprised by the polymer and nanofiller blend [16]. Nanosized fillers in bionanocomposites make them appropriate for drug conveyance, as they generally present an agonizing dispersion way for typified little particles/drugs forming powerful boundaries and supported conveyance [17]. Moreover, drug-delivering bionanocomposites are exceptionally appropriate for wound dressing applications, as they have high water take-up and non-cytotoxicity together, high mucoadhesion, and tear obstruction, making them ideal as a wound dressing [14]. The advancements of bionanocomposites give new roads to satisfying specific requirements of the arising innovations in matrix formation, tissue recovery, drug conveyance, and wound dressing and will be instrumental in speeding up the development of new therapeutics [18].

9.2 BIOMARKER DISCOVERY AND VALIDATION

The discovery and validation of biomarkers are pivotal in the estimation of disease progression and inform the therapeutic treatment in the clinical settings. Closely examining scientific journals and articles, it becomes apparent that numerous techniques, such as genomics, proteomics, and metabolomics, are employed to identify potential biomarkers [19]. This progress holds the commitment to more accurate diagnostics, designated treatments, and improved prognosis. The excursion from biomarker discovery to clinical application requires a joint effort between scientists, clinicians, and administrative bodies to guarantee that these molecular insights convert into unmistakable advantages for patients and the medical healthcare system. However, the path to validation is challenging, requiring rigorous testing in large cohorts to ensure their reliability and clinical utility [20].

9.2.1 Types of Biomarkers

Biomarkers come in different structures, including proteins, nucleic acids (like DNA and RNA), lipids, metabolites, and cellular networks. They are often found in body fluids like blood, urine, saliva, and cerebrospinal liquid and inside tissues themselves [21]. These markers can be utilized for many purposes, including early disease detection, disease classification, monitoring treatment efficacy, and predicting patient outcomes. Understanding biomarkers' diverse nature, their potential applications can be better appreciated [22].

Biomarkers are essential in medical research and diagnostics, providing valuable insights into various diseases and conditions [23]. They are measurable indicators, often found in biological samples, that can be used to detect and monitor the progression of a disease, assess treatment efficacy, and predict patient outcomes. The meaning of biomarkers in clinical examination and practice is irrefutable. There are different types of biomarkers, each serving a specific purpose and providing unique information [24].

To comprehend the implications of bionanocomposites in biomarker development, it is essential to understand the different types of biomarkers. Biomarkers can be classified into various categories based on their origin, function, and structure [25]. Some common types include genetic, protein, imaging, and metabolomic biomarkers. Bionanocomposites have gained attention due to their unique properties and versatility in improving these biomarkers' sensitivity, selectivity, and stability [26].

9.2.1.1 Pharmacodynamic Biomarkers

These biomarkers provide information about the effects of a drug or other therapeutic intervention on an organism. These biomarkers are used to monitor the direct biological effects of therapies, such as drug-target engagement, target inhibition, or downstream pathway modulation [27]. Pharmacodynamic biomarkers help determine the optimal dosage and timing of drug administration for individual patients. They can help researchers understand the mechanism of action for new medications and determine optimal dosages or treatment durations. For instance, blood concentrations of a drug can guide safe dosage adjustments for achieving therapeutic success, including Ki67 expression levels in breast cancer patients undergoing treatment with aromatase inhibitors [28].

9.2.1.2 Predictive Biomarkers

Predictive biomarkers determine the likelihood of an individual's response to a specific therapy or treatment regimen. They are instrumental in developing personalized medicine strategies that tailor treatments based on individual patient characteristics [29]. One example is epidermal growth factor receptor (EGFR) mutations in non-small cell lung cancer patients associated with responsiveness to EGFR-targeted therapies [30].

Predictive biomarkers play a critical role in advancing personalized medicine by enabling the identification of individuals who are more likely to respond to specific treatments or develop certain diseases. In recent years, the emergence of bionanocomposites has revolutionized the field of predictive biomarkers, providing new avenues for diagnosis, prognosis, and therapeutic monitoring [31].

Understanding the fundamentals of predictive biomarkers and their significance in clinical practice is important. Predictive biomarkers are molecular indicators that can be measured objectively and reliably to predict a patient's response to a particular therapy or the likelihood of developing a specific disease [32]. By identifying individuals more likely to benefit from particular treatments or at an increased risk of certain diseases, clinicians can tailor interventions to individual patients, maximizing efficacy and minimizing side effects. This personalized approach to medicine has the potential to revolutionize patient care and improve outcomes [33].

Bionanocomposites, at the intersection of nanotechnology and biology, have shown immense promise as predictive biomarkers. These innovative materials combine the unique properties of nanoparticles with biological molecules, such as DNA or proteins, to create hybrid structures that exhibit enhanced diagnostic capabilities [34]. Bionanocomposites can be engineered to detect specific biomarkers, such as genetic mutations or protein expression levels, which are indicative of disease onset or treatment response. The ability to precisely measure and monitor these biomarkers in real time enables proactive interventions and personalized treatment strategies [35].

One of the key advantages of bionanocomposites as predictive biomarkers is their ability to provide clinical correlation. Integrating bionanocomposites with clinical data provides a comprehensive understanding of disease progression, treatment response, and patient outcomes. By analyzing the correlation between bionanocomposite-based biomarkers and clinical parameters, such as patient demographics, treatment modalities, and disease progression, researchers and clinicians can gain valuable insights into these biomarkers' predictive power and clinical relevance [36].

In summary, bionanocomposites offer a promising avenue for developing predictive biomarkers with clinical correlation. By combining nanotechnology with biology, these innovative materials enable the precise detection of biomarkers, facilitating personalized medicine and improving patient outcomes.

9.2.1.3 Safety Biomarkers

Safety biomarkers are indicators to evaluate adverse effects or toxicity associated with a particular treatment. Monitoring safety biomarkers allows for early identification and mitigation of potential patient harm, enhancing patient safety and optimizing treatment efficacy. An example of a safety biomarker is alanine aminotransferase (ALT), which can indicate elevated liver damage [32].

Safety biomarkers are essential in clinical medicine as they allow for the early detection and monitoring of various conditions and diseases. In recent years, there has been a growing interest in developing bionanocomposites as potential safety biomarkers due to their unique properties and potential clinical correlation [37].

Safety biomarkers play a crucial role in ensuring the well-being of patients by providing early indications of adverse effects and potential risks associated with therapeutic interventions [38]. These biomarkers can be used to evaluate the safety and efficacy of new drugs, diagnostics, and medical devices. By monitoring specific molecular signatures or physiological changes, safety biomarkers allow healthcare professionals to assess the impact of interventions on patient health and adjust treatment strategies accordingly [39].

Bionanocomposites have emerged as a promising platform for developing safety biomarkers in recent years. Bionanocomposites are nanoscale materials composed of biological and non-biological components, offering unique properties such as high stability, biocompatibility, and multifunctionality. These materials can be engineered to carry specific molecular markers or imaging agents, allowing for targeted and sensitive detection of disease-related biomarkers [40].

Clinical correlation is critical when considering safety biomarkers, as it determines the reliability and relevance of these markers in real-world medical settings. Bionanocomposites offer the opportunity for clinical correlation through their ability to interact with biological systems and produce measurable responses [41]. By designing bionanocomposites that target specific diseases or conditions, researchers can establish a strong correlation between the presence of these biomarkers and the underlying pathology. This correlation enhances safety biomarkers' diagnostic accuracy and predictive value, improving patient outcomes and personalized medicine approaches [42].

Safety biomarkers, particularly bionanocomposites, hold great potential in clinical medicine due to their unique properties and clinical correlation. These biomarkers allow for early detection, monitoring, and evaluation of therapeutic interventions, ensuring patient safety and optimizing treatment strategies. As researchers continue to explore the possibilities of bionanocomposites, it is crucial to investigate further their biocompatibility, long-term safety, and clinical applicability [43].

9.2.1.4 Monitoring Biomarkers

These types of biomarkers focus on tracking a disease progression or regression, providing valuable information for evaluating a chosen therapy's effectiveness and long-term outcomes. Identifying and successfully monitoring biomarkers play a crucial role in the early detection, diagnosis, and effective treatment of various diseases [44]. Biomarkers are measurable substances or indicators in the human body that reflect normal or pathological processes. Monitoring biomarkers can transform healthcare by enabling medical professionals to detect disease progression or response to therapy non-invasively and timely [45].

Bionanocomposites, a novel branch of nanotechnology, have shown great promise in biomarker monitoring. These materials possess unique properties such as high surface area, enhanced reactivity, and tunability, making them excellent candidates for biomarker detection and analysis [46]. By incorporating bionanocomposites into diagnostic assays, researchers can further improve the sensitivity and selectivity of biomarker detection, thereby allowing for earlier and more accurate disease diagnosis [47].

The scientific literature reveals many studies demonstrating the potential of bionanocomposites in clinical biomarker monitoring. For example, nanoparticles functionalized with specific antibodies have been used to detect cancer biomarkers in patient samples with remarkable accuracy [48]. Additionally, bionanocomposite-based biosensors have been developed to detect cardiac biomarkers, aiding in the early diagnosis of heart disease. These findings highlight the versatility and efficacy of bionanocomposites in various disease-monitoring applications [46].

9.2.1.5 Nucleic Acid-Based Biomarkers

One type of biomarker commonly used in bionanocomposites is nucleic acid-based biomarkers. These biomarkers, such as DNA or RNA, offer immense potential in molecular diagnostics (Hasnat et al., 2023). They can be utilized to detect specific genetic mutations or alterations associated with various diseases, including cancer. By incorporating nucleic acid-based biomarkers into bionanocomposites, researchers can develop highly sensitive and specific diagnostic tools, enabling early detection and personalized treatment strategies [49].

In conjunction with bionanocomposites, nucleic acid biomarkers have exhibited a remarkable potential to revolutionize clinical diagnostics. Their correlation opens new horizons for early disease detection, personalized medicine, and precise treatment monitoring [50]. However, several challenges, including standardization, regulatory obstacles, and ethical concerns, must be addressed to unlock their clinical utility fully. Despite these challenges, ongoing research and technological advancements promise a bright future for bionanocomposite-assisted nucleic acid biomarkers in healthcare settings.

In recent years, nucleic acid biomarkers have gained significant attention in personalized medicine. The ability to analyze an individual's genetic makeup has opened up new avenues for targeted therapies and precision medicine [51]. Healthcare professionals can make accurate diagnoses and develop personalized treatment plans by identifying specific nucleic acid biomarkers associated with certain diseases [52].

Nucleic acid biomarkers offer valuable insights into genetic variations, gene expression patterns, and disease progression. They play a significant role in personalized medicine and contribute to the development of targeted therapies [53].

9.2.1.6 Challenges and Limitations

1. Standardizing and validating bionanocomposite-based assays for clinical use [54].
2. Ethical considerations surrounding the implementation of nucleic acid biomarkers and bionanocomposites in patient care [55].
3. Regulatory hurdles and commercialization barriers in translating bionanocomposites into clinical settings [56].

9.2.1.7 Future Prospects and Implications

1. Promising innovations and advancements in bionanocomposite technology for improved nucleic acid biomarker analysis [57].
2. Integration of artificial intelligence and machine learning algorithms for efficient nucleic acid biomarker detection using bionanocomposites [58].
3. Potential applications of bionanocomposites in non-invasive diagnostics and point-of-care testing [59].

9.2.1.8 Protein-Based Biomarkers

Another type of biomarker frequently employed in bionanocomposites is protein-based biomarkers. Proteins are vital in numerous biological processes and often indicate specific diseases or conditions [60]. By incorporating protein-based biomarkers into bionanocomposites, researchers can develop diagnostic platforms capable of detecting and quantifying these proteins with high precision [61].

Protein-based biomarkers are essential tools in medical research and clinical diagnostics. These biomarkers serve as indicators of various physiological and pathological processes, aiding in identifying and monitoring diseases [62]. These biomarkers can be found in bodily fluids such as blood, urine, and cerebrospinal fluid. Protein biomarkers play a crucial role in disease diagnosis and prognosis. For example, prostate-specific antigen (PSA) is a protein biomarker to detect and monitor prostate cancer [63].

The use of protein-based biomarkers in healthcare has revolutionized the diagnosis and treatment of numerous diseases. One prominent example is the detection of tumor-specific antigens in cancer patients. These biomarkers can provide valuable information on cancer progression, treatment response, and prognosis [64].

Protein-based biomarkers play a vital role in medical research and clinical diagnostics. They offer valuable insights into detecting, monitoring, and managing various diseases [65].

9.2.1.9 Cellular Biomarkers

Cellular biomarkers (specific to certain cells or cell types) also hold great promise in bionanocomposites. Researchers can create innovative and personalized diagnostic tools by incorporating cells, such as circulating tumor cells or immune cells, into bionanocomposite platforms [66]. These biomarkers can be used to identify and characterize different cell populations in tissues or fluids. These cellular biomarkers offer valuable insights into cellular processes, disease progression, and treatment response, enhancing our understanding of diseases, particularly useful in cancer research, as they can help classify tumors and predict treatment responses, enabling more effective therapeutic interventions [67].

9.2.1.10 Metabolic Biomarkers

Metabolic biomarkers play a significant role in understanding and monitoring various metabolic pathways and disorders. These biomarkers are measurable indicators of the physiological state of an organism and provide valuable insights into metabolic processes, such as energy production, nutrient utilization, and waste elimination [68]. Metabolic biomarkers, on the other hand, provide insights into metabolic pathways and biochemical processes occurring in the body. These biomarkers can be measured in blood or urine samples and help diagnose and manage metabolic disorders such as diabetes and cardiovascular diseases (CVDs) [69].

Metabolic biomarkers are molecules or compounds that reflect specific metabolic activities in the body. They can be found in various biological samples, including blood, urine, and tissue extract [70]. These biomarkers are often identified through advanced analytical techniques, such as metabolomics, which comprehensively analyze small molecules present in biological systems [71].

Metabolic biomarkers have proven to be invaluable in clinical research. They can provide early detection of metabolic dysfunctions, enabling timely interventions and treatment strategies [72]. For instance, abnormal levels of specific biomarkers, such as glucose or insulin, can indicate the presence of diabetes or pre-diabetic conditions. By monitoring these biomarkers, clinicians can implement appropriate lifestyle modifications, prescribe medications, and prevent disease progression [73].

Moreover, metabolic biomarkers have expanded the possibilities of personalized medicine. With the advancements in genomic technologies, it is now possible to analyze an individual's genetic makeup and identify specific biomarkers associated with certain metabolic pathways [74]. This information can facilitate the development of tailored treatment plans, optimizing patient care and outcomes [75]. For example, identifying genetic biomarkers can help determine an individual's response to specific medications, allowing healthcare providers to select the most effective therapeutic options [37].

The use of metabolic biomarkers extends beyond clinical settings. Researchers and pharmaceutical companies utilize biomarker profiling to evaluate the efficacy of drugs and interventions during clinical trials [76]. Researchers can assess drug metabolism, toxicity, and therapeutic effectiveness by monitoring changes in biomarker levels. This information is crucial in drug development, patient safety, and drug therapy optimization [77].

Metabolic biomarkers are powerful tools that provide valuable insights into metabolic processes, aid in early disease detection, and drive advancements in personalized medicine. These biomarkers, identified through various analytical techniques, allow for more targeted and practical clinical research and practice interventions [78]. As further research continues to uncover new biomarkers and refine measurement techniques, their potential applications will expand, promising exciting opportunities for improved healthcare and disease management.

9.2.1.11 Imaging Biomarkers

Imaging biomarkers are vital in medical imaging as they provide essential information about various diseases and conditions. These biomarkers are objective measures obtained from different imaging modalities, such as magnetic resonance imaging (MRI), computed tomography (CT), or positron emission tomography (PET). They help diagnose, monitor, and predict the progression and response to treatment of various diseases [79].

One of the primary applications of imaging biomarkers is in oncology, where they are used for cancer detection, staging, and treatment response evaluation [80]. For example, in breast cancer, imaging biomarkers like tumor size, lymph node involvement, and the presence of distant metastases are essential for determining the stage of the disease and planning appropriate treatment strategies. Additionally, biomarkers like tumor vascularity and metabolic activity can provide valuable insights into the tumor's aggressiveness and potential response to therapy [81].

Neurology also extensively utilizes imaging biomarkers to study and characterize various neurological disorders. In conditions like Alzheimer's, biomarkers like brain atrophy, amyloid plaque accumulation, and glucose metabolism changes can aid in early diagnosis and disease monitoring [82]. These biomarkers help researchers and clinicians understand the underlying pathology and develop targeted therapeutic interventions [83].

In cardiovascular imaging, biomarkers such as coronary artery calcium score and myocardial perfusion can assist in assessing the risk of cardiovascular events and determining appropriate interventions. These biomarkers provide valuable information about the integrity and function of the heart and blood vessels, aiding in diagnosing and managing CVDs [84].

The use of imaging biomarkers extends beyond traditional medical specialties. In musculoskeletal imaging, biomarkers like bone mineral density and muscle volume can help evaluate the effects of aging, disease, and treatment on the musculoskeletal system. These biomarkers enable clinicians to assess bone strength, muscle mass, and overall functional capacity, guiding treatment decisions and interventions [85].

Overall, imaging biomarkers revolutionize medicine by providing objective and quantitative measures of disease burden, treatment response, and prognosis. They enhance diagnostic accuracy, facilitate personalized medicine, and contribute to developing novel therapeutic approaches. As the field of medical imaging continues to advance, the discovery and validation of new imaging biomarkers hold immense potential to revolutionize patient care and improve outcomes [86].

9.2.1.12 Cardiovascular Biomarkers

CVDs are a main source of morbidity and mortality worldwide. Early findings and successful administration of CVDs are essential for working on persistent results and lessening healthcare costs. Cardiovascular biomarkers have arisen as significant instruments for disease determination, risk delineation, and treatment checking [87, 88].

Cardiovascular biomarkers are quantifiable marks of biological processes that mirror the presence or seriousness of CVDs. These biomarkers can be arranged into various classifications in view of their origin, capability, and clinical utility. For instance, cardiovascular troponins are biomarkers of myocardial injury and are broadly utilized to determine acute myocardial infarction (AMI). Brain natriuretic peptide (BNP) and N-terminal pro-BNP (NT-proBNP) [88].

9.2.1.13 Troponin Detection

Troponin biomarkers are a crucial tool for diagnosing and prognosing various cardiac conditions. These biomarkers are proteins released into the bloodstream when cardiac muscle cells are damaged [89]. By measuring the troponin levels in a patient's blood, healthcare professionals can assess the extent of cardiac injury and determine the appropriate treatment course [90].

In the correlation between troponin levels and the severity of myocardial infarction, higher troponin levels indicate larger infarct sizes and increased mortality rates. This information can greatly aid in risk stratification and decision-making in clinical practice [91].

Furthermore, troponin biomarkers have demonstrated great accuracy and sensitivity in diagnosing acute coronary syndromes, such as unstable angina and myocardial infarction [92]. Troponin assays have consistently shown high diagnostic accuracy, especially when combined with other clinical and electrocardiographic findings [93].

In addition to their diagnostic value, troponin biomarkers also have prognostic significance. The predictive role of troponin levels in heart failure patients revealed that elevated troponin levels are strongly associated with adverse outcomes, including increased hospitalizations and mortality rates [94]. Accordingly, monitoring troponin levels can assist healthcare professionals in evaluating the effectiveness of therapeutic interventions and adjusting treatment plans accordingly [95].

To summarize, troponin biomarkers play a crucial role in cardiology. These proteins, released into the bloodstream during cardiac injury, provide valuable information regarding various cardiac conditions' diagnosis, prognosis, and risk stratification [96]. Through the extensive use of high-sensitivity troponin assays and their correlation with clinical and electrocardiographic findings, healthcare professionals can effectively manage patients and optimize treatment outcomes [97].

9.2.1.14 Lipid Profiling

Bionanocomposites work with the recognition of lipid biomarkers related to cardiovascular infections. By coordinating lipid-restricting proteins with nanoparticles, they empower the measurement of lipid concentrations, supporting risk assessment and disease management [98].

Lipid profiling biomarkers are essential tools for diagnosing and monitoring various diseases. These biomarkers are specific lipid molecules that can be detected and quantified in biological samples such as blood or tissue. By analyzing the lipid profile, clinicians can gain valuable insights into the patient's metabolic health and identify potential risk factors for disease development [99].

The importance of lipid profiling biomarkers lies in their ability to provide a comprehensive overview of an individual's lipid metabolism. Lipids play diverse roles in our bodies, including serving as energy sources, structural components of cell membranes, and signaling molecules [100]. Any imbalance or alteration in lipid metabolism can profoundly affect overall health and contribute to the development of certain diseases, such as cardiovascular disorders, diabetes, and obesity [101].

Scientists and clinicians rely on advanced technologies and methods to accurately analyze lipid profiles. Mass spectrometry and liquid chromatography are commonly used techniques that identify and quantify individual lipid species within a sample [102]. These techniques provide valuable data on lipid composition, saturation levels, and molecular structure, allowing for a more detailed understanding of lipid-related diseases [103].

Lipid profiling biomarkers have revolutionized the diagnosis and monitoring of diseases by providing valuable insights into an individual's lipid metabolism. Through the analysis of lipid profiles, clinicians can identify potential risk factors, enabling timely intervention and personalized treatment strategies [104].

9.2.1.15 Molecular Biomarkers

Molecular biomarkers are classified on the basis of their application such as diagnostic biomarkers, staging biomarkers, diagnostic biomarkers.

Biomarkers are used to monitor the onset and progression of disease or the effectiveness of treatment. The best biomarkers for this purpose should be specific to a particular form of cancer (Figure 9.1) and not be found in healthy people or normal tissues. The most common method for determining cancer biomarkers is measuring biomolecule concentrations such as proteins, peptides, biochemicals, DNA, and RNA.

9.2.1.15.1 Genetic Biomarkers

One type of biomarker is genetic biomarkers derived from an individual's genetic material. These biomarkers include genetic mutations, polymorphisms, and gene expression profiles that can be

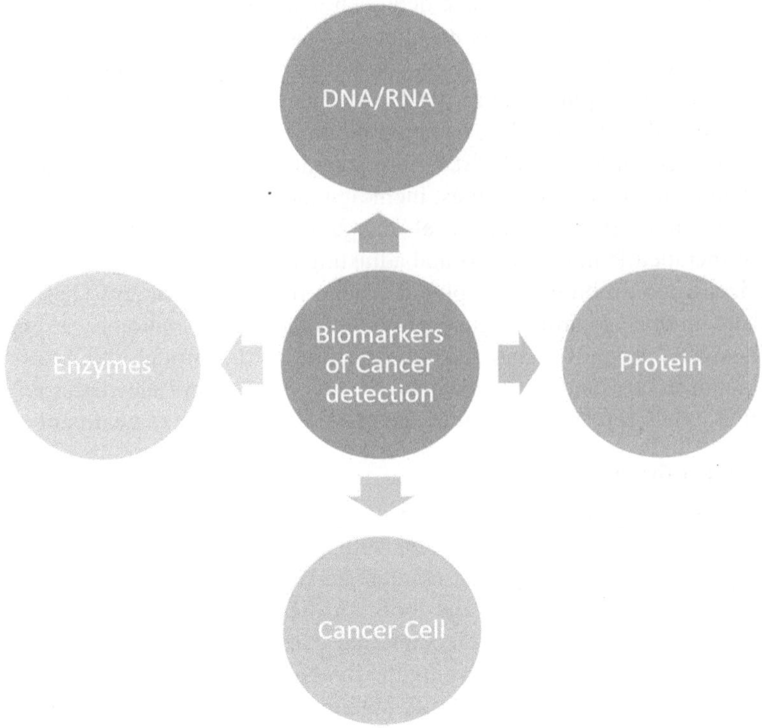

FIGURE 9.1 Biomarkers of cancer detection.

associated with specific diseases or conditions [105]. Genetic biomarkers have revolutionized personalized medicine, allowing targeted therapies based on an individual's genetic makeup [106, 107].

Genetic biomarkers consist of DNA sequences altered or mutated due to environmental factors or genetic predisposition. Examples include single nucleotide polymorphisms (SNPs), microRNAs (miRNAs), and copy number variations (CNVs). Also, mutations in the BRCA1 and BRCA2 genes are associated with a higher risk for breast and ovarian cancers. Preventative measures can be implemented by identifying high-risk populations through genomic markers [108].

A genetic biomarker is a measurable indicator found in an individual's genetic material that can be used to identify or predict various biological traits or disease conditions to understand the underlying principles of genetic biomarkers [109]. These biomarkers are specific DNA sequences or genetic variations associated with certain characteristics or conditions. They can be classified into different types, such as SNPs, CNVs, or structural variants [110].

Genetic biomarkers are crucial in various areas of genetics research and clinical practice. One of their critical applications is in the field of personalized medicine [111]. By analyzing an individual's genetic profile, researchers can identify biomarkers associated with drug response, disease susceptibility, or the likelihood of developing certain conditions. This information can then be used to tailor treatment plans and interventions to each patient's specific needs, leading to more effective and personalized healthcare [112].

Moreover, genetic biomarkers have proven to be invaluable in the early detection and prevention of diseases. By identifying biomarkers indicative of a particular condition, healthcare professionals can screen individuals at risk and initiate proactive measures to mitigate the development or progression of the disease [113]. This has significant implications for the individual and the healthcare system, as early detection often leads to better outcomes and reduced healthcare costs [114].

Furthermore, genetic biomarkers have contributed to understanding complex genetic traits and disorders. Researchers can identify biomarkers associated with specific traits or conditions by analyzing large datasets and combining information from genetic studies [115]. This knowledge enhances our understanding of the underlying genetic mechanisms and opens avenues for developing targeted therapies and interventions [116].

To further explore the concept of genetic biomarkers, it is essential to consult reliable and up-to-date scientific journals. These sources will provide in-depth information about the latest research findings, methodologies, and applications of genetic biomarkers [117]. By reviewing relevant literature, researchers and healthcare professionals can stay informed about the advancements in the field and make informed decisions regarding the use of genetic biomarkers in their respective disciplines [111].

Genetic biomarkers hold immense potential in the field of genetics and medicine. Their ability to identify and predict various biological traits or disease conditions has revolutionized personalized medicine, early detection, and our understanding of complex genetic traits [118].

9.2.1.15.2 Epigenetic Biomarkers

These biomarkers involve changes in gene expression that do not affect the underlying DNA sequence (e.g., DNA methylation and histone modifications). Epigenetic modifications might be associated with cancer and neurodegenerative disorders [119].

Epigenetic biomarkers are a crucial area of study in genetics and genomics. These biomarkers are significant in regulating gene expression and have been recognized as important indicators of various diseases and conditions [120]. It is essential to understand the basic principles of epigenetics. Epigenetics refers to the study of heritable changes in gene expression that do not involve alterations in the DNA sequence itself [121]. Instead, epigenetic modifications involve modifications to the DNA structure or the associated proteins, thus influencing gene activity. These modifications can be influenced by both genetic and environmental factors, making them an intriguing field to explore [122].

Epigenetic biomarkers, in particular, are specific epigenetic modifications that can indicate various biological processes and disease states. These biomarkers can be found in different biological samples, such as blood, saliva, or tissues [123]. They provide valuable insights into the molecular mechanisms of diseases, potentially leading to earlier detection, improved diagnosis, and personalized treatment strategies [124].

One area where epigenetic biomarkers have shown great potential is cancer research. DNA methylation, a common epigenetic modification, has been associated with various types of cancer, including breast, lung, and colorectal cancer [125]. By studying specific DNA methylation patterns in cancer cells, researchers can identify potential biomarkers that can aid in cancer diagnosis, prognosis, and treatment selection. These biomarkers can also provide information about the therapy response, helping tailor treatment plans for individual patients [126].

Apart from cancer, epigenetic biomarkers have also been implicated in neurological disorders, CVD, and other conditions. Identifying and validating these biomarkers can contribute to a better understanding of disease mechanisms, uncover potential therapeutic targets, and ultimately improve patient outcomes [127].

Epigenetic biomarkers represent a fascinating area of study within genetics and genomics. These biomarkers have significant implications for diagnosing, treating, and understanding various diseases [128]. Through extensive research and technological advancements, epigenetic biomarkers hold great potential to revolutionize personalized medicine. By harnessing the power of epigenetic modifications, researchers can unlock new insights into disease mechanisms and develop targeted therapies for improved patient care [129].

9.2.1.15.3 Proteomic Biomarkers

Proteomic biomarkers are proteins or peptides that reflect specific cellular processes associated with a disease state or physiological change. They are often used as diagnostic tools for cancer. For example, the PSA test is a well-known proteomic biomarker for early cancer detection [130].

Proteomic biomarkers are molecules that can be found in biological specimens and are indicative of various diseases or conditions. These biomarkers hold great potential in diagnostics and can provide valuable insight into the underlying mechanisms of diseases and aid in developing targeted therapies [131].

To understand the concept of proteomic biomarkers, it is essential first to grasp the fundamentals of proteomics. Proteomics studies the entire set of proteins an organism, tissue, or cell expresses at a given time. It involves identifying, quantifying, and functionalizing proteins in different biological contexts [132].

Identifying proteomic biomarkers usually involves using high-throughput techniques such as mass spectrometry or protein microarrays. These methods allow for the simultaneous analysis of many proteins, providing comprehensive data on protein expression and modification patterns [133].

One of the primary applications of proteomic biomarkers is in the field of clinical diagnostics. Researchers can identify specific biomarkers associated with certain diseases or conditions by analyzing the protein profiles in biological samples [134]. For example, elevated levels of a particular protein may indicate the presence of cancer, while a decrease in the expression of another protein may suggest the onset of neurodegenerative disorders [135].

Proteomic biomarkers have emerged as potent tools in diagnostics and personalized medicine. These biomarkers offer valuable information on disease diagnosis, prognosis, and therapeutic response by analyzing protein expression profiles [136]. With the continuous advancements in proteomic technologies and the availability of scientific knowledge through journals, the identification and validation of biomarkers will continue to contribute to the advancement of medical research and patient care [137].

9.2.1.15.4 Transcriptomic Biomarkers

Transcriptomic biomarkers involve the study of gene expression patterns (mRNA) as indicators of function or dysfunction. A prominent example of a transcriptomic biomarker is the Oncotype DX test for early-stage breast cancer patients [138]. This test analyzes the expression patterns of 21 genes to determine the probability of cancer recurrence and the need for chemotherapy treatment [139].

A transcriptomic biomarker is a type of biomarker that is derived from the analysis of gene expression patterns in an organism. It involves the study of the transcriptome, which is the complete set of RNA molecules produced by an organism's genome [140]. Transcriptomic biomarkers provide valuable insights into the functional state of cells, tissues, and organisms and have numerous applications in basic research and clinical settings [31].

One of the key advantages of transcriptomic biomarkers is their ability to reflect the dynamic nature of gene expression. By analyzing changes in gene expression levels, researchers can gain a deeper understanding of biological processes and identify potential targets for therapeutic interventions [141]. For example, in cancer research, transcriptomic biomarkers can classify tumors into different subtypes, predict treatment responses, and monitor disease progression [142].

Researchers rely on various high-throughput technologies, such as microarray analysis and RNA sequencing, to study transcriptomic biomarkers. These techniques enable the simultaneous measurement of thousands of genes, providing a comprehensive view of gene expression patterns [143]. In addition to these experimental approaches, bioinformatics tools, and computational algorithms are used to analyze and interpret transcriptomic data. These tools help researchers identify differentially expressed genes, perform functional enrichment analysis, and construct gene regulatory networks [144].

In recent years, transcriptomic biomarkers have gained increasing attention in precision medicine. By analyzing gene expression profiles, clinicians can identify patients more likely to respond to certain treatments or develop specific diseases [145]. This personalized approach allows for more targeted and effective therapies, minimizing side effects and improving patient outcomes. Moreover, transcriptomic biomarkers have the potential to revolutionize the field of diagnostics, enabling early detection and accurate diagnosis of diseases [146].

In conclusion, transcriptomic biomarkers offer a powerful tool for understanding gene expression patterns and their implications in various biological processes. By leveraging high-throughput technologies and bioinformatics tools, researchers can uncover valuable insights that can be applied in basic and clinical research [147]. The use of transcriptomic biomarkers in precision medicine holds great promise for improving patient care and driving advancements in personalized therapies. As the field continues to evolve, staying updated with the latest scientific findings and technological advancements is essential to harness the full potential of transcriptomic biomarkers [148].

9.2.1.16 Role of Bionanocomposites in Biomarker Development

Biomarkers play a critical role in identifying and diagnosing diseases. However, their detection and quantification can often be challenging due to their low abundance levels. In recent years, nanotechnology has emerged as a promising approach to improving the sensitivity and reliability of biomarker detection [149].

Bionanocomposites show uncommon sensing mechanisms and signal amplification because of their high surface region, increased binding sites, and productive electron movement. These traits empower the identification of biomarkers at super-low focuses, adding to early disease detection and monitoring [3].

9.2.1.17 Sensing Mechanisms

Bionanocomposites have stood out lately because of their unique properties and likely applications in different fields, including biomedical engineering [150]. These materials are made from a blend of natural and nanomaterials, which bring about original properties that can be taken advantage of for different applications. One of the most encouraging uses of bionanocomposites is their utilization as sensing systems for identifying biomarkers [151].

In the realm of biomarker improvements, bionanocomposites have shown tremendous potential. Biomarkers are measurable indicators of biological states or conditions, and their accurate detection plays a crucial role in medical diagnosis, disease monitoring, and personalized medicine [45]. However, traditional biomarker detection methods often face sensitivity, specificity, and real-time monitoring limitations [152].

By incorporating nanoparticles into bionanocomposites, researchers have developed sensing mechanisms that overcome these limitations. These nanoparticles provide unique optical, electrical, and magnetic properties that can be finely tuned for specific biomarkers [153]. Combining biological components and nanoparticles enables the bionanocomposites to interact with and detect biomarkers with high precision and sensitivity [46].

One example of a sensing mechanism in bionanocomposites is using gold nanoparticles. These nanoparticles can be functionalized with specific biological molecules, such as antibodies or aptamers, that selectively bind to target biomarkers [154]. When the biomarker interacts with the functionalized gold nanoparticles, a detectable signal is generated, which can be quantified and analyzed [155].

Incorporating bionanocomposites in biomarker improvements also opens up new possibilities for real-time monitoring. Traditional biomarker detection methods often involve time-consuming and labor-intensive processes [156]. In contrast, bionanocomposite-based sensing mechanisms can provide rapid and on-site detection, allowing for more efficient and timely medical interventions [157].

In summary, bionanocomposites offer a promising avenue for biomarker improvements through their unique sensing mechanisms. Researchers can develop highly sensitive, specific, and real-time detection systems by combining biological components with nanoparticles [158].

9.2.1.18 Signal Amplification

Incorporating metallic nanoparticles into bionanocomposites has shown substantial improvements in signal amplification. Metallic nanoparticles, such as gold nanoparticles, possess unique optical properties that enhance signal generation and detection [154]. This intensification upgrades the sensitivity and accuracy of biomarker detection, even inside complex biological matrices [159]. Additionally, the surface chemistry of these nanoparticles can be modified to selectively bind with specific biomarkers, further enhancing their detection specificity [160].

Another noteworthy study highlights the importance of bionanocomposite design in achieving optimal signal amplification. By carefully engineering the composition and structure of bionanocomposites, researchers have successfully achieved susceptible and selective detection of biomarkers [161]. Nanomaterials, such as carbon nanotubes and quantum dots, have been extensively investigated for their signal amplification capabilities [162].

9.2.1.19 Biomarkers in Disease Diagnosis

One of the primary applications of biomarkers lies in disease diagnosis. They are useful in detecting diseases early when clinical symptoms are not apparent [163]. Examples include blood glucose levels for diabetes mellitus diagnosis and PSA levels for prostate cancer detection as its well-known diagnostic biomarker [164]. Moreover, scientific journals and articles provide evidence of the successful implementation of biomarkers in various diseases, including cancer, cardiovascular disorders, and neurological conditions [165]. For instance, carcinoembryonic antigen (CEA) has been widely utilized as a biomarker in diagnosing colorectal cancer, exhibiting high sensitivity and specificity [166].

9.2.1.20 Biomarkers in Prognosis and Treatment Monitoring

Biomarkers are also crucial in predicting disease outcomes and monitoring treatment efficacy. Prognostic biomarkers predict the likelihood of disease progression or recurrence and help clinicians determine the most appropriate treatment plan, allowing for timely intervention and improving patient outcomes [167]. These biomarkers help assess the likely course of disease in patients diagnosed with the condition. Prognostic biomarkers consider disease stage, aggressiveness, and potential responsiveness to treatment [168]. For example, PSA is widely used as a biomarker for prostate cancer prognosis and monitoring treatment effectiveness. Some common examples are the presence of specific gene mutations in cancer patients that indicate a higher risk of metastasis or poor survival rates, including estrogen receptor status in breast cancer patients and tumor grade in colon cancer patients [169].

9.2.1.21 Personalized Medicine

Personalized medicine, or precision medicine, is a progressive way to deal with healthcare that tailors clinical decisions and mediations to the individual characteristics of every patient [170]. This approach perceives that every individual's genetic makeup, way of living, and environmental factors are important in deciding their response to disease and therapeutic agents [171]. Biomarkers, which are quantifiable signs of biological processes, have arisen as fundamental apparatuses in the field of personalized medicine. They empower healthcare professionals to distinguish, analyze, and treat diseases successfully by giving insights into an individual's unique biological characteristics [172].

By investigating a patient's genetic and molecular profile, medical services suppliers can fit therapies to match the individual's unique characteristics, improving the probability of progress and lessening adverse effects [173].

Utilizing personalized medicine in biomarkers has significantly advanced our understanding and management of various diseases [174]. By identifying specific biomarkers associated with particular disease states, healthcare practitioners can better assess an individual's risk of developing certain conditions. For example, genetic biomarkers can help identify individuals predisposed to inheritable diseases, allowing for proactive interventions or preventive measures [175].

In summary, personalized medicine in biomarkers has transformed the healthcare industry by offering tailored and precise treatment plans for individual patients. Using biomarkers allows healthcare practitioners to make accurate diagnoses, predict disease outcomes, and design personalized interventions [176].

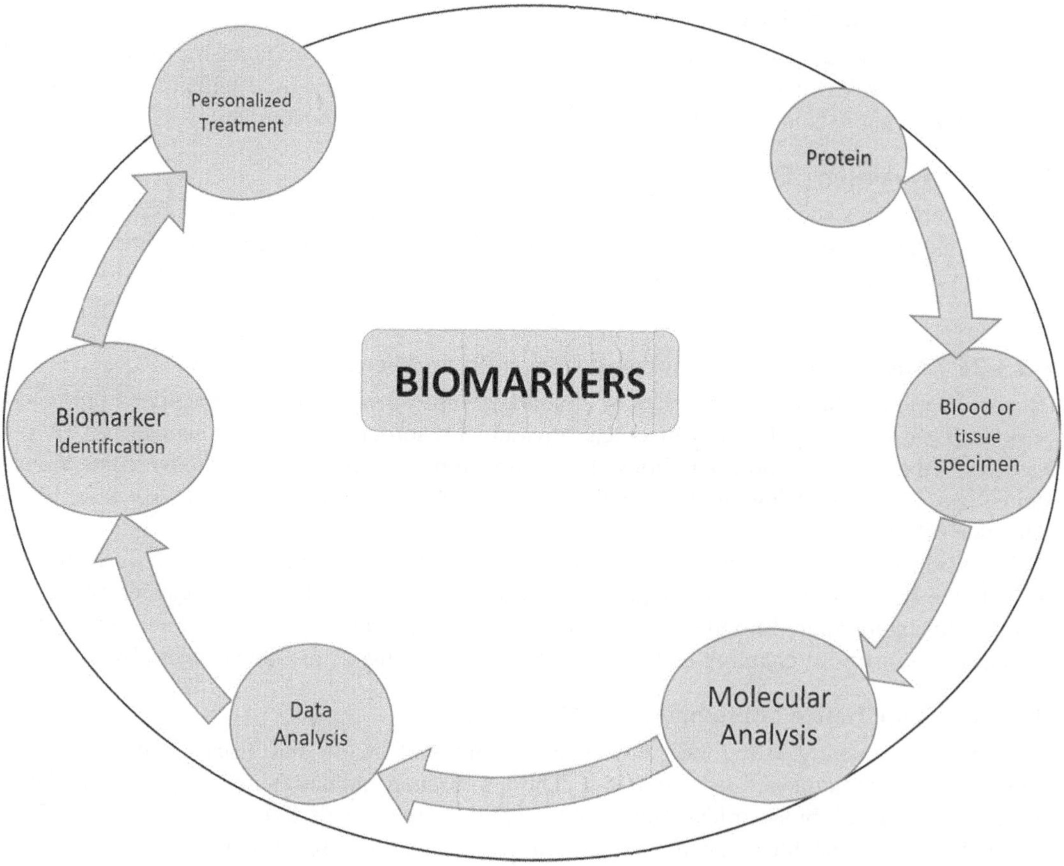

FIGURE 9.2 Biomarker testing.

For biomarker testing, a sample of cells from tumor is required (Figure 9.2). It can be collected by biopsy (tissue specimen) or blood. When the samples have been collected, they are sent to a pathologist, a doctor who focuses on examining cells to identify disease. Specific treatment alternatives may be considered when a certain trait is discovered through thorough biomarker testing.

9.2.1.22 Treatment Monitoring

Bionanocomposites help with checking treatment adequacy by identifying biomarkers characteristic of therapeutic reaction. For example, they can be utilized to measure levels of explicit proteins or nucleic acids, mirroring the adequacy of targeted therapies [177].

9.2.1.23 Neurological Disorders

Neurological disorders envelop an expansive scope of conditions that influence the sensory system, including the brain, spinal cord, and peripheral nerves [178]. These disorders can prompt different cognitive, sensory, and motor impairments. Early and accurate diagnosis of neurological disorders is critical for viable administration and treatment [178]. Biomarkers, quantifiable signs of biological processes, are essential in diagnosing and observing these disorders. Bionanocomposites, a mix of nanomaterials and biological components, are extraordinarily committed to upgrading the sensitivity and specificity of biomarker-based diagnostics for neurological issues [179].

9.2.1.24 Alzheimer's Disease

Bionanocomposites are used to recognize biomarkers related to neurodegenerative problems like Alzheimer's disease. Functionalized nanoparticles can tie to beta-amyloid plaques, which are normal for Alzheimer's, empowering harmless imaging and early diagnosis [180].

9.2.1.25 Parkinson's Disease

Bionanocomposites add to the recognizable proof of biomarkers for Parkinson's disease, including alpha-synuclein aggregates. Nanoparticles functionalized with antibodies well defined for alpha-synuclein work with detecting these aggregates, supporting early-stage diagnosis and disease monitoring [181].

9.2.1.26 Application of Bionanocomposites in Biomarker Improvements

The application of bionanocomposites in biomarker improvements holds tremendous promise for various disease areas, including cancer, cardiovascular disorders, and infectious diseases [25]. By harnessing the amplification capabilities of bionanocomposites, researchers can overcome the limitations associated with low-abundance biomarkers, enabling earlier and more accurate disease detection [182].

For instance, in a study conducted by Ratajczak et al. (2020), bionanocomposites were utilized to amplify the signals from PSA, a biomarker commonly associated with prostate cancer. By incorporating gold nanoparticles into the bionanocomposite, the study achieved a remarkable enhancement in detection sensitivity, enabling early diagnosis and monitoring of prostate cancer [183].

9.2.1.27 Importance of Biomarkers in Healthcare

Biomarkers, frequently called the "molecular signatures of health and disease," are fundamental apparatuses in medicine and research [184]. These molecular indicators give important knowledge of the physiological, biochemical, and pathological processes inside living organisms. Biomarkers are vital in modern healthcare, enabling early disease detection, diagnosis, and prognosis [44].

Biomarkers, measurable and quantifiable indicators of biological processes, are crucial in diagnosing diseases, monitoring treatment effectiveness, and predicting patient outcomes [185]. Biomarkers are measurable substances or indicators found in blood, urine, or tissues that can offer valuable insights into various physiological processes and abnormalities. Hence, the importance of biomarkers in healthcare cannot be overstated [186].

9.2.2 Nanotechnology and Bionanocomposites

Nanotechnology, manipulating matter on an atomic and molecular scale, has emerged as a revolutionary field of study with promising applications in various sectors. It refers to the science, engineering, and application of materials at the nanoscale, typically between 1 and 100 nanometers [187]. It has recently gained significant attention and recognition due to its potential capabilities in various fields, including medicine, electronics, and energy. One particularly intriguing aspect of nanotechnology is its integration with the field of bionanocomposites [188]. Bionanocomposites, which combine biological components with nanomaterials, hold immense potential for advancing fundamental concepts, making significant impacts, and unlocking new clinical applications in biomarker research [189].

9.2.2.1 Fundamental Concepts

The concept of bionanocomposites revolves around the fundamental principles of nanotechnology and biomaterial science. Nanoscale materials exhibit distinct properties compared to their bulk counterparts, such as high surface area, quantum confinement, and superior mechanical strength. These characteristics can be leveraged to enhance the performance of biological materials when integrated into composites [190]. Biopolymers, derived from renewable sources, are the matrix material in bionanocomposites. These polymers possess unique mechanical, thermal, and biological properties, making them desirable for various applications.

Meanwhile, nanomaterials, such as nanoparticles and nanofibers, are incorporated into the biopolymer matrix to enhance specific properties like mechanical strength, electrical conductivity, and drug delivery capabilities [191]. By incorporating nanoscale materials, such as nanoparticles, nanotubes, or nanofibers, with biological macromolecules like proteins, polysaccharides, or DNA, researchers can create bionanocomposites with unique properties tailored for specific applications [192]. For example, for tissue engineering scaffolds, bionanocomposites can be engineered to exhibit improved biocompatibility, drug delivery capabilities, or enhanced mechanical strength. This unique combination allows for harnessing the desirable properties of both entities, creating hybrid materials with enhanced functionalities [193]. The fundamental understanding of how these materials interact and their synthesis methods form the basis for developing bionanocomposites. The interaction between the biopolymer and nanomaterials plays a pivotal role in determining the overall performance of the bionanocomposites [194].

9.2.2.2 Impacts

The impact of bionanocomposites spans various fields, ranging from medicine to environmental sustainability. In materials science, bionanocomposites offer a renewable and eco-friendly alternative to traditional materials [195]. Their enhanced properties make them suitable for various applications, including packaging materials, sensors, membranes, and biomedical devices. Bionanocomposites have demonstrated immense potential in drug delivery systems, tissue engineering, and diagnostic applications in the medical field [196]. By incorporating nanoparticles or nanofibers into biologically compatible matrices, researchers have enhanced drug delivery efficiency, promoted tissue regeneration, and improved diagnostic techniques [197]. Moreover, the environmental sector has also experienced the ripple effects of bionanocomposites, with innovations in water purification, pollutant removal, and renewable energy. Bionanocomposites have proven highly effective in removing contaminants from water sources and catalyzing chemical reactions to produce sustainable energy [198]. Furthermore, biocompatibility and mechanical robustness in bionanocomposites provide new opportunities in tissue engineering and regenerative medicine. By mimicking the structure and properties of native tissues, bionanocomposites hold great potential in promoting tissue repair and regeneration [199].

9.2.2.3 Clinical Applications

The clinical applications of bionanocomposites are particularly intriguing as they offer novel approaches to address pressing healthcare challenges. Controlled drug release systems based on bionanocomposites offer personalized medicine approaches with improved therapeutic outcomes [2]. The ability to modulate drug release rates by manipulating the biopolymer matrix and nanomaterial properties opens new doors for targeted and sustained drug delivery [199]. Additionally, bionanocomposites with antibacterial properties can combat microbial infections, reducing the risk of complications in various medical procedures. The versatility of bionanocomposites also allows for the development of bioactive coatings on implantable devices, promoting better integration and reducing the likelihood of rejection [200].

Clinical applications of bionanocomposites are also becoming increasingly prevalent. For instance, nanocomposites fabricate dental restorations that closely resemble natural teeth in color and strength [201]. Therefore, bionanocomposites are being explored for their antimicrobial properties, which can help combat infections and improve the success rate of implants and prosthetics [202].

The utilization of bionanocomposites has significant impacts across different fields. In materials science, the development of bionanocomposites has opened doors for creating lightweight and high-strength materials [198]. These materials can revolutionize the aerospace, automotive, and construction industries by providing stronger and more durable components [203].

In the medical field, bionanocomposites have shown great promise in drug delivery systems, tissue engineering, and bioimaging. The ability to precisely control the release of drugs through nanoscale carriers has revolutionized drug therapy, making treatments more targeted and effective [55]. Furthermore, bionanocomposites can be engineered to mimic the structure and functionality of natural tissues, enabling the creation of artificial organs and scaffolds for tissue regeneration [2].

In the end, nanotechnology has opened up new avenues for developing bionanocomposites with remarkable properties. Researchers have created materials with enhanced mechanical, electrical, and biocompatible properties by integrating biological macromolecules with nanoscale materials [204]. These advancements can potentially impact several fields, including biomedicine, electronics, and energy. Using bionanocomposites in clinical applications holds great promise for improving patient care and personalized medicine. Scientific research and advancements in this field continue to unlock new possibilities, offering a promising future for bionanocomposites [205].

9.2.2.4 Challenges and Future Perspectives

Despite their immense potential, the utilization of biomarkers in personalized medicine faces challenges, for example, standardization of testing strategies, approval of biomarker utility, and protection concerns connected with genetic information. Moreover, improving multilayered biomarker profiles integrating genetic, genomic, proteomic, and different information is an area of continuous exploration [206].

9.2.3 Bionanocomposites as Biomarkers

Bionanocomposites, a combination of biomaterials and nanoparticles, are emerging as potential biomarkers in healthcare. These nanocomposites possess unique physical and chemical properties that enhance their detectability and specificity [192]. The nanoparticles used in bionanocomposites can be metallic, magnetic, or polymeric and are functionalized with biomolecules such as antibodies or DNA aptamers. By utilizing these bionanocomposites, the detection and quantification of biomarkers can be achieved with exceptional precision [207]. By engineering bionanocomposites, researchers can develop highly sensitive and selective biomarkers for various diseases, such as cancer, cardiovascular disorders, and infectious diseases [208].

Bionanocomposites have a few properties that make them suitable for biomarker applications. First and foremost, they show improved sensitivity and selectivity for target biomolecules [209]. This is because of the great surface area-to-volume proportion of nanoparticles, which empowers a higher number of biomolecules to collaborate with the surface of the composite. Furthermore, the surface of the nanoparticles can be functionalized with specific ligands to capture and distinguish target biomolecules selectively.

Bionanocomposites refer to hybrid materials made of nanomaterials (for instance, nanoparticles) and biological molecules (like antibodies, proteins, or DNA) [210].

The applications of bionanocomposites in neurological disorder diagnosis are early recognition and treatment of Alzheimer's disease, Parkinson's disease, and multiple sclerosis [211].

9.2.3.1 Fundamental Concepts of Bionanocomposites in Biomarker Development

The development of bionanocomposites as biomarkers involves several fundamental concepts. First, it is crucial to understand the physicochemical properties of nanoparticles and their interactions with biomaterials [212]. This knowledge aids in designing bionanocomposites that combine biological components with nanoscale materials, enhancing properties and functionalities. These innovative materials have transformed the field of biomarkers by providing more accurate and sensitive detection methods [213]. Second, selecting appropriate biomarkers for specific diseases is essential for accurate diagnosis and targeted therapy. Lastly, integrating bionanocomposites with advanced detection techniques, such as nanosensors and imaging modalities, enables real-time monitoring of

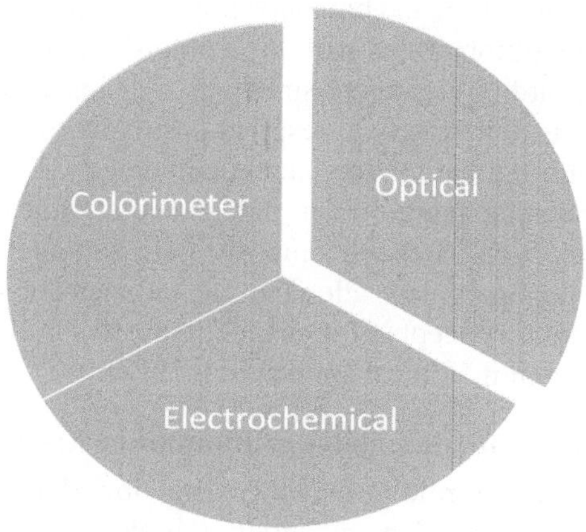

FIGURE 9.3 Characterization of bionanocomposites.

biomarkers in clinical settings. The biocompatibility and biodegradability of bionanocomposites make them suitable for biomedical applications [192].

The success of bionanocomposites in biomarker research lies in their ability to bind to target biomarkers and amplify detection signals specifically. For instance, by immobilizing nanoparticle antibodies, bionanocomposites facilitate the recognition and binding of specific biomarkers, leading to highly sensitive detection. Moreover, the incorporation of different types of nanoparticles enables multivariate analysis, allowing simultaneous detection of multiple biomarkers within a single assay [9].

Bionanocomposites are created when biodegradable biopolymers and nanofibrils (NFs) extensively interweave (Figure 9.3). Biopolymers serve as the matrix, and NFs act as reinforcement. As a result, robust, ecologically friendly materials are produced for various uses, including packaging and biomedical fields.

9.2.3.2 Impacts of Bionanocomposites in Healthcare

The utilization of bionanocomposites as biomarkers has significant impacts on healthcare. First, these biomarkers enable the early detection of diseases, leading to timely interventions and improved treatment outcomes. Second, bionanocomposites facilitate personalized medicine by enabling the selection of targeted therapies based on individual patient characteristics [211]. Moreover, these biomarkers aid in monitoring treatment response and disease progression, ensuring timely adjustments in treatment plans. Integrating bionanocomposites into clinical practice ultimately enhances patient care and promotes better healthcare outcomes [214].

The impacts of bionanocomposites in biomarker research are far-reaching. For instance, these materials allow for detecting biomarkers at extremely low concentrations, opening up possibilities for early disease diagnosis. Furthermore, bionanocomposites can be engineered to bind selectively to specific biomarkers, leading to improved specificity in diagnostic tests [215].

9.2.3.3 Clinical Applications of Bionanocomposites as Biomarkers

Bionanocomposites have found clinical applications in various fields of medicine. These biomarkers detect cancer-specific genetic mutations in oncology and facilitate personalized treatment selection. In cardiology, bionanocomposites aid in the early detection of cardiac biomarkers, allowing for timely interventions and prevention of adverse cardiac events. Additionally, bionanocomposites can detect specific pathogen biomarkers in infectious disease management, enabling rapid and accurate diagnosis [216].

In clinical applications, biomarkers and bionanocomposites work hand in hand to improve patient care. With the ability to detect biomarkers with high precision, healthcare professionals can make more informed decisions regarding treatment strategies. For instance, biomarker-based diagnostic tests can help identify patients more likely to respond positively to a particular treatment, minimizing unnecessary interventions and optimizing patient outcomes [214].

One specific area of biomarker research that has gained significant attention is using bionanocomposites in biomarker detection. Bionanocomposites are nanomaterials reinforced with biologically active molecules or nanoparticles, allowing for enhanced biomarker sensing capabilities. Understanding the fundamental concepts of bionanocomposites in biomarker detection is essential for unlocking their full potential in clinical applications [217].

9.2.3.4 Advantages of Bionanocomposites in Biomarker Research

Biomarker research plays a crucial role in the early detection, diagnosis, and treatment of various diseases. Bionanocomposites, defined as integrating biological and nanoscale materials, offer numerous advantages that enhance biomarker research [218]. One of the key advantages of bionanocomposites in biomarker research is their enhanced sensitivity. Incorporating nanoparticles into biological matrices allows for improved detection and quantification of biomarkers [219]. Nanoparticles possess unique physical and chemical properties, such as high surface area-to-volume ratio and surface plasmonic resonance, which enable them to interact efficiently with target biomolecules. This heightened sensitivity facilitates the early detection of diseases, enabling timely and effective interventions [158].

Furthermore, bionanocomposites offer enhanced selectivity in biomarker research. The surface functionalization of nanoparticles with specific ligands or antibodies allows for the selective binding and identification of target biomarkers [220]. By tailoring the surface properties of bionanocomposites, researchers can create highly specific and sensitive biosensors. This selectivity minimizes false-positive results and improves the accuracy of biomarker detection, leading to more reliable diagnostics and personalized medicine approaches [192].

Bionanocomposites also possess excellent stability and durability. Combining biological and nanoscale materials results in a robust and long-lasting platform for biomarker research. This stability ensures consistent performance and reproducibility of results over extended periods [192]. Moreover, bionanocomposites can withstand harsh experimental conditions, making them suitable for various applications in clinical settings.

In addition to these advantages, bionanocomposites offer versatility in terms of their fabrication and functionalization. Researchers can customize the composition, size, and shape of bionanocomposites to suit specific biomarker research needs [147]. This adaptability allows for the development of diverse sensing platforms, including electrochemical sensors, optical sensors, and MRI contrast agents. Bionanocomposites can also be integrated into various biomedical devices, such as lab-on-a-chip systems and implantable biosensors, further expanding their clinical applications [192].

Fundamentally, bionanocomposites are designed to harness the unique properties of both biological molecules and nanomaterials. By combining the specificity and selectivity of biomolecules with the enhanced properties of nanomaterials, such as high surface area and conductivity, researchers can develop innovative approaches for biomarker detection and quantification. Using bionanocomposites enables precise and sensitive analysis, overcoming many limitations associated with traditional biomarker research techniques [221].

Bionanocomposites possess unique optical, electrical, and magnetic properties, which can be exploited for various diagnostic and therapeutic applications. For instance, nanomaterials integrated into bionanocomposites can act as labels or probes, enabling visualization and tracking of biomarkers within biological samples. This capability opens new avenues for non-invasive disease progression monitoring and treatment efficacy assessment [39].

9.2.3.5 Challenges and Future Perspectives

While the capability of bionanocomposites in neurological disorder biomarker detection is encouraging, there are challenges to address, including regulatory approval, standardization of tests, and potential toxicity of nanomaterials. Also, investigating the advancement of painless strategies for biomarker identification utilizing bionanocomposites is an exciting path [222].

9.2.4 Fabrication and Synthesis of Bionanocomposites

Bionanocomposites, as the name suggests, are composite materials composed of biological elements and nanomaterials. The fabrication and synthesis of bionanocomposites have garnered significant attention in recent years due to their potential applications in various fields, including biomarker technology [150]. It is crucial to delve into the concept to understand the fabrication and synthesis of bionanocomposites. Bionanocomposites combine biological materials, such as proteins, DNA, or cells, with nanomaterials, such as nanoparticles or nanofibers. The aim is to harness the advantageous properties of both components and create a material with enhanced functionality and performance [192].

Several methods exist for the fabrication and synthesis of bionanocomposites. One widely used approach involves bottom-up assembly, where the nanomaterials are carefully integrated with the biological components [223]. This might be achieved through layer-by-layer assembly, where alternating nanomaterials and biomolecules are deposited, creating a multilayered structure. Other methods include self-assembly, where the constituents spontaneously arrange themselves into a desired structure, and template-assisted synthesis, where the biological components are deposited onto a pre-existing template [224].

The fabrication process of bionanocomposites involves the dispersion of nanomaterials within the matrix material, followed by a series of steps to achieve a homogeneous distribution. Various techniques, such as solution blending, melt compounding, and in situ polymerization, have been employed to fabricate bionanocomposites with tailored properties [209]. The choice of fabrication method depends on factors such as the final product's desired properties, scalability, and cost-effectiveness [225].

The synthesis of bionanocomposites involves the preparation of nanomaterials and their subsequent incorporation into the matrix material. Nanoparticles, for instance, can be synthesized through various techniques, including the sol-gel method, hydrothermal synthesis, or chemical vapor deposition. Once synthesized, these nanoparticles are mixed with the matrix material to form bionanocomposites [226].

The choice of fabrication method depends on several factors, including the desired properties of the bionanocomposite, the intended application, and the compatibility of the materials used. Furthermore, proper characterization techniques, such as transmission electron microscopy and spectroscopy, are employed to analyze the structure and properties of the fabricated bionanocomposites [227].

The impacts of bionanocomposites on biomarkers are significant and far-reaching. By combining the unique properties of nanomaterials with the biological functionality of biomolecules, bionanocomposites hold immense potential for diagnostic and therapeutic applications [228]. For instance, bionanocomposites can be tailored to deliver drugs to specific sites in the body, enhancing efficacy and minimizing side effects. Additionally, they can be utilized for targeted imaging and sensing, allowing for early disease detection and accurate monitoring of treatment progress [229].

In the clinical realm, bionanocomposites have shown immense potential in regenerative medicine, tissue engineering, and biosensing. Incorporating biological components into nanomaterials provides a platform for developing advanced biomarkers to reorganize healthcare practices. From 3D-printed scaffolds for tissue regeneration to biosensors for rapid disease diagnosis, the potential applications of bionanocomposites are vast and exciting [230]. The unique properties of these materials, such as tunable optical and magnetic properties, have paved the way for advanced bioimaging techniques, such as MRI and fluorescence imaging. Additionally, bionanocomposites have been used in biosensors to detect diseases, toxins, and biomarkers, enabling early diagnosis and personalized medicine [231].

The fabrication and synthesis of bionanocomposites have opened up new avenues in biomarker technology. Combining biological elements with nanomaterials has resulted in materials with exceptional properties and functionalities. From tissue engineering to drug delivery and clinical diagnostics, bionanocomposites have demonstrated their significance in various applications [43].

9.2.4.1 Bionanocomposites Based on Biosensors for Biomarker Detection

Bionanocomposites, a combination of biological and nanomaterial components, have gained significant attention in biosensors for biomarker detection and biosensing technology. To understand the significance of bionanocomposites in biomarker detection, it is essential first to define biosensors [232]. Biosensors are scientific devices incorporating a biological recognition component with a physicochemical transducer to recognize and evaluate explicit analytes. In the case of bionanocomposites, the recognition element is typically a biomolecule, such as an antibody or DNA aptamer, which specifically binds to the target biomarker of interest [233]. Conversely, the transducer converts the binding event into a measurable signal, often using nanomaterials such as carbon nanotubes or quantum dots. With the increasing demand for rapid and accurate biomarker detection in various fields, including medical diagnostics and environmental monitoring, the development of bionanocomposites-based biosensors holds great potential [234]. This interdisciplinary research area combines the principles of biology, nanotechnology, and materials science to develop innovative strategies for detecting and analyzing biomarkers by combining the specificity of biological recognition elements and the enhanced transduction capabilities of nanomaterials [225]. Integrating biomaterials and nanotechnology has created highly sensitive and selective biosensors that can detect and quantify biomarkers with high precision and accuracy. These biosensors have the potential to revolutionize the field of biomarker detection by providing real-time and non-invasive monitoring of various diseases and conditions, leading to improved healthcare and environmental analysis [235].

An integrated receptor-transducer device known as a biosensor "can provide selective quantitative or semi-quantitative analytical information using a biological recognition element." These are divided into many categories based on the transducer used or the type of biological recognition components used, such as colorimetric, optical, and electrochemical biosensors.

9.2.4.2 Advantages of Biosensors

Bionanocomposites have found various applications in biomarker detection, revolutionizing disease diagnosis and monitoring. For example, in cancer diagnostics, bionanocomposites detect specific protein biomarkers, allowing early detection and precise monitoring of tumor progression [236]. Similarly, in infectious disease diagnostics, bionanocomposites enable the rapid and sensitive detection of pathogenic agents, facilitating timely and targeted treatment. Furthermore, bionanocomposites have been utilized in detecting cardiac biomarkers, neurodegenerative disease markers, and environmental pollutants, showcasing their versatility in diverse fields [237, 238]. The incorporation of nanoparticles enhances the surface area of the biosensor, facilitating increased biomolecule immobilization, improving sensor sensitivity, and enabling the detection of biomarkers at low concentrations, and the hybrid structure of bionanocomposites ensures the stability and biocompatibility of biosensors, ensuring long-term performance and minimizing false-positive results [238].

To begin with, bionanocomposites offer several advantages in biosensing applications. Integrating biological elements such as enzymes, antibodies, or nucleic acids with nanomaterials provides enhanced sensitivity, selectivity, and stability [239]. These attributes are crucial for accurately detecting and quantifying biomarkers, indicators of various physiological and pathological conditions. Biosensors based on bionanocomposites can be tailored to specific targets, making them ideal for early disease diagnosis, drug screening, and environmental monitoring [240].

The integration of nanomaterials into bionanocomposites offers several advantages in terms of signal transduction. Nanomaterials, with their unique optical, electrical, and magnetic properties, can facilitate signal amplification, leading to improved sensitivity and detection limits [241]. For example, noble metal nanoparticles exhibit localized surface plasmon resonance, which generates a highly detectable signal upon binding to biomarkers. Carbon-based nanomaterials, such as graphene or carbon nanotubes, possess excellent electrical conductivity, enabling direct electrical readouts of biomarker binding events [242].

One of the key advantages of using bionanocomposites in biosensors is their high surface area-to-volume ratio. This enhances the interaction between the biomarker of interest and the sensing elements, improving sensitivity. Furthermore, the composition and structure of bionanocomposites can be tailored to achieve optimal sensing performance, making them highly versatile in detecting a wide range of biomarkers [192].

9.2.4.3 Challenges in Bionanocomposites-Based Biosensors

Despite their immense potential, bionanocomposites-based biosensors face challenges that must be addressed. First, the nanomaterial-biomolecule interface needs careful optimization to ensure effective immobilization and minimize nonspecific binding, which could lead to false-positive results [243]. Additionally, the synthesis and functionalization of nanomaterials require expertise in nanotechnology and may involve costly and time-consuming processes. Furthermore, the long-term stability and biocompatibility of bionanocomposites need to be thoroughly investigated to ensure their reliability and safety for practical applications [244].

However, using bionanocomposites in biosensors for biomarker detection also presents certain challenges. One of the major challenges is properly integrating the biosensing elements into the composite matrix while maintaining their bioactivity. Any loss or alteration of the sensing elements' activity can significantly impact the sensor's performance [245]. Therefore, carefully selecting compatible materials and fabrication techniques is crucial to ensure the integrity and functionality of the biosensing platform [246].

9.2.5 Applications of Bionanocomposites in Early Disease Detection

Bionanocomposites, composed of biological and nanomaterial components, have emerged as a promising technology in early disease detection [49]. By incorporating nanomaterials into the composite matrix, these materials exhibit enhanced properties, such as improved sensitivity and selectivity, making them ideal for early disease detection. This innovative approach utilizes nanomaterials' unique properties to enhance diagnostic tests' sensitivity and specificity, preparing for further developed medical services results. By integrating biological molecules with nanoparticles, bionanocomposites offer a wide range of applications in the early detection of diseases such as cancer, cardiovascular disorders, and infectious diseases. In recent years, scientific research has focused on utilizing bionanocomposites for medical diagnostics, particularly in detecting diseases at their earliest stages [247].

Bionanocomposites, imaginative hybrid materials containing biological molecules and nanomaterials, stand out in different fields, especially biomarker applications. Biomarkers, quantifiable signs of biological processes or conditions, are crucial in disease diagnosis, prognosis, and therapeutic observation [248]. Utilizing the exceptional properties of bionanocomposites, scientists have opened many utilizations in the domain of biomarkers, going from malignant growth diagnostics to irresistible disease monitoring and neurodegenerative disorder detection. This exposition investigates the different utilizations of bionanocomposites in biomarkers, featuring their effect on healthcare and personalized medicine [211].

Bionanocomposites have introduced another period of biomarker applications, offering extraordinary open doors in disease discovery, treatment observation, and personalized medicine. Their versatility, sensitivity, and specificity enable analysts and clinicians to foster creative analytic stages

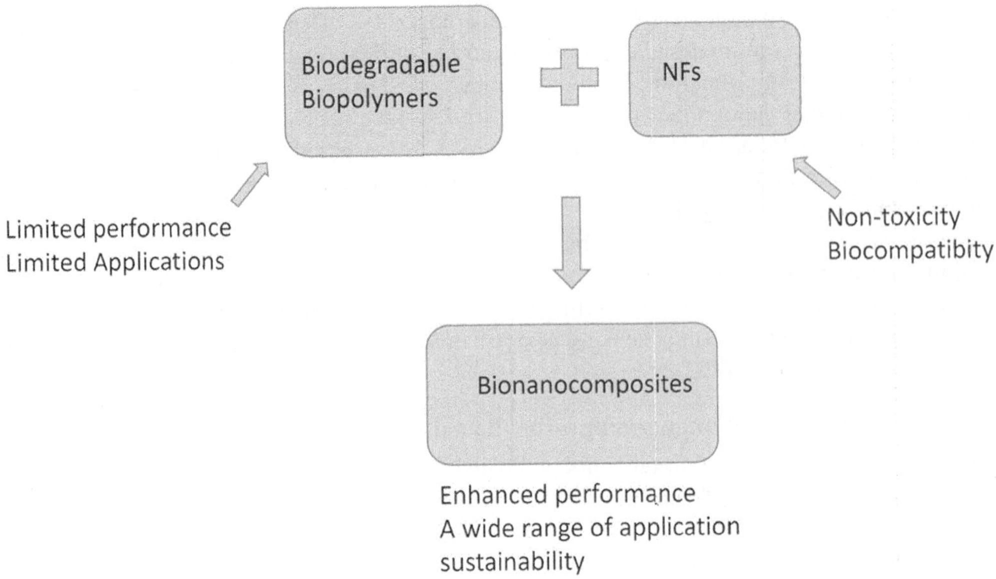

FIGURE 9.4 Applications of biomarkers.

above traditional limitations. As these applications keep on advancing, bionanocomposites hold the possibility to alter healthcare, work on persistent results, and add to the acknowledgment of the accuracy of medication's maximum capacity [249].

Biomarkers play a pivotal role in early disease detection, clinical diagnosis, prediction of disease, risk assessment, grading tumors, monitoring vaccine efficacy, staging cancer, disease prognosis, and many more (Figure 9.4).

9.2.5.1 Disease Diagnostics and Therapeutics

9.2.5.1.1 Early Detection

Bionanocomposites assume a basic part in improving early disease discovery. By forming growth-explicit antibodies with nanoparticles, they make delicate biosensors for distinguishing disease-related antigens in blood, urine, or tissue tests. These biosensors empower the analysis of malignant growth at its beginning stages, considering ideal mediation and working on prognosis [250].

9.2.5.1.2 Circulating Tumor Cells (CTCs)

The discovery of CTCs, shed by essential growths into the circulatory system, helps check disease movement and treatment reaction. Bionanocomposites furnished with attractive nanoparticles work with the separation and enhancement of CTCs from blood tests. This segregation empowers downstream examination, like genetic profiling, offering valuable insights into tumor heterogeneity and metastasis potential [251].

9.2.5.1.3 Therapeutic Delivery

Bionanocomposites act as vehicles for designated drug delivery to cancer cells. Functionalized nanoparticles stacked with restorative specialists can be intended to specifically tie to disease cells and deliver drugs in light of explicit upgrades, limiting off-target impacts and improving treatment adequacy [252].

9.2.5.2 Infectious Disease Monitoring

9.2.5.2.1 *Point-of-Care Diagnostics*

Bionanocomposites add to the advancement of fast, point-of-care symptomatic stages for irresistible infections. By coordinating biological recognition components with nanoparticles, these stages empower sensitive and specific detection of microorganisms, viruses, and microbial biomarkers in understanding examples, empowering timely diagnosis and control of outbreaks [253].

9.2.5.2.2 *Multiplex Detection*

Irresistible infections frequently include the presence of numerous microbes. Bionanocomposite-based multiplex measures grant the synchronous discovery of different biomarkers, working with the ID of co-diseases and giving thorough symptomatic data in a solitary examination [254].

9.2.5.2.3 *Antimicrobial Treatment*

Bionanocomposites can be utilized in antimicrobial treatment by filling in as transporters for antimicrobial specialists or improving the antimicrobial properties of existing medications. This approach offers the possibility to battle drug-safe microbes and upgrade antitoxins viability [255].

In summary, bionanocomposites offer tremendous potential in the early detection of diseases by combining the unique properties of nanomaterials with the specificity of biological molecules [256]. Integrating bionanocomposites with advanced technologies and the extensive research reported in scientific journals underscore their significance in improving healthcare outcomes. By harnessing the power of bionanocomposites, we can pave the way for more accurate and timely disease diagnosis, ultimately leading to improved patient care and better overall health outcomes [257].

9.2.5.2.4 *Application*

One of the critical applications of bionanocomposites in early disease detection is the development of targeted drug delivery systems. Bionanocomposites can be functionalized with ligands or targeting agents that specifically recognize and bind to diseased cells or tissues [3]. This allows for the selective delivery of drugs to the affected areas, minimizing side effects and improving the efficacy of the treatment. Furthermore, bionanocomposites can be designed to release the drugs in a controlled manner, ensuring sustained drug release and long-lasting therapeutic effects [258].

Moreover, bionanocomposites can also be used in early disease detection imaging techniques. By incorporating nanomaterials with imaging capabilities, such as quantum dots or iron oxide nanoparticles, into the composite matrix, researchers can develop contrast agents for various imaging modalities, including CT, MRI, and fluorescence imaging [259]. These bionanocomposite-based contrast agents can provide enhanced imaging resolution and sensitivity, allowing for the early detection and characterization of diseases [260].

One notable application of bionanocomposites in early disease detection is their use in biosensors. Bionanocomposites, with enhanced properties such as high surface area and biocompatibility, can be incorporated into biosensors to improve their sensitivity and selectivity. For example, nanoparticles of silver or gold can be embedded in a polymer matrix to create a bionanocomposite film that enhances the signal transduction and detection limits of biosensors [261]. This allows for the early detection of disease-specific biomarkers, enabling timely intervention and improved treatment outcomes. Moreover, the integration of bionanocomposites with portable devices, such as smartphones, could revolutionize point-of-care diagnostics with cost-effective biosensors and enable widespread access to advanced biomarker detection technologies [262].

Furthermore, bionanocomposites have been explored to develop targeted drug delivery systems. Traditional drug delivery methods often lack specificity, leading to poor efficacy and adverse side effects. Bionanocomposites offer a unique solution by incorporating nanoparticles or nanofibers capable of carrying therapeutic agents and targeting specific diseased tissues. By functionalizing the surface of these nanoparticles with disease-specific ligands, bionanocomposites can selectively deliver drugs to affected areas while minimizing off-target effects [263]. This targeted drug delivery approach has the potential to revolutionize early disease detection and treatment, as it allows for the precise administration of therapeutics to specific sites of interest [264].

One of the key advantages of bionanocomposites is their ability to detect biomarkers with higher precision and accuracy. These materials can be functionalized with specific biological molecules, such as antibodies or DNA probes that recognize and bind to disease-specific biomarkers [265]. When combined with nanomaterials, such as gold nanoparticles or quantum dots, these functionalized bionanocomposites enable sensitive and selective detection of target biomarkers in biological samples [219]. This enhanced detection capability is crucial in the early stages of the disease, where biomarker concentrations are often low, making traditional diagnostic methods less reliable [266].

Several studies have reported successful utilization of bionanocomposites in detecting cancer biomarkers, such as PSA or CEA, with high sensitivity and specificity. Furthermore, the integration of bionanocomposites with emerging technologies, such as microfluidics and biosensors, has shown promising results in the detection of infectious diseases, such as the Zika virus or Ebola virus, enabling rapid and point-of-care diagnostics [267].

9.2.5.3 Challenges in Utilizing Bionanocomposites for Biomarker Detection

Biomarker detection is integral to various biomedical applications, enabling the early diagnosis and treatment of diseases. In recent years, using bionanocomposites has shown promising potential in enhancing the sensitivity and specificity of biomarker detection platforms [268]. However, integrating bionanocomposites into such platforms poses several challenges and obstacles, focusing on stability, scalability, and biocompatibility, that must be addressed for successful implementation [45].

Bionanocomposites, which consolidate biological macromolecules and nanomaterials, have arisen as promising materials for biomarker applications. Like any innovation, joining bionanocomposites into biomarker research accompanies its arrangement of difficulties [192].

9.2.5.3.1 Stability

One of the major challenges faced in integrating bionanocomposites into biomarker detection platforms is the stability of these materials. These materials must maintain structural integrity and functionality over time, especially when exposed to various environmental conditions. Factors such as degradation, aggregation, and activity loss can hinder their performance, leading to unreliable and inconsistent results. The stability issue becomes particularly important when considering biomarker detection devices' long-term storage and transport. Ensuring the stability of bionanocomposites requires careful selection of materials, appropriate encapsulation techniques, and control over environmental conditions. Furthermore, understanding the degradation mechanisms and developing strategies to inhibit or minimize degradation can enhance the stability of bionanocomposite-based biomarker detection platforms [269].

9.2.5.3.1.1 Long-Term Stability and Degradation Bionanocomposites, as different materials, may degrade after some time, influencing their exhibition and dependability in biomarker applications. Understanding the degradation mechanisms and designing materials with controlled degradation profiles are basic to guaranteeing reliable and long-lasting functionality. The stability of these composites in various physiological conditions should be entirely examined to avoid untimely disappointment and off-base biomarker detection [270].

9.2.5.3.2 Scalability

Scalability is another significant obstacle associated with using bionanocomposites for biomarker detection. Scaling up the production of bionanocomposites while maintaining their desired properties can be complex [192]. The synthesis methods used to produce bionanocomposites often involve intricate procedures and require precise control over reaction parameters. Additionally, the production cost can be limiting, especially when considering large-scale applications. Overcoming these challenges requires the development of scalable and cost-effective synthesis approaches that ensure consistent and reliable production of bionanocomposites for biomarker detection platforms [271].

9.2.5.3.2.1 Scalability and Cost-Adequacy While research center scale combination of bionanocomposites is practical, interpreting these cycles to modern scale creation presents difficulties. The scalability of union strategies while keeping up with predictable material quality postures challenges. Moreover, the expense of creating bionanocomposites, which includes costly unrefined substances and specialized equipment, can obstruct broad reception. Developing cost-effective and scalable production techniques is basic to making these materials open for indicative and helpful applications [272].

9.2.5.3.3 Biocompatibility

The biocompatibility of bionanocomposites is critical when integrating them into biomarker detection platforms. Bionanocomposites should not induce any adverse reactions when in contact with biological systems to ensure their safe and effective use. However, the interaction between these composites and biological components may lead to cytotoxicity, immunogenicity, or instability in complex biological environments [273]. Overcoming these challenges requires a thorough understanding and control of the physicochemical properties of bionanocomposites, such as surface charge, size, and functionalization. Only through meticulous design and optimization can biocompatible bio-nanocomposite-based biomarker detection platforms be achieved [274].

Utilizing bionanocomposites for biomarker detection presents exciting opportunities and significant challenges [150]. Addressing the limitations and obstacles related to stability, scalability, and biocompatibility is crucial for successfully integrating these composites into biomarker detection platforms. Through interdisciplinary research and advancements in synthesis methodologies, bionanocomposites have the potential to revolutionize biomarker detection, leading to improved diagnostics and personalized medicine applications. However, further studies and collaborations are needed to overcome the current challenges and unlock the full potential of bionanocomposites in biomarker detection [275].

9.2.5.3.3.1 Biocompatibility and Safety One of the principal challenges in utilizing bionanocomposites for biomarker applications is guaranteeing their biocompatibility and security profiles. As these composites are frequently expected for use in vivo, evaluating their potential toxicity, immunogenicity, and long-haul impacts on living frameworks is fundamental. The connections between the nanomaterials and biological components can prompt potentially negative side effects, such as inflammation, cell damage, or impedance with cellular functions. Far-reaching biocompatibility studies should be led to assess the effect of these materials on various cell types and creatures, guaranteeing negligible damage [276].

9.2.6 Standardization of Synthesis and Characterization

The blend of bionanocomposites includes many-sided techniques that require cautious command over boundaries, such as nanoparticle size, shape, surface chemistry, and the coupling of biological molecules. The absence of normalized conventions for the synthesis and characterization of bionanocomposites prompts varieties in material properties, upsetting reproducibility and equivalence across studies. Laying out prominent conventions that can be taken on generally is critical for propelling the field and making an interpretation of examination discoveries into pragmatic applications [277].

9.2.6.1 Regulatory Considerations

Incorporating bionanocomposites into clinical settings for biomarker applications expects adherence to severe regulatory guidelines. Contingent upon the planned use, these materials might fall under various administrative characterizations, like clinical gadgets or drugs. Exploring the administrative scene can be complicated and tedious, requesting huge assets to get vital endorsements and guaranteeing consistency with safety and efficacy standards. Regulatory harmonization is fundamental to working with the turn of events and interpreting bionanocomposites in the clinic [278].

9.2.6.2 Interdisciplinary Collaboration

The effective combination of bionanocomposites in biomarker research requires cooperative endeavors across different fields, including materials science, biology, medicine, engineering, and ethics. Successful correspondence and joint effort between experts from these disciplines are fundamental to beating difficulties connected with material design, functionalization, characterization, and clinical interpretation. Cultivating interdisciplinary organizations will speed progress and lead to all-encompassing arrangements [192].

In summary, although bionanocomposites offer numerous biomarker detection possibilities, various challenges must be addressed. The stability, scalability, and biocompatibility of bionanocomposites are vital issues that require focused research and development [279]. By understanding the limitations and obstacles faced in the utilization of bionanocomposites, researchers can focus on developing innovative strategies to overcome these challenges and unlock the full potential of bionanocomposites in biomarker detection applications as biomarker detection, enabling early disease diagnosis, personalized medicine, and improved healthcare outcomes.

9.2.6.3 Ethical Considerations in Biomarker Research

Biomarker research is vital in advancing medical knowledge and improving patient care. In recent years, the development of bionanocomposites has introduced new possibilities in biomarker research, particularly in clinical applications [280]. However, the ethical considerations surrounding using bionanocomposites as biomarkers cannot be overlooked. Biomarker research is a rapidly growing field that holds great promise for improving diagnostic and treatment options in healthcare. As new technologies and techniques are developed, it is crucial to consider the ethical implications of using biomarkers in clinical applications, particularly those involving bionanocomposites. Biomarker research holds great promise for improving diagnostic and therapeutic approaches in medicine. However, using bionanocomposites in biomarker research raises important ethical considerations that must be carefully addressed [281].

Combining bionanocomposites into biomarker applications raises moral and cultural worries that warrant cautious thought. As these materials become more refined, questions emerge regarding potentially negative results, ecological effects, and the equitable distribution of benefits. Moral structures should be laid out to resolve issues connected with protection, data ownership, and the capable utilization of biomarker data, guaranteeing that headway in innovation aligns with cultural qualities [40].

To begin, it is essential to define bionanocomposites and their role in biomarker research. Bionanocomposites are materials that combine biological molecules with nanotechnology to create innovative diagnostic tools and therapeutic agents [282]. These materials have the potential to revolutionize healthcare by enhancing the sensitivity and specificity of biomarker detection, facilitating targeted drug delivery, and enabling personalized medicine. However, using bionanocomposites in biomarker research raises several ethical concerns that must be carefully considered.

A crucial ethical consideration in biomarker research lies in conducting thorough risk assessments and ensuring the safety of patients and research participants. When developing bionanocomposites, evaluating their potential adverse effects and addressing associated health risks is imperative [281].

One of the primary ethical considerations is the safety of using bionanocomposites in clinical settings. These materials are relatively new, but their long-term effects on human health and the environment are not yet fully understood. Conducting rigorous testing to assess potential risks and ensure patient safety is essential. Additionally, proper disposal methods for bionanocomposites must be established to prevent environmental harm [150]. Ethical guidelines and regulations should be in place to govern the development, testing, and use of bionanocomposites in biomarker research.

Informed consent also plays a critical role in ethical biomarker research involving bionanocomposites. Patients must clearly understand the purpose, risks, and potential benefits of participating in studies that utilize bionanocomposites [283]. Informed consent should be obtained transparently and comprehensively, allowing individuals to make autonomous decisions about their involvement in biomarker research. Additionally, vulnerable populations, such as children or individuals with cognitive impairments, require special attention to protect their rights and well-being.

Another ethical concern is the equitable distribution and access to biomarker research utilizing bionanocomposites because equity and accessibility are ethical concerns that should not be overlooked. These advanced technologies may be costly to develop, leading to potential inequalities in healthcare if they are only available to specific populations or healthcare systems. It is essential to address these disparities and ensure that biomarker research using bionanocomposites benefits everyone, regardless of socioeconomic status or geographic location [284]. Collaboration between researchers, policymakers, and healthcare providers is necessary to promote equitable access and prevent further healthcare disparities [285].

Furthermore, the potential impact of biomarker research using bionanocomposites on privacy and data protection must be considered. Collecting and analyzing biomarker data raises concerns about patient confidentiality and privacy. Safeguards should be in place to protect sensitive information and ensure that data is used ethically and responsibly. Clear guidelines for data storage, access, and sharing should be established to maintain patient trust and protect their autonomy [286].

In summary, using bionanocomposites in biomarker research presents exciting opportunities for improving healthcare outcomes. However, addressing the ethical considerations associated with their use is crucial. Safety, informed consent, equitable access, and data protection are essential factors that must be carefully considered and addressed to ensure the responsible and ethical implementation of biomarker research using bionanocomposites [287]. By upholding these ethical principles, we can leverage the potential of bionanocomposites to advance healthcare while ensuring the well-being and autonomy of patients.

9.2.6.4 Future Perspectives and Trends in Biomarker Clinical Applications and Impact

In recent years, the field of bionanocomposites has garnered significant attention in the field of biomarkers for clinical applications [218]. These innovative materials have shown immense potential in enhancing the sensitivity and specificity of biomarker detection, thereby revolutionizing clinical applications.

One of the key future perspectives of bionanocomposites in biomarker research is their ability to enable rapid and accurate diagnostics. With advancements in nanotechnology, bionanocomposites can offer enhanced sensitivity and selectivity for detecting various biomarkers [269]. This opens up new avenues for early disease diagnosis, improving patient outcomes. Additionally, the versatility of bionanocomposites allows for integrating different functionalities, such as multi-modal imaging and therapeutic capabilities, further enhancing their potential in clinical applications.

Moreover, bionanocomposites hold promise in the development of point-of-care testing devices. These portable and user-friendly platforms can provide real-time results, eliminating the need for time-consuming laboratory analyses. Such devices can be particularly valuable in resource-limited settings and emergency scenarios where prompt and accurate diagnosis is crucial [288].

9.2.6.5 Trends in Bionanocomposite-Based Biomarker Detection

The utilization of bionanocomposites in biomarker research is witnessing several emerging trends. One such trend is the incorporation of nanosensors within bionanocomposites [289]. These nanosensors can interact with specific biomarkers, triggering a measurable response that can be easily quantified. This allows for the sensitive and quantitative detection of biomarkers, aiding in disease diagnosis and monitoring. Furthermore, integrating novel nanomaterials, such as carbon-based nanomaterials and metallic nanoparticles, into bionanocomposites has improved overall biomarker detection sensitivity and specificity.

Additionally, advanced imaging techniques, such as fluorescence imaging and surface-enhanced Raman scattering (SERS), combined with bionanocomposites, have gained traction in biomarker detection [290]. These techniques can provide real-time and non-invasive imaging of biomarkers, allowing for accurate diagnosis and monitoring of diseases. Moreover, the ability to customize the surface properties of bionanocomposites enables the incorporation of targeting ligands, facilitating the specific recognition and capture of biomarkers, further enhancing their detection capabilities.

Recently, there has been an increasing interest in utilizing bionanocomposites to detect and monitor various diseases through biomarkers. These composite materials, consisting of a matrix phase reinforced with nanoparticles, offer unique properties such as enhanced sensitivity, increased selectivity, and improved stability [291]. Such advancements have opened the doors to a wide range of clinical applications.

One future perspective for bionanocomposites in biomarker research is their potential to revolutionize early disease detection. These materials can be engineered to have high affinity and specificity toward specific biomarkers associated with various diseases. By utilizing these specific interactions, bionanocomposites can enable the development of highly sensitive biosensing platforms capable of detecting diseases in their early stages. This early detection can significantly improve patient outcomes and reduce healthcare costs [269].

Another promising trend in the field of bionanocomposites is the integration of multifunctional properties into these materials. By incorporating diverse functionalities, such as fluorescence, magnetic properties, or drug delivery capabilities, bionanocomposites can be designed to perform multiple tasks simultaneously [292]. This integration opens up new avenues for personalized medicine, where targeted therapies can be delivered precisely to affected areas while monitoring treatment response using the same bionanocomposite-based biomarkers.

Furthermore, bionanocomposites have the potential to address current challenges in clinical diagnosis. By utilizing their unique properties, these materials can enhance the sensitivity and reliability of diagnostic techniques such as imaging and immunoassay methods. This advancement may lead to more accurate diagnoses, enabling clinicians to make informed decisions and tailor treatments based on individual patient needs [46].

9.2.6.5.1 Advancements in Bionanocomposite Design and Synthesis

Bionanocomposites, which refer to the combination of biomolecules and nanomaterials, offer a wide range of possibilities for biomarker development. Due to their high surface area, biocompatibility, and customizable properties, these nanocomposites can enhance the sensitivity and selectivity of biomarker detection assays [293]. Recent advancements in nanotechnology have enabled the development of novel bionanocomposites with improved stability, controlled release properties, and targeted delivery capabilities. This opens up new avenues for the diagnosis and treatment of various diseases.

9.2.6.5.2 Clinical Applications of Bionanocomposites in Biomarker Detection

The integration of bionanocomposites in biomarker detection has the potential to revolutionize clinical diagnostics. These nanocomposites can be used in various diagnostic platforms, including immunoassays, molecular diagnostics, and biosensors [294]. The enhanced sensitivity and specificity offered by bionanocomposites enable the detection of biomarkers at lower concentrations, leading to early disease diagnosis, as in the case of cancer diagnostics, CVD monitoring, infectious disease detection, and neurological disorder diagnosis with improved patient outcomes. Furthermore, integrating bionanocomposites in point-of-care devices can facilitate rapid and on-site diagnosis, reducing the need for complex laboratory infrastructure [295].

9.2.6.5.3 Impact on Healthcare

The utilization of bionanocomposites in biomarker clinical applications has the potential to transform healthcare in several ways. First, the early detection and accurate diagnosis facilitated by these nanocomposites can lead to the timely initiation of treatment, ultimately improving patient survival rates [296]. Second, the development of personalized medicine can be accelerated with the use of bionanocomposites, allowing for tailored treatment strategies based on individual biomarker profiles. Additionally, integrating bionanocomposites in therapeutic interventions, such as drug delivery systems, can enhance efficacy and minimize the side effects of treatments [49]. Overall, the impact of bionanocomposites on healthcare is promising, paving the way for more effective and efficient clinical practices.

In summary, bionanocomposites have immense potential to shape the future of biomarker research and clinical diagnostics. The ability of these materials to enhance sensitivity, selectivity, and portability makes them a promising candidate for developing next-generation diagnostic devices [297]. The emerging trends, such as nanosensors and advanced imaging techniques, further augment their capabilities. As research advances, bionanocomposites are poised to revolutionize biomarker-based clinical applications, ultimately leading to improved patient outcomes such as early disease detection, personalized medicine, and improved clinical diagnosis [42].

9.3 CONCLUSION

In conclusion, bionanocomposites have emerged as a promising tool in the field of biomarkers. By integrating nanotechnology and biocompatible materials, these innovative composites have demonstrated great potential in developing advanced diagnostic and therapeutic strategies. Using bionanocomposites in biomarker research offers numerous advantages, including enhanced sensitivity, improved accuracy, and multifunctionality.

Biomarkers are essential medical research and diagnostic tools, providing invaluable information about diseases and conditions. Genetic, protein, metabolic, imaging, and cellular biomarkers offer unique insights and contribute to our understanding of various diseases [298]. Researchers can develop more targeted and personalized treatment strategies by studying and utilizing these biomarkers, leading to improved patient outcomes.

Overall, bionanocomposites hold immense promise for the future of biomarker studies. By continuously exploring and refining their properties, bionanocomposites will undoubtedly contribute to advancements in diagnosing and treating various diseases [204].

Bionanocomposites based on biosensors offer immense potential for biomarker detection in various biomedical applications. Their high surface area-to-volume ratio and biocompatibility contribute to improved sensitivity and specificity for biomarker detection. However, challenges such as properly integrating biosensing elements and understanding physicochemical properties must be addressed to successfully develop and implement bionanocomposites in the biosensing platform. Further research and development are needed to optimize the manufacturing processes, ensure biocompatibility, and enable their integration into portable devices. With continued advancements, bionanocomposites hold tremendous potential for revolutionizing healthcare and environmental analysis [204].

Biomarkers are basic devices in customized medication, empowering healthcare professionals to settle on informed decisions and give modified treatments to patients. As how we might interpret genetics and disease mechanisms keeps evolving, the reconciliation of biomarkers into clinical practice will become progressively refined, prompting work on understanding results and more compelling healthcare interventions [47].

Integrating bionanocomposites into biomarker-based diagnostics for neurological disorders holds enormous potential for right-on-time and accurate infection discovery. These inventive materials can alter neurological diagnostics by upgrading sensitivity, specificity, and multiplexing capacities. As exploration advances, bionanocomposites will probably assume a remarkable part in improving patient outcomes and propelling comprehension as we might interpret complex neurological disorders [299].

The reconciliation of bionanocomposites in biomarker applications holds a gigantic commitment for upsetting disease diagnosis, therapy checking, and personalized biomarkers. Nonetheless, tending to the difficulties related to biocompatibility, standardization, regulatory compliance, scalability, ethical considerations, interdisciplinary collaboration, and material stability is fundamental to saddling their potential completely. As scientists, policymakers, and stakeholders team up to conquer these difficulties, bionanocomposites can genuinely arise as groundbreaking apparatuses in propelling healthcare and working on patient outcomes [60].

Bionanocomposites address a state-of-the-art approach in biomarker research, offering creative answers for disease detection and monitoring. Their novel properties and flexibility make them an incredible asset in improving cutting-edge symptomatic stages. As exploration in this field advances and difficulties are tended to, bionanocomposites can alter personalized medicine and work on understanding results [300].

These bionanocomposites offer immense potential in biomarker monitoring, with significant clinical correlation. Their unique properties and enhanced reactivity make them ideal candidates for biomarker detection, enabling early disease diagnosis and effective patient monitoring. By harnessing the power of bionanocomposites, healthcare professionals can pave the way for personalized medicine and improved patient care. As the field advances, further research is needed to exploit the benefits of bionanocomposites in clinical settings fully. By embracing this innovative technology, we can enhance disease detection and monitoring, leading to a healthier society [45].

9.4 SUGGESTION

To overcome these challenges, extensive research and development are required to enhance the stability, scalability, and biocompatibility of bionanocomposites. Strategies to improve the stability involve surface modification techniques, such as functionalizing the nanomaterials with bioinert molecules or using protective coatings to prevent aggregation or degradation. Optimizing synthesis techniques, process engineering, and quality control measures can address the scalability issue. Techniques like encapsulation or surface modification can also enhance the biocompatibility of bionanocomposites, ensuring their safe interaction with biological systems.

REFERENCES

[1] F. Mushtaq et al., "Preparation, properties, and applications of gelatin-based hydrogels (GHs) in the environmental, technological, and biomedical sectors," *International Journal of Biological Macromolecules*, vol. 218, pp. 601–633, 2022.

[2] E. M. Fernandes, R. A. Pires, J. F. Mano, and R. L. Reis, "Bionanocomposites from lignocellulosic resources: Properties, applications and future trends for their use in the biomedical field," *Progress in Polymer Science*, vol. 38, no. 10–11, pp. 1415–1441, 2013.

[3] H. Daraee, A. Eatemadi, E. Abbasi, S. Fekri Aval, M. Kouhi, and A. Akbarzadeh, "Application of gold nanoparticles in biomedical and drug delivery," *Artificial Cells, Nanomedicine, and Biotechnology*, vol. 44, no. 1, pp. 410–422, 2016.

[4] M. J. Limo et al., "Interactions between metal oxides and biomolecules: From fundamental understanding to applications," *Chemical Reviews*, vol. 118, no. 22, pp. 11118–11193, 2018.
[5] R. R. Costa, M. Alatorre-Meda, and J. F. Mano, "Drug nano-reservoirs synthesized using layer-by-layer technologies," *Biotechnology Advances*, vol. 33, no. 6, pp. 1310–1326, 2015.
[6] F. Arduini et al., "Electrochemical biosensors based on nanomodified screen-printed electrodes: Recent applications in clinical analysis," *TrAC Trends in Analytical Chemistry*, vol. 79, pp. 114–126, 2016.
[7] L. W. C. Ho, Y. Liu, R. Han, Q. Bai, and C. H. J. Choi, "Nano–cell interactions of non-cationic bionanomaterials," *Accounts of Chemical Research*, vol. 52, no. 6, pp. 1519–1530, 2019.
[8] M. Gandhi and K. Amreen, "Emerging trends in nanomaterial-based biomedical aspects," *Electrochem*, vol. 4, no. 3, pp. 365–388, 2023.
[9] L. N. Thwala, S. C. Ndlovu, K. T. Mpofu, M. Y. Lugongolo, and P. Mthunzi-Kufa, "Nanotechnology-based diagnostics for diseases prevalent in developing countries: Current advances in point-of-care tests," *Nanomaterials*, vol. 13, no. 7, p. 1247, 2023.
[10] V. B. Kraus et al., "Application of biomarkers in the development of drugs intended for the treatment of osteoarthritis," *Osteoarthritis and Cartilage*, vol. 19, no. 5, pp. 515–542, 2011.
[11] M. S. García-Gutiérrez, F. Navarrete, F. Sala, A. Gasparyan, A. Austrich-Olivares, and J. Manzanares, "Biomarkers in psychiatry: Concept, definition, types and relevance to the clinical reality," *Frontiers in Psychiatry*, vol. 11, p. 432, 2020.
[12] S. Qiu et al., "Small molecule metabolites: Discovery of biomarkers and therapeutic targets," *Signal Transduction and Targeted Therapy*, vol. 8, no. 1, p. 132, 2023.
[13] R. A. M. Osmani, E. Singh, U. Hani, S. Chavan, H. Kazi, and M. Menon, "Bionanocomposite hydrogels for regenerative medicine and biomedical applications," in *Bionanocomposites in Tissue Engineering and Regenerative Medicine*: Elsevier, 2021, pp. 91–118.
[14] M. A. Abourehab et al., "Chondroitin sulfate-based composites: A tour d'horizon of their biomedical applications," *Journal of Materials Chemistry B*, vol. 10, no. 44, pp. 9125–9178, 2022.
[15] J. Pires, C. D. D. Paula, V. G. L. Souza, A. L. Fernando, and I. Coelhoso, "Understanding the barrier and mechanical behavior of different nanofillers in chitosan films for food packaging," *Polymers*, vol. 13, no. 5, p. 721, 2021.
[16] A. D. Štiglic, *Preparation of Three Dimensional Structures of Polysaccharide Derivatives for Application in Regenerative Medicine*: Univerza v Mariboru (Slovenia), 2022.
[17] M. M. Reddy, S. Vivekanandhan, M. Misra, S. K. Bhatia, and A. K. Mohanty, "Biobased plastics and bionanocomposites: Current status and future opportunities," *Progress in Polymer Science*, vol. 38, no. 10–11, pp. 1653–1689, 2013.
[18] R. K. Saini, A. K. Bajpai, and E. Jain, "13 Advances in bionanocomposites for biomedical applications," *Biodegradable and Biocompatible Polymer Composites: Processing, Properties and Applications*, vol. 379, 2017.
[19] R. M. Sallam, "Proteomics in cancer biomarkers discovery: Challenges and applications," *Disease Markers*, vol. 2015, p. 321370, 2015.
[20] H. Hampel et al., "Blood-based biomarkers for Alzheimer disease: Mapping the road to the clinic," *Nature Reviews Neurology*, vol. 14, no. 11, pp. 639–652, 2018.
[21] G. G. Shetgaonkar, S. M. Marques, C. E. DCruz, R. Vibhavari, L. Kumar, and R. K. Shirodkar, "Exosomes as cell-derivative carriers in the diagnosis and treatment of central nervous system diseases," *Drug Delivery and Translational Research*, vol. 12, no. 5, pp. 1047–1079, 2022.
[22] D. Bauer et al., "Classification of osteoarthritis biomarkers: A proposed approach," *Osteoarthritis and Cartilage*, vol. 14, no. 8, pp. 723–727, 2006.
[23] J. Montaner et al., "Multilevel omics for the discovery of biomarkers and therapeutic targets for stroke," *Nature Reviews Neurology*, vol. 16, no. 5, pp. 247–264, 2020.
[24] J. P. O'Connor, A. Jackson, G. J. Parker, and G. C. Jayson, "DCE-MRI biomarkers in the clinical evaluation of antiangiogenic and vascular disrupting agents," *British Journal of Cancer*, vol. 96, no. 2, pp. 189–195, 2007.
[25] S. Yasri and V. Wiwanitkit, "Carbon nanotorous for advanced therapeutic applications," in *Carbon Nanostructures in Biomedical Applications*: Springer, 2023, pp. 123–144.
[26] V. Kumar and K. Arora, "Trends in nano-inspired biosensors for plants," *Materials Science for Energy Technologies*, vol. 3, pp. 255–273, 2020.

[27] M. Panda, E. Kalita, S. Singh, K. Kumar, A. Rao, and V. K. Prajapati, "MiRNA-SARS-CoV-2 dialogue and prospective anti-COVID-19 therapies," *Life Sciences*, vol. 305, p. 120761, 2022.

[28] T. Tuntland et al., "Implementation of pharmacokinetic and pharmacodynamic strategies in early research phases of drug discovery and development at Novartis Institute of Biomedical Research," *Frontiers in Pharmacology*, vol. 5, p. 174, 2014.

[29] R. Hu, X. Wang, and X. Zhan, "Multi-parameter systematic strategies for predictive, preventive and personalised medicine in cancer," *EPMA Journal*, vol. 4, pp. 1–12, 2013.

[30] P. T. Harrison, S. Vyse, and P. H. Huang, "Rare epidermal growth factor receptor (EGFR) mutations in non-small cell lung cancer," in *Seminars in Cancer Biology*, vol. 61: Elsevier, 2020, pp. 167–179.

[31] M. Lu and X. Zhan, "The crucial role of multiomic approach in cancer research and clinically relevant outcomes," *EPMA Journal*, vol. 9, no. 1, pp. 77–102, 2018.

[32] N. A. Alymani, M. D. Smith, D. J. Williams, and R. D. Petty, "Predictive biomarkers for personalised anti-cancer drug use: Discovery to clinical implementation," *European Journal of Cancer*, vol. 46, no. 5, pp. 869–879, 2010.

[33] M. G. Shlipak et al., "The case for early identification and intervention of chronic kidney disease: Conclusions from a kidney disease: Improving global outcomes (KDIGO) controversies conference," *Kidney International*, vol. 99, no. 1, pp. 34–47, 2021.

[34] Y. Wang, Y. Liu, J. Li, Y. Chen, S. Liu, and C. Zhong, "Engineered living materials (ELMs) design: From function allocation to dynamic behavior modulation," *Current Opinion in Chemical Biology*, vol. 70, p. 102188, 2022.

[35] V. V. Konopelniuk et al., "Efficacy of Fenugreek-based bionanocomposite on renal dysfunction and endogenous intoxication in high-calorie diet-induced obesity rat model—Comparative study," *EPMA Journal*, vol. 8, pp. 377–390, 2017.

[36] T. C. Fuchs and P. Hewitt, "Biomarkers for drug-induced renal damage and nephrotoxicity—An overview for applied toxicology," *The AAPS Journal*, vol. 13, pp. 615–631, 2011.

[37] K. D. Davis et al., "Discovery and validation of biomarkers to aid the development of safe and effective pain therapeutics: Challenges and opportunities," *Nature Reviews Neurology*, vol. 16, no. 7, pp. 381–400, 2020.

[38] P. A. Andreux et al., "The mitophagy activator urolithin A is safe and induces a molecular signature of improved mitochondrial and cellular health in humans," *Nature Metabolism*, vol. 1, no. 6, pp. 595–603, 2019.

[39] M. P. Nikolova and M. S. Chavali, "Metal oxide nanoparticles as biomedical materials," *Biomimetics*, vol. 5, no. 2, p. 27, 2020.

[40] D. Olvera and M. G. Monaghan, "Electroactive material-based biosensors for detection and drug delivery," *Advanced Drug Delivery Reviews*, vol. 170, pp. 396–424, 2021.

[41] A. J. Vargas and C. C. Harris, "Biomarker development in the precision medicine era: Lung cancer as a case study," *Nature Reviews Cancer*, vol. 16, no. 8, pp. 525–537, 2016.

[42] A. Sadana and N. Sadana, *Biomarkers and Biosensors: Detection and Binding to Biosensor Surfaces and Biomarkers Applications*: Newnes, 2014.

[43] A. N. Simpkins et al., "Biomarker application for precision medicine in stroke," *Translational Stroke Research*, vol. 11, pp. 615–627, 2020.

[44] K. K. Jain and K. K. Jain, *The Handbook of Biomarkers*: Springer, 2010.

[45] R. P. Singh, "Prospects of nanobiomaterials for biosensing," *International Journal of Electrochemistry*, vol. 2011, p. 125487, 2011.

[46] A. Mohammadpour-Haratbar, Y. Zare, and K. Y. Rhee, "Electrochemical biosensors based on polymer nanocomposites for detecting breast cancer: Recent progress and future prospects," *Advances in Colloid and Interface Science*, vol. 309, p. 102795, 2022.

[47] R. Singla, A. Guliani, A. Kumari, and S. K. Yadav, "Metallic nanoparticles, toxicity issues and applications in medicine," *Nanoscale Materials in Targeted Drug delivery, Theragnosis and Tissue Regeneration*, pp. 41–80, 2016. https://doi.org/10.1007/978-981-10-0818-4

[48] T. Khan and A. Chauhan, "Polymer-based bionanomaterials for biomedical applications," in *Bionanotechnology: Emerging Applications of Bionanomaterials*: Elsevier, 2022, pp. 187–225.

[49] A. K. Mishra, "Application of nanotechnology in diagnosis, drug dissolution, drug discovery, and drug carrier," *Nanobiotechnology in Bioformulations*: Springer, pp. 449–475, 2019.

[50] Y. Y. Li and S. J. Jones, "Drug repositioning for personalized medicine," *Genome Medicine*, vol. 4, pp. 1–14, 2012.

[51] N. Jain, U. Nagaich, M. Pandey, D. K. Chellappan, and K. Dua, "Predictive genomic tools in disease stratification and targeted prevention: A recent update in personalized therapy advancements," *EPMA Journal*, vol. 13, no. 4, pp. 561–580, 2022.

[52] L. Mancinelli, M. Cronin, and W. Sadée, "Pharmacogenomics: The promise of personalized medicine," *AAPS Pharmsci*, vol. 2, pp. 29–41, 2000.

[53] S. Gopi, A. Amalraj, S. Jude, S. Thomas, and Q. Guo, "Bionanocomposite films based on potato, tapioca starch and chitosan reinforced with cellulose nanofiber isolated from turmeric spent," *Journal of the Taiwan Institute of Chemical Engineers*, vol. 96, pp. 664–671, 2019.

[54] D. Tao et al., "Development of a label-free electrochemical aptasensor for the detection of Tau381 and its preliminary application in AD and non-AD patients' sera," *Biosensors*, vol. 9, no. 3, p. 84, 2019.

[55] R. Misra, S. Acharya, and S. K. Sahoo, "Cancer nanotechnology: Application of nanotechnology in cancer therapy," *Drug Discovery Today*, vol. 15, no. 19–20, pp. 842–850, 2010.

[56] X. Chen, A. Ghorbani, L. Quan, and D. Toghraie, "Application of microfluidics in sports and tumor biomarker detection: Advancing the identification of physiological disorders," *Journal of Molecular Liquids*, vol. 387, p. 122706, 2023.

[57] K. P. Das, "Nanoparticles and convergence of artificial intelligence for targeted drug delivery for cancer therapy: Current progress and challenges," *Frontiers in Medical Technology*, vol. 4, p. 1067144, 2023.

[58] A. Sanati et al., "Recent advancement in electrode materials and fabrication, microfluidic designs, and self-powered systems for wearable non-invasive electrochemical glucose monitoring," *Applied Materials Today*, vol. 26, p. 101350, 2022.

[59] Z. Zhao et al., "Advancements in electrochemical biosensing for respiratory virus detection: A review," *TrAC Trends in Analytical Chemistry*, vol. 139, p. 116253, 2021.

[60] S. Er et al., "Amino acids, peptides, and proteins: Implications for nanotechnological applications in biosensing and drug/gene delivery," *Nanomaterials*, vol. 11, no. 11, p. 3002, 2021.

[61] Z. Khurshid, M. S. Zafar, R. S. Khan, S. Najeeb, P. D. Slowey, and I. U. Rehman, "Role of salivary biomarkers in oral cancer detection," *Advances in Clinical Chemistry*, vol. 86, pp. 23–70, 2018.

[62] O. Beylerli, I. Gareev, A. Sufianov, T. Ilyasova, and Y. Guang, "Long noncoding RNAs as promising biomarkers in cancer," *Non-coding RNA Research*, vol. 7, no. 2, pp. 66–70, 2022.

[63] T. M. Gorges and K. Pantel, "Circulating tumor cells as therapy-related biomarkers in cancer patients," *Cancer Immunology, Immunotherapy*, vol. 62, pp. 931–939, 2013.

[64] Y. Shen, T. B. Anwar, and A. Mulchandani, "Current status, advances, challenges and perspectives on biosensors for COVID-19 diagnosis in resource-limited settings," *Sensors and Actuators Reports*, vol. 3, p. 100025, 2021.

[65] S. Pillozzi et al., "Soft tissue sarcoma: An insight on biomarkers at molecular, metabolic and cellular level," *Cancers*, vol. 13, no. 12, p. 3044, 2021.

[66] P. Ramburrun, R. A. Khan, and Y. E. Choonara, "Design, preparation, and functionalization of nanobiomaterials for enhanced efficacy in current and future biomedical applications," *Nanotechnology Reviews*, vol. 11, no. 1, pp. 1802–1826, 2022.

[67] V. Iacobazzi, A. Castegna, V. Infantino, and G. Andria, "Mitochondrial DNA methylation as a next-generation biomarker and diagnostic tool," *Molecular Genetics and Metabolism*, vol. 110, no. 1–2, pp. 25–34, 2013.

[68] G. Lucarelli et al., "Metabolomic insights into pathophysiological mechanisms and biomarker discovery in clear cell renal cell carcinoma," *Expert Review of Molecular Diagnostics*, vol. 19, no. 5, pp. 397–407, 2019.

[69] O. Beckonert et al., "Metabolic profiling, metabolomic and metabonomic procedures for NMR spectroscopy of urine, plasma, serum and tissue extracts," *Nature Protocols*, vol. 2, no. 11, p. 2692, 2007.

[70] B. C. Muthubharathi, T. Gowripriya, and K. Balamurugan, "Metabolomics: Small molecules that matter more," *Molecular Omics*, vol. 17, no. 2, pp. 210–229, 2021.

[71] M. A. Karsdal et al., "Biochemical markers of ongoing joint damage in rheumatoid arthritis-current and future applications, limitations and opportunities," *Arthritis Research & Therapy*, vol. 13, pp. 1–20, 2011.

[72] J. T. Warshauer, J. A. Bluestone, and M. S. Anderson, "New frontiers in the treatment of type 1 diabetes," *Cell Metabolism*, vol. 31, no. 1, pp. 46–61, 2020.

[73] M. Olivier, R. Asmis, G. A. Hawkins, T. D. Howard, and L. A. Cox, "The need for multi-omics biomarker signatures in precision medicine," *International Journal of Molecular Sciences*, vol. 20, no. 19, p. 4781, 2019.
[74] M. S. McCabe, A. H. Partridge, E. Grunfeld, and M. M. Hudson, "Risk-based health care, the cancer survivor, the oncologist, and the primary care physician," *Seminars in Oncology*, vol. 40, no. 6, pp. 804–812, 2013.
[75] M. P. Quinones and R. Kaddurah-Daouk, "Metabolomics tools for identifying biomarkers for neuropsychiatric diseases," *Neurobiology of Disease*, vol. 35, no. 2, pp. 165–176, 2009.
[76] J. L. Cummings, "Biomarkers in Alzheimer's disease drug development," *Alzheimer's & Dementia*, vol. 7, no. 3, pp. e13–e44, 2011.
[77] R. D. Beger et al., "Metabolomics enables precision medicine: "A white paper, community perspective"," *Metabolomics*, vol. 12, pp. 1–15, 2016.
[78] J. W. Prescott, "Quantitative imaging biomarkers: The application of advanced image processing and analysis to clinical and preclinical decision making," *Journal of Digital Imaging*, vol. 26, pp. 97–108, 2013.
[79] M. Filippi and F. Agosta, "Imaging biomarkers in multiple sclerosis," *Journal of Magnetic Resonance Imaging: An Official Journal of the International Society for Magnetic Resonance in Medicine*, vol. 31, no. 4, pp. 770–788, 2010.
[80] I. S. Haldorsen, N. Lura, J. Blaakær, D. Fischerova, and H. M. Werner, "What is the role of imaging at primary diagnostic work-up in uterine cervical cancer?," *Current Oncology Reports*, vol. 21, pp. 1–15, 2019.
[81] T. L. Benzinger et al., "Regional variability of imaging biomarkers in autosomal dominant Alzheimer's disease," *Proceedings of the National Academy of Sciences*, vol. 110, no. 47, pp. E4502–E4509, 2013.
[82] P. T. Murray et al., "Potential use of biomarkers in acute kidney injury: Report and summary of recommendations from the 10th acute dialysis quality Initiative consensus conference," *Kidney International*, vol. 85, no. 3, pp. 513–521, 2014.
[83] A. Mangla, E. Oliveros, K. A. Williams Sr, and D. K. Kalra, "Cardiac imaging in the diagnosis of coronary artery disease," *Current Problems in Cardiology*, vol. 42, no. 10, pp. 316–366, 2017.
[84] T. A. Soomro, L. Zheng, A. J. Afifi, A. Ali, M. Yin, and J. Gao, "Artificial intelligence (AI) for medical imaging to combat coronavirus disease (COVID-19): A detailed review with direction for future research," *Artificial Intelligence Review*, pp. 1–31, 2022.
[85] S. Ranjbar and J. R. Mitchell, "An introduction to radiomics: An evolving cornerstone of precision medicine," in *Biomedical Texture Analysis*: Elsevier, 2017, pp. 223–245.
[86] A. D. Bowry, J. Lewey, S. B. Dugani, and N. K. Choudhry, "The burden of cardiovascular disease in low- and middle-income countries: Epidemiology and management," *Canadian Journal of Cardiology*, vol. 31, no. 9, pp. 1151–1159, 2015.
[87] J. Viereck and T. Thum, "Circulating noncoding RNAs as biomarkers of cardiovascular disease and injury," *Circulation Research*, vol. 120, no. 2, pp. 381–399, 2017.
[88] K. M. Aakre and T. Omland, "Physical activity, exercise and cardiac troponins: Clinical implications," *Progress in Cardiovascular Diseases*, vol. 62, no. 2, pp. 108–115, 2019.
[89] H. V. Lakhani et al., "Detecting early onset of anthracyclines-induced cardiotoxicity using a novel panel of biomarkers in West-Virginian population with breast cancer," *Scientific Reports*, vol. 11, no. 1, p. 7954, 2021.
[90] A. M. Ranchord et al., "High-concentration versus titrated oxygen therapy in ST-elevation myocardial infarction: A pilot randomized controlled trial," *American Heart Journal*, vol. 163, no. 2, pp. 168–175, 2012.
[91] J. H. Greenslade et al., "Diagnostic accuracy of a new high-sensitivity troponin I assay and five accelerated diagnostic pathways for ruling out acute myocardial infarction and acute coronary syndrome," *Annals of Emergency Medicine*, vol. 71, no. 4, pp. 439–451, 2018.
[92] Z. Zhelev et al., "Diagnostic accuracy of single baseline measurement of Elecsys Troponin T high-sensitive assay for diagnosis of acute myocardial infarction in emergency department: Systematic review and meta-analysis," *BMJ*, vol. 350, 2015. https://doi.org/10.1136/bmj.h15
[93] L. Babuin and A. S. Jaffe, "Troponin: The biomarker of choice for the detection of cardiac injury," *CMAJ*, vol. 173, no. 10, pp. 1191–1202, 2005.

[94] G. Curigliano et al., "Management of cardiac disease in cancer patients throughout oncological treatment: ESMO consensus recommendations," *Annals of Oncology*, vol. 31, no. 2, pp. 171–190, 2020.
[95] S. M. Wells and M. Sleeper, "Cardiac troponins," *Journal of Veterinary Emergency and Critical Care*, vol. 18, no. 3, pp. 235–245, 2008.
[96] D. Corcoran, P. Grant, and C. Berry, "Risk stratification in non-ST elevation acute coronary syndromes: Risk scores, biomarkers and clinical judgment," *IJC Heart & Vasculature*, vol. 8, pp. 131–137, 2015.
[97] M. Panteghini, "Role and importance of biochemical markers in clinical cardiology," *European Heart Journal*, vol. 25, no. 14, pp. 1187–1196, 2004.
[98] I. Riedmaier and M. W. Pfaffl, "Transcriptional biomarkers–high throughput screening, quantitative verification, and bioinformatical validation methods," *Methods*, vol. 59, no. 1, pp. 3–9, 2013.
[99] V. V. Arslanov, E. V. Ermakova, D. I. Krylov, and O. O. Popova, "On the relationship between the properties of planar structures of non-ionic surfactants and their vesicular analogues–Niosomes," *Journal of Colloid and Interface Science*, vol. 640, pp. 281–295, 2023.
[100] V. Rani, G. Deep, R. K. Singh, K. Palle, and U. C. Yadav, "Oxidative stress and metabolic disorders: Pathogenesis and therapeutic strategies," *Life Sciences*, vol. 148, pp. 183–193, 2016.
[101] Y.-Y. Zhao, S.-P. Wu, S. Liu, Y. Zhang, and R.-C. Lin, "Ultra-performance liquid chromatography–mass spectrometry as a sensitive and powerful technology in lipidomic applications," *Chemico-Biological Interactions*, vol. 220, pp. 181–192, 2014.
[102] L. Vigh et al., "The significance of lipid composition for membrane activity: New concepts and ways of assessing function," *Progress in Lipid Research*, vol. 44, no. 5, pp. 303–344, 2005.
[103] Y.-Y. Zhao, X.-L. Cheng, and R.-C. Lin, "Lipidomics applications for discovering biomarkers of diseases in clinical chemistry," *International Review of Cell and Molecular Biology*, vol. 313, pp. 1–26, 2014.
[104] M. Jenab, N. Slimani, M. Bictash, P. Ferrari, and S. A. Bingham, "Biomarkers in nutritional epidemiology: Applications, needs and new horizons," *Human Genetics*, vol. 125, pp. 507–525, 2009.
[105] D. F. Hayes, H. S. Markus, R. D. Leslie, and E. J. Topol, "Personalized medicine: Risk prediction, targeted therapies and mobile health technology," *BMC Medicine*, vol. 12, pp. 1–8, 2014.
[106] C. Fenoglio, "Genetics and epigenetics: Basic concepts," *Neurodegenerative Diseases: Clinical Aspects, Molecular Genetics and Biomarkers*, pp. 1–15, 2014. https://doi.org/10.1007/978-3-319-72938-1
[107] R. Ottman, "Gene–environment interaction: Definitions and study design," *Preventive Medicine*, vol. 25, no. 6, pp. 764–770, 1996.
[108] C. Jones and C. B. Nemeroff, "Precision psychiatry: Biomarker-guided tailored therapy for effective treatment and prevention in major depression," *Major Depressive Disorder: Rethinking and Understanding Recent Discoveries*, pp. 535–563, 2021.
[109] S. H. Almal and H. Padh, "Implications of gene copy-number variation in health and diseases," *Journal of Human Genetics*, vol. 57, no. 1, pp. 6–13, 2012.
[110] L. Hu et al., "Fluorescence in situ hybridization (FISH): An increasingly demanded tool for biomarker research and personalized medicine," *Biomarker Research*, vol. 2, pp. 1–13, 2014.
[111] G. S. Ginsburg and H. F. Willard, "Genomic and personalized medicine: Foundations and applications," *Translational Research*, vol. 154, no. 6, pp. 277–287, 2009.
[112] O. Gassmann, G. Reepmeyer, and M. Von Zedtwitz, *Leading Pharmaceutical Innovation*, vol. 1007: Springer, p. 978, 2008.
[113] P. Maresova et al., "Consequences of chronic diseases and other limitations associated with old age – A scoping review," *BMC Public Health*, vol. 19, pp. 1–17, 2019.
[114] C. Giambartolomei et al., "Bayesian test for colocalisation between pairs of genetic association studies using summary statistics," *PLoS Genetics*, vol. 10, no. 5, p. e1004383, 2014.
[115] J. C. Polanco, C. Li, L.-G. Bodea, R. Martinez-Marmol, F. A. Meunier, and J. Götz, "Amyloid-β and tau complexity—Towards improved biomarkers and targeted therapies," *Nature Reviews Neurology*, vol. 14, no. 1, pp. 22–39, 2018.
[116] J. Vamathevan et al., "Applications of machine learning in drug discovery and development," *Nature Reviews Drug discovery*, vol. 18, no. 6, pp. 463–477, 2019.
[117] R. Khamisy-Farah, L. B. Furstenau, J. D. Kong, J. Wu, and N. L. Bragazzi, "Gynecology meets big data in the disruptive innovation medical era: State-of-art and future prospects," *International Journal of Environmental Research and Public Health*, vol. 18, no. 10, p. 5058, 2021.

[118] S. Ramazi, A. Allahverdi, and J. Zahiri, "Evaluation of post-translational modifications in histone proteins: A review on histone modification defects in developmental and neurological disorders," *Journal of Biosciences*, vol. 45, pp. 1–29, 2020.
[119] N. M. Qadir Nanakali et al., "The role of dietary polyphenols in alternating DNA methylation in cancer," *Critical Reviews in Food Science and Nutrition*, vol. 63, pp. 1–14, 2022.
[120] R. Jaenisch and A. Bird, "Epigenetic regulation of gene expression: How the genome integrates intrinsic and environmental signals," *Nature Genetics*, vol. 33, no. 3, pp. 245–254, 2003.
[121] J. D. Sweatt, "The epigenetic basis of individuality," *Current Opinion in Behavioral Sciences*, vol. 25, pp. 51–56, 2019.
[122] S. Horvath and K. Raj, "DNA methylation-based biomarkers and the epigenetic clock theory of ageing," *Nature Reviews Genetics*, vol. 19, no. 6, pp. 371–384, 2018.
[123] D. M. Chiorean et al., "New insights into genetics of endometriosis—A comprehensive literature review," *Diagnostics*, vol. 13, no. 13, p. 2265, 2023.
[124] M. S. Kim, J. Lee, and D. Sidransky, "DNA methylation markers in colorectal cancer," *Cancer and Metastasis Reviews*, vol. 29, pp. 181–206, 2010.
[125] T. Witte, C. Plass, and C. Gerhauser, "Pan-cancer patterns of DNA methylation," *Genome Medicine*, vol. 6, pp. 1–18, 2014.
[126] C. Costa et al., "MicroRNAs alteration as early biomarkers for cancer and neurodegenerative diseases: New challenges in pesticides exposure," *Toxicology Reports*, vol. 7, pp. 759–767, 2020.
[127] L. Pinilla, F. Barbe, and D. de Gonzalo-Calvo, "MicroRNAs to guide medical decision-making in obstructive sleep apnea: A review," *Sleep Medicine Reviews*, vol. 59, p. 101458, 2021.
[128] L. Chin, J. N. Andersen, and P. A. Futreal, "Cancer genomics: From discovery science to personalized medicine," *Nature Medicine*, vol. 17, no. 3, pp. 297–303, 2011.
[129] E. Posadas, F. Simpkins, L. Liotta, C. MacDonald, and E. Kohn, "Proteomic analysis for the early detection and rational treatment of cancer—Realistic hope?" *Annals of Oncology*, vol. 16, no. 1, pp. 16–22, 2005.
[130] N. A. Ghallab, "Diagnostic potential and future directions of biomarkers in gingival crevicular fluid and saliva of periodontal diseases: Review of the current evidence," *Archives of Oral Biology*, vol. 87, pp. 115–124, 2018.
[131] A. Bayés and S. G. Grant, "Neuroproteomics: Understanding the molecular organization and complexity of the brain," *Nature Reviews Neuroscience*, vol. 10, no. 9, pp. 635–646, 2009.
[132] A. Panchaud, M. Affolter, P. Moreillon, and M. Kussmann, "Experimental and computational approaches to quantitative proteomics: Status quo and outlook," *Journal of Proteomics*, vol. 71, no. 1, pp. 19–33, 2008.
[133] A. Zhang, H. Sun, P. Wang, and X. Wang, "Salivary proteomics in biomedical research," *Clinica Chimica Acta*, vol. 415, pp. 261–265, 2013.
[134] L. Migliore and F. Coppedè, "Genetic and environmental factors in cancer and neurodegenerative diseases," *Mutation Research/Reviews in Mutation Research*, vol. 512, no. 2–3, pp. 135–153, 2002.
[135] A. Amir-Aslani and V. Mangematin, "The future of drug discovery and development: Shifting emphasis towards personalized medicine," *Technological Forecasting and Social Change*, vol. 77, no. 2, pp. 203–217, 2010.
[136] H. Mischak et al., "Implementation of proteomic biomarkers: Making it work," *European Journal of Clinical Investigation*, vol. 42, no. 9, pp. 1027–1036, 2012.
[137] M. Tsakiroglou, A. Evans, and M. Pirmohamed, "Leveraging transcriptomics for precision diagnosis: Lessons learned from cancer and sepsis," *Frontiers in Genetics*, vol. 14, p. 1100352, 2023.
[138] L. J. Van't Veer and R. Bernards, "Enabling personalized cancer medicine through analysis of gene-expression patterns," *Nature*, vol. 452, no. 7187, pp. 564–570, 2008.
[139] H. J. Kim, P. Koedrith, and Y. R. Seo, "Ecotoxicogenomic approaches for understanding molecular mechanisms of environmental chemical toxicity using aquatic invertebrate, Daphnia model organism," *International Journal of Molecular Sciences*, vol. 16, no. 6, pp. 12261–12287, 2015.
[140] B. Hwang, J. H. Lee, and D. Bang, "Single-cell RNA sequencing technologies and bioinformatics pipelines," *Experimental & Molecular Medicine*, vol. 50, no. 8, pp. 1–14, 2018.
[141] O. Menyhárt and B. Győrffy, "Multi-omics approaches in cancer research with applications in tumor subtyping, prognosis, and diagnosis," *Computational and Structural Biotechnology Journal*, vol. 19, pp. 949–960, 2021.

[142] X. Yang et al., "High-throughput transcriptome profiling in drug and biomarker discovery," *Frontiers in Genetics*, vol. 11, p. 19, 2020.

[143] J. Reimand et al., "Pathway enrichment analysis and visualization of omics data using g: Profiler, GSEA, Cytoscape and EnrichmentMap," *Nature Protocols*, vol. 14, no. 2, pp. 482–517, 2019.

[144] J. Rello et al., "Towards precision medicine in sepsis: A position paper from the European Society of Clinical Microbiology and Infectious Diseases," *Clinical Microbiology and Infection*, vol. 24, no. 12, pp. 1264–1272, 2018.

[145] I. I. Wistuba, J. G. Gelovani, J. J. Jacoby, S. E. Davis, and R. S. Herbst, "Methodological and practical challenges for personalized cancer therapies," *Nature Reviews Clinical Oncology*, vol. 8, no. 3, pp. 135–141, 2011.

[146] I. Ullah et al., "Multi-omics approaches in colorectal cancer screening and diagnosis, recent updates and future perspectives," *Cancers*, vol. 14, no. 22, p. 5545, 2022.

[147] G. Cammarota et al., "Gut microbiome, big data and machine learning to promote precision medicine for cancer," *Nature Reviews Gastroenterology & Hepatology*, vol. 17, no. 10, pp. 635–648, 2020.

[148] C. I. Justino, A. C. Freitas, R. Pereira, A. C. Duarte, and T. A. R. Santos, "Recent developments in recognition elements for chemical sensors and biosensors," *TrAC Trends in Analytical Chemistry*, vol. 68, pp. 2–17, 2015.

[149] S. Ray, P. J. Reddy, R. Jain, K. Gollapalli, A. Moiyadi, and S. Srivastava, "Proteomic technologies for the identification of disease biomarkers in serum: Advances and challenges ahead," *Proteomics*, vol. 11, no. 11, pp. 2139–2161, 2011.

[150] M. Azmana, S. Mahmood, A. R. Hilles, A. Rahman, M. A. B. Arifin, and S. Ahmed, "A review on chitosan and chitosan-based bionanocomposites: Promising material for combatting global issues and its applications," *International Journal of Biological Macromolecules*, vol. 185, pp. 832–848, 2021.

[151] M. Primožič, Ž. Knez, and M. Leitgeb, "(Bio) Nanotechnology in food science—food packaging," *Nanomaterials*, vol. 11, no. 2, p. 292, 2021.

[152] X. Chen, L. Wang, and J. Lou, "Nanotechnology strategies for the analysis of circulating tumor DNA: A review," *Medical Science Monitor: International Medical Journal of Experimental and Clinical Research*, vol. 26, pp. e921040–e921041, 2020.

[153] L. Zhou et al., "Size-tunable synthesis of lanthanide-doped Gd_2O_3 nanoparticles and their applications for optical and magnetic resonance imaging," *Journal of Materials Chemistry*, vol. 22, no. 3, pp. 966–974, 2012.

[154] J. Wang, "Electrochemical biosensing based on noble metal nanoparticles," *Microchimica Acta*, vol. 177, pp. 245–270, 2012.

[155] F. Li et al., "Multiplexed chemiluminescence determination of three acute myocardial infarction biomarkers based on microfluidic paper-based immunodevice dual amplified by multifunctionalized gold nanoparticles," *Talanta*, vol. 207, p. 120346, 2020.

[156] Z. Karimzadeh, M. Mahmoudpour, M. de la Guardia, J. E. N. Dolatabadi, and A. Jouyban, "Aptamer-functionalized metal organic frameworks as an emerging nanoprobe in the food safety field: Promising development opportunities and translational challenges," *TrAC Trends in Analytical Chemistry*, vol. 152, p. 116622, 2022.

[157] A. Srivastava and G. Agarwal, "Research aspects and strategies for the development of biosensors for renal disease diagnosis," in *BioSensing, Theranostics, and Medical Devices: From Laboratory to Point-of-Care Testing*: Springer, 2021, pp. 165–183.

[158] M. Mahmoudpour et al., "Aptamer functionalized nanomaterials for biomedical applications: Recent advances and new horizons," *Nano Today*, vol. 39, p. 101177, 2021.

[159] S. Yadav, N. Sawarni, T. Dahiya, J. Rana, M. Sharma, and B. Batra, "Nanoagriculture: Advantages and drawbacks," in *Agricultural and Environmental Nanotechnology: Novel Technologies and their Ecological Impact*: Springer, 2023, pp. 3–42.

[160] B. Shan, Y. Pu, Y. Chen, M. Liao, and M. Li, "Novel SERS labels: Rational design, functional integration and biomedical applications," *Coordination Chemistry Reviews*, vol. 371, pp. 11–37, 2018.

[161] H. Moulahoum, F. Ghorbanizamani, E. Guler Celik, and S. Timur, "Nano-scaled materials and polymer integration in biosensing tools," *Biosensors*, vol. 12, no. 5, p. 301, 2022.

[162] D. Du, W. Chen, W. Zhang, D. Liu, H. Li, and Y. Lin, "Covalent coupling of organophosphorus hydrolase loaded quantum dots to carbon nanotube/Au nanocomposite for enhanced detection of methyl parathion," *Biosensors and Bioelectronics*, vol. 25, no. 6, pp. 1370–1375, 2010.

[163] Y.-H. Lee and D. T. Wong, "Saliva: An emerging biofluid for early detection of diseases," *American Journal of Dentistry*, vol. 22, no. 4, p. 241, 2009.

[164] A. R. Lima, J. Pinto, F. Amaro, M. D. L. Bastos, M. Carvalho, and P. Guedes de Pinho, "Advances and perspectives in prostate cancer biomarker discovery in the last 5 years through tissue and urine metabolomics," *Metabolites*, vol. 11, no. 3, p. 181, 2021.

[165] J. Lin et al., "Exosomes: Novel biomarkers for clinical diagnosis," *The Scientific World Journal*, vol. 2015, p. 657086, 2015.

[166] J. Tiernan et al., "Carcinoembryonic antigen is the preferred biomarker for in vivo colorectal cancer targeting," *British Journal of Cancer*, vol. 108, no. 3, pp. 662–667, 2013.

[167] K. Kourou, T. P. Exarchos, K. P. Exarchos, M. V. Karamouzis, and D. I. Fotiadis, "Machine learning applications in cancer prognosis and prediction," *Computational and Structural Biotechnology Journal*, vol. 13, pp. 8–17, 2015.

[168] R. Huss, "Biomarkers," in *Translational Regenerative Medicine*: Elsevier, 2015, pp. 235–241.

[169] N. Mottet et al., "EAU-EANM-ESTRO-ESUR-SIOG guidelines on prostate cancer—2020 update. Part 1: Screening, diagnosis, and local treatment with curative intent," *European Urology*, vol. 79, no. 2, pp. 243–262, 2021.

[170] O. Golubnitschaja, V. Costigliola, and EPMA Olga, "General report & recommendations in predictive, preventive and personalised medicine 2012: White paper of the European Association for Predictive, Preventive and Personalised Medicine," *EPMA Journal*, vol. 3, pp. 1–53, 2012.

[171] A. Di Paolo, F. Sarkozy, B. Ryll, and U. Siebert, "Personalized medicine in Europe: Not yet personal enough?" *BMC Health Services Research*, vol. 17, no. 1, pp. 1–9, 2017.

[172] J. W. Lee et al., "Method validation and measurement of biomarkers in nonclinical and clinical samples in drug development: A conference report," *Pharmaceutical Research*, vol. 22, pp. 499–511, 2005.

[173] M. A. Myszczynska et al., "Applications of machine learning to diagnosis and treatment of neurodegenerative diseases," *Nature Reviews Neurology*, vol. 16, no. 8, pp. 440–456, 2020.

[174] M. Kalia, "Personalized oncology: Recent advances and future challenges," *Metabolism*, vol. 62, pp. S11–S14, 2013.

[175] R. Nabbout and M. Kuchenbuch, "Impact of predictive, preventive and precision medicine strategies in epilepsy," *Nature Reviews Neurology*, vol. 16, no. 12, pp. 674–688, 2020.

[176] R. Mayeux, "Biomarkers: Potential uses and limitations," *NeuroRx*, vol. 1, pp. 182–188, 2004.

[177] J. M. Dennison, *Chemistry and Measurement at Aqueous Nanoscale Interfaces*, 2018.

[178] Y. Wu, Y. Lan, J. Mao, J. Shen, T. Kang, and Z. Xie, "The interaction between the nervous system and the stomatognathic system: From development to diseases," *International Journal of Oral Science*, vol. 15, no. 1, p. 34, 2023.

[179] C. C. B. Ventura, *In Vitro Genotoxic and Epigenotoxic Effects of Occupational Exposure to Nanofibres*, 2019.

[180] T. Bhattacharya et al., "Applications of phyto-nanotechnology for the treatment of neurodegenerative disorders. Materials 2022, 15, 804," *Preparation, Physico Chemical Properties and Biomedical Applications of Nanoparticles*, p. 121, 2022.

[181] P. Mittal et al., "A review on natural antioxidants for their role in the treatment of Parkinson's disease," *Pharmaceuticals*, vol. 16, no. 7, p. 908, 2023.

[182] L. Ding and H. Ju, "Biofunctionalization of nanoparticles for cytosensing and cell surface carbohydrate assay," *Journal of Materials Chemistry*, vol. 21, no. 45, pp. 18154–18173, 2011.

[183] K. Ratajczak and M. Stobiecka, "High-performance modified cellulose paper-based biosensors for medical diagnostics and early cancer screening: A concise review," *Carbohydrate Polymers*, vol. 229, p. 115463, 2020.

[184] B. L. Miller, "Strategy for the future of health 297 RG Bushko (Ed.) IOS Press, 2009© 2009 Renata G. Bushko. All rights reserved," *Strategy for the Future of Health*, vol. 3, p. 297, 2009.

[185] R. B. Walter et al., "Measurable residual disease as a biomarker in acute myeloid leukemia: Theoretical and practical considerations," *Leukemia*, vol. 35, no. 6, pp. 1529–1538, 2021.

[186] A. Bodaghi, N. Fattahi, and A. Ramazani, "Biomarkers: Promising and valuable tools towards diagnosis, prognosis and treatment of Covid-19 and other diseases," *Heliyon*, vol. 9, 2023.

[187] A. Haleem, M. Javaid, R. P. Singh, S. Rab, and R. Suman, "*Applications of Nanotechnology in Medical Field*," *Global Health Journal*, vol. 7, pp. 70–77, 2023.

[188] O. Gohardani, M. C. Elola, and C. Elizetxea, "Potential and prospective implementation of carbon nanotubes on next generation aircraft and space vehicles: A review of current and expected applications in aerospace sciences," *Progress in Aerospace Sciences*, vol. 70, pp. 42–68, 2014.
[189] Y. Khan et al., "Classification, synthetic, and characterization approaches to nanoparticles, and their applications in various fields of nanotechnology: A review," *Catalysts*, vol. 12, no. 11, p. 1386, 2022.
[190] Y. Wang, S. E. Naleway, and B. Wang, "Biological and bioinspired materials: Structure leading to functional and mechanical performance," *Bioactive Materials*, vol. 5, no. 4, pp. 745–757, 2020.
[191] E. Jamróz, P. Kulawik, and P. Kopel, "The effect of nanofillers on the functional properties of biopolymer-based films: A review," *Polymers*, vol. 11, no. 4, p. 675, 2019.
[192] R. Xiong, A. M. Grant, R. Ma, S. Zhang, and V. V. Tsukruk, "Naturally-derived biopolymer nanocomposites: Interfacial design, properties and emerging applications," *Materials Science and Engineering: R: Reports*, vol. 125, pp. 1–41, 2018.
[193] Z. H. Mohammad, F. Ahmad, S. A. Ibrahim, and S. Zaidi, "Application of nanotechnology in different aspects of the food industry," *Discover Food*, vol. 2, no. 1, p. 12, 2022.
[194] K. Y. Perera, S. Jaiswal, and A. K. Jaiswal, "A review on nanomaterials and nanohybrids based bionanocomposites for food packaging," *Food Chemistry*, vol. 376, p. 131912, 2022.
[195] B. Prakash, R. Soman, S. A. Sasi, and M. Mohan, "Impact of bionanocomposites on the environment," in *Bionanocomposites for Food Packaging Applications*: Elsevier, 2022, pp. 435–452.
[196] A. Inamuddin and A. Mohammad, *Applications of Nanocomposite Materials in Drug Delivery*: Elsevier, 2018.
[197] S. Ediyilyam et al., "Synthesis, characterization and physicochemical properties of biogenic silver nanoparticle-encapsulated chitosan bionanocomposites," *Polymers*, vol. 14, no. 3, p. 463, 2022.
[198] I. D. Ibrahim et al., "Biopolymer composites and bionanocomposites for energy applications," *Green Biopolymers and Their Nanocomposites*, pp. 313–341, 2019.
[199] M. Abbas, M. S. Alqahtani, and R. Alhifzi, "Recent developments in polymer nanocomposites for bone regeneration," *International Journal of Molecular Sciences*, vol. 24, no. 4, p. 3312, 2023.
[200] R. G. Araújo et al., "Recent advances in prodigiosin as a bioactive compound in nanocomposite applications," *Molecules*, vol. 27, no. 15, p. 4982, 2022.
[201] F. M. Al-Oqla, M. H. Alaaeddin, M. E. Hoque, and V. K. Thakur, "Biopolymers and biomimetic materials in medical and electronic-related applications for environment–health–development nexus: Systematic review," *Journal of Bionic Engineering*, vol. 19, no. 6, pp. 1562–1577, 2022.
[202] N. Hossain, M. A. Islam, M. A. Chowdhury, and A. Alam, "Advances of nanoparticles employment in dental implant applications," *Applied Surface Science Advances*, vol. 12, p. 100341, 2022.
[203] N. Shahrubudin, T. C. Lee, and R. Ramlan, "An overview on 3D printing technology: Technological, materials, and applications," *Procedia Manufacturing*, vol. 35, pp. 1286–1296, 2019.
[204] A. H. Anwer et al., "State-of-the-art advances in nanocomposite and bio-nanocomposite polymeric materials: A comprehensive review," *Advances in Colloid and Interface Science*, p. 102955, 2023.
[205] J. R. A. Pires, C. Rodrigues, I. Coelhoso, A. L. Fernando, and V. G. L. Souza, "Current applications of bionanocomposites in food processing and packaging," *Polymers*, vol. 15, no. 10, p. 2336, 2023.
[206] K. Bensalah, F. Montorsi, and S. F. Shariat, "Challenges of cancer biomarker profiling," *European Urology*, vol. 52, no. 6, pp. 1601–1609, 2007.
[207] S. Kizhepat, A. S. Rasal, J.-Y. Chang, and H.-F. Wu, "Development of two-dimensional functional nanomaterials for biosensor applications: Opportunities, challenges, and future prospects," *Nanomaterials*, vol. 13, no. 9, p. 1520, 2023.
[208] T. Kalyani, A. Sangili, A. Nanda, S. Prakash, A. Kaushik, and S. K. Jana, "Bio-nanocomposite based highly sensitive and label-free electrochemical immunosensor for endometriosis diagnostics application," *Bioelectrochemistry*, vol. 139, p. 107740, 2021.
[209] C. I. Idumah, "Novel trends in conductive polymeric nanocomposites, and bionanocomposites," *Synthetic Metals*, vol. 273, p. 116674, 2021.
[210] O. Hosu, A. Florea, C. Cristea, and R. Sandulescu, "Functionalized advanced hybrid materials for biosensing applications," in *Advanced Biosensors for Health care Applications*: Elsevier, 2019, pp. 171–207.
[211] A. U. Khan, M. Khan, M. H. Cho, and M. M. Khan, "Selected nanotechnologies and nanostructures for drug delivery, nanomedicine and cure," *Bioprocess and Biosystems Engineering*, vol. 43, pp. 1339–1357, 2020.

[212] F. Lebre et al., "Nanosafety: An evolving concept to bring the safest possible nanomaterials to society and environment," *Nanomaterials*, vol. 12, no. 11, p. 1810, 2022.
[213] B. Sharma, S. Tiwari, K. C. Kumawat, and M. Cardinale, "Nano-biofertilizers as bio-emerging strategies for sustainable agriculture development: Potentiality and their limitations," *Science of The Total Environment*, vol. 860, p. 160476, 2023.
[214] S. Deng et al., "Application of nanotechnology in the early diagnosis and comprehensive treatment of gastrointestinal cancer," *Journal of Nanobiotechnology*, vol. 20, no. 1, p. 415, 2022.
[215] Y. Zhang et al., "Programmable and multifunctional DNA-based materials for biomedical applications," *Advanced Materials*, vol. 30, no. 24, p. 1703658, 2018.
[216] M. L. Sin, K. E. Mach, P. K. Wong, and J. C. Liao, "Advances and challenges in biosensor-based diagnosis of infectious diseases," *Expert Review of Molecular Diagnostics*, vol. 14, no. 2, pp. 225–244, 2014.
[217] N. A. Dahlan et al., "Role of nanomaterials in the fabrication of bioNEMS/MEMS for biomedical applications and towards pioneering food waste utilisation," *Nanomaterials*, vol. 12, no. 22, p. 4025, 2022.
[218] G. Maduraiveeran, "Bionanomaterial-based electrochemical biosensing platforms for biomedical applications," *Analytical Methods*, vol. 12, no. 13, pp. 1688–1701, 2020.
[219] A. Atapour et al., "Gold nanoparticle-based aptasensors: A promising perspective for early-stage detection of cancer biomarkers," *Materials Today Communications*, vol. 30, p. 103181, 2022.
[220] Z. Ren, L. Xu, L. Yang, and Y. Cui, "Minimizing cross-reactivity for the chemiluminescent lateral flow immunoassay of cardiac troponin I based on PEGylation of gold nanoparticles," *Analytical Chemistry*, vol. 95, no. 16, pp. 6646–6654, 2023.
[221] R. Kottappara, S. C. Pillai, and B. K. Vijayan, "Copper-and iron-based bio-nanocomposites for green applications," *Biobased Nanotechnology for Green Applications*, pp. 41–72, 2021.
[222] P. B. Chouke et al., "Bioinspired metal/metal oxide nanoparticles: A road map to potential applications," *Materials Today Advances*, vol. 16, p. 100314, 2022.
[223] K. C. Lai, L. Y. Lee, B. Y. Z. Hiew, S. Thangalazhy-Gopakumar, and S. Gan, "Environmental application of three-dimensional graphene materials as adsorbents for dyes and heavy metals: Review on ice-templating method and adsorption mechanisms," *Journal of Environmental Sciences*, vol. 79, pp. 174–199, 2019.
[224] X. Zhang, H. Chen, and H. Zhang, "Layer-by-layer assembly: From conventional to unconventional methods," *Chemical Communications*, no. 14, pp. 1395–1405, 2007.
[225] U. Chadha et al., "Current trends and future perspectives of nanomaterials in food packaging application," *Journal of Nanomaterials*, vol. 2022, pp. 1–32, 2022.
[226] Z. Aguilar, *Nanomaterials for Medical Applications*: Newnes, 2012.
[227] M. Abniki, A. Moghimi, and F. Azizinejad, "Fabrication of bionanocomposite based on LDH using biopolymer of gum arabic and chitosan-coating for sustained drug-release," *Journal of the Serbian Chemical Society*, vol. 85, no. 9, pp. 1223–1235, 2020.
[228] L. N. Ribeiro, A. C. Alcântara, M. Darder, P. Aranda, F. M. Araújo-Moreira, and E. Ruiz-Hitzky, "Pectin-coated chitosan–LDH bionanocomposite beads as potential systems for colon-targeted drug delivery," *International Journal of Pharmaceutics*, vol. 463, no. 1, pp. 1–9, 2014.
[229] D.-Y. Fu et al., "Polymer-metal-organic framework hybrids for bioimaging and cancer therapy," *Coordination Chemistry Reviews*, vol. 456, p. 214393, 2022.
[230] Z. Zheng, S. Zhu, M. Lv, Z. Gu, and H. Hu, "Harnessing nanotechnology for cardiovascular disease applications-A comprehensive review based on bibliometric analysis," *Nano Today*, vol. 44, p. 101453, 2022.
[231] K. Y. Goud et al., "Electrochemical diagnostics of infectious viral diseases: Trends and challenges," *Biosensors and Bioelectronics*, vol. 180, p. 113112, 2021.
[232] A. Baranwal et al., "Chitosan: An undisputed bio-fabrication material for tissue engineering and biosensing applications," *International Journal of Biological Macromolecules*, vol. 110, pp. 110–123, 2018.
[233] S. Guo and S. Dong, "Biomolecule-nanoparticle hybrids for electrochemical biosensors," *TrAC Trends in Analytical Chemistry*, vol. 28, no. 1, pp. 96–109, 2009.
[234] S. Pandit, D. Dasgupta, N. Dewan, and A. Prince, "Nanotechnology based biosensors and its application," *The Pharma Innovation*, vol. 5, no. 6, Part A, p. 18, 2016.
[235] X. Zheng et al., "Smart biosensors and intelligent devices for salivary biomarker detection," *TrAC Trends in Analytical Chemistry*, vol. 140, p. 116281, 2021.
[236] A. Nilghaz, S. M. Mousavi, J. Tian, R. Cao, R. M. Guijt, and X. Wang, "Noble-metal nanoparticle-based colorimetric diagnostic assays for point-of-need applications," *ACS Applied Nano Materials*, vol. 4, no. 12, pp. 12808–12824, 2021.

[237] E. Lahiff, C. Lynam, N. Gilmartin, R. O'Kennedy, and D. Diamond, "The increasing importance of carbon nanotubes and nanostructured conducting polymers in biosensors," *Analytical and Bioanalytical Chemistry*, vol. 398, pp. 1575–1589, 2010.

[238] S. Tiwari, V. Sharma, M. Mujawar, Y. K. Mishra, A. Kaushik, and A. Ghosal, "Biosensors for epilepsy management: State-of-art and future aspects," *Sensors*, vol. 19, no. 7, p. 1525, 2019.

[239] P. Pashazadeh, A. Mokhtarzadeh, M. Hasanzadeh, M. Hejazi, M. Hashemi, and M. de la Guardia, "Nanomaterials for use in sensing of salmonella infections: Recent advances," *Biosensors and Bioelectronics*, vol. 87, pp. 1050–1064, 2017.

[240] V. Chaudhary, S. Punia Bangar, N. Thakur, and M. Trif, "Recent advancements in smart biogenic packaging: Reshaping the future of the food packaging industry," *Polymers*, vol. 14, no. 4, p. 829, 2022.

[241] Y. He, C. Hu, Z. Li, C. Wu, Y. Zeng, and C. Peng, "Multifunctional carbon nanomaterials for diagnostic applications in infectious diseases and tumors," *Materials Today Bio*, vol. 14, p. 100231, 2022.

[242] K. Rambabu et al., "Biocompatible nanomaterials for sensing and remediation of nitrites and fluorides from polluted water," in *Advances in Nano and Biochemistry*: Elsevier, 2023, pp. 57–84.

[243] M. Hasanzadeh and N. Shadjou, "Electrochemical and photoelectrochemical nano-immunesensing using origami paper based method," *Materials Science and Engineering: C*, vol. 61, pp. 979–1001, 2016.

[244] C. M. Leung et al., "A guide to the organ-on-a-chip," *Nature Reviews Methods Primers*, vol. 2, no. 1, p. 33, 2022.

[245] A. Othman, A. Karimi, and S. Andreescu, "Functional nanostructures for enzyme based biosensors: Properties, fabrication and applications," *Journal of Materials Chemistry B*, vol. 4, no. 45, pp. 7178–7203, 2016.

[246] R. Ahmad, O. S. Wolfbeis, Y.-B. Hahn, H. N. Alshareef, L. Torsi, and K. N. Salama, "Deposition of nanomaterials: A crucial step in biosensor fabrication," *Materials Today Communications*, vol. 17, pp. 289–321, 2018.

[247] E. Ruiz-Hitzky et al., "Nanotechnology responses to COVID-19," *Advanced Healthcare Materials*, vol. 9, no. 19, p. 2000979, 2020.

[248] R. Pathak, V. D. Punetha, S. Bhatt, and M. Punetha, "Carbon nanotube-based biocompatible polymer nanocomposites as an emerging tool for biomedical applications," *European Polymer Journal*, vol. 196, p. 112257, 2023.

[249] S. Hua, E. Marks, J. J. Schneider, and S. Keely, "Advances in oral nano-delivery systems for colon targeted drug delivery in inflammatory bowel disease: Selective targeting to diseased versus healthy tissue," *Nanomedicine: Nanotechnology, Biology and Medicine*, vol. 11, no. 5, pp. 1117–1132, 2015.

[250] E. Sadiku et al., "Biological, biomedical, and medical applications of graphene and graphene-based materials (G-bMs)," *Handbook of Graphene Set*, vol. 1, pp. 1–41, 2019.

[251] B. Sharma, S. Shekhar, A. Kumar, and S. Sharma, "Biomimetic nanosystems in theranostics," in *Advanced Nanoformulations*: Elsevier, 2023, pp. 637–660.

[252] R. Umapathi, S. M. Ghoreishian, S. Sonwal, G. M. Rani, and Y. S. Huh, "Portable electrochemical sensing methodologies for on-site detection of pesticide residues in fruits and vegetables," *Coordination Chemistry Reviews*, vol. 453, p. 214305, 2022.

[253] A. Ascherio and K. L. Munger, "Environmental risk factors for multiple sclerosis. Part I: The role of infection," *Annals of Neurology*, vol. 61, no. 4, pp. 288–299, 2007.

[254] H. Qamar et al., "CuO bionanocomposite with enhanced stability and antibacterial activity against extended-spectrum beta-lactamase strains," *Materials*, vol. 14, no. 21, p. 6336, 2021.

[255] S. Ning, M. Jorfi, S. R. Patel, D. Y. Kim, and R. E. Tanzi, "Neurotechnological approaches to the diagnosis and treatment of Alzheimer's disease," *Frontiers in Neuroscience*, vol. 16, p. 854992, 2022.

[256] S. A. Ansari and Q. Husain, "Potential applications of enzymes immobilized on/in nano materials: A review," *Biotechnology Advances*, vol. 30, no. 3, pp. 512–523, 2012.

[257] K. Hu, D. D. Kulkarni, I. Choi, and V. V. Tsukruk, "Graphene-polymer nanocomposites for structural and functional applications," *Progress in Polymer Science*, vol. 39, no. 11, pp. 1934–1972, 2014.

[258] M. Ekrami, Z. Emam-Djomeh, P. Joolaei-Ahranjani, S. Mahmoodi, and S. Khaleghi, "Eco-friendly UV protective bionanocomposite based on Salep-mucilage/flower-like ZnO nanostructures to control photo-oxidation of kilka fish oil," *International Journal of Biological Macromolecules*, vol. 168, pp. 591–600, 2021.

[259] J. Pellico, C. M. Ellis, and J. J. Davis, "Nanoparticle-based paramagnetic contrast agents for magnetic resonance imaging," *Contrast Media & Molecular Imaging*, vol. 2019, 2019.

[260] B. Wang et al., "Early diagnosis and treatment for Sjögren's syndrome: Current challenges, redefined disease stages and future prospects," *Journal of Autoimmunity*, vol. 117, p. 102590, 2021.

[261] M. Dervisevic, E. Dervisevic, E. Çevik, and M. Şenel, "Novel electrochemical xanthine biosensor based on chitosan–polypyrrole–gold nanoparticles hybrid bio-nanocomposite platform," *journal of Food and Drug Analysis*, vol. 25, no. 3, pp. 510–519, 2017.

[262] K. Wang, R. Shen, T. Meng, F. Hu, and H. Yuan, "Nano-drug delivery systems based on different targeting mechanisms in the targeted therapy of colorectal cancer," *Molecules*, vol. 27, no. 9, p. 2981, 2022.

[263] K. Ying, B. Bai, X. Gao, Y. Xu, H. Wang, and B. Xie, "Orally administrable therapeutic nanoparticles for the treatment of colorectal cancer," *Frontiers in Bioengineering and Biotechnology*, vol. 9, p. 670124, 2021.

[264] R. Eivazzadeh-Keihan et al., "Functionalized magnetic nanoparticles for the separation and purification of proteins and peptides," *TrAC Trends in Analytical Chemistry*, vol. 141, p. 116291, 2021.

[265] F. Martinelli et al., "Advanced methods of plant disease detection. A review," *Agronomy for Sustainable Development*, vol. 35, no. 1, pp. 1–25, 2015.

[266] A. Bekmurzayeva, M. Sypabekova, and D. Kanayeva, "Tuberculosis diagnosis using immunodominant, secreted antigens of Mycobacterium tuberculosis," *Tuberculosis*, vol. 93, no. 4, pp. 381–388, 2013.

[267] K. K. Alharbi and Y. A. Al-Sheikh, "Role and implications of nanodiagnostics in the changing trends of clinical diagnosis," *Saudi Journal of Biological Sciences*, vol. 21, no. 2, pp. 109–117, 2014.

[268] R. Zhou et al., "Recent advances in food-derived nanomaterials applied to biosensing," *TrAC Trends in Analytical Chemistry*, vol. 127, p. 115884, 2020.

[269] F. Sharifianjazi et al., "Biosensors and nanotechnology for cancer diagnosis (lung and bronchus, breast, prostate, and colon): A systematic review," *Biomedical Materials*, vol. 17, no. 1, p. 012002, 2021.

[270] H. Ahari et al., "Bio-nanocomposites as food packaging materials; the main production techniques and analytical parameters," *Advances in Colloid and Interface Science*, vol. 310, p. 102806, 2022.

[271] E. O. Wilson, *Sociobiology: The New Synthesis*: Harvard University Press, 2000.

[272] N. Dubey, C. S. Kushwaha, and S. Shukla, "A review on electrically conducting polymer bionanocomposites for biomedical and other applications," *International Journal of Polymeric Materials and Polymeric Biomaterials*, vol. 69, no. 11, pp. 709–727, 2020.

[273] M. Goldberg, R. Langer, and X. Jia, "Nanostructured materials for applications in drug delivery and tissue engineering," *Journal of Biomaterials Science, Polymer Edition*, vol. 18, no. 3, pp. 241–268, 2007.

[274] S. Ullah et al., "MXene-based aptasensors: Advances, challenges, and prospects," *Progress in Materials Science*, vol. 129, p. 100967, 2022.

[275] R. de Sousa Victor, A. Marcelo da Cunha Santos, B. Viana de Sousa, G. de Araújo Neves, L. Navarro de Lima Santana, and R. Rodrigues Menezes, "A review on Chitosan's uses as biomaterial: Tissue engineering, drug delivery systems and cancer treatment," *Materials*, vol. 13, no. 21, p. 4995, 2020.

[276] A. D. Pomogailo and G. I. Dzhardimalieva, *Nanostructured Materials Preparation via Condensation Ways*: Springer, 2014.

[277] R. Dewar and J. Werbel, "Universalistic and contingency predictions of employee satisfaction and conflict," *Administrative Science Quarterly*, pp. 426–448, 1979.

[278] J. A. Malik and M. J. S. Mohamed, *Modern Nanotechnology: Volume 1: Environmental Sustainability and Remediation*: Springer Nature, 2023.

[279] H. Liu et al., "Application of biodegradable and biocompatible nanocomposites in electronics: Current status and future directions," *Nanomaterials*, vol. 9, no. 7, p. 950, 2019.

[280] D. W. Kimmel, G. LeBlanc, M. E. Meschievitz, and D. E. Cliffel, "Electrochemical sensors and biosensors," *Analytical Chemistry*, vol. 84, no. 2, pp. 685–707, 2012.

[281] P. R. Srinivas et al., "Nanotechnology research: Applications in nutritional sciences," *The Journal of Nutrition*, vol. 140, no. 1, pp. 119–124, 2010.

[282] R. Zafar, K. M. Zia, S. Tabasum, F. Jabeen, A. Noreen, and M. Zuber, "Polysaccharide based bionanocomposites, properties and applications: A review," *International Journal of Biological Macromolecules*, vol. 92, pp. 1012–1024, 2016.

[283] M. G. D. Morais, V. G. Martins, D. Steffens, P. Pranke, and J. A. V. da Costa, "Biological applications of nanobiotechnology," *Journal of Nanoscience and Nanotechnology*, vol. 14, no. 1, pp. 1007–1017, 2014.

[284] P. V. Tawade and K. L. Wasewar, "Nanotechnology in biological science and engineering," in *Environmental Applications of Microbial Nanotechnology*: Elsevier, 2023, pp. 43–64.

[285] R. Bawa, "Patents and nanomedicine," 2007. https://doi.org/10.2217/17435889.2.3.351

[286] M.-A. Baucher, R. Scott, C. Cannizzaro, S. Standridge, E. Nesbitt, and T. Fadel, *Symposium on Assessing the Economic Impact of Nanotechnology: Synthesis Report*, 2013.

[287] M. Boenink, T. Swierstra, and D. Stemerding, "Anticipating the interaction between technology and morality: A scenario study of experimenting with humans in bionanotechnology," *Studies in Ethics, Law, and Technology*, vol. 4, no. 2, pp. 1–38, 2010.

[288] T. Adam and S. C. Gopinath, "Nanosensors: Recent perspectives on attainments and future promise of downstream applications," *Process Biochemistry*, vol. 117, pp. 153–173, 2022.

[289] N. Pradhan et al., "Facets of nanotechnology as seen in food processing, packaging, and preservation industry," *BioMed Research International*, vol. 2015, 2015. https://doi.org/10.1155/2015/365672

[290] M. N. F. Norrrahim et al., "The frontiers of functionalized nanocellulose-based composites and their application as chemical sensors," *Polymers*, vol. 14, no. 20, p. 4461, 2022.

[291] B. L. Peng, N. Dhar, H. Liu, and K. Tam, "Chemistry and applications of nanocrystalline cellulose and its derivatives: A nanotechnology perspective," *The Canadian Journal of Chemical Engineering*, vol. 89, no. 5, pp. 1191–1206, 2011.

[292] A. Kalsoom Khan et al., "Carrageenan based bionanocomposites as drug delivery tool with special emphasis on the influence of ferromagnetic nanoparticles," *Oxidative Medicine and Cellular Longevity*, vol. 2017, p. 8158315, 2017.

[293] M. Rizwan, M. Hazmi, S. A. Lim, and M. U. Ahmed, "A highly sensitive electrochemical detection of human chorionic gonadotropin on a carbon nano-onions/gold nanoparticles/polyethylene glycol nanocomposite modified glassy carbon electrode," *Journal of Electroanalytical Chemistry*, vol. 833, pp. 462–470, 2019.

[294] L. M. T. Phan et al., "Nanomaterial-based optical and electrochemical biosensors for amyloid beta and tau: Potential for early diagnosis of Alzheimer's disease," *Expert Review of Molecular Diagnostics*, vol. 21, no. 2, pp. 175–193, 2021.

[295] A. Parihar et al., "Internet-of-medical-things integrated point-of-care biosensing devices for infectious diseases: Toward better preparedness for futuristic pandemics," *Bioengineering & Translational Medicine*, vol. 8, p. e10481, 2023.

[296] N. M. Noah and P. M. Ndangili, "Current trends of nanobiosensors for point-of-care diagnostics," *Journal of Analytical Methods in Chemistry*, vol. 2019, p. 2179718, 2019.

[297] S. Solanki, C. M. Pandey, R. K. Gupta, and B. D. Malhotra, "Emerging trends in microfluidics based devices," *Biotechnology Journal*, vol. 15, no. 5, p. 1900279, 2020.

[298] E. Drucker and K. Krapfenbauer, "Pitfalls and limitations in translation from biomarker discovery to clinical utility in predictive and personalised medicine," *EPMA Journal*, vol. 4, pp. 1–10, 2013.

[299] F. S. Rodrigues Ribeiro Teles, L. A. Pires de Tavora Tavira, and L. J. Pina da Fonseca, "Biosensors as rapid diagnostic tests for tropical diseases," *Critical Reviews in Clinical Laboratory Sciences*, vol. 47, no. 3, pp. 139–169, 2010.

[300] I. M. Buhazi et al., "Polydopamine conjugated SiO_2 nanoparticles as potential drug carriers for melanoma treatment," *Therapeutic Delivery*, vol. 14, no. 2, pp. 157–173, 2023.

10 Seaweed-Based Bionanocomposite for Biomedical Applications

Jeba Sweetly Dharmadhas, Rajiv Periakaruppan, Gomathi Renga Raj, Issac Abraham Sybiya Vasantha Packiavathy, Aminu Abdullahi and Selva Kumar T.

10.1 INTRODUCTION

The fascinating field of bionanocomposite science combines biology, nanotechnology, and material sciences. We can describe bionanocomposites as hybrid materials in recent years. Because they are effective substitutes for petroleum-based products in a variety of applications, researchers' interest in bionanocomposites has impressively increased. Bionanocomposites exhibit good physical, mechanical, and chemical properties, a high surface area, and a reasonable cost because of their nanoscale size [1, 2]. Green composites, or bionanocomposites, are materials that are entirely biodegradable and can be made by mixing in a natural or biopolymer. The characteristics of bionanocomposite materials are determined by their modules, which consist of organic, inorganic, and biopolymer nanoparticles (NPs). In recent decades, a variety of biopolymeric materials have been converted into bionanocomposites, and these materials are essential to our daily existence. The primary benefit of bionanocomposites, also known as green composites, is their easy environmental degradation due to their eco-friendliness [3]. The highly valuable, newly developed hybrid nanostructured materials known as bionanocomposites are created when biopolymers are combined, assembled, or mixed using nanoscale organic or inorganic substances. The mechanical and thermal stability of the biopolymer, as well as several other properties (biocompatibility and biodegradability), are improved by this combination. They are environmentally friendly materials with numerous applications in tissue manipulation, cancer diagnosis, dressing for wounds (artificial skin), medication delivery systems, and other areas [4].

The first application of nanotechnology to improve a drug's therapeutic effect was made around 1965. Various techniques, including adsorption and physical or chemical conjugation, are used to encapsulate or load drug molecules into nanocarriers [5]. Pharmaceutical researchers have introduced many benefits (longer systemic circulation, precise drug targeting, controlled sustained release, and enhanced drug solubility) for the purpose of treating different infectious infections using nanocarriers [6]. Therefore, to increase the effectiveness of treatment for currently available antibiotics or medications, the usage of liposomes, polymeric NPs, dendrimers, and other inorganic NPs as drug delivery platforms has increased. The scientific discipline of this technology holds abundant capacity for producing novel as well as inventive materials. The use of nanotechnology in the biological sciences has been expanding quickly with a great deal of fresh and original content throughout the previous few years [7]. It entails the investigation, synthesis, creation, and characterization of materials at the nanoscale, or those containing at least one dimension on the scale of B1100 nm. This skill is still expanding quickly throughout the world and has greatly advanced medical research. Nanomaterials have distinct physical and chemical properties that set them apart from their bulk material due to their specific qualities (small size and huge surface area-to-volume ratio).

DOI: 10.1201/9781003650812-10

Today, because polymeric materials are nontoxic, nonallergenic, biodegradable, and biocompatible, researchers from a variety of fields are working to create environmentally friendly polymeric materials. In general, bionanocomposites are made of inexpensive materials. Nanoscale inorganic fillers are added to or blended with biopolymers to address their shortcomings [8].

Polysaccharides are thought to be appealing materials for the creation of cutting-edge bioapplication systems, like tissue engineering and medication delivery, because they incorporate a variety of functionalities into their structures, exhibit intriguing physical and chemical characteristics, and have important biological activities [9, 10]. In this instance, natural carbohydrates are being used more and more, either in their original state or following chemical modification, to provide customized materials for particular uses [11]. Compared to polysaccharides derived from animals, those from marine algae are thought to be safer and non-immunogenic [12, 13]. Numerous green algae species are globally distributed and are valued as vital components of the human diet, commonly referred to as marine vegetables, in numerous regions. Algal biomass is a sustainable and renewable waste material that can be used to produce fine chemicals and biopolymers. It is typically collected from marine-eutrophicated coastal areas. Simultaneously, green algae can be grown in open cages near coasts or in land-based tanks, where they can act as a biofilter to improve the quality of the seawater and guarantee enough of their polysaccharides for industrial use. Researchers have announced several strategies to replace the synthetic material with amazing biopolymers (alginate, heparin, cellulose, carboxymethyl cellulose, starch, collagen, pectin, keratin, dextran sulfate, albumin, nanoclay, polylactic-co-glycolic acid, pullulan, chitosan, xanthan, fibroin, gelatin, hyaluronic acid, etc.) [14]. Bionanocomposites have numerous biomedical uses, including drug delivery, antibacterial agents, wound dressings, and other medical devices. Because of its antimicrobial activity, chitosan-based nanocomposite in particular demonstrated very positive applications in tissue engineering, medicine, wound healing, and medication delivery [15–17]. Since the 1960s, various surgical fixation instruments, such as PGLAs, PGA, and PLA, have been used to make sutures, bone plates, clips, and pins. These days, biodegradable polymers, copolymers, and biocomposites come in over forty varieties and serve as great substitutes for metal implants. The drawbacks of metal implants are also addressed by the bionanocomposite material, which eliminates the need for an implant removal procedure. Thanks to developments in bionanocomposites, hard and soft scaffolds for tissue engineering and tissue culture are now possible. Currently, scientists are creating and altering biobased materials with a range of uses across diverse domains.

Carrageenan is a type of seaweed-based bionanocomposites that has drawn a great deal of interest in recent years due to its many characteristics, which include biodegradability, nontoxicity, and biocompatibility. Moreover, by utilizing various nanofillers, these composites can be customized to serve the intended purpose [18]. Material chemists have created sophisticated medications with enhanced biological, magnetic, and electrical properties in the last few years. A range of medication administration methods, including targeted drug release, have been investigated using NPs [19].

The main components used in the synthesis of bionanocomposites are biopolymers. They are separated into four groups: DNA, proteins, polysaccharides, and poly(hydroxyalkanoates). The most preferred of these are proteins and carbohydrates. Natural polymers called biopolymers are sourced from renewable resources like microbes, algae, and plants. In dental research, biopolymers are essential as a supportive material for regeneration. For use in dentistry in periodontal, prosthodontic, orthodontic, and endodontic applications, biopolymers have been developed extensively. These applications include scaffolds and biomembranes (e.g., hydrogels, barrier membranes, nanofibers, bioink, guided bone regeneration, and guided tissue regeneration are all used in 3D printing). Since the beginning of time, various biopolymers have been used. These include hyaluronic acid, collagen, and chitosan, all of which are challenging and non-versatile to obtain and not economically viable in such an environment. Biopolymers, namely ulvan, alginate, carrageenan, fucoidan, and agar, remain useful in dental applications. Seaweed biopolymers are readily accessible and have the same properties as other biopolymers when it comes to material creation. As with other biopolymers, it is possible to blend antibiotics and NPs for slow release with seaweed polymers. Moreover, osteogenic processes, cytocompatibility, and biocompatibility in nature are supported by seaweed biopolymers. Its strong gel strength and excellent resorbability make it an excellent option for dental applications because of its favorable mechanical and physical attributes. Seaweed-derived biopolymers also have strong structural integrity, biocompatibility, and the capacity to encourage the growth and division of cells. Seaweed biopolymers have antimicrobial, antioxidant, and anti-inflammatory properties [20].

Natural biomaterials derived from seaweeds are becoming more and more significant in the medical industry, particularly for use in dentistry. Agar, carrageenan, alginate, and ulvan are examples of biopolymers that are widely used in various fields. Particularly in dental applications, biopolymers are either irreversible (alginate) or reversible (agar and carrageenan). Common applications in the dental field include impression creation and scaffold preparation. In addition to dental applications, these polymers are used in food and drug delivery applications [21].

Seaweeds are macroalgae that fall into three different categories according to their outward appearance: red (Rhodophyta), green (Chlorophyta), and brown (Phaeophyceae). Seaweeds are abundant in biopolymers, pigments, and other bioactive substances (such as polyphenols). Together with biopolymers, seaweeds are rich sources of bioactive pigments, including phycobiliproteins, carotenoids, and some polyphenols. These substances have numerous medicinal applications and are physiologically active. Biopolymers are finding increasing use in medicine for a range of purposes, especially in scaffold applications related to cancer and dental impressions. Biopolymers, hydrocolloids, and polysaccharides make up the majority of seaweeds (50–70%), with proteins (5–47%), pigments, lipids, and polyphenols [22].

Seaweeds are the best option for generating biopolymers because they have a number of benefits over other biological sources, such as increased biomass productivity, abundance, cultivability, and year-round availability. The main bioactive component of hydrocolloid-rich seaweeds is polysaccharides, which also include lipids, polyphenols, carotenoids, and chlorophylls. Seaweeds are widely recognized for providing important raw materials for a range of industries, including textile, fertilizer, food, and pharmaceutical. As per their economic worth, ulvan, fucoidan, laminarin, agar-agar, alginate, carrageenan, etc. are some of the hydrocolloids from seaweeds that are commonly extracted. It is commonly known that carrageenan, a polysaccharide obtained from seaweed that was isolated from *Kappaphycus alvarezii*, possesses remarkable properties that are similar to those of plant-based biopolymers. Carrageenan is frequently employed in the food and packaging industries due to its high swelling and exceptional gel-forming capabilities. Because of their poor mechanical qualities (brittle and fragile) and hydrophilic (water-permeable) character, biopolymers outlast man-made plastics even if they are superior alternatives. Because of this, mixing biopolymers derived from seaweed with other polymeric materials (such as agar and alginate) may be a useful way to alter their surface characteristics. Plasticizers are also commonly utilized for surface modification for a variety of purposes in many different sectors. These include PEG, sorbitol, glutaraldehyde, KCl, glycerol, etc. This enhances the mechanical strength, optical, physical, thermal, and biological properties of the biopolymers as well as their moisture retention. They also get stronger mechanically [23].

10.2 STRUCTURE OF POLYSACCHARIDES

Polysaccharides are an extremely intricate category of biopolymers that are essential for all living things. They are composed of uronic acids linked to α-(1,4)-glycosidic linkages and homo- or heteromonosaccharides as in Figure 10.1 [24]. They are generally present in a wide range of flora, animals, algae, fungi, and bacteria, and they are essential to many physiological processes in life [25]. Furthermore, because polysaccharides are naturally occurring biomaterials with unique bioactivities and properties, cellular physiology is an excellent fit for their possession [26]. Carbohydrates are the conventional term for polysaccharides, also called glycans. The standard formula for

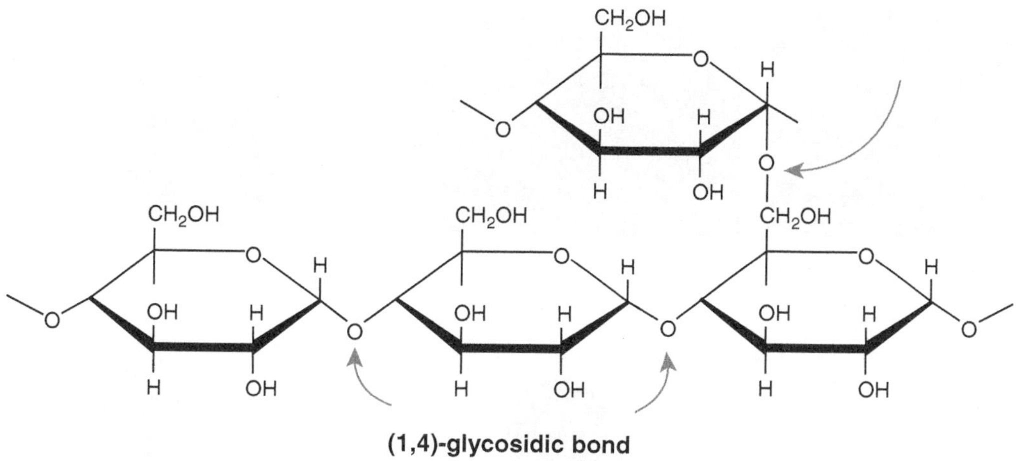

FIGURE 10.1 Schematic representation of a seaweed polysaccharide.

polysaccharides is Cx (H_2O) y, where x might be between 200 and 2500. Ketones and hydroxy aldehydes are examples of monosaccharide units that make up the polysaccharide [27]. These monosaccharides typically include five carbon atoms (furanose) or six carbon atoms (pyrenees). The hydroxyl (OH) groups found in monosaccharides cause hydrogen bonds to form between polymer chains [28]. Specifically, spiral structures like coils or helices can form in polysaccharides as a result of hydrogen bonding between neighboring monosaccharide molecules. The hydroxyl groups (OH) on nearby glucose units produced a hydrogen bond, which strengthened and stabilized the contact between the two monomers [29]. The glucose units can form a long chain that is twisted according to where the glucose units came from by repeating this pattern of hydrogen bonding between the units. One important component of a plant's cell wall, cellulose, has a helical structure that gives it its mechanical strength. Because of hydrogen bonds between neighboring monomers, spiral structures are also seen in other polysaccharides, such as chitin and glycogen [30]. These polysaccharides' special qualities—like their stiffness or capacity to store glucose for energy—come from their structural makeup. In addition to serving a variety of physiological purposes, polysaccharides are being thoroughly researched to create innovative goods in a variety of industries, including food, medicine, cosmetics, and more [31].

Some of the most commonly produced nanocomposites from brown algae are metallic ones, such as copper (CuNPs), silver (AgNPs), and gold (AuNPs) [32–34]. Over 50% of the published information found in the literature concerning various metallic nanocomposites deals with the synthesis of silver particles from various strains of algae. This happens due to the reason that AgNPs have better physical and chemical properties than their bulk forms, which makes them very helpful in a variety of industries, including wound healing, paints, jewelry, textiles, dental alloys, and drug delivery [35–37].

10.3 SYNTHESIS OF NANOCOMPOSITES

From Figure 10.2, it seems that in green synthesis, algae are becoming more and more common because they are abundant in proteins, peptides, pigments, and secondary metabolites that operate as tiny biofactories [38]. Because of their rapid growth rate, simplicity of harvesting, and economical scale-up, they are also attractive candidates for the biological synthesis of NPs [39]. The most rudimentary creatures on Earth, algae are the predominant photosynthetic organisms and inhabit a variety of environments [40]. Algae are the ideal material for green synthesis since they can hyperaccumulate metals and convert them into NPs [41]. As illustrated in Figure 10.3 [42, 43], many types

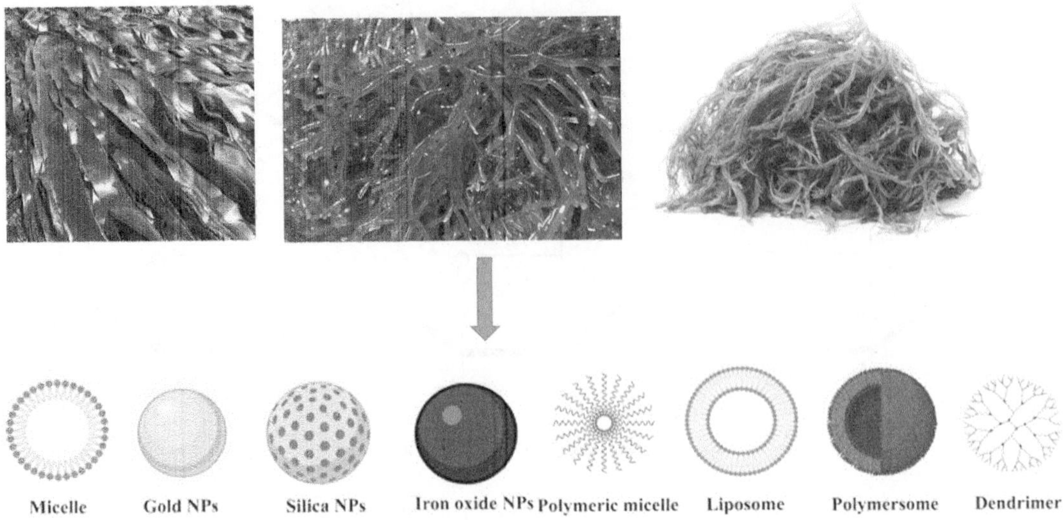

FIGURE 10.2 Graphical representation of marine seaweed-mediated biosynthesis.

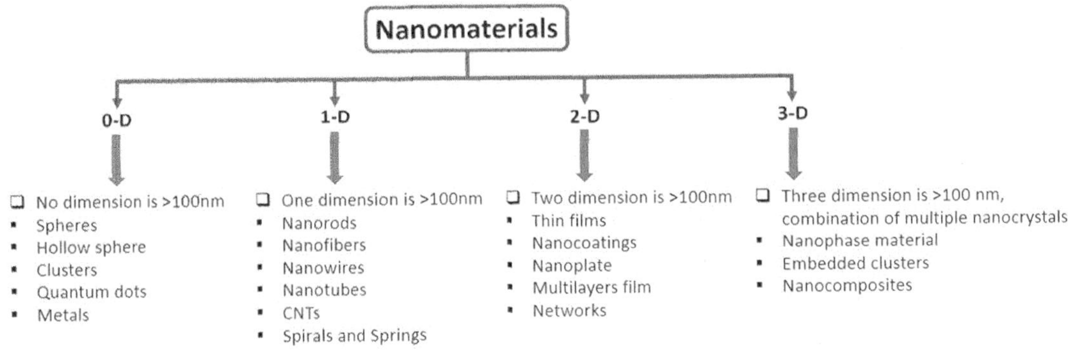

FIGURE 10.3 Illustrates the 0D, 1D, 2D, and 3D structures of nanocomposites.

of algae, such as blue-green algae (Cyanophyceae), brown algae (Phaeophyceae), green algae (Chlorophyceae), and red algae (Rhodophyceae), are used to produce metallic and metal oxide NPs.

Nanomaterials can be categorized using dimensionality, which is the number of dimensions with a length longer than 100 nm, as Figure 10.3 shows: 0D, 1D, 2D, and 3D. Metals, hollow spheres, spheres, clusters, and quantum dots are examples of particles with zero dimension (0D), which are all defined by a single dimension that is either zero or more than 100 nm at the nanoscale. One-dimensional (1D) nanomaterials, like nanorods, nanowires, nanofibers, and nanotubes, have one dimension that is not in the nanoscale (>100 nm) and the other two are in the nanoscale. Two-dimensional (2D) nanomaterials, like thin films, nanocoatings, nanoplates, and nanolayers, have two dimensions—one not in the nanoscale and another in the nanoscale. Combining nanocrystals with varying dimensions above 100 nm in different directions creates three-dimensional (3D) structures. According to dimensionality, nanomaterials are categorized in Figure 10.3 [44–46].

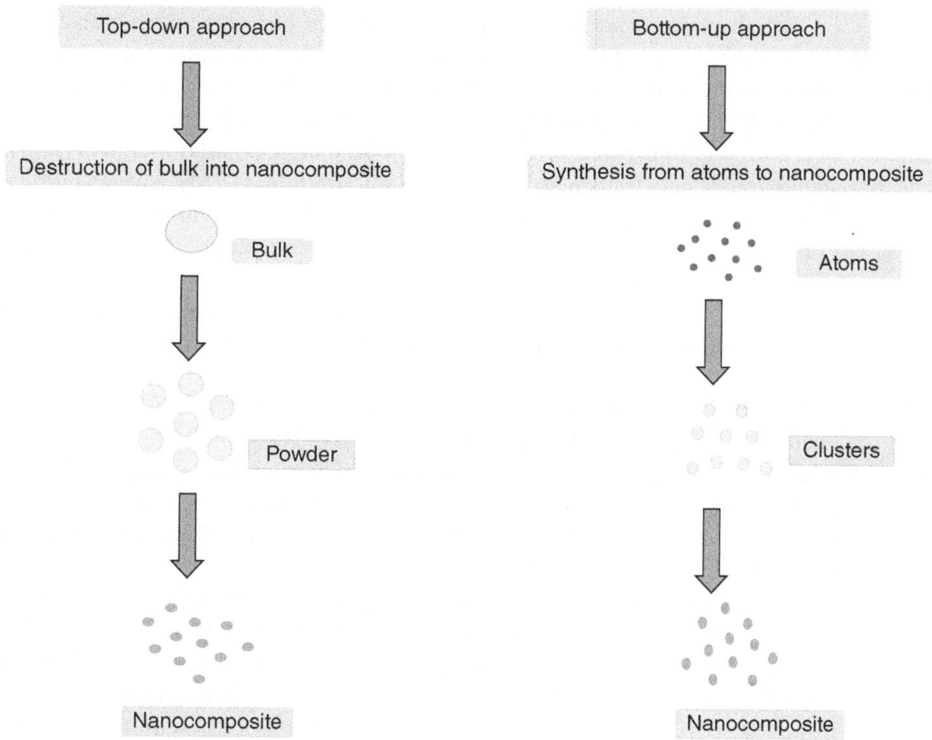

FIGURE 10.4 Shows various methods for synthesizing nanomaterials.

10.3.1 Synthesis Methods of Nanocomposites

There are two methods for synthesizing nanomaterials: top-down and bottom-up (Figure 10.4). The top-down approach uses lithography, ball milling, grinding, polishing, and other techniques to restructure the bulk material into nanomaterials. According to ref. [44, 45], the bottom-up approach involves assembling nanomaterials from molecules, particles, or nanoclusters in the atomic range employing a range of methods, including vapor phase deposition, spinning, molecular self-assembly, pyrolysis and condensation, and sol–gel method.

10.3.2 Characterization of Nanocomposites

The distinct qualities of nanomaterials have expanded their application in numerous scientific domains and spawned a market for goods incorporating nano-objects. Many characterization techniques are employed in order to comprehend the physicochemical properties of synthesized bionanomaterials. When creating the bionanomaterials, a few things like the stabilizing and reducing agent and the solvent medium must be taken into account. Characterization methods are primarily used to assess and improve the synthetic bionanomaterials unique molecular weight, size, shape, purity, solubility, and chemical makeup. These properties are important because they enable the determination of the applications of the materials across numerous domains, such as biomedical, sensing, agricultural, and environmental [47–49].

Chemical and structural characterization are the two categories into which the characterization procedures are separated. The application of structural characterization is to determine a bionanomaterial's structural morphology, size, shape, and crystallinity, whereas different surface and chemical atoms are identified as well as the spatial conjugation using chemical characterization. One method for structural characterization is electron spectroscopy, or X-ray photoelectron spectroscopy, or XPS. It is necessary to look into the chemical and physical characteristics of the nanomaterials and is typically used in chemical analysis. The photoionization principle is the basis for XPS's operation, and it is frequently used to examine the surface characteristics of bionanomaterials, which aids in the investigation of their chemical state and energy distribution [50].

Because they are so easy to use and convenient, two of the most popular methods for examining synthetic bionanomaterials are transmission electron microscopy (TEM) and scanning electron microscopy (SEM). They are employed in the examination of green synthetic bionanomaterials' morphological properties, such as size, distribution, and shape. Because it provides information about the material's chemical composition and generates a clear picture with a high resolution within the atomic range, TEM has been regarded as a more advanced technique. Apart from sample thickness and methods of material data collection, there aren't many differences between SEM and TEM.

TEM and SEM can be used in conjunction with X-ray spectroscopy to investigate in-depth details regarding the chemical composition of bionanomaterials [51]. The morphological analysis of several bionanomaterials, including silver, copper, and nickel, has been done using TEM [52]. A commonly used method for examining the composition of bionanomaterials is energy dispersive X-ray (EDX). The elemental composition, microstructure, and spectra can be effectively detected by combining EDX, SEM, and TEM with EDX [53].

EDX maps the spatial distribution of components to provide qualitative, quantitative, or semi-quantitative analysis. When it comes to examining the different physical, chemical, and compositional properties of green bionanomaterials, including NPs made of gold and silver, EDX is regarded as one of the most effective instruments [54]. One of the key methods in the field of nanotechnology is the X-ray diffraction (XRD) method, which is used to ascertain the crystalline material's atomic spacing, crystallinity, defects, and crystal structure. Many green synthesized bionanoparticles, such as silver NPs, are characterized by XRD [55].

A variety of methods are utilized to look at the composition of the green synthesized bionanomaterials, such as UV-visible spectroscopy, a fundamental method used to characterize all biochemical compounds both quantitatively and qualitatively. It is typically employed to examine chemical and physical characteristics like concentration, size, and aggregation. It is utilized to investigate the structural conformation and optoelectronic characteristics of bionanomaterials. The Beer-Lambert Law serves as the foundation for UV-visible spectroscopy, which uses linear connections between absorbance and concentrations. Several green bionanomaterials have been produced and described, such as silver, gold, copper, cerium, selenium, and others. The structural properties of green bionanomaterials have been studied using these materials. In contrast, it is believed that the fastest and most accurate analytical technique for characterizing bionanomaterials is Fourier transform infrared spectroscopy, or FTIR. It examines specific vibration patterns of individual molecules to determine the functional groups—such as aldehydes, ketones, alcohols, carboxylic acid, and terpenoids—present in the bionanomaterial. It is therefore used in the quantitative and qualitative examination of solid and watery materials. It is also used to determine the structural composition, aggregation, dynamics, and stability. With the aid of FTIR, a number of environmentally friendly synthesized bionanomaterials, including iron oxide, gold, nickel, and silver NPs, have been examined [56]. A variety of bionanomaterial characterization techniques are displayed in Figure 10.5.

10.4 BIOMEDICAL APPLICATIONS OF SEAWEED BIONANOCOMPOSITES

Over the past 20 years (Figure 10.6), bionanocomposites have made a substantial contribution to biotechnology with the advancement of nanotechnology [57]. Three types of multiphasic nanocomposites are metal, polymer, and ceramic nanocomposites. They consist of an organic matrix covered in solid inorganic materials. Polymer-based nanocomposites, or simply nanocomposites, are a new class of biomaterials that exhibit much superior performance than their monophasic counterparts when inorganic components are combined with an organic matrix [58]. Bionanocomposites have

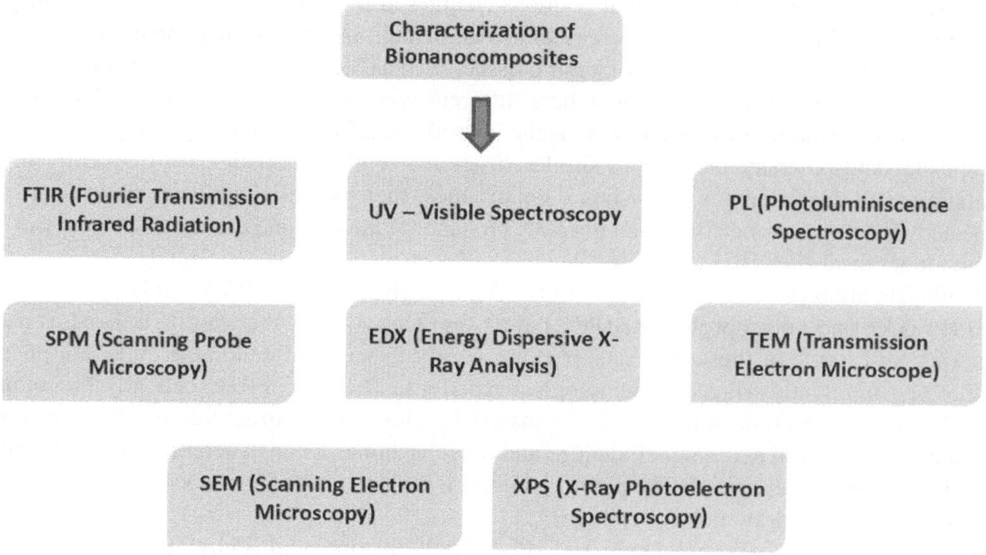

FIGURE 10.5 Characterization of bionanocomposites.

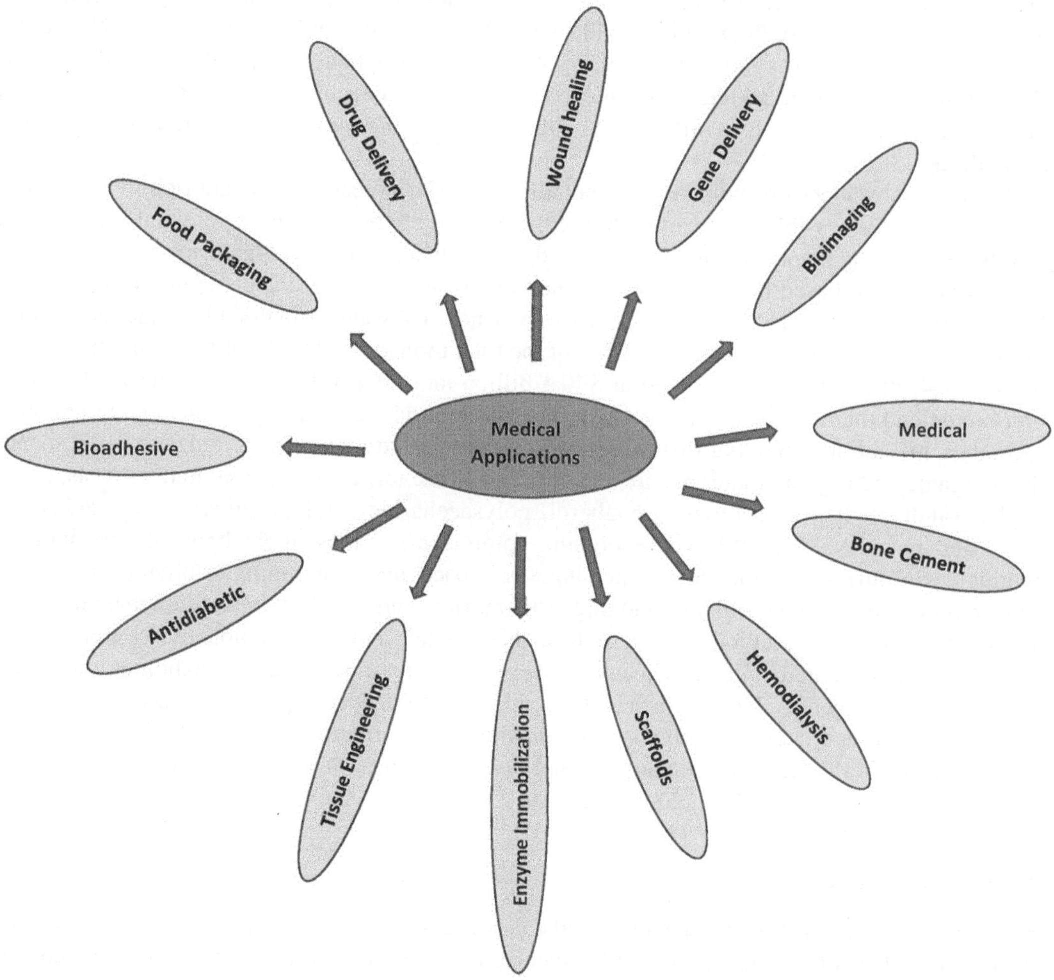

FIGURE 10.6 Various applications of bionanocomposites.

been used for marked dentistry, primarily due to changes in formulation and polymer/ceramic/metal manipulation techniques that have increased interest in their use [59]. Dental materials that replicate the composition and characteristics of natural tissue, such as bionanocomposites, can withstand high biting forces and harsh environments where different types of food can cause sudden changes in temperature or osmotic pressure, as well as the invasion of different pathogens [60]. Since bionanocomposites and other materials with similar structures or characteristics are frequently found in dental enamel, dentin, and alveolar bone, for instance, their potential applications in dentistry are expected. The polymer matrix is used to create bionanocomposites and can act as a biological stimulus to attract local cells [61].

Collagen, alginate, silk, polylactic acid (PLA), polyglycolic acid (PGA), polylactic-co-glycolic acid (PLGA), and polycaprolactone (PCL) are a few biopolymers that can be utilized as a matrix material. Still, some of these materials perform poorly in terms of cellular activity, are physically brittle, and frequently trigger immunological reactions. They are also excellently biocompatible [61]. Since bionanocomposites and other materials with similar structures or characteristics are frequently found in dental enamel, dentin, and alveolar bone, for instance, their potential applications in dentistry are expected. The polymer matrix is used to create bionanocomposites and can act as a living carrier to draw in local cells [61].

Collagen, alginate, silk, polylactic acid (PLA), polyglycolic acid (PGA), polylactic-co-glycolic acid (PLGA), and polycaprolactone (PCL) are examples of biopolymers that are extremely biocompatible and can be utilized as a matrix material; however, certain materials have poor cellular activity, are often immunologically stimulating, and are mechanically fragile. These inorganic compounds include graphene oxide (GO), titanium oxide, silica NPs, magnetic NPs, bioactive glass NPs, carbon nanotubes (CNTs), hydroxyapatite, silver or gold NPs, and graphene oxide (GO), according to [62]. The primary purpose of adding inorganic components to the polymer matrix is to improve its mechanical properties, such as stiffness, Young's modulus, hardness, tensile strength, and flexural strength [63].

The medical sciences heavily rely on metallic NPs. Marine ecosystems are rich in biodiversity; this makes them a possible source of cutting-edge bioactive substances with potential uses in human health [64]. Marine plants, sponges, micro- and macroalgae, and microorganisms are only a few of the several marine-based bioactive component sources. Each of these sources has a distinct set of biomolecules of its own [65]. When it comes to marine, freshwater, and brackish water aquaculture, macroalgae, or seaweed, account for 23.4% of the total tonnage and 9.7% of the value of the industry. In 2004, the industry was valued at \$70.3 billion and 59.4 million tons, respectively [66]. In order to defend themselves against herbivory and biofouling, seaweeds generate a large number of secondary metabolites, making them frequently vulnerable to microbial colonization [67]. Among the inorganic and organic materials present in seaweed are terpenoids, carotenoids, sterols, chlorophylls, xanthophylls, phycobilins, tocopherol, polysaccharides, polyunsaturated fatty acids, vitamins, and phycocyanins [68]. These organic components act as allelochemicals, mediating in benthic environments, competing for exchanges for space, and functioning as phytochemist attractants, bioprotectants, biostimulants, and microbial nutrient sources [69]. In addition to being utilized as food, feed, fertilizer, and fodder, macroalgae also produce a number of bioactive components that may be useful in the medical field. The undiscovered diversity of secondary metabolites, particularly terpenes and acerogenins, has drawn scientists' attention to seaweed species in the genus *Laurencia* [70]. Using seaweeds such as *Codium capitatum* and *Fucus gardeneri* [71, 72], *Turbinaria conoides* [34], seaweeds of the Gulf of Mannar [73], and *Padina gymnospora* seaweed extract [74], a variety of biosynthetic nanomaterials, including Ag, Au, ZnO, and Ag-ZnO composite (Table 10.1).

10.4.1 Dental Care

According to ref. [108], a new wave of hybrid nanostructured materials represents a developing area at the intersection of nanotechnology, life science, and materials science. The term "bionanocomposites" has gained widespread usage in recent years. An emerging class of hybrid materials with

TABLE 10.1
Biological Applications of Seaweed Bionanocomposites

S. No.	Seaweed	Applications	References
1	*Laurencia dendroidea*	Antiprotozoal	[75]
2	*Gelidiella acerosa*	Antifungal	[76]
3	*Dictyota bartayresiana*	Antifungal	[77]
4	*Gracilaria corticata*	Antifungal activity	[78]
5	*Laurencia aldingensis*	Cytotoxic activities	[79]
6	*Laurencia dendroidea*	Biocidal activity	[80]
7	*Laurencia dendroidea*	Biological activity	[81]
8	*Laurencia dendroidea*	Biological activity	[82]
9	*Chaetomorpha linum.*	Biological activity	[71]
10	Marine macro algae	Biological activity	[83]
11	*Laurenciella sp.*	Cytotoxic activities	[79]
12	*Turbinaria conoides*	Antibacterial activity	[32]
13	*Turbinaria ornata*	Antibacterial activity	[83]
14	*Sargassum muticum*	Mosquito vectors and bacterial pathogens	[84]
15	*Sargassum muticum*	Antioxidant and antibacterial	[85]
16	*Laurencia species*	Antibacterial activity	[86]
17	*Laurencia catarinensis*	Bactericidal efficacy	[87]
18	*Padina tetrastromatical*	Antibacterial	[88]
19	*Padina gymnospora*	Antibacterial	[89]
20	*Sargassum cinereum*	Antibacterial	[90]
21	*Ulva lactuca*	Antimicrobials activity	[91]
22	Alginate fiber	Antimicrobial properties	[92]
23	*Gracilaria edulis*	Antimicrobial	[93]
24	*Galaxaura elongate*	Antibacterial	[94]
25	*Lemanea fluviatilis*	Antioxidant	[95]
26	*Gracilaria corticata*	Antimicrobial and antioxidant	[96]
27	*Gracilaria dura*	antibacterial	[97]
28	*Gelidiella sp.*	Anticancer activity	[98]
29	*Gracilaria birdiae*	Antibacterial	[99]
30	*Acanthophora specifera*	Antimicrobial activity	[100]
31	*Amphiroa fragilissima*	Antibacterial	[101]
32	*Ulva lactuca*	Antimicrobial activity	[102]
33	*Caulerpa racemosa*	Antibacterial	[103]
34	*Enteromorpha flexuosa*	Antimicrobial activity	[104]
35	*Caulerpa serrulata*	Antibacterial activity	[105]
36	*Urospora sp.*	Antibacterial activity	[106]
37	*Ulva lactuca*	Antimicrobials activity	[107]
38	*Turbinaria conoides*	Antibacterial activity	[32]

nanostructures is called bionanocomposites. They have at least one nanometer-scale dimension and are created by combining inorganic solids with natural polymers. These biohybrid materials have enhanced structural and functional qualities that are highly desirable for various applications, much like conventional nanocomposites that contain synthetic polymers [109].

A National Institutes of Health report on denture materials states that more than 100 million people are toothless, highlighting the urgent need for implant dentistry. In the last 50 years,

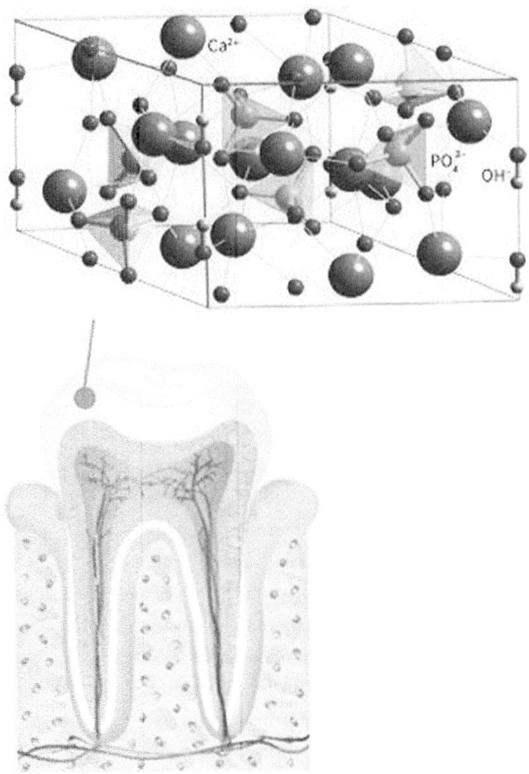

FIGURE 10.7 Microstructure of enamel represented schematically.

researchers have focused on developing biomaterials that can interact with biological systems to evaluate, treat, improve, or replace any organ, tissue, or function in the body. These biomaterials include medical and dental implants, which are used to treat millions of patients annually. The hardest substance in our body is called hydroxyapatite, or Ca_5 $(PO_4)_3(OH)$, which makes up teeth (Figure 10.7).

The National Bureau of Standards of the United States government has set criteria for the selection and grading of dental amalgam implants. According to ref. [110], it is easily formulated to meet specific needs. Composite resin is used in adhesive dental restorations such as cavity liners, restorative materials, pit and fissure sealants, cores and buildups, inlays, onlays, crowns, provisional restorations, cements for single or multiple tooth prostheses and orthodontic devices, endodontic sealers, and root canal posts. These materials, which have superior mechanical qualities and proven lower shrinkage than conventional dimethacrylate-based resins, serve as the foundation for universal self-adhesive composites. This is most likely due to the epoxide curing process, which is now recommended for liners and minor repairs and includes opening an oxiranering [111, 112].

10.4.2 Drug Delivery

Drugs can be safely and effectively delivered to their intended sites without causing any toxicity when they are delivered through controlled and long-term delivery networks. Numerous bionanocomposite materials have been used in drug delivery systems due to growing concerns regarding safety, biodegradability, and compatibility [113]. The toxicity risks can be decreased by using methods for delivering drugs based on bionanocomposite technology. Additionally, their drug-loading capacity is higher. In the field of delivering drugs, numerous novel bionanocomposites, or biohybrids, have recently been added. They have great potential for loading, releasing, and targeting drugs in an efficient manner. Because of its cationic nature, biocompatibility, capacity to bind certain organic compounds, and presence of a primary amino group that enables controlled drug release and mucoadhesion, among other properties, chitosan finds widespread application in the pharmaceutical industry as a drug carrier, in wound healing, and in biomedical fields. One of the more expansive fields of science that uses a multidisciplinary scientific approach and advances human health care is drug delivery technology. For many years, patients have received medication in order to treat either acute or chronic illnesses [114].

The characteristics of the administration site (pH, surface area, presence of enzymes, active transport mechanisms, etc.) and the drug (solubility, charge, molecular size, etc.) impact the rate of drug uptake that results from standard drug administration techniques and routes. The application of polymer nanotechnology and nanocomposites to potential biomedical and biotechnological applications is a fast-expanding field. Certain bionanocomposites' biocompatibility and nanoscale dimensions are highly advantageous properties for drug delivery applications. The torturous diffusion path that polymer bionanocomposites typically present for compressed small molecules/drugs, forming an effective barrier and enabling sustained delivery with little to no burst release, is one benefit of using them for drug delivery [113].

Nanoscale dimensions can be achieved in fucoidan-based drug delivery systems, leading to the creation of nanogels [115]. The fucoidan extracted from Turbinaria decurrens and the fucoidan-coated AgNPs showed great antibacterial activity against clinical pathogens, with a stronger effect against Gram-negative bacteria (namely, Escherichia coli MTCC 40 and Pseudomonas aeruginosa MTCC 2642) than against Gram-positive bacteria (namely, Streptococcus mutans MTCC 896 and Staphylococcus aureus MTCC 96) [116].

The pharmacological activity of carrageenan, which is extracted from marine seaweeds, includes anticancer, anticoagulant, antihyperlipidemic, and immunomodulatory effects [117, 118]. Furthermore, other research reported that carrageenan efficiently inhibits a wide variety of human papillomaviruses that are transmitted through sexual activity [119]. Furthermore, antioxidant activity has been observed in polysaccharides derived from red and brown seaweeds [120]. This demonstrates a clever "collaboration" between various carrageenan types with the drug delivery system. Longer drug delivery is also possible when carrageenan and NPs are combined, although the effects of the various types of NPs vary. For instance, adding gold nanofillers reduces the model drug's release rate [121].

Carrageenan-based formulations have found many uses in recent years: they can be used as local anesthetics to treat oral mucositis, as well as antimicrobial and anti-inflammatory medications for efficient wound healing [122, 123], and as carrageenan-based polyelectrolyte complexes for tissue engineering [124], ophthalmic delivery [125], and vaginal drug delivery systems [126], among other applications. The development of pH/temperature-sensitive medication delivery systems is aided by carrageenan. The desired drug release characteristics, like pH independence and zero-order release, cannot be achieved when carrageenan is the only matrix material used to control drug release [127]. Carrageenan has been used in drug delivery in a variety of forms, including NPs, gelling agents, nano- and micro-stabilizers, beads, microspheres, and microcapsules [128]. One medicine for treating hypercholestrolemia is fluvastatin, which comes in a sustained-release version [129]. The study therefore showed that the NPs can behave as nanocarriers for the delivery of medications and growth factors for tissue engineering applications, according to ref. [130] (Table 10.2).

Formulations based on carrageenan are specifically used for extended drug release, meaning that the drug is released over many days or hours [145, 146]. Carrageenan has some intriguing properties that give it an extra edge in extending drug release in mucosal and epithelial tissues, such as both its positive surface charge and adhesiveness [147]. Carrageenan interacts with other polymers to achieve the optimal profile for drug release. According to research, fast degeneration causes κ-carrageenan to release quickly [148]. Combining different forms of carrageenan also appears to be an effective way to extend the release of the medication, even though SEM investigations found that some carrageenan is not miscible in blends [149].

TABLE 10.2
Algae-Mediated Biosynthesis of Bionanocomposites for Drug Delivery and Wound Healing

S. No.	Seaweed	Application	References
1.	*Kappaphycus sp., Gracilaria sp., Gelidium sp.*	Oral drug delivery	[131–135]
2.	*Laminaria sp., Ascophyllum sp., Sargassum sp., Fucus sp., Turbinaria sp.*	Drug delivery	[136–138]
3.	*Sargassum sp., Fucus sp., Turbinaria sp., Laminaria sp., Ascophyllum sp.*	Wound healing/dressing for oral cavity	[139–141]
4.	Alginate	Antibacterial wound dressings as they are breathable	[142]
5.	Alginate	Wound healing	[143]
6.	Sodium alginate oligosaccharides	Wound dressing material	[144]

TABLE 10.3
Algae-Mediated Biosynthesis of Bionanocomposites for Tissue Engineering

S. No.	Seaweed	Application	References
1.	*Kappaphycus sp., Gracilaria sp., Gelidium sp.*	Bone tissue engineering	[151–156]
2.	*Sargassum sp., Laminaria sp., Fucus sp., Ascophyllum sp., Turbinaria sp.*	Bone tissue engineering	[157–159]
3.	*Ulva sp.*	Scaffolds for tissue engineering	[160, 161]
4.	Seaweed alginate	Chubbiness and type 2 diabetes	[162]
5.	Seaweed alginate	Dental impression materials	[163]
6.	Alginate gels	Tissue engineering	[164, 165]
7.	Injectable biomaterial carrageenan	Bone surgery	[166]

10.4.3 Tissue Engineering

According to Ahn et al. [150], hydroxyapatite-fucoidan nanocomposites were evaluated for bioactivity using an in vivo biomimetic procedure, and no negative effects were seen on stem cells generated from adipose tissue. Furthermore, collagen type-1, osteocalcin, osteopontin, and Runx2 were among the early and terminal stage indicators of osteogenic differentiation that were significantly increased by hydroxyapatite-fucoidan nanocomposites, which also caused mineralization (Table 10.3) for bone production.

Additionally, in rabbits with tibia defects, hydroxyapatite-fucoidan nanocomposites stimulated the formation of bone, indicating that this biomaterial is suitable for bone tissue engineering [150]. We deal with the potential applications of alginate and its nanocomposite in bone tissue engineering in our earlier article [167].

10.4.4 Anticoagulant Activity

Hemostasis's natural mechanism for preventing blood loss from wounds is coagulation. Long used as an anticoagulant, heparin is a highly sulfated polysaccharide found in mammalian tissues that is a member of the glycosaminoglycan family. However, heparin can cause thrombocytopenia and excessive bleeding, among other side effects [168]. It is known that fucoidan, a substance found in marine macroalgae, is a successful substitute for anticoagulants. The recovered fucoidan was used to manufacture silver nanoparticles (AgNPs), which showed improved anticoagulant action [167] in comparison to the fucoidan polymer. *Turbinaria decurrens*, a brown seaweed, contains a fucoidan that has been isolated and shown to have anticoagulant qualities.

10.4.5 Anticancer Properties of Seaweed Nanocomposites

Cancer is a disease marked by aberrant tissue growth. It has a severe impact on the patient and can result in complications and severities that could be fatal [169]. According to ref. [170], cancer is the second most common cause of death in the United States, accounting for about 2 million diagnoses annually. Modern treatments like radiation and chemotherapy, while useful, have serious side effects that include anemia, immunosuppression, illness, and even death. They are also not entirely effective. Indeed, it has been documented that certain cancer cells have developed resistance to certain treatments, resulting in the development of tumors resistant to chemotherapy, rendering those treatments unfeasible for this type of patient [171]. As per ref. [172], various nanocomposites have demonstrated the ability to efficiently encapsulate chemotherapy drugs and transport them straight to the tumor site, thereby reducing or even eliminating the potential side effects. Furthermore, compared to free drugs, the use of nanocomposites enables a more effective permeability to the tumor site [173, 174]. By adding various biomolecules, they can also be functionalized to target particular cancerous cells because the nanocomposites can bind to the carcinogenic structures specifically [175].

One of the most active areas of nanobiotechnology research is the use of NPs for cancer therapy and targeted delivery of anticancer drugs [176]. Recent years have seen the publication of numerous studies on the anticancerous properties of NPs mediated by algae. In a study [177], AgNPs (10 nm) produced by *Sargassum vulgare* showed a substantial anticancerous effect against HeLa cells and human myeloblastic leukemic cells HL60. Using silver nano-triangles coated in chitosan polymers made from algae, the non-small human lung cancer cell line (NCI-H460) was treated photothermally (Chit-AgNPs) [178].

Additionally, AgNPs mediated by *S. muticum* have demonstrated cytotoxic results against the breast cancer cell line MCF7 in vitro. The MCF7 cell line was treated with AgNPs at different concentrations ranging from 3 µg/mL to 50 µg/mL for approximately 48 hours. The concentration of 12.5 µg/mL showed the greatest viability rate of 100.36%. These AgNPs have caused intracellular ROS generation, which causes cancer cells to undergo apoptosis and ultimately die [179]. In an additional investigation, the cytotoxic potential of AgNPs generated by *S. myriocystum* against the HeLa cell line was evaluated through the use of MTT assay at different dosages starting from 0 to 512 µg/mL.

AgNP treatment resulted in 50% inhibitory and apoptotic activities in the HeLa cell line, and the concentration of AgNPs in the media increased the cell line's overall cytotoxic potential [180]. Similarly, the in vitro cytotoxicity capability of algal-mediated AgNPs against the breast cancer MCF-7 cell line was assessed at varying concentrations (0–100 µg/mL) during intervals of 24, 36, and 48 hours. AgNPs have the potential to be antitumorous; their highest inhibitory concentration value against breast cancer cells was found to be 20 µg/mL, as evidenced by nuclear fragmentation, apoptosis, and cell death [181].

AuNPs mediated by the marine algae *Chaetomorpha linum* were the subject of another investigation, wherein the HCT-116 colon cancer cell line was shown in Table 10.4 to exhibit anticancerous potential in vitro. After being incubated with these NPs, colon cancer cell lines demonstrated the deadly effects of AuNPs at different doses. Without a doubt, the AuNPs produced by algae are powerful anticancer agents [192]. A number of apoptotic inductions were noted, resulting in the decrease of anti-apoptotic proteins such as Bcl-xl and Bcl-2 as well as the activation of apoptotic caspases 3 and 9.

TABLE 10.4
Algae-Mediated Biosynthesis of Bionanocomposites for Anticancer Activity

S. No.	Seaweed	Application	References
1.	*Cystoseira baccata*	Colon cancer cells	[182]
2.	*Sargassum polycystum*	Antibacterial and anticancer	[183]
3.	*Corallina officinalis*	Breast cancer	[184]
4.	*Codium capitatum*	Anticancer activity	[185]
5.	*Sargassum muticum*	HepG2, liver	[186]
6.	*Sargassum muticum*	Pancreas, ovarian, colon, leukemia, and murine leukemia	[187]
7.	*Gracilaria edulis*	Cervical, murine leukemia, ovarian, colon, and leukemia	[188]
8.	Carrageenan	Antitumor and immunomodulation activities, antiviral activity, antioxidant activity, anticoagulant, and antithrombotic activities	[120, 189]
9.	*Sargassum muticum*	HepG2, liver	[186]
10.	*Sargassum muticum*	Pancreas, ovarian, colon, leukemia, and murine leukemia	[187]
11.	*Gracilaria edulis*	Cervical, murine leukemia pancreas, ovarian, colon, and leukemia	[188]
12.	*Laurencia spp.*	Antibiotic, Antiviral, Antileishmanial, Antimalarial, Antitrypanosomal, Anticancer, and Anti-diabetic activities	[70, 190]
13.	*Laurencia dendroidea*	Anticancer	[75]
14.	*Sargassum vulgare*	Anticancer activity	[191]

10.5 APPLICATIONS OF NANOCOMPOSITES WITH COMMERCIALLY AVAILABLE PRODUCTS

Amazing research on nanocomposite materials has been obtained recently, moving the field from its theoretical underpinnings to clinical application. There are currently many different dental subspecialties using nanomaterials (Table 10.2) [193, 194]. There will be a notable expansion in the selection of dental items in the near future, which is anticipated as a result of continuing studies to create novel nanoproducts (Table 10.5).

TABLE 10.5
Applications of Nanocomposites with Commercially Available Products

S. No.	Discipline	Available Materials
1	Restorative dentistry	Ketac™, Nano-primer, Premise™, Ketac N100, Filtek Supreme XT, Adper™ Single bond plus Adhesive, Fuji IX GP, and Ceram X™.
2	Regenerative dentistry and tissue engineering	Ostim®, VITOSSO™, and Nano-Bone®.
3	Periodontics	Arestin® and Nanogen®.
4	Preventive dentistry Orthodontics	NanoCare® Gold, Nano-Ionomers, and Ketac™ N100 Light Curing Filtek Supreme Plus Universal.
5	Prosthodontics	Nanotech elite H-D plus, GC OPTIGLAZE color® (GC).
6	Oral implantology	Nanotite™ Nano-coated implant.

10.6 CONCLUSION

The process of using marine materials has been lengthy. Because marine biological materials may possess novel characteristics and distinctive biochemical properties, they have emerged as a hotspot for materials science and biomedicine research. This focus is also ascribed to the advancements in technology and research in the extraction and processing of materials. The effects of marine biological materials on blood lipid levels, immunity enhancement, antitumor activity, antioxidation, and anticoagulation have all been thoroughly studied. Nevertheless, there aren't many products targeted at the market because many of these compounds aren't extracted and purified on an industrial scale. The application of marine materials' clinical potential will take time and effort because they must pass strict regulations, similar to those that apply to medical devices and advanced therapy medications. It's exciting to think that as science and technology advance and new technologies are applied, marine biological materials will likely industrialize, lead to the development of medications, medical devices, and nutraceuticals, and acknowledge the highly beneficial uses of marine biology. In addition to promoting the research, development, and use of marine biomedical materials, safety is a concern. Active biological macromolecules with uncertain immunogenicity make up the majority of marine biomedical materials. Their safety and usefulness are also influenced by their molecular structure and content. Strict biosafety rules make the applications of these biomaterials in the biomedical industry difficult. Therefore, we need to create physicochemical characterization methods suitable for medical devices and marine biomaterials, taking into account factors like the biomaterial's anticipated use, mode of contact, and duration of contact. It has a significant impact on how marine materials are developed and used. As continued study on the oceans has revealed a wide range of biomedical materials with great qualities, we should keep optimizing the exploitation of marine resources to ensure the sustainability of the identified biomedical material production. The improvement of new resources established on the fusion of cutting-edge techniques as well as biology, along with careful consideration of current clinical needs, will make marine biomedical materials research more beneficial to humanity.

REFERENCES

[1] J. K. Kim, K. Pal, V. Sridhar, "Role of different nanoparticles in elastomeric nanocomposites". *Recent advances in elastomeric nanocomposites*. Springer, p. 355, 2011.

[2] M. Liu, Y. Zhang, C. Wu, S. Xiong, C. Zhou, "Chitosan/halloysite nanotubes bionanocomposites: structure, mechanical properties and biocompatibility", *Int J Biol Macromol*, 51: 565–575, 2012.

[3] P. Dwivedi, S. S. Narvi, R. P. Tewari, "Application of polymer nanocomposites in the nanomedicine landscape: envisaging strategies to combat implant associated infections", *J Appl Biomater Funct Mater*, 11: 12942, 2013.

[4] M. Barikani, E. Oliaei, H. Seddiqi, H. Honarkar, "Preparation and application of chitin and its derivatives: a review", *Iran Polym J*, 23: 307–326, 2014.

[5] R. A. Petros, J. M. DeSimone, "Strategies in the design of nanoparticles for therapeutic applications", *Nat Rev Drug Discov*, 9: 615, 2010.

[6] M. E. Davis, D. M. Shin, "Nanoparticle therapeutics: an emerging treatment modality for cancer", *Nat Rev Drug Discov*, 7: 771, 2008.

[7] J. A. Rodriguez, M. Fernandez-Garcia, *Synthesis, properties, and applications of oxide nanomaterials*. John Wiley & Sons, 2007.

[8] N. Bitinis, M. Hernandez, R. Verdejo, J. M. Kenny, M. Lopez-Manchado, "Recent advances in clay/polymer nanocomposites", *Adv Mater*, 23: 522936, 2011.

[9] S. Patel, "Therapeutic importance of sulphated polysaccharides from seaweeds: updating the recent findings", *Biotech*, 2: 171–185, 2012.

[10] N. B. Shelke, R. James, C. T. Laurencin, S. G. Kumbar, "Polysaccharide biomaterials materials for drug delivery and regenerative engineering" *Polym Adv Technol*, 25: 448–460, 2014.

[11] M. J. Cardoso, R. R. Costa, J. F. Mano, "Marine origin polysaccharides in drug delivery systems" *Mar Drugs*, 14: 34, 2016.

[12] J. Venkatesan, S. Anil, S. K. Kim, *Seaweed polysaccharides. Isolation, biological and biomedical applications*, Netherlands: Elsevier, 2017.

[13] J. Venkatesan, S. Anil, S. K. Kim, M. S. Shim, "Seaweed polysaccharide-based nanoparticles: preparation and applications for drug delivery", *Polymer*, 8: 30–54, 2016.

[14] T. Jiang, Z. Zhang, Y. Zhou, Y. Liu, Z. Wang, H. Tong, "Surface functionalization of titanium with chitosan/gelatin via electrophoretic deposition: characterization and cell behavior", *Biomacromolecules*, 11: 1254–1260, 2010.

[15] H. Li, L. H. Greene, "Sequence and structural analysis of the chitinase insertion domain reveals two conserved motifs involved in chitin-binding", *PLoS One*, 5: e8654, 2010.

[16] A. Mohandas, S. Deepthi, R. Biswas, R. Jayakumar, "Chitosan based metallic nanocomposite scaffolds as antimicrobial wound dressings", *Bioact Mater*, 3: 267–277, 2017.

[17] M. A. Nazeer, E. Yilgör, I. Yilgör, "Intercalated chitosan/hydroxyapatite nanocomposites: promising materials for bone tissue engineering applications", *Carbohydr Polym*, 175: 38–46, 2017.

[18] Abida Kalsoom Khan, Ain Us Saba, Shamyla Nawazish, Fahad Akhtar, Rehana Rashid, Sadullah Mir, Bushra Nasir, Furqan Iqbal, Samina Afzal, Fahad Pervaiz, Ghulam Murtaza, "Carrageenan based bionanocomposites as drug delivery tool with special emphasis on the influence of ferromagnetic nanoparticles", *Hindawi Oxid Med Cell Longev*, Article ID 8158315, 13, 2017, doi: 10.1155/2017/8158315

[19] S. L. Iconaru, A. M. Prodan, M. Motelica-Heino, S. Sizaret, D. Predoi, "Synthesis and characterization of polysaccharide-maghemite composite nanoparticles and their antibacterial properties", *Nanoscale Res Lett*, 7: 1–8, 2012.

[20] M. P. Sudhakar, V. Deepak Nallasamy, G. Dharani, Alejandro H. Buschmann, "Applications of seaweed biopolymers and its composites in dental applications", *J Appl Biol Biotechnol*, 12(1), pp. 62–68, 2024, doi: 10.7324/JABB.2024.143201

[21] A. Rasool, S. Ata, A. Islam, R. U. Khan, "Fabrication of novel carrageenan based stimuli responsive injectable hydrogels for controlled release of cephradine", *RSC Adv*, 9: 12282–12290, 2019.

[22] J. Fleurence, M. Morançais, J. Dumay, "Seaweed proteins". In: Yada, R. Y., editor. *Proteins in food processing*, 2nd ed. United Kingdom: Woodhead Publishing, pp. 245–262, 2018.

[23] Muthiyal Prabakaran Sudhakar, Srinivas Venkatnarayanan, Gopal Dharani, "Fabrication and characterization of bio-nanocomposite films using κ-Carrageenan and Kappaphycus alvarezii seaweed for multiple industrial applications", *Int J Biol Macromol*, 219: 138–149, 2022.

[24] S. Li, Q. Xiong, X. Lai, "Molecular modification of polysaccharides and resulting bioactivities", *Compr Rev Food Sci Food Saf*. 15: 237–250, 2016.

[25] J. Wang, S. Hu, S. Nie, Q. Yu, M. Xie, "Reviews on mechanisms of in vitro antioxidant activity of polysaccharides", *Oxid Med Cell Longev*, 2016: 13, 2016.

[26] A. M. Stephen, G. O. Phillips. *Food polysaccharides and their applications*. CRC Press, 2016.

[27] M. Q. Guo, X. Hu, C. Wang, L. Ai, Solubility of polysaccharides, 2: 8, 2017.

[28] S. S. Ferreira, C. P. Passos, P. Madureira, M. Vilanova, M. A. Coimbra, "Structure–function relationships of immunostimulatory polysaccharides: a review". *Carbohydr Polym*, 132: 378–396, 2015.

[29] B. Tanna and A. Mishra, "Nutraceutical potential of seaweed polysaccharides: structure, bioactivity, safety, and toxicity", *Compr Rev Food Sci Food Saf*, 18: 817–831, 2019.

[30] S. Y. Xu, X. Huang, K. L. Cheong, "Recent advances in marine algae polysaccharides: isolation, structure, and activities", *Mar Drugs*, 15: 388, 2017.

[31] M. E. El-Naggar, S. I. Othman, A. A. Allam, O. M. Morsy, "Synthesis, drying process and medical application of polysaccharide-based aerogels". *Int J Biol Macromol*, 145: 1115–1128, 2020.

[32] S. Rajeshkumar, C. Kannan, G. Annadurai, "Green synthesis of silver nanoparticles using marine brown algae *Turbinaria conoides* and its antibacterial activity", *Int J Pharma Bio Sci.*, 3: 502–510, 2012.

[33] G. Ghodake, D. S. Lee, "Biological synthesis of gold nanoparticles using the aqueous extract of the brown algae *Laminaria japonica*", *J Nanoelectron Optoelectron*, 6: 268–271, 2011.

[34] S. Rajeshkumar, C. Malarkodi, G. Gnanajobitha, K. Paulkumar, M. Vanaja, C. Kannan, G. Annadurai, "Seaweed-mediated synthesis of gold nanoparticles using Turbinaria conoides and its characterization", *J Nanostructure Chem*, 3: 44, 2013.

[35] P. Mohanpuria, N. K. Rana, S. K. Yadav, "Biosynthesis of nanoparticles: technological concepts and future applications", *J Nanopart Res*, 10: 507–517, 2008.

[36] R. Vaidyanathan, K. Kalishwaralal, S. Gopalram, S. Gurunathan, Nanosilver—the burgeoning therapeutic molecule and its green synthesis (Retraction of vol 27, pg 924, 2009), *Biotechnol Adv*, 28: 940, 2010.

[37] T. Maneerung, S. Tokura, R. Rujiravanit, Impregnation of silver nanoparticles into bacterial cellulose for antimicrobial wound dressing, *Carbohydr Polym*, 72: 43–51, 2008.
[38] V. Patel, D. Berthold, P. Puranik, M. Gantar, "Screening of cyanobacteria and microalgae for their ability to synthesize silver nanoparticles with antibacterial activity", *Biotechnol. Rep.*, 5: 112–119, 2015.
[39] P. R. Chandran, M. Naseer, N. Udupa, N. Sandhyarani, "Size controlled synthesis of biocompatible gold nanoparticles and their activity in the oxidation of NADH", *Nanotechnology*, 23: 015602, 2011.
[40] D. Fawcett, J. J. Verduin, M. Shah, S. B. Zharma, G. E. J. Poinern, "A review of current research into the biogenic synthesis of metal and metal oxide nanoparticles via marine algae and seagrasses", *J Nanosci*, 2017: 1–15, 2017.
[41] G. S. Dhillon, S. K. Brar, S. Kaur, M. Verma, "Green approach for nanoparticle biosynthesis by fungi: current trends and applications". *Crit Rev Biotechnol*, 32: 49–73, 2012.
[42] P. C. Sahoo, F. Kausar, J. H. Lee, J. I. Han, "Facile fabrication of silver nanoparticle embedded $CaCO_3$ microspheres via microalgae-templated CO_2 biomineralization: application in antimicrobial paint development", *RSC Adv*, 4: 32562–32569, 2014.
[43] S. Agnihotri, S. Mukherji, S. Mukherji, "Size-controlled silver nanoparticles synthesized over the range 5–100 nm using the same protocol and their antibacterial efficacy", *RSC Adv*, 4: 3974–3983, 2014.
[44] C. Ngo and M. H. Van de Voorde, "Nanomaterials: doing more with less". In: Ngô, C., Van de Voorde, M., editors. *Nanotechnology in a nutshell: from simple to complex systems*. Paris, France: Atlantis Press, pp. 55–70, 2014, ISBN 978-94-6239-012-6.
[45] T. A. Saleh, "Nanomaterials: classification, properties, and environmental toxicities", *Environ Technol Innov*, 20: 101067, 2020.
[46] V. Singh, P. Yadav, V. Mishra, "Recent advances on classification, properties, synthesis, and characterization of nanomaterials." In: *Green synthesis of nanomaterials for bioenergy applications*. Hoboken, NJ, USA: John Wiley & Sons, Ltd., pp. 83–97, 2020, ISBN 978-1-119-57678-5.
[47] C. Zeppa, F. Gouanvé, E. Espuche, "Effect of a plasticizer on the structure of biodegradable starch/clay nanocomposites: thermal, water-sorption, and oxygen-barrier properties", *J Appl Polym Sci*, 112: 2044–2056, 2009.
[48] N. Magalhães, C. Andrade "Thermoplastic corn starch/clay hybrids: effect of clay type and content on physical properties", *Carbohydr Polym*, 75: 712–718, 2009.
[49] M. Huang, J. Yu, "Structure and properties of thermoplastic corn starch/montmorillonite biodegradable composites", *J Appl Polym Sci*, 99: 170–176 2006.
[50] V. P. Cyras, L. B. Manfredi, M. T. Ton-That, A. Vázquez, "Physical and mechanical properties of thermoplastic starch/montmorillonite nanocomposite films", *Carbohydr Polym*, 73: 55–63, 2008.
[51] S. M. Ibrahim, "Characterization, mechanical, and thermal properties of gamma irradiated starch films reinforced with mineral clay", *J Appl Polym Sci*, 119: 685–692, 2011.
[52] L. M. Famá, V. Pettarin, S. N. Goyanes and C. R. Bernal, "Starch/multi-walled carbon nanotubes composites with improved mechanical properties", *Carbohydr Polym*, 83: 1226–1231, 2011.
[53] X. Ma, J. Yu, N. Wang "Glycerol plasticized-starch/multiwall carbon nanotube composites for electroactive polymers", *Compos Sci Technol*, 68: 268–273, 2008.
[54] B. S. Harrison, A. Atala, "Carbon nanotube applications for tissue engineering", *Biomaterials*, 28: 344–353, 2007.
[55] J. Wang, "Carbon-nanotube based electrochemical biosensors: a review", *Electroanalysis*, 17: 7–14, 2005.
[56] M. G. Valdés, A. C. V. González, J. A. G. Calzón and M. E. Díaz-García, "Analytical nanotechnology for food analysis", *Microchim Acta*, 166: 1–19, 2009.
[57] J. K. Carrow, A. K. Gaharwar, "Bioinspired polymeric nanocomposites for regenerative medicine", *Macromol Chem Phys*, 216(3): 248–264, 2015.
[58] A. K. Gaharwar, N. A. Peppas, A. Khademhosseini, "Nanocomposite hydrogels for biomedical applications", *Biotechnol Bioeng*, 111(3): 441–453, 2014.
[59] V. Ojijo, S. Sinha Ray, "Processing strategies in bionanocomposites", *Prog Polym Sci*, 38(10–11): 1543–1589, 2013.
[60] M.-H. Chen, "Update on dental nanocomposites", *J Dent Res*, 89(6): 549–560, 2010.
[61] K. M. Galler, R. N. D'Souza, J. D. Hartgerink, G. Schmalz, "Scaffolds for dental pulp tissue engineering", *Adv Dent Res*, 23(3): 333–339, 2011.
[62] D. R. Paul, L. M. Robeson, "Polymer nanotechnology: nanocomposites", *Polymer*, 49(15): 3187–3204, 2008.

[63] J. J. Park, E. J. Yu, W.-K. Lee, C.-S. Ha, "Mechanical properties and degradation studies of poly(D,L-lactide-co-glycolide) 50:50/graphene oxide nanocomposite films", *Polym Adv Technol*, 25(1): 48–54, 2014.

[64] F. Ameen, S. AlNadhari, A. A. Al-Homaidan, "Marine microorganisms as an untapped source of bioactive compounds", *Saudi J Biol Sci*, 28(1): 224–231 2021, doi: 10.1016/j.sjbs.2020.09.052

[65] H. Malve, "Exploring the ocean for new drug developments: marine pharmacology", *J Pharm Bioallied Sci*, 8(2): 83–91, 2016, doi: 10.4103/0975-7406.171700

[66] R. Ghosh, K. Banerjee, A. Mitra, *Eco-biochemical studies of common seaweeds in the lower Gangetic Delta*. New York: John Wiley & Sons, Ltd, 2012.

[67] R. B. Mrid, B. Benmrid, J. Hafsa, H. Boukcim, M. Sobeh, A. Yasri "Secondary metabolites as biostimulant and bioprotectant agents: a review", *Sci Total Environ*, 777: 146–204, 2021, doi: 10.1016/j.scitotenv.2021.146204

[68] B. Das, S. K. Dash, D. Mandal, T. Ghosh, S. Chattopadhyay, S. Tripathy, S. Das, S. K. Dey, D. Das, C. L. F. De Almeida, S. H. De Falcao, G. R. M. De Lima, A. C. De Montenegro, N. S. Lira, P. F. De Athayde-Filho, L. C. Rodrigues, M. F. V. De Souza, J. M. Barbosa-Filho, L. M. Batista, "Bioactivities from marine algae of the genus *Gracilaria*", *Int J Mol Sci*, 12(7): 4550–4573, 2011, doi: 10.3390/ijms12074550

[69] S. Kadam, P. Prabhasankar, "Marine foods as functional ingredients in bakery and pasta products", *Food Res Int*, 43(8): 1975–1980, 2010, doi: 10.1016/j.foodres.2010.06.007

[70] A. M. Cikos, M. Jurin, R. Coz-Rakovac, D. Gaso-Sokac, S. Jokic, I. Jerkovic, "Update on sesquiterpenes from red macroalgae of the *Laurencia* genus and their biological activities (2015–2020)", *Algal Res*, 56: 1023–1030, 2021, doi: 10.1016/j.algal.2021.102330

[71] R. Kannan, R. Arumugam, D. Ramya, K. Manivannan, P. Anantharaman, "Green synthesis of silver nanoparticles using marine macroalga *Chaetomorpha linum*", *Appl Nanosci*, 3(3): 229–233, 2013. doi: 10.1007/s13204-012-0125-5

[72] K. F. Princy, A. Gopinath, "Green synthesis of silver nanoparticles using polar seaweed Fucus gardeneri and its catalytic efficacy in the reduction of nitrophenol", *Polar Sci*, 30: 100692, 2021, doi: 10.1016/j.polar.2021.100692

[73] S. Nagarajan, K. Arumugam Kuppusamy, "Extracellular synthesis of zinc oxide nanoparticle using seaweeds of Gulf of Mannar, India", *J Nanobiotechnol*, 11(1): 1–1, 2013, doi: 10.1186/1477-3155-11-1

[74] S. Rajaboopathi, S. Thambidurai, "Enhanced photocatalytic activity of Ag-ZnO nanoparticles synthesized by using *Padina gymnospora* seaweed extract", *J Mol Liq*, 262: 148–160, 2018, doi: 10.1016/j.molliq.2018.04.073

[75] M. Amina, N. M. Al Musayeib, S. F. Alterary. M. A. El-Tohamy, S. Alhwaiti, "Advanced polymeric metal/metal oxide bionanocomposite using seaweed Laurencia dendroidea extract for antiprotozoal, anticancer, and photocatalytic applications", *PeerJ*, 11: e15004, 2023, doi: 10.7717/peerj.15004

[76] M. Vivek, P. S. Kumar, S. Steffi, S. Sudha, "Biogenic silver nanoparticles by *Gelidiella acerosa* extract and their antifungal effects", *Avicenna J Med Biotechnol* 2011, 3: 143.

[77] S. Varun, S. Sudha, P. Senthil Kumar, "Biosynthesis of gold nanoparticles from aqueous extract of *Dictyota bartayresiana* and their anti-fungal activity", *Indian J Adv Chem Sci*, 2: 190–193, 2014.

[78] N. González-Ballesteros, J. González-Rodríguez, M. Rodríguez-Argüelles, M. Lastra, "New application of two Antarctic macroalgae *Palmaria decipiens* and *Desmarestia menziesii* in the synthesis of gold and silver nanoparticles". *Polar Sci*, 15: 49–54, 2018.

[79] A. P. Vieira, E. M. Stein, D. X. Andreguetti, P. Colepicolo, A. M. Da Costa Ferreira, "Preparation of silver nanoparticles using aqueous extracts of the red algae *Laurencia aldingensis* and *Laurenciella sp.* and their cytotoxic activities", *J Appl Phycol*, 28(4): 2615–2622, 2016, doi: 10.1007/s10811-015-0757-4

[80] L. S. De Oliveira, D. A. Tschoeke, A. S. De Oliveira, L. J. Hill, W. C. Paradas, L. T. Salgado, C. C. Thompson, R. C. Pereira, F. L. Thompson, "New insights on the terpenome of the red seaweed *Laurencia dendroidea* (Florideophyceae, Rhodophyta)", *Mar Drugs*, 13(2): 879–902, 2015, doi: 10.3390/md13020879

[81] K. G. Goncalves, L. L. Da Silva, A. R. Soares, N. C. Romeiro, Acetylcholinesterase as a target of halogenated marine natural products from *Laurencia dendroidea*, *Algal Res*, 52: 102130, 2020, doi: 10.1016/j.algal.2020.102130

[82] M. M. Barcellos, D. W. Rodrigues, D. M. F. Lacerda, R. L. I. Correa, S. A. Ribeiro, K. M. Masahiko, M. M. Frazao, "Cytotoxic activity of halogenated sesquiterpenes from Laurencia dendroidea", *Phytother Res*, 32(6): 1119–1125, 2018, doi: 10.1002/ptr.6052

[83] M. M. Khalil, E. H. Ismail, K. Z. El-Baghdady, D. Mohamed, "Green synthesis of silver nanoparticles using olive leaf extract and its antibacterial activity", *Arab J Chem*, 7: 1131–1139, 2014.

[84] P. Madhiyazhagan, K. Murugan, A. N. Kumar, T. Nataraj, D. Dinesh, C. Panneerselvam, J. Subramaniam, P. M. Kumar, U. Suresh, M. Roni, "*Sargassum muticum*-synthesized silver nanoparticles: an effective control tool against mosquito vectors and bacterial pathogens", *Parasitol Res*, 114: 4305–4317, 2015.

[85] N. González-Ballesteros, M. Rodríguez-Argüelles, M. Lastra-Valdor, G. González-Mediero, S. Rey-Cao, M. Grimaldi, A. Cavazza, F. Bigi, "Synthesis of silver and gold nanoparticles by *Sargassum muticum* biomolecules and evaluation of their antioxidant activity and antibacterial properties", *J Nanostructure Chem*, 10: 1–14, 2020.

[86] C. S. Vairappan, M. Suzuki, T. Abe, M. Masuda, "Halogenated metabolites with antibacterial activity from the *Okinawan Laurencia* species", *Phytochemistry*, 58(3): 517–523, 2001, doi: 10.1016/S0031-9422(01)00260-6

[87] N. Abdel-Raouf, N. M. Al-Enazi, I. B. Ibraheem, "Green biosynthesis of gold nanoparticles using *Galaxaura elongata* and characterization of their antibacterial activity", *Arab J Chem*, 10: S3029–S3039, 2017.

[88] P. Bhuyar, M. H. A. Rahim, S. Sundararaju, R. Ramaraj, G. P. Maniam, N. Govindan, "Synthesis of silver nanoparticles using marine macroalgae Padina sp. and its antibacterial activity towards pathogenic bacteria", *Beni-Suef Univ J Basic Appl Sci*, 9: 3, 2020.

[89] P. Shiny, A. Mukherjee, N. Chandrasekaran, "Marine algae mediated synthesis of the silver nanoparticles and its antibacterial efficiency", *Int J Pharm Pharm Sci*, 5: 239–241, 2013.

[90] C. Mohandass, A. Vijayaraj, R. Rajasabapathy, S. Satheeshbabu; S. Rao, C. Shiva, I. De-Mello, "Biosynthesis of silver nanoparticles from marine seaweed *Sargassum cinereum* and their antibacterial activity", *Indian J Pharm Sci*, 75: 606, 2013.

[91] R. Ishwarya, B. Vaseeharan, S. Kalyani, B. Banumathi, N. S. Marimuthu Govindarajan, S. K. Alharbi, M. N. Al-Anbr, J. M. Khaled, G. Benelli, "Facile green synthesis of zinc oxide nanoparticles using *Ulva lactuca* seaweed extract and evaluation of their photocatalytic, antibiofilm and insecticidal activity", *J Photochem Photobiol B*, 178: 249–258, 2018.

[92] Marguerite Rinaudo, "Biomaterials based on a natural polysaccharide, alginate", *TIP Rev Espec en Cienc Quím-Biol*, 17: 92–96, 2014.

[93] A. Pugazhendhi, D. Prabakar, J. M. Jacob, I. Karuppusamy, R. G. Saratale, "Synthesis and characterization of silver nanoparticles using *Gelidium amansii* and its antimicrobial property against various pathogenic bacteria", *Microb Pathog*, 114: 41–45, 2018.

[94] E. Ayranci, S. Tunc, "A method for the measurement of the oxygen permeability and the development of edible films to reduce the rate of oxidative reactions in fresh foods", *Food Chem*, 80: 423–431, 2003.

[95] L. Castro, M. L. Blázquez, J. A. Muñoz, F. González, A. Ballester, "Biological synthesis of metallic nanoparticles using algae", *IET Nanobiotechnol*, 7: 109–116, 2013.

[96] B. Sharma, D. D. Purkayastha, S. Hazra, M. Thajamanbi, C. R. Bhattacharjee, N. N. Ghosh, J. Rout, "Biosynthesis of fluorescent gold nanoparticles using an edible freshwater red alga, *Lemanea fluviatilis* (L.) C. Ag. and antioxidant activity of biomatrix loaded nanoparticles", *Bioprocess Biosyst Eng*, 37: 2559–2565, 2014.

[97] M. K. Shukla, R. P. Singh, C. Reddy, B. Jha, "Synthesis and characterization of agar-based silver nanoparticles and nanocomposite film with antibacterial applications", *Bioresour Technol*, 107: 295–300, 2012.

[98] J. S. Devi, B. V. Bhimba, K. Ratnam, "In vitro anticancer activity of silver nanoparticles synthesized using the extract of *Gelidiella sp*", *Int J Pharm Pharm Sci*, 4: 710–715, 2012.

[99] A. P. de Aragao, T. M. de Oliveira, P. V. Quelemes, M. L. G. Perfeito, M. C. Araujo, J. D. A. S. Santiago, V. S. Cardoso, P. Quaresma, J. R. D. S. de Almeida, D. A. da Silva, "Green synthesis of silver nanoparticles using the seaweed *Gracilaria birdiae* and their antibacterial activity", *Arab J Chem*, 12: 4182–4188, 2019.

[100] I. Ibraheem, B. Abd-Elaziz, W. Saad, W. Fathy, "Green biosynthesis of silver nanoparticles using marine Red Algae *Acanthophora specifera* and its antimicrobial activity", *J Nanomed Nanotechnol*, 7: 6, 2016.

[101] K. Sajidha Parveen, D. Lakshmi, "Biosynthesis of silver nanoparticles using red algae, Amphiroa fragilissima and its antibacterial potential against gram positive and gram negative bacteria", *Int J Curr Sci*, 19: 93–100, 2016.

[102] B. Bhimba, P. Kumari, "Phytosynthesis of silver nanoparticles from the extracts of seaweed *Ulva lactuca* and its antimicrobial activity", *Int J Pharm Bio Sci*, 5: 666–677, 2014.

[103] T. Kathiraven, A. Sundaramanickam, N. Shanmugam, T. Balasubramanian, "Green synthesis of silver nanoparticles using marine algae *Caulerpa racemosa* and their antibacterial activity against some human pathogens", *Appl Nanosci*, 5: 499–504, 2015.

[104] M. Yousefzadi, Z. Rahimi, V. Ghafori, "The green synthesis, characterization and antimicrobial activities of silver nanoparticles synthesized from green alga *Enteromorpha flexuosa* (wulfen) J. Agardh", *Mater Lett*, 137: 1–4, 2014.

[105] E. F. Aboelfetoh, R. A. El-Shenody, M. M. Ghobara, "Eco-friendly synthesis of silver nanoparticles using green algae (*Caulerpa serrulata*): reaction optimization, catalytic and antibacterial activities", *Environ Monit Assess*, 189: 349, 2017.

[106] J. Suriya, S. B. Raja, V. Sekar, R. Rajasekaran, "Biosynthesis of silver nanoparticles and its antibacterial activity using seaweed *Urospora sp*", *Afr J Biotechnol*, 11: 12192–12198, 2012.

[107] D. S. Cha, J. H. Choi, M. S. Chinnan, H. J. Park, Antimicrobial films based on Na-alginate and κ-carrageenan. *Lebensm-Wiss u-Technol*, 35: 715–719, 2002.

[108] G. Ozin, A. Arsenault, *Nanochemistry: a chemical approach to nanomaterials*. Cambridge, UK: Royal Society of Chemistry, 2005, Ch. 10.

[109] Margarita Darder, Pilar Aranda, Eduardo Ruiz-Hitzky, "Bionanocomposites: a new concept of ecological, bioinspired, and functional hybrid materials", *Adv Mater*, 19: 1309–1319, 2007.

[110] M. Sun-Hong, J. L. Ferracane, L. In-Bog, *Dental Mater*, 26: 1024–1033, 2010.

[111] W. Weinmann, C. Thalacker, R. Guggenberger, Dental materials: official publication of the academy, *Dental Mater*, 21: 68–74, 2005.

[112] N. Ilie, R. Hickel, Silorane-based dental composite: behavior and abilities, *Dental Mater J*, 25: 445–454, 2006.

[113] M. H. Mousa, Y. Dong, I. J. Davies, "Recent advances in bionanocomposites: preparation, properties, and applications". *Int J Polym Mater Polym Biomater*, 65: 225–254, 2016.

[114] D. F. Emerich, C. Thanos, "The pinpoint promise of nanoparticle-based drug delivery and molecular diagnosis", *Biomol Eng*, 23(4): 171–184, 2006, doi: 10.1016/j.bioeng.2006.05.026

[115] A. M. Ramos-de-la-Peña, J. C. Contreras-Esquivel, O. Aguilar, J. González-Valdez, "Structural and bioactive roles of fucoidan in nanogel delivery systems. A review". *Carbohydr Polym Technol Appl*, 4: 100235, 2022.

[116] N. Shanthi, P. Arumugam, M. Murugan, M. P. Sudhakar, K. Arunkumar, "Extraction of fucoidan from *Turbinaria decurrens* and the synthesis of fucoidan-coated AgNPs for anticoagulant application", *ACS Omega*, 6: 30998–31008, 2021.

[117] V. L. Campo, D. F. Kawano, D. B. D. Silva Jr., I. Carvalho, "Carrageenans: biological properties, chemical modifications and structural analysis—a review", *Carbohydr Polym*, 77(2): 167–180, 2009.

[118] I. Wijesekara, R. Pangestuti, S.-K. Kim, "Biological activities and potential health benefits of sulfated polysaccharides derived from marine algae", *Carbohydr Polym*, 84(1): 14–21, 2011.

[119] C. B. Buck, C. D. Thompson, J. N. Roberts, M. Muller, D. R. Lowy, J. T. Schiller, "Carrageenan is a potent inhibitor of papillomavirus infection", *PLoS Pathogens*, 2(7): article e69, 2006.

[120] M. C. Rocha De Souza, C. T. Marques, C. M. Guerra Dore, F. R. Ferreira Da Silva, H. A. Oliveira Rocha, E. L. Leite, "Antioxidant activities of sulfated polysaccharides from brown and red seaweeds", *J Appl Phycol*, 19(2): 153–160, 2007.

[121] A. M. Salgueiro, A. L. Daniel-Da-Silva, S. Fateixa, T. Trindade, "κ-Carrageenan hydrogel nanocomposites with release behavior mediated by morphological distinct Au nanofillers", *Carbohydr Polym*, 91(1): 100–109, 2013.

[122] J. S. Boateng, H. V. Pawar, J. Tetteh, "Polyox and carrageenan based composite film dressing containing antimicrobial and anti-inflammatory drugs for effective wound healing", *Int J Pharm*, 441(1–2): 181–191, 2013.

[123] J. V. Araujo, N. Davidenko, M. Danner, R. E. Cameron, S. M. Best, "Novel porous scaffolds of pH responsive chitosan/carrageenan-based polyelectrolyte complexes for tissue engineering", *J Biomed Mater Res A*, 102(12): 4415–4426, 2014.

[124] K. Tomoda, M. Asahiyama, E. Ohtsuki et al., "Preparation and properties of carrageenan microspheres containing allopurinol and local anesthetic agents for the treatment of oral mucositis", *Colloids Surf B Biointerfaces*, 71(1): 27–35, 2009.

[125] M. C. Bonferoni, P. Chetoni, P. Giunchedi et al., "Carrageenan gelatin mucoadhesive systems for ion-exchange based ophthalmic delivery: in vitro and preliminary in vivo studies", *Eur J Pharm Biopharm*, 57(3): 465–472, 2004.

[126] Y. Liu, Y.-Y. Zhu, G. Wei, W.-Y. Lu, "Effect of carrageenan on poloxamer-based in situ gel for vaginal use: improved in vitro and in vivo sustained-release properties", *Eur J Pharm Sci*, 37(3–4): 306–312, 2009.
[127] C. Maderuelo, A. Zarzuelo, J. M. Lanao, "Critical factors in the release of drugs from sustained release hydrophilic matrices", *J Control Release*, 154(1): 2–19, 2011.
[128] L. Li, R. Ni, Y. Shao, S. Mao, "Carrageenan, and its applications in drug delivery", *Carbohydr Polym*, 103: 1–11, 2014.
[129] E. Karavas, E. Koutris, A. G. Papadopoulos, M. Sigalas, et al., "Application of density functional theory in combination with FTIR and DSC to characterise polymer drug interactions for the preparation of sustained release formulations between fluvastatin and carrageenans", *Int J Pharm*, 466: 211–222, 2014.
[130] Y.-C. Huang, T.-J. Liu, "Mobilization of mesenchymal stem cells by stromal cell-derived factor-1 released from chitosan/tripolyphosphate/fucoidan nanoparticles", *Acta Biomater*, 2012, 8: 1048–1056.
[131] S. Saedi, M. Shokri, J. W. Rhim, "Preparation of carrageenan-based antimicrobial films incorporated with sulfur nanoparticles", *Korean J Pack Sci Technol*, 26: 125–131, 2020.
[132] K. Alba, V. Kontogiorgos, "Seaweed polysaccharides (agar, alginate carrageenan)". In: Melton, L., Shahidi, F., Varelis, P., editors. *Encyclopedia of food chemistry*. Netherlands: Elsevier, pp. 240–250, 2018.
[133] S. Manna, S. Jana, "Carrageenan-based nanomaterials in drug delivery applications". In: *Biopolymer-based nanomaterials in drug delivery and biomedical applications*. Netherlands: Elsevier, pp. 365–382, 2021.
[134] T. Brenner, R. Tuvikene, A. Parker, S. Matsukawa, K. Nishinari, "Rheology and structure of mixed kappa-carrageenan/iota-carrageenan gels", *Food Hydrocoll*, 39: 272–279, 2014.
[135] J. W. Rhim, L. F. Wang, "Preparation and characterization of carrageenan based nanocomposite films reinforced with clay mineral and silver nanoparticles", *Appl Clay Sci*, 97–98: 174–181, 2014.
[136] M. Suhail, Y. H. Hsieh, A. Khan, M. U. Minhas, P. C. Wu, "Preparation and in vitro Evaluation of aspartic/alginic acid based semi-interpenetrating network hydrogels for controlled release of ibuprofen", *Gels*, 7: 68–107, 2021.
[137] M. L. Amin, D. Mawad, S. Dokos, P. Koshy, P. J. Martens, C. C. Sorrell, "Fucoidan- and carrageenan-based biosynthetic poly(vinyl alcohol) hydrogels for controlled permeation", *Mater Sci Eng C Mater Biol Appl*, 121: 111821, 2021.
[138] R. Rajesh, Y. D. Ravichandran, Y. C. Kuo, Alginate in bone tissue engineering. In: Venkatesan, J., Anil, S., Kim, S. K., editors. *Seaweed polysaccharides: isolation, biological and biomedical applications*. Netherlands: Elsevier Inc., pp. 349–368, 2017.
[139] M. H. Kim, Y. W. Lee, W. K. Jung, J. Oh, S. Y. Nam, "Enhanced rheological behaviors of alginate hydrogels with carrageenan for extrusion-based bioprinting", *J Mech Behav Biomed Mater*, 98: 187–194, 2019.
[140] L. Muthulakshmi, U. Pavithra, V. Sivaranjani, N. Balasubramanian, K. M. Sakthivel, C. I. Pruncu, "A novel Ag/carrageenan-gelatin hybrid hydrogel nanocomposite and its biological applications: preparation and characterization", *J Mech Behav Biomed Mater*, 115: 104257, 2021.
[141] B. Li, Y. Liu, Y. Zhou, P. You, M. Wang, L. Tang, "Development of a novel extracellular matrix membrane with an asymmetric structure for guided bone regeneration", *Mater Lett*, 274: 127926, 2020.
[142] K. Suzuki, Y. Suzuki, M. Tanihara, T. Hashimoto, K. Endo, "Reconstruction of rat peripheral nerve gap without sutures using freeze dried alginate gel", *J Biomed Mater Res*, 49: 528–533, 2000.
[143] Y. L. Kuen, J. David, "Mooney, alginate, properties and biomedical applications", *Prog Polym Sci*, 37: 106–126, 2012.
[144] K. Murakami, H. Aoki, S. Nakamura, S. Nakamura, M. Takikawa, M. Hanzawa, S. Kishimoto, H. Hattori, Y. Tanaka, "Hydrogel blends of chitin/chitosan, fucoidan and alginate as healing-impaired wound dressings", *Biomaterials*, 31: 83–90, 2010.
[145] A. Grenha, M. E. Gomes, M. Rodrigues et al., "Development of new chitosan/carrageenan nanoparticles for drug delivery applications", *J Biomed Mater Res A*, 92(4): 1265–1272, 2010.
[146] M. Pavli, F. Vrecer, S. Baumgartner, "Matrix tablets based on carrageenans with dual controlled release of doxazosin mesylate", *Int J Pharm*, 400(1–2):15–23, 2010.
[147] F. Kianfar, M. Antonijevic, B. Chowdhry, J. S. Boateng, "Lyophilized wafers comprising carrageenan and pluronic acid for buccal drug delivery using model soluble and insoluble drugs", *Colloids Surf B: Biointerfaces*, 103: 99–106, 2013.
[148] D. Ghanam, P. Kleinebudde, "Suitability of κ-carrageenan pellets for the formulation of multiparticulate tablets with modified release", *Int J Pharm*, 409(1–2): 9–18, 2011.
[149] S. Nanaki, E. Karavas, L. Kalantzi, D. Bikiaris, "Miscibility study of carrageenan blends and evaluation of their effectiveness as sustained release carriers", *Carbohydr Polym*, 79(4): 1157–1167, 2010.

[150] T. Y. Ahn, J. H. Kang, D. J. Kang, J. Venkatesan, H. K. Chang, I. Bhatnagar, K. Y. Chang, J. H. Hwang, Z. Salameh, S. K. Kim, "Interaction of stem cells with nano hydroxyapatite-fucoidan bionanocomposites for bone tissue regeneration", *Int J Biol Macromol*, 93: 1488–1491, 2016.

[151] V. D. Alves, R. Castelló, A. R. Ferreira, N. Costa, I. M. Fonseca, I. M. Coelhoso, "Barrier properties of carrageenan/pectin biodegradable composite films", *Procedia Food Sci*, 1: 240–245, 2011.

[152] V. E. Santo, A. M. Frias, M. Carida, R. Cancedda, M. E. Gomes, J. F. Mano, "Carrageenan-based hydrogels for the controlled delivery of PDGF-BB in bone tissue engineering applications", *Biomacromolecules*, 10: 1392–1401, 2009.

[153] L. Y. Madruga, R. M. Sabino, E. C. Santos, K. C. Popat, R. C. Balaban, M. J. Kipper, "Carboxymethyl-kappa-carrageenan: a study of biocompatibility, antioxidant and antibacterial activities", *Int J Biol Macromol*, 152: 483–491, 2020.

[154] A. A. Oun, J. W. Rhim, "Carrageenan-based hydrogels and films: effect of ZnO and CuO nanoparticles on the physical, mechanical, and antimicrobial properties", *Food Hydrocoll*, 67: 45–53, 2017.

[155] J. W. Rhim, L. F. Wang. Mechanical and water barrier properties of agar/κ-carrageenan/konjac glucomannan ternary blend biohydrogel films, *Carbohydr Polym*, 96: 71–81, 2013.

[156] E. Tavassoli-Kafrani, H. Shekarchizadeh, M. Masoudpour-Behabadi, "Development of edible films and coatings from alginates and carrageenans", *Carbohydr Polym*, 137: 360–374, 2016.

[157] L. Dou, B. Li, K. Zhang, X. Chu, H. Hou, "Physical properties and antioxidant activity of gelatin-sodium alginate edible films with tea polyphenols", *Int J Biol Macromol*, 118: 1377–1383, 2018.

[158] F. Menaa, P. A. Wijesinghe, G. Thiripuranathar, B. Uzair, H. Iqbal, B. A. Khan, B. Menaa "Ecological and industrial implications of dynamic seaweed-associated microbiota interactions", *Marine Drugs*, 18(12): 641, 2020, doi: 10.3390/md18120641.1377-83

[159] K. Senthilkumar, G. Ramajayam, J. Venkatesan, S. K. Kim, B. C. Ahn, Biomedical applications of fucoidan, seaweed polysaccharides. In: Anil, S., editor. *Seaweed polysaccharides: isolation, biological and biomedical applications*. Netherlands: Elsevier Inc., pp. 269–281, 2017.

[160] C. Ben Amor, M. A. Jmel, P. Chevallier, D. Mantovani, I. Smaali, "Efficient extraction of a high molecular weight ulvan from stranded *Ulva sp.* biomass: application on the active biomembrane synthesis", *Biomass Conv Bioref*, 13: 3975–3985, 2023.

[161] A. Alves, R. A. Sousa, R. L. Reis, "A practical perspective on ulvan extracted from green algae", *J Appl Phycol*, 25: 407–424, 2012.

[162] N. Yavorska, "Sodium alginate, A potential tool for weight management: effect on subjective appetite, food intake, and glycemic and insulin regulation", *Journal of Undergraduate Life Sciences*, 6: 66–69, 2012.

[163] S. Madhavan, "Abirami: a review on hydrocolloids-agar and alginate", *J Pharm Sci Res*, 7: 704–707, 2015.

[164] T. Andersen, C. Markussen, M. Dornish, "In situ gelation for cell immobilization and culture in alginate foam scaffolds", *Tissue Eng A*, 20: 600–610, 2014.

[165] X. Xu, X. Wu, Q. Wang, "Immunomodulatory effects of alginate oligosaccharides on murine macrophage RAW264.7 cells and their structure-activity relationships", *J Agric Food Chem*, 62: 3168–3176, 2014.

[166] S. L. Gan, Q. L. Feng, "Preparation and characterization of a new injectable bone substitutecarrageenan/nano-hydroxyapatite/collagen", *Acta Acad Med Sin*, 28: 710–713, 2006.

[167] J. Venkatesan, I. Bhatnagar, P. Manivasagan, K. H. Kang, S. K. Kim, "Alginate composites for bone tissue engineering: a review", *Int J Biol Macromol*, 72: 269–281, 2015.

[168] T. Vo, S. Kim, "Fucoidans as a natural bioactive ingredient for functional foods", *J Funct Foods*, 5: 16–27, 2012.

[169] (US), National Institutes of Health, and Biological Sciences Curriculum Study, 2007, *Understanding cancer*, NIH curriculum supplement series (available at: www.ncbi.nlm.nih.gov/books/NBK20362/)

[170] R. L. Siegel, K. D. Miller, A. Jemal, "Cancer statistics, 2019 CA", *Cancer J Clin*, 69: 7–34, 2019.

[171] A. Pavlopoulou, Y. Oktay, K. Vougas, M. Louka, C. E. Vorgias, A. G. Georgakilas, "Determinants of resistance to chemotherapy and ionizing radiation in breast cancer stem cells", *Cancer Lett*, 380: 485–493, 2016.

[172] S. E. Ahmed, N. Awad, V. Paul, H. G. Moussa, G. A. Husseini, "Improving the efficacy of anticancer drugs via encapsulation and acoustic release", *Curr Top Med Chem*, 18: 857–880, 2018.

[173] Y. L. Su, S. H. Hu, "Functional nanoparticles for tumor penetration of therapeutics", *Pharmaceutics*, 10: E193, 2018.

[174] N. Asadi, N. Annabi, E. Mostafavi, M. Anzabi, R. Khalilov, S. Saghfi, M. Mehrizadeh and A. Akbarzadeh, "Synthesis, characterization and in vitro evaluation of magnetic nanoparticles modified with PCL–PEG–PCL for controlled delivery of 5FU Artif. Cells", *Nanomed Biotechnol*, 46: 938–945, 2018.

[175] Z. Vahed, N. F. Sepideh, M. Samiei, S. M. Dizaj, S. Sharifi, "Targeted cancer drug delivery with aptamer-functionalized polymeric nanoparticles", *J Drug Target*, 27: 292–299, 2019.

[176] R. C. F. Cheung, T. B. Ng, J. H. Wong, W. Y. Chan, "Chitosan: an update on potential biomedical and pharmaceutical applications", *Mar Drugs*, 13: 5156–5186, 2015.

[177] F. Lewis-Oscar, S. Vismaya, M. Arunkumar, N. Thajuddin, D. Dhanasekaran, C. Nithya, "Algal nanoparticles: synthesis and biotechnological potentials", *Algae Org Imminent Biotechnol*, 7: 157–182, 2016.

[178] K. J. Prashob Peter, "Multi-functional silver nanoparticles for drug delivery: a review", *Int J Curr Pharm Rev Res*, 9: 1–5, 2017.

[179] N. Supraja, T. Prasad, M. Soundariya, R. Babujanarthanam, "Synthesis, characterization and dose dependent antimicrobial and anti-cancerous activity of phycogenic silver nanoparticles against human hepatic carcinoma (HepG2) cell line", *AIMS Bioeng*, 3: 425–440, 2016.

[180] P. Balaraman, B. Balasubramanian, D. Kaliannan, M. Durai, H. Kamyab, S. Park, S. Chelliapan, C. T. Lee, V. Maluventhen, A. Maruthupandian, "Phyco-synthesis of silver nanoparticles mediated from marine algae *Sargassum myriocystum* and its potential biological and environmental applications", *Waste Biomass Valori*, 11: 5255–5271, 2020.

[181] M. Gopu, P. Kumar, T. Selvankumar, B. Senthilkumar, C. Sudhakar, M. Govarthanan, R. S. Kumar, K. Selvam, "Green biomimetic silver nanoparticles utilizing the red algae *Amphiroa rigida* and its potent antibacterial, cytotoxicity and larvicidal efficiency", *Bioprocess Biosyst Eng*, 44: 1–7, 2020.

[182] N. González-Ballesteros, S. Prado-López, J. Rodríguez-González, M. Lastra, M. Rodríguez-Argüelles, "Green synthesis of gold nanoparticles using brown algae *Cystoseira baccata*: its activity in colon cancer cells", *Colloids Surf B Biointerfaces*, 153: 190–198, 2017.

[183] N. Thangaraju, R. Venkatalakshmi, A. Chinnasamy, P. Kannaiyan, "Synthesis of silver nanoparticles and the antibacterial and anticancer activities of the crude extract of *Sargassum polycystum* C. Agardh", *Nano Biomed Eng*, 4" 89–94, 2012.

[184] H. Y. El-Kassas, M. M. El-Sheekh, "Cytotoxic activity of biosynthesized gold nanoparticles with an extract of the red seaweed *Corallina officinalis* on the MCF-7 human breast cancer cell line", *Asian Pac J Cancer Prev*, 15: 4311–4317, 2014.

[185] R. I. Priyadharshini, G. Prasannaraj, N. Geetha, P. Venkatachalam, "Microwave-mediated extracellular synthesis of metallic silver and zinc oxide nanoparticles using macro-algae (*Gracilaria edulis*) extracts and its anticancer activity against human PC3 cell lines", *Appl Biochem Biotechnol*, 174: 2777–2790, 2014.

[186] Z. Sanaeimehr, I. Javadi, F. Namvar, "Antiangiogenic and antiapoptotic effects of green-synthesized zinc oxide nanoparticles using *Sargassum muticum* algae extraction", *Cancer Nanotechnol*, 9: 3, 2018.

[187] F. Namvar, S. Azizi, H. S. Rahman, R. Mohamad, A. Rasedee, M. Soltani, R. A. Rahim "Green synthesis, characterization, and anticancer activity of hyaluronan/zinc oxide nanocomposite", *Onco Targets Ther*, 9: 4549–4559, 2016.

[188] R. Mohamed Asik, B. Gowdhami, M. S. Mohamed Jaabir, G. Archunan, N. Suganthy "Anticancer potential of zinc oxide nanoparticles against cervical carcinoma cells synthesized via biogenic route using aqueous extract of *Gracilaria edulis*", *Mater Sci Eng C*, 103: 109840, 2019.

[189] H. Yuan, J. Song, X. Li, N. Li, J. Dai, "Immunomodulation and antitumor activity of κcarrageenan oligosaccharides", *Cancer Lett*, 243: 228–234, 2006.

[190] Y. Minamida, H. Matsuura, T. Ishii, K. Sato, T. Kamada, A. Kato, Y. Yamagishi, T. Abe, N. Kikuchi, M. Suzuki, "Chemical composition of *Laurencia* spp. collected from the Seto Inland Sea of Japan", *Biochem Syst Ecol*, 96: 104259, 2021, doi: 10.1016/j.bse.2021.104259

[191] K. Govindaraju, K. Krishnamoorthy, S. A. Alsagaby, G. Singaravelu, M. Premanathan, "Green synthesis of silver nanoparticles for selective toxicity towards cancer cells", *IET Nanobiotechnol*, 9: 325–330, 2015.

[192] D. Acharya, S. Satapathy, P. Somu, U. K. Parida, G. Mishra, "Apoptotic effect and anticancer activity of biosynthesized silver nanoparticles from marine algae *Chaetomorpha linum* extract against human colon cancer cell HCT-116", *Biol Trace Elem Res*, 199: 1–11, 2020.

[193] R. Kanaparthy, A. Kanaparthy, "The changing face of dentistry: nanotechnology", *Int J Nanomed*, 6: 2799–2804, 2011.

[194] R. Chandki, M. Kala, K. N. Kumar, B. Brigit, B. Banthia, R. Banthia, "Nanodentistry": exploring the beauty of miniature, *J Clin Exp Dent*, 4: e119, 2012.

11 Biopolymer-Nanoparticle Hybrid Systems for Advanced Drug Delivery and Therapeutics

Polaki Suman, Pushpalatha Ganesh, B. Rabi Prasad and Ghanistha Prusty

11.1 INTRODUCTION

In modern medicine, advanced drug delivery systems offer hope for revolutionizing how therapeutic agents are administered, distributed, and targeted within the human body. This introduction serves as a gateway to explore the multifaceted realm of advanced drug delivery systems, focusing on the pivotal roles of biopolymers and nanoparticles in shaping the future of therapeutic interventions [1].

Advanced drug delivery systems are designed to overcome the limitations of conventional drug administration methods [2]. Traditional drug delivery methods often have limitations such as poor bioavailability, non-specific targeting, and quick clearance from the body. On the other hand, advanced drug delivery systems offer a more refined approach, allowing for precise control of drug release kinetics, better targeting capabilities, and improved therapeutic outcomes [3].

Biopolymers are essential in drug delivery applications as they offer diverse materials with unique properties. These materials are inspired by nature's resources [4]. Biopolymers, such as proteins, polysaccharides, and nucleic acids derived from natural sources, offer inherent benefits, including biocompatibility, biodegradability, and low immunogenicity [5, 6]. These inherent qualities make biopolymers attractive candidates for encapsulating, protecting, and delivering therapeutic agents with precision and efficacy.

Similarly, nanoparticles have emerged as indispensable tools in the arsenal of drug delivery scientists, offering unparalleled control over the physicochemical properties of drug carriers and enabling precise modulation of drug release profiles [7]. Nanoparticles, characterized by their nanoscale dimensions ranging from 1 to 1000 nanometers, exhibit unique behaviors dictated by quantum size effects, high surface area-to-volume ratios, and tunable surface properties. Through meticulous engineering, nanoparticles can be tailored to optimize drug loading capacities, enhance stability, and facilitate targeted delivery to specific tissues or cells within the body [8–10].

However, the truly transformative potential of drug delivery systems is realized through the synergy achieved by combining biopolymers and nanoparticles into hybrid constructs. These hybrid systems represent a convergence of nature-inspired materials and cutting-edge nanotechnology, harnessing the strengths of both components to address the multifaceted challenges of drug delivery [11]. By integrating biopolymers with nanoparticles, hybrid systems offer many advantages, including enhanced drug-loading capacities, prolonged circulation times, and targeted delivery to disease sites [12].

Moreover, combining biopolymers and nanoparticles enables precise control over drug release kinetics, enabling tailored therapeutic interventions suited to individual patient needs [13]. Hybrid

DOI: 10.1201/9781003650812-11

systems can be fine-tuned through surface modification, encapsulation, or co-polymerization techniques to achieve desired release profiles, responsiveness to environmental stimuli, and compatibility with specific disease microenvironments [14].

Advanced drug delivery systems have become increasingly significant in the field of therapeutics. These systems represent a paradigm shift in healthcare with far-reaching implications for patient care and treatment outcomes. By integrating biopolymers and nanoparticles, hybrid systems can address longstanding challenges in drug delivery, paving the way for more effective, targeted, and personalized therapeutic interventions. As we embark on a journey to explore the intricacies of biopolymer-nanoparticle hybrid systems, we stand poised at the forefront of a new era in drug delivery science, driven by innovation, collaboration, and a commitment to advancing human health and well-being.

11.2 CLASSIFICATION AND SOURCES OF BIOPOLYMERS

Biopolymers represent a diverse class of materials derived from natural sources or synthesized by living organisms. They possess unique properties such as biodegradability, renewability, and biocompatibility, making them attractive alternatives to conventional synthetic polymers in various applications [15]. Understanding the classification and sources of biopolymers is essential for exploring their wide-ranging potential across industries. Here, we delve into a detailed examination of these aspects.

11.2.1 Classification Based on Origin

11.2.1.1 Plant-Derived Biopolymers

Plants serve as abundant sources of biopolymers, offering a rich array of materials with diverse properties and functionalities.

11.2.1.1.1 Cellulose

Cellulose stands out as the most abundant biopolymer on Earth, constituting the primary component of plant cell walls. Comprised of linear chains of glucose molecules, cellulose provides structural support to plants and is a fundamental building block for various industries. Its applications span traditional papermaking to advanced nanocomposites for aerospace and biomedical applications [16, 17]. Plant cell walls contain cellulose, a highly versatile polysaccharide in biopolymer-nanoparticle hybrid systems for drug delivery and therapeutics. Due to its biocompatibility, mechanical strength, and ability to be processed into various nanostructures, it is an ideal candidate for improving drug delivery efficacy.

Nanocellulose derived from cellulose nanocrystals or nanofibers can be an effective drug carrier [18] due to its high surface area, tunable porosity, and chemical modifiability. Nanocellulose particles that have been functionalized can encapsulate therapeutic agents and enable targeted delivery to specific tissues or cells. Hydrogels that incorporate nanocellulose particles offer benefits in controlled drug release and tissue engineering applications. The hydrophilic nature of cellulose enhances the water retention capacity of hydrogels, which prolongs drug release kinetics and promotes cellular adhesion and proliferation.

11.2.1.1.2 Starch

Starch represents another prominent plant-derived biopolymer, a central energy reserve. Composed of glucose units arranged in amylose and amylopectin molecules, starch finds extensive use in food, pharmaceuticals, and biodegradable packaging materials. Its versatility and biocompatibility make it an attractive candidate for sustainable solutions in various sectors [19–22]. Starch-based biopolymer-nanoparticle hybrid systems represent promising drug delivery and therapeutics platforms, leveraging starch's biodegradability, biocompatibility, and versatility in nanoparticle formulations.

Starch nanoparticles, fabricated through techniques such as nanoprecipitation or emulsification, can encapsulate hydrophobic drugs within their core or adsorb hydrophilic drugs onto their surface. These starch-based nanocarriers offer controlled release profiles and enhanced stability for various therapeutic agents. Surface modification of starch nanoparticles with targeting ligands or stimuli-responsive moieties enables site-specific drug delivery and controlled release in response to physiological cues or external stimuli. This allows for personalized therapeutic interventions with minimized off-target effects.

11.2.1.1.3 Lignin

Lignin is a complex aromatic polymer found in the cell walls of plants, contributing to their rigidity and impermeability. Although traditionally considered a byproduct of the paper and pulp industry, lignin is gaining attention as a valuable renewable resource for producing bio-based materials, chemicals, and fuels. Its inherent structural diversity and abundance offer potential avenues for valorization in diverse applications [23–26].

Lignin-derived biopolymer-nanoparticle hybrid systems show great potential in revolutionizing drug delivery and therapeutics. This is due to lignin's structural diversity, biocompatibility, and potential for functionalization. Lignin nanoparticles, which can be obtained through nanoprecipitation or self-assembly techniques, offer a versatile platform for drug delivery. This is because they are amphiphilic and can encapsulate hydrophobic drugs within their hydrophobic core. The specificity and efficacy of lignin nanoparticles in targeted drug delivery applications can be enhanced through surface modification with targeting ligands or imaging agents. In addition, lignin-based biopolymer-nanoparticle hybrids have emerged as promising theranostic platforms. They can deliver drugs and imaging by incorporating contrast agents or fluorescent probes into lignin nanoparticles. These theranostic systems enable real-time monitoring of drug distribution and therapeutic efficacy in vivo.

11.2.1.1.4 Natural Rubber

Natural rubber, derived from the latex sap of certain plants, such as the rubber tree (*Hevea brasiliensis*), is a unique biopolymer with exceptional elasticity and resilience. Natural rubber is used to manufacture tires, adhesives, and medical devices. It offers superior mechanical properties and biodegradability compared to synthetic counterparts, making it an environmentally friendly choice in various sectors [26].

Natural rubber-based biopolymer-nanoparticle hybrid systems offer innovative drug delivery and therapeutic solutions, leveraging natural rubber's elasticity, biocompatibility, and potential for surface modification. Natural rubber nanoparticles, prepared via emulsion polymerization or solvent evaporation techniques, exhibit excellent colloidal stability and drug-loading capacity. Surface modification with biopolymers or targeting ligands enhances their biocompatibility and specificity for targeted drug delivery applications. Natural rubber-based biopolymer-nanoparticle hybrids demonstrate mucoadhesive properties, facilitating prolonged residence time and enhanced drug absorption at mucosal surfaces. These systems are particularly advantageous for delivering drugs to mucosal tissues, such as the gastrointestinal or respiratory tract, for localized therapeutic interventions.

11.2.1.2 Animal-Derived Biopolymers

Animals provide a rich source of biopolymers, particularly proteins, which exhibit diverse structures and functionalities.

11.2.1.2.1 Collagen

Collagen is the most abundant protein [27] in the animal kingdom, constituting the structural framework of connective tissues, skin, and bones. With its remarkable biocompatibility and biodegradability, collagen finds widespread applications in biomedical fields [28], such as tissue engineering, wound healing, and cosmetic surgery. Its ability to mimic the extracellular matrix makes it indispensable in regenerative medicine and drug delivery systems [29–31].

The most abundant protein forms the structural framework of connective tissues, skin, and bones. Its remarkable biocompatibility and biodegradability make it invaluable in various biomedical applications. Collagen-based scaffolds mimic the extracellular matrix, providing a conducive environment for cell adhesion, proliferation, and tissue regeneration. These scaffolds are used in regenerative medicine for repairing damaged tissues and organs. Collagen dressings promote wound healing by facilitating cell migration, angiogenesis, and extracellular matrix deposition. They are used to treat burns, ulcers, and traumatic injuries. Collagen fillers and implants are employed in cosmetic procedures to restore volume, contour, and elasticity to aging or damaged tissues.

11.2.1.2.2 Gelatin

Gelatin, derived from the partial hydrolysis of collagen, represents a versatile biopolymer with gelling properties. It is widely used in the food, pharmaceutical, and photographic industries; gelatin is a natural thickener, stabilizer, and encapsulating agent [32]. Its ability to form thermoreversible gels and complex bioactive compounds makes it a valuable ingredient in drug delivery systems and nutraceutical formulations [33–35].

Gelatin, derived from the partial hydrolysis of collagen, is a versatile biopolymer with gelling properties. It finds applications in the food, pharmaceutical, and photographic industries. Gelatin is a natural thickener, stabilizer, and gelling agent in different food products such as desserts, confectionery, and dairy products. It imparts texture, viscosity, and mouthfeel to food formulations. Gelatin capsules are widely used for oral drug delivery due to their biocompatibility, dissolution properties, and ease of manufacturing. Gelatin microspheres and nanoparticles are also utilized for targeted drug delivery and controlled release. Gelatin emulsions are used as light-sensitive coatings in photographic films and papers. Gelatin's ability to form stable colloidal dispersions and undergo controlled gelation makes it suitable for producing high-quality photographic images.

11.2.1.2.3 Silk Fibroin

Silk fibroin, produced by silkworms and spiders, stands out as a remarkable protein-based biopolymer with exceptional mechanical properties. Renowned for its strength, flexibility, and biocompatibility, silk fibroin finds applications in tissue engineering, drug delivery, and textile industries. Its unique structure and biodegradability make it a promising candidate for advanced biomaterials with tailored properties and functionalities [36–38].

Silk fibroin scaffolds offer a biocompatible and mechanically robust platform for tissue engineering applications. They support cell attachment, proliferation, and differentiation, making them suitable for constructing artificial tissues and organs.

Silk fibroin-based nanoparticles and microparticles are employed as carriers for drug delivery due to their biodegradability, sustained release kinetics, and tunable mechanical properties. These drug delivery systems enhance therapeutic efficacy and minimize side effects. Silk fibroin fibers are used in the textile industry to produce high-quality fabrics and garments with luxurious texture, sheen, and durability. Silk-based textiles are prized for their softness, breathability, and hypoallergenic properties.

11.2.1.3 Microbial-Derived Biopolymers

Microorganisms offer a promising avenue for producing biopolymers through fermentation processes, presenting opportunities for sustainable biomanufacturing.

11.2.1.3.1 Polyhydroxyalkanoates (PHAs)

PHAs represent a class of biodegradable polyesters synthesized by various microorganisms as intracellular carbon and energy storage compounds. With their biocompatibility, thermoplasticity, and biodegradability, PHAs have immense potential as eco-friendly alternatives to petroleum-based plastics. Their diverse properties and tunable characteristics make them suitable for various applications, including packaging, biomedical devices, and agricultural materials [39–41].

PHAs are increasingly utilized as biodegradable packaging materials due to their barrier properties, mechanical strength, and compostability. They offer a sustainable alternative to conventional plastics, reducing environmental pollution and reliance on non-renewable resources. PHAs are compatible with biological systems and can be processed into implants, sutures, and drug delivery systems. Their biocompatibility and biodegradability make them suitable for applications in tissue engineering, wound healing, and controlled drug release. PHA-based materials such as mulch films, seed coatings, and biodegradable pots can be used in agricultural applications. These materials contribute to soil health and reduce plastic waste in agricultural ecosystems.

11.2.1.3.2 Xanthan Gum

Xanthan gum is a microbial polysaccharide produced by Xanthomonas bacteria through the fermentation of carbohydrates. With its unique rheological properties and stability, xanthan gum is a versatile thickening, stabilizing, and suspending agent in food, pharmaceutical, and cosmetic formulations. Its pseudoplastic behavior and shear-thinning properties make it an ideal additive for enhancing texture, viscosity, and shelf stability in various products [42–44].

Xanthan gum is widely used as a thickening and stabilizing agent in food products such as sauces, dressings, and dairy alternatives. It improves texture, mouthfeel, and shelf stability while providing a gluten-free alternative in food formulations. Xanthan gum is a suspending agent and viscosity enhancer in pharmaceutical formulations such as oral suspensions, topical gels, and ophthalmic solutions. It improves drug stability, bioavailability, and patient compliance in dosage forms. As a stabilizer and emulsifier, xanthan gum is incorporated into cosmetic formulations such as creams, lotions, and hair care products. It imparts smoothness, viscosity control, and hydration to cosmetic formulations, enhancing their performance and sensory attributes.

11.2.1.3.3 Alginate

Alginate, extracted from brown seaweeds and certain bacteria, represents a polysaccharide with remarkable gelling and film-forming properties. It is widely used in food, pharmaceutical, and biomedical industries as a natural hydrogel for encapsulating cells, drugs, and bioactive compounds. Its biocompatibility, biodegradability, and ability to form complex structures make it attractive for tissue engineering, wound dressing, and drug delivery applications [45, 46].

Alginate hydrogels are scaffolds for cell encapsulation and three-dimensional (3D) bioprinting in tissue engineering applications. They provide a supportive matrix for cell growth, differentiation, and tissue regeneration in vitro and in vivo. Alginate-based dressings are employed for wound management due to their moisture-retentive properties, biocompatibility, and hemostatic effects. They facilitate wound healing by promoting granulation tissue formation and epithelialization, minimizing pain and infection. Due to their high loading capacity and controlled release properties, alginate nanoparticles and microcapsules are utilized as carriers in the drug delivery process. They protect encapsulated drugs from degradation and enable targeted delivery to specific sites within the body, improving therapeutic efficacy and minimizing side effects.

11.3 BIOPOLYMERS IN DRUG DELIVERY

Biopolymers stand at the forefront of innovation in drug delivery, offering a diverse array of materials derived from natural sources and endowed with unique properties ideally suited for therapeutic applications. This section delves into the intricate world of biopolymers, exploring their properties, applications, and advantages in drug delivery. Biopolymers represent a class of polymers derived from natural sources such as proteins, polysaccharides, and nucleic acids. Unlike synthetic polymers, often derived from petroleum-based sources, biopolymers offer distinct advantages, including biocompatibility, biodegradability, and low immunogenicity. These inherent properties stem from their natural origins, making them well-suited for biomedical applications [47, 48].

Proteins, the building blocks of life, serve as one of the most versatile biopolymer classes for drug delivery. With diverse structures and functionalities, proteins offer precise control over drug encapsulation, release, and targeting. Polysaccharides, such as chitosan and alginate, possess unique physicochemical properties that enable them to form stable matrices or hydrogels for sustained drug release. Nucleic acids, including DNA and RNA, exhibit programmable properties that can be harnessed for gene delivery and therapeutic applications.

11.3.1 Overview of Commonly Used Biopolymers in Drug Delivery

Several biopolymers have garnered significant attention in drug delivery due to their unique properties [49] and versatile applications, as shown in Table 11.1. Chitosan, a chitin derivative found in crustaceans' exoskeleton, offers mucoadhesive properties that enhance drug absorption across mucosal membranes [50–52]. Alginate, extracted from seaweed, forms gel-like matrices in the presence of divalent cations, enabling the controlled release of encapsulated drugs [53, 54]. Gelatin, derived from collagen, offers biocompatibility and ease of modification for specific drug delivery applications. Other commonly used biopolymers include hyaluronic acid, derived from connective tissues, which exhibits excellent biocompatibility and viscoelastic properties ideal for intra-articular drug delivery [55, 56]. Similarly, albumin, a protein found in blood plasma, is a versatile carrier for a wide range of therapeutic agents, owing to its biocompatibility, prolonged circulation time, and ability to bind various drugs via non-covalent interactions.

11.3.2 Advantages of Using Biopolymers

Using biopolymers in drug delivery systems offers several distinct advantages over synthetic polymers. Biopolymers are derived from natural sources, making them biocompatible and biodegradable. This reduces the risk of side effects or long-term toxicity associated with synthetic polymers, making biopolymers ideal candidates for biomedical applications [57]. Furthermore, these biopolymers can be tailored to exhibit specific properties such as stimuli responsiveness, allowing controlled drug release in response to physiological cues [58, 59]. Their natural origins also minimize the risk of immunogenicity or inflammatory responses, ensuring compatibility with biological systems. Additionally, the abundance and diversity of natural sources for biopolymers offer scalability and sustainability, making them attractive options for large-scale production and clinical translation [60].

11.3.3 Examples of Biopolymer-Based Drug Delivery Systems

Many biopolymer-based drug delivery systems have been developed, spanning a spectrum of therapeutic modalities and disease indications. Liposomal formulations, such as Doxil® and AmBisome®, exemplify the clinical translation of biopolymer-based delivery systems, offering improved pharmacokinetics and reduced systemic toxicity compared to conventional formulations [61, 62]. Polymeric nanoparticles, presented by Abraxane®, showcase the potential of biopolymers in enhancing the delivery of chemotherapeutic agents, prolonging circulation times, and improving tumor targeting [63, 64]. Moreover, hydrogels based on biopolymers like hyaluronic acid have been developed for localized drug delivery applications, enabling sustained release of therapeutics at specific sites within the body [58, 65]. Similarly, implantable devices incorporating biopolymers, such as drug-eluting stents and intraocular implants, offer controlled release of drugs over extended periods, reducing the need for frequent dosing and improving patient compliance.

TABLE 11.1
Overview of Biopolymer-Based Drug Delivery Systems

Biopolymer	Properties	Common Sources	Formulation Methods	Drug Payloads	Release Kinetics	Targeted Applications	Reference
Chitosan	Biocompatible, biodegradable, mucoadhesive	Chitin (crustacean shells)	Nanoparticle fabrication (emulsification, nanoprecipitation)	Small molecule drugs, proteins, nucleic acids	Controlled release (sustained, stimuli-responsive)	Oral delivery, mucosal delivery, gene therapy	Mohammed et al. (2017) [66]
Alginate	Biocompatible, biodegradable, gel-forming	Seaweed (algae)	Encapsulation (droplet extrusion, ionotropic gelation)	Small molecule drugs, cells, growth factors	Sustained release, diffusion-controlled release	Wound dressings, tissue engineering, cell therapy	Sahoo and Biswal, (2021) [67]
Gelatin	Biocompatible, biodegradable, gel-forming	Collagen (animal tissues)	Crosslinking (chemical crosslinking, physical gelation)	Small molecule drugs, peptides, growth factors	Degradation-mediated release (enzymatic, hydrolytic)	Controlled release implants, tissue regeneration, wound healing	Naomi et al. (2021) [68]
Hyaluronic Acid	Biocompatible, biodegradable, hydrophilic	Animal tissues, biosynthesis	Self-assembly (hyaluronate derivatives, crosslinked hydrogels)	Small molecule drugs, proteins, nanoparticles	Diffusion-controlled release, matrix degradation	Ophthalmic delivery, osteoarthritis therapy, tissue engineering	Dovedytis et al. (2020) [69]

11.4 NANOPARTICLES IN DRUG DELIVERY

Nanoparticles serve as dynamic entities within the realm of drug delivery, offering myriad capabilities that enhance therapeutic efficacy and precision [70]. This section delves into the fundamental aspects of nanoparticles in drug delivery systems, elucidating their definition, characteristics, diverse typologies, benefits, and exemplary applications [71]. At its essence, understanding the meaning and characteristics of nanoparticles is paramount. Nanoparticles are particles characterized by nanoscale dimensions, typically ranging from 1 to 1000 nanometers. This diminutive size imparts nanoparticles with unique physicochemical properties, including a high surface area-to-volume ratio, quantum size effects, and enhanced reactivity [72]. These distinctive characteristics endow nanoparticles with exceptional functionalities that diverge from their bulk counterparts, making them indispensable tools in drug delivery systems [73].

Various types of nanoparticles find application in drug delivery, each offering tailored properties and functionalities to meet specific therapeutic objectives [74, 75]. Notable examples include liposomes, polymeric nanoparticles, and dendrimers, as shown in Table 11.2. Liposomes, lipid bilayer vesicles, offer versatility in encapsulating hydrophobic and hydrophilic drugs, facilitating their delivery to target sites. Polymeric nanoparticles, constructed from synthetic or natural polymers, afford tunable properties for controlled drug release and enhanced bioavailability [76]. Dendrimers, highly branched macromolecules, provide precise control over drug loading and release kinetics, enabling tailored therapeutic interventions [77–79].

The benefits of nanoparticles in drug delivery are wide-ranging and profound, encompassing targeted delivery, controlled release, and enhanced stability of therapeutic agents. Nanoparticles enable precise delivery of drugs to specific tissues or cells within the body, minimizing off-target effects and maximizing therapeutic efficacy [80, 81]. Moreover, nanoparticles facilitate the controlled release of encapsulated drugs, prolonging their circulation time and optimizing pharmacokinetics. Additionally, the nanoscale dimensions of nanoparticles allow for precise modulation of drug release kinetics, offering tailored therapeutic interventions suited to individual patient needs.

TABLE 11.2
Characteristics and Applications of Nanoparticles in Drug Delivery Systems

Nanoparticle Type	Characteristics	Various Types Used in Drug Delivery	Benefits of Drug Delivery	Examples of Drug Delivery Systems	References
Liposomes	Phospholipid bilayer vesicles; versatile encapsulation system	Encapsulation of hydrophilic and hydrophobic drugs, targeted delivery	Enhanced bioavailability, targeted delivery, controlled release	Doxil®, AmBisome®	Lai et al. (2021), Farooq and Trevaskis [82, 83]
Polymeric Nanoparticles	Synthetic or natural polymer-based particles	PLGA, PCL, PNIPAM, etc.; diverse applications	Tailored drug release kinetics, enhanced stability, targeted delivery	Abraxane®, Estrasorb®, Vivagel®	Zielińska et al. (2020), Perumal (2022) [84, 85]
Dendrimers	Highly branched macromolecules with precise structure	Controlled size and shape, functionalization capabilities	Accurate drug loading, targeted delivery, combination therapy	VivaGel®, PAMAM dendrimers	Abbasi et al. (2014), Pérez-Ferreiro et al., 2023 [86, 87]

Examples of nanoparticle-based drug delivery systems abound, highlighting the versatility and efficacy of nanoparticles across a spectrum of therapeutic applications. From liposomal formulations such as Doxil® and AmBisome® to polymeric nanoparticles exemplified by Abraxane®, these systems underscore the transformative potential of nanoparticles in enhancing drug delivery outcomes. Furthermore, dendrimer-based platforms such as VivaGel® showcase the versatility and adaptability of nanoparticles in combating infectious diseases through targeted drug delivery and potent antimicrobial activity.

11.5 HYBRID SYSTEMS: BIOPOLYMER-NANOPARTICLE COMBINATIONS

The fusion of biopolymers and nanoparticles in hybrid systems represents a groundbreaking approach to drug delivery, offering unique advantages that transcend the capabilities of individual components. This section delves into the rationale behind combining biopolymers and nanoparticles, elucidates the synergistic effects achieved, explores integration methods, and showcases exemplary case studies demonstrating the efficacy of biopolymer-nanoparticle hybrid systems, as shown in Figure 11.1 [88].

The rationale behind combining biopolymers and nanoparticles lies in leveraging the complementary properties of these components to address the limitations of conventional [89] drug delivery methods. Biopolymers, derived from natural sources such as proteins, polysaccharides, and nucleic acids, offer inherent advantages, including biocompatibility, biodegradability, and low immunogenicity. Meanwhile, nanoparticles provide precise control over drug release kinetics, targeted delivery, and enhanced stability of therapeutic agents. By integrating biopolymers with nanoparticles, hybrid systems can harness the strengths of both components to optimize drug loading, release profiles, and pharmacokinetics [6, 90].

The synergistic effects of biopolymer-nanoparticle hybrids in drug delivery are profound and multifaceted. These hybrid constructs offer enhanced drug-loading capacities, prolonged circulation times, and targeted delivery to specific sites within the body. Moreover, integrating biopolymers with nanoparticles enables precise control over drug release kinetics, responsiveness to environmental stimuli, and compatibility with disease microenvironments. Hybrid systems can be fine-tuned through surface modification, encapsulation, or co-polymerization techniques to achieve desired release profiles and therapeutic outcomes.

Integrating biopolymers with nanoparticles encompasses a range of techniques tailored to achieve specific objectives and desired properties. Surface modification techniques, such as covalent or non-covalent conjugation, enable the functionalization of nanoparticles with biopolymers to impart targeting ligands, improve stability, or enhance biocompatibility [91, 92]. Encapsulation methods, including emulsification, solvent evaporation, or self-assembly, facilitate the incorporation of nanoparticles within biopolymer matrices, enabling controlled release and protection of encapsulated drugs. Alternatively, blending or co-polymerizing biopolymers with nanoparticle precursors can yield hybrid constructs with tunable properties suited for specific drug delivery applications [93].

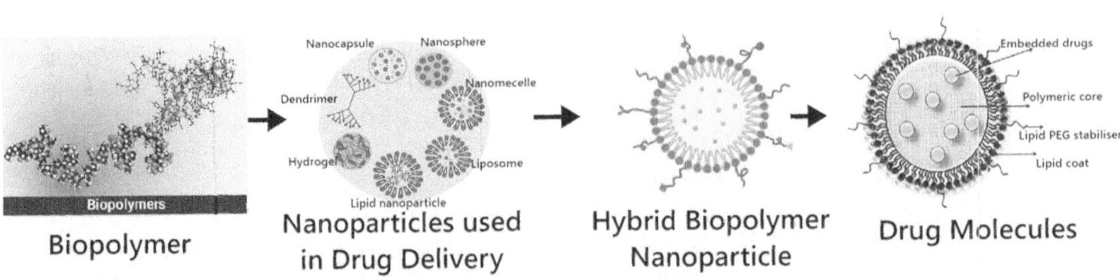

FIGURE 11.1 Schematic diagram of biopolymer-nanoparticle hybrid systems in drug delivery.

Case studies or examples demonstrating the efficacy of biopolymer-nanoparticle hybrid systems abound, showcasing their versatility and potential across a spectrum of therapeutic applications. From targeted delivery of anticancer drugs using chitosan-coated nanoparticles to sustained release of antibiotics from gelatin-based hydrogels, these case studies underscore the transformative impact of hybrid systems in enhancing drug delivery outcomes. Furthermore, integrating biopolymer-nanoparticle hybrids into commercial products such as Abraxane® and VivaGel® highlights their clinical relevance and significant potential for widespread adoption in clinical practice [94, 95].

11.6 APPLICATIONS OF BIOPOLYMER-NANOPARTICLE HYBRID SYSTEMS

Biopolymer-nanoparticle hybrid systems herald a new era in drug delivery, offering a versatile platform for a myriad of applications aimed at enhancing therapeutic outcomes. This section explores the diverse applications these hybrid constructs enable, including targeted drug delivery, improved stability and bioavailability, tailored release kinetics for personalized medicine, and the potential for combination therapy and multifunctional drug delivery systems.

11.6.1 Drug Delivery to Specific Target Sites

One of the primary applications of biopolymer-nanoparticle hybrid systems lies in the precise delivery of therapeutics to specific target sites within the body. By leveraging the targeting capabilities of both biopolymers and nanoparticles, these hybrid constructs can navigate biological barriers and selectively accumulate at desired sites, such as cancer cells or brain tissues. Functionalizing hybrid systems with targeting ligands or antibodies further enhances their specificity, enabling localized drug delivery while minimizing systemic toxicity and off-target effects [96].

Biopolymer-nanoparticle hybrid systems possess inherent properties that enable them to target specific cells or tissues within the body. Biopolymers such as peptides, proteins, or polysaccharides can interact with cell surface receptors [97] or extracellular matrix components, facilitating cellular uptake or tissue penetration. Nanoparticles provide a versatile platform for incorporating targeting ligands or antibodies that recognize molecular markers overexpressed on diseased cells, enabling selective accumulation at target sites.

Functionalizing hybrid systems targeting ligands or antibodies enhances their specificity for particular cell types or tissues. Targeting moieties such as antibodies, aptamers, or small molecules can recognize and bind to specific antigens or receptors present on the surface of target cells, promoting selective internalization and intracellular drug release. This targeted approach minimizes systemic exposure to the therapeutic agent, reducing the risk of adverse effects on healthy tissues and organs.

Biopolymer-nanoparticle hybrid systems enable localized drug delivery to specific anatomical sites or pathological regions within the body. By accumulating preferentially at target sites, these constructs can achieve therapeutic concentrations of drugs while minimizing systemic distribution. This localized drug delivery approach improves the efficacy of therapeutics by maximizing their concentration at the site of action, leading to enhanced therapeutic outcomes and reduced dosage requirements.

Targeted drug delivery with biopolymer-nanoparticle hybrid systems offers significant advantages in minimizing systemic toxicity and off-target effects. By selectively delivering therapeutics to diseased tissues or cells, these systems reduce exposure of healthy tissues to cytotoxic drugs, thereby mitigating adverse effects such as organ toxicity, immunogenicity, and drug resistance. This targeted approach enhances the safety profile of therapeutics and improves patient compliance with treatment regimens.

The precise delivery of therapeutics to specific target sites has profound implications for treating various diseases, including cancer, neurological disorders, and infectious diseases. Biopolymer-nanoparticle hybrid systems promise to overcome biological barriers and deliver drugs across physiological barriers [98], such as the blood-brain barrier or tumor microenvironment. By optimizing the design and functionality of hybrid systems, researchers can develop personalized and effective therapeutic strategies tailored to individual patient needs.

11.6.2 Enhancement of Drug Stability and Bioavailability

Biopolymer-nanoparticle hybrid systems offer a robust platform for increasing the bioavailability and stability of encapsulated drugs [99]. Biopolymers provide a protective shield around nanoparticles, shielding encapsulated drugs from degradation and enzymatic metabolism. Moreover, nanoparticles facilitate drug-controlled release, prolonging their circulation time and enhancing their bioavailability. This synergistic interaction between biopolymers and nanoparticles ensures efficient delivery of therapeutics to target sites while maximizing their therapeutic efficacy [100].

Biopolymers act as a protective shield around nanoparticles, shielding encapsulated drugs from degradation and enzymatic metabolism. This protective barrier prevents premature drug release and degradation in biological fluids, thereby preserving the stability and efficacy of the therapeutic agent during circulation in the body.

Nanoparticles facilitate controlled drug release, allowing for sustained and controlled release kinetics over an extended period. By modulating the physicochemical properties of nanoparticles, such as size, shape, and surface charge, researchers can tailor the release kinetics of encapsulated drugs to achieve optimal therapeutic outcomes.

Biopolymer-nanoparticle hybrid systems prolong the circulation time of encapsulated drugs in the bloodstream, enhancing their bioavailability. The biocompatible nature of biopolymers and the stealth properties of nanoparticles reduce recognition and clearance by the reticuloendothelial system, leading to prolonged systemic exposure and enhanced therapeutic efficacy.

Nanoparticles enhance the absorption and distribution of encapsulated drugs within the body, improving their bioavailability and pharmacokinetic profile. By encapsulating drugs within nanoparticles, researchers can overcome barriers to drug absorption, such as poor solubility, instability, and rapid metabolism, thereby increasing the concentration of therapeutics at target sites.

The synergy between biopolymers and nanoparticles ensures efficient delivery of therapeutics to target sites while maximizing their therapeutic efficacy. Biopolymers provide a biocompatible and biodegradable matrix for nanoparticle formulation, while nanoparticles offer a versatile platform for drug encapsulation and controlled release. This synergistic combination enhances encapsulated drugs' stability, bioavailability, and therapeutic potential, improving patient outcomes.

11.6.3 Tailoring Release Kinetics for Personalized Medicine

The tunable properties of biopolymer-nanoparticle hybrid systems enable precise control over drug release kinetics, paving the way for personalized medicine approaches. By modulating factors such as polymer composition, nanoparticle size, and surface functionalization, the release profile of encapsulated drugs can be tailored to match individual patient needs and disease characteristics. This customization allows for optimized therapeutic outcomes, minimization of adverse effects, and improved patient compliance, thereby advancing the paradigm of personalized drug delivery [101].

Biopolymer-nanoparticle hybrid systems offer a versatile platform with tunable properties that can be adjusted to achieve specific drug release kinetics. By varying parameters such as polymer composition, nanoparticle size, and surface chemistry, researchers can precisely control the rate and duration of drug release, tailoring it to match the therapeutic requirements of individual patients.

Tailoring release kinetics enables the implementation of precision medicine approaches, where treatment strategies are customized based on individual patient characteristics and disease profiles. By matching the release profile of encapsulated drugs to each patient's pharmacokinetic and pharmacodynamic properties, personalized therapeutic regimens can be designed to optimize efficacy and minimize adverse effects.

Customizing drug release kinetics allows for optimized therapeutic outcomes by ensuring therapeutic agents are delivered at the correct dose, concentration, and duration to achieve the desired clinical effect. By synchronizing drug release with the physiological needs of patients, personalized drug delivery systems enhance treatment efficacy and patient outcomes across a wide range of diseases and clinical conditions.

Tailoring release kinetics also minimizes the adverse effects of drug therapy [102] by controlling the rate and duration of drug release; personalized drug delivery systems can reduce systemic exposure to therapeutic agents, thereby mitigating the risk of toxicity, side effects, and drug interactions. This targeted approach enhances the safety profile of therapeutics and improves patient tolerance and compliance with treatment regimens.

Personalized drug delivery systems enhance patient compliance by providing tailored treatment regimens that align with individual preferences and lifestyle factors. By optimizing the release kinetics of encapsulated drugs to match patient needs, these systems reduce the frequency of dosing, simplify treatment schedules, and improve convenience, leading to greater patient satisfaction and adherence to therapy.

11.6.4 Potential for Combination Therapy and Multifunctional Drug Delivery Systems

Biopolymer-nanoparticle hybrid systems offer a versatile platform for combination therapy and developing multifunctional drug delivery systems. By encapsulating multiple therapeutic agents within a single hybrid construct, these systems enable synergistic interactions between drugs, enhanced therapeutic efficacy, and the potential for overcoming drug resistance. Furthermore, integrating diagnostic agents or imaging probes into hybrid systems facilitates real-time drug delivery and disease progression monitoring, thereby enabling personalized treatment strategies and precision medicine approaches [103].

Biopolymer-nanoparticle hybrid systems allow for the encapsulation of multiple therapeutic agents, enabling combination therapy approaches. Combining drugs with complementary mechanisms of action promotes synergistic interactions between therapeutic agents, enhancing therapeutic efficacy and improving treatment outcomes. Combination therapy offers the potential to overcome drug resistance, minimize adverse effects, and target multiple pathways involved in disease progression.

Multifunctional drug delivery systems enable the targeted delivery of multiple therapeutic agents to specific sites within the body. Researchers can achieve optimal drug ratios and release profiles by co-encapsulating drugs within a single hybrid construct, maximizing therapeutic efficacy while minimizing systemic exposure and off-target effects. This targeted approach enhances drug bioavailability and tissue penetration, improving treatment outcomes in various disease conditions.

Combination therapy with biopolymer-nanoparticle hybrid systems holds promise for overcoming drug resistance, a significant challenge in cancer and infectious disease treatment. By targeting multiple signaling pathways or employing synergistic drug combinations, these systems can circumvent resistance mechanisms that enhance drug-resistant cells' sensitivity to therapeutic agents. This approach increases the likelihood of achieving durable responses and preventing disease recurrence.

Multifunctional drug delivery systems can integrate diagnostic agents or imaging probes into hybrid constructs, enabling real-time drug delivery and disease progression monitoring. By incorporating contrast agents, fluorescent probes, or magnetic nanoparticles, researchers can visualize drug distribution, monitor therapeutic responses, and assess disease status non-invasively. This real-time feedback facilitates personalized treatment strategies and enables clinicians to adjust therapeutic regimens based on individual patient responses.

Integrating diagnostic capabilities into biopolymer-nanoparticle hybrid systems enables personalized treatment strategies tailored to individual patient characteristics and disease profiles. By combining therapeutic agents with diagnostic agents or imaging probes, these systems support precision medicine approaches that optimize treatment selection, dosing, and timing based on real-time patient data. This personalized approach improves treatment outcomes, minimizes adverse effects, and enhances patient satisfaction and compliance with therapy.

11.7 CHALLENGES AND FUTURE PERSPECTIVES

The development of biopolymer-nanoparticle hybrid systems holds immense promise for advancing drug delivery paradigms, yet it is not challenging. This section delves into the field's current hurdles, regulatory considerations, emerging trends, future directions, and further research and innovation opportunities.

11.7.1 Current Challenges in Developing Biopolymer-Nanoparticle Hybrid Systems

Several challenges impede the seamless integration of biopolymers and nanoparticles into hybrid drug delivery systems. These challenges include achieving optimal compatibility between biopolymers and nanoparticles, ensuring controlled drug release kinetics, maintaining stability during formulation and storage, and scaling up production processes to meet commercial demand. Additionally, challenges related to reproducibility, batch-to-batch variability, and regulatory compliance pose significant hurdles that must be addressed to translate laboratory innovations into clinically viable products [104, 105].

11.7.2 Regulatory Considerations and Safety Concerns

As with any novel therapeutic modality, regulatory considerations and safety concerns loom large in developing biopolymer-nanoparticle hybrid systems. Regulatory agencies worldwide scrutinize drug delivery systems' safety, efficacy, and quality, necessitating rigorous preclinical and clinical evaluation. Safety concerns such as immunogenicity, toxicity, and off-target effects must be assessed to ensure patient safety and regulatory approval. Moreover, problems regarding the long-term fate and biocompatibility of nanoparticles within the body underscore the need for comprehensive safety assessments and risk mitigation strategies [106–108].

11.7.3 Emerging Trends and Future Directions in the Field

Despite the challenges, the field of biopolymer-nanoparticle hybrid systems is rife with emerging trends and promising avenues for future exploration. Emerging trends include the development of stimuli-responsive hybrid systems capable of on-demand drug release in response to physiological cues, the integration of advanced imaging modalities for real-time monitoring of drug delivery, and the exploration of novel biopolymer-nanoparticle combinations to unlock new therapeutic possibilities. Furthermore, the convergence of nanotechnology with other disciplines, such as artificial intelligence, gene editing, and tissue engineering, holds immense potential for driving innovation in drug delivery and personalized medicine [109].

11.7.4 Opportunities for Further Research and Innovation

Opportunities abound for further research and innovation in biopolymer-nanoparticle hybrid systems. Areas ripe for exploration include the development of biocompatible and biodegradable nanoparticles, elucidating mechanisms governing nanoparticle-cell interactions, and optimizing targeted drug delivery strategies for specific disease indications. Moreover, interdisciplinary collaborations between researchers, clinicians, and industry stakeholders are crucial to unlocking new insights and accelerating the translation of benchtop discoveries into clinical applications. By harnessing these opportunities, the field stands poised to overcome current challenges and chart a course toward transformative drug delivery and therapeutics advancements [110–112].

11.8 CONCLUSION

In conclusion, integrating biopolymers and nanoparticles into hybrid systems represents a paradigm shift in the landscape of advanced drug delivery. Throughout this discourse, we have underscored the pivotal role of biopolymer-nanoparticle hybrid systems in overcoming critical challenges associated with conventional drug delivery methods and unlocking new possibilities for precision therapeutics. These hybrid systems offer a versatile platform for enhancing drug stability, bioavailability, and targeted delivery to specific tissues or cells within the body. By combining the unique advantages of biopolymers and nanoparticles, these hybrid constructs enable precise control over drug release kinetics, tailored targeting strategies, and enhanced therapeutic efficacy. Our exploration has revealed many applications for biopolymer-nanoparticle hybrid systems, from cancer therapy to infectious disease treatment. By recapitulating the importance of these hybrid systems in advancing drug delivery, we emphasize their potential to revolutionize the field of therapeutics and improve patient outcomes.

In summary, the synergy achieved by combining biopolymers and nanoparticles holds immense promise for addressing current healthcare challenges and paving the way for personalized medicine. As we look to the future, continued research, collaboration, and innovation will be crucial in harnessing the full potential of these hybrid systems and translating laboratory discoveries into clinical realities. In closing, we envision a future where biopolymer-nanoparticle hybrid systems play a central role in shaping the landscape of drug delivery, offering tailored solutions for individual patient needs and ushering in a new era of precision therapeutics.

REFERENCES

[1] T. C. Ezike et al., "Advances in drug delivery systems, challenges and future directions," *Heliyon*, vol. 9, no. 6, p. e17488, 2023.

[2] M. S. Alqahtani, M. Kazi, M. A. Alsenaidy, and M. Z. Ahmad, "Advances in oral drug delivery," *Front. Pharmacol.*, vol. 12, 2021.

[3] S. Adepu and S. Ramakrishna, "Controlled drug delivery systems: Current status and future directions," *Molecules*, vol. 26, no. 19, p. 5905, 2021.

[4] O. Opris, C. Mormile, I. Lung, A. Stegarescu, M.-L. Soran, and A. Soran, "An overview of biopolymers for drug delivery applications," *Appl. Sci. (Basel)*, vol. 14, no. 4, p. 1383, 2024.

[5] R. Gheorghita, L. Anchidin-Norocel, R. Filip, M. Dimian, and M. Covasa, "Applications of biopolymers for drugs and probiotics delivery," *Polymers (Basel)*, vol. 13, no. 16, p. 2729, 2021.

[6] M. C. Biswas et al., "Recent advancement of biopolymers and their potential biomedical applications," *J. Polym. Environ.*, vol. 30, no. 1, pp. 51–74, 2022.

[7] S. Nasra, D. Bhatia, and A. Kumar, "Recent advances in nanoparticle-based drug delivery systems for rheumatoid arthritis treatment," *Nanoscale Adv.*, vol. 4, no. 17, pp. 3479–3494, 2022.

[8] P. Velavan, C. Karuppusamy, and P. Venkatesan, "Nanoparticles as drug delivery systems," *J. Pharm. Sci. Res.*, vol. 7, no. 12, pp. 1118–1122, 2015.

[9] J. K. Patra et al., "Nano-based drug delivery systems: Recent developments and future prospects," *J. Nanobiotechnol.*, vol. 16, no. 1, 2018.

[10] A. A. H. Abdellatif and A. F. Alsowinea, "Approved and marketed nanoparticles for disease targeting and applications in COVID-19," *Nanotechnol. Rev.*, vol. 10, no. 1, pp. 1941–1977, 2021.

[11] S. Salel and B. Iyisan, "Polymer–lipid hybrid nanoparticles as potential lipophilic anticancer drug carriers," *Discov. Nano*, vol. 18, no. 1, 2023.

[12] R. Rajan et al., "Polymeric nanoparticles in hybrid catalytic processing and drug delivery system," *Top. Catal.*, vol. 65, no. 19–20, pp. 1860–1884, 2022.

[13] N. S. Heredia et al., "Comparative statistical analysis of the release kinetics models for nanoprecipitated drug delivery systems based on poly(lactic-co-glycolic acid)," *PLoS One*, vol. 17, no. 3, p. e0264825, 2022.

[14] I. Gholamali and M. Yadollahi, "Bio-nanocomposite polymer hydrogels containing nanoparticles for drug delivery: A review," *Regen. Eng. Transl. Med.*, vol. 7, no. 2, pp. 129–146, 2021.

[15] P. S. Shasiya, K. Simi Pushpan, and A. B. Nair, "Biopolymers as engineering materials," in *Handbook of Biopolymers*, Singapore: Springer Nature Singapore, 2022, pp. 1–27.

[16] T. Aziz et al., "A review on the modification of cellulose and its applications," *Polymers (Basel)*, vol. 14, no. 15, p. 3206, 2022.
[17] H. Seddiqi et al., "Cellulose and its derivatives: Towards biomedical applications," *Cellulose*, vol. 28, no. 4, pp. 1893–1931, 2021.
[18] A. Divsalar, A. A. Saboury, M. Nabiuni, Z. Zare, M. E. Kefayati, and A. Seyedarabi, "Characterization and side effect analysis of a newly designed nanoemulsion targeting human serum albumin for drug delivery," *Colloids Surf. B Biointerfaces*, vol. 98, pp. 80–84, 2012.
[19] A. Surendren, A. K. Mohanty, Q. Liu, and M. Misra, "A review of biodegradable thermoplastic starches, their blends and composites: Recent developments and opportunities for single-use plastic packaging alternatives," *Green Chem.*, vol. 24, no. 22, pp. 8606–8636, 2022.
[20] O. Peter Adigwe, H. O. Egharevba, and M. Ochubiojo Emeje, "Starch: A veritable natural polymer for economic revolution," in *Starch - Evolution and Recent Advances*, IntechOpen, 2022.
[21] S. M. Amaraweera et al., "Development of starch-based materials using current modification techniques and their applications: A review," *Molecules*, vol. 26, no. 22, p. 6880, 2021.
[22] H. Onyeaka, K. Obileke, G. Makaka, and N. Nwokolo, "Current research and applications of starch-based biodegradable films for food packaging," *Polymers (Basel)*, vol. 14, no. 6, p. 1126, 2022.
[23] O. Yu and K. H. Kim, "Lignin to materials: A focused review on recent novel lignin applications," *Appl. Sci. (Basel)*, vol. 10, no. 13, p. 4626, 2020.
[24] J. H. Lora and W. G. Glasser, "Recent industrial applications of lignin: A sustainable alternative to non-renewable materials," *J. Polym. Environ.*, vol. 10, no. 1/2, pp. 39–48, 2002.
[25] C. Ma, T.-H. Kim, K. Liu, M.-G. Ma, S.-E. Choi, and C. Si, "Multifunctional lignin-based composite materials for emerging applications," *Front. Bioeng. Biotechnol.*, vol. 9, 2021.
[26] A. Beaucamp et al., "Lignin for energy applications – State of the art, life cycle, technoeconomic analysis and future trends," *Green Chem.*, vol. 24, no. 21, pp. 8193–8226, 2022.
[27] M. Arias and P. J. van Dijk, "What is natural rubber and why are we searching for new sources?," *Front. Young Minds*, vol. 7, p. 100, 2019.
[28] C. Xu, *Nanostructure and Nanomechanics of Collagen Self-assemblies*, Memorial University of Newfoundland, 2014.
[29] N. Yin et al., "Fabrication and characterization of hydroxyapatite nanocomposites based on bacterial cellulose with surface modification," *Adv. Mat. Res.*, vol. 476–478, pp. 457–460, 2012.
[30] Y.-S. Lim, Y.-J. Ok, S.-Y. Hwang, J.-Y. Kwak, and S. Yoon, "Marine collagen as a promising biomaterial for biomedical applications," *Mar. Drugs*, vol. 17, no. 8, p. 467, 2019.
[31] E. Rezvani Ghomi, N. Nourbakhsh, M. Akbari Kenari, M. Zare, and S. Ramakrishna, "Collagen-based biomaterials for biomedical applications," *J. Biomed. Mater. Res. B Appl. Biomater.*, vol. 109, no. 12, pp. 1986–1999, 2021.
[32] I. N. Amirrah, Y. Lokanathan, I. Zulkiflee, M. F. M. R. Wee, A. Motta, and M. B. Fauzi, "A comprehensive review on collagen type I development of biomaterials for tissue engineering: From biosynthesis to bioscaffold," *Biomedicines*, vol. 10, no. 9, p. 2307, 2022.
[33] D. Abbey, *Improving the Utilisation and Quality of Low Value Fish (Brachydeuters auritus and Dactylopterus volitans) by Processing*, 2018.
[34] M. I. Said, "Role and function of gelatin in the development of the food and non-food industry: A review," *IOP Conf. Ser. Earth Environ. Sci.*, vol. 492, no. 1, p. 012086, 2020.
[35] J. Alipal et al., "A review of gelatin: Properties, sources, process, applications, and commercialisation," *Mater. Today*, vol. 42, pp. 240–250, 2021.
[36] M. J. Dille, I. J. Haug, and K. I. Draget, "Gelatin and collagen," in *Handbook of Hydrocolloids*, Elsevier, 2021, pp. 1073–1097.
[37] H. Zheng and B. Zuo, "Functional silk fibroin hydrogels: Preparation, properties and applications," *J. Mater. Chem. B Mater. Biol. Med.*, vol. 9, no. 5, pp. 1238–1258, 2021.
[38] G. Carissimi, M. G. Montalbán, M. G. Fuster, and G. Víllora, "Silk fibroin nanoparticles: Synthesis and applications as drug nanocarriers," in *21st Century Nanostructured Materials - Physics, Chemistry, Classification, and Emerging Applications in Industry, Biomedicine, and Agriculture*, IntechOpen, 2022.
[39] M. T. Sultan et al., "Silk fibroin-based biomaterials for hemostatic applications," *Biomolecules*, vol. 12, no. 5, p. 660, 2022.
[40] P. Poltronieri and P. Kumar, "Polyhydroxyalkanoates (PHAs) in industrial applications," in *Handbook of Ecomaterials*, Cham: Springer International Publishing, 2019, pp. 2843–2872.

[41] L. Addagada, P. Pathak, M. K. Shahid, and P. R. Rout, "Microbial polyhydroxyalkanoates (PHAs): A brief overview of their features, synthesis, and agro-industrial applications," in *Advances in Agricultural and Industrial Microbiology*, Singapore: Springer Nature Singapore, 2022, pp. 217–236.
[42] V. C. Kalia, S. K. S. Patel, and J.-K. Lee, "Exploiting polyhydroxyalkanoates for biomedical applications," *Polymers (Basel)*, vol. 15, no. 8, p. 1937, 2023.
[43] F. García-Ochoa, V. E. Santos, J. A. Casas, and E. Gómez, "Xanthan gum: Production, recovery, and properties," *Biotechnol. Adv.*, vol. 18, no. 7, pp. 549–579, 2000.
[44] A. Kumar, K. M. Rao, and S. S. Han, "Application of xanthan gum as polysaccharide in tissue engineering: A review," *Carbohydr. Polym.*, vol. 180, pp. 128–144, 2018.
[45] I. M. Bhat, S. M. Wani, S. A. Mir, and F. A. Masoodi, "Advances in xanthan gum production, modifications and its applications," *Biocatal. Agric. Biotechnol.*, vol. 42, no. 102328, p. 102328, 2022.
[46] R. Gheorghita Puscaselu, A. Lobiuc, M. Dimian, and M. Covasa, "Alginate: From food industry to biomedical applications and management of metabolic disorders," *Polymers (Basel)*, vol. 12, no. 10, p. 2417, 2020.
[47] S. Ahmed, *Alginates: Applications in the Biomedical and Food Industries*, Wiley-Scrivener, 2019.
[48] Y. A. Skorik, "Biopolymers in drug and gene delivery systems 2.0," *Int. J. Mol. Sci.*, vol. 24, no. 23, p. 17099, 2023.
[49] M. Harun-Or-Rashid et al., "Recent advances in micro- and nano-drug delivery systems based on natural and synthetic biomaterials," *Polymers (Basel)*, vol. 15, no. 23, p. 4563, 2023.
[50] P. K. Prabhakar et al., *Revolutionizing Herbal Medicine: Exploring Nano Drug Delivery Systems*, 2023.
[51] B. K. Heragh, S. Javanshir, G. R. Mahdavinia, and M. R. N. Jamal, "Hydroxyapatite grafted chitosan/laponite RD hydrogel: Evaluation of the encapsulation capacity, pH-responsivity, and controlled release behavior," *Int. J. Biol. Macromol.*, vol. 190, pp. 351–359, 2021.
[52] J. Varshosaz, "The promise of chitosan microspheres in drug delivery systems," *Expert Opin. Drug Deliv.*, vol. 4, no. 3, pp. 263–273, 2007.
[53] E. Fakhri et al., "Chitosan biomaterials application in dentistry," *Int. J. Biol. Macromol.*, vol. 162, pp. 956–974, 2020.
[54] J. P. Paques, E. van der Linden, C. J. M. van Rijn, and L. M. C. Sagis, "Preparation methods of alginate nanoparticles," *Adv. Colloid Interface Sci.*, vol. 209, pp. 163–171, 2014.
[55] P. Severino, C. F. da Silva, L. N. Andrade, D. de Lima Oliveira, J. Campos, and E. B. Souto, "Alginate nanoparticles for drug delivery and targeting," *Curr. Pharm. Des.*, vol. 25, no. 11, pp. 1312–1334, 2019.
[56] G. A. Martău, M. Mihai, and D. C. Vodnar, "The use of chitosan, alginate, and pectin in the biomedical and food sector-biocompatibility, bioadhesiveness, and biodegradability," *Polymers (Basel)*, vol. 11, no. 11, p. 1837, 2019.
[57] D.-Q. Li, S.-Y. Wang, Y.-J. Meng, Z.-W. Guo, M.-M. Cheng, and J. Li, "Fabrication of self-healing pectin/chitosan hybrid hydrogel via Diels-Alder reactions for drug delivery with high swelling property, pH-responsiveness, and cytocompatibility," *Carbohydr. Polym.*, vol. 268, p. 118244, 2021.
[58] H. Omidian, S. Dey Chowdhury, and N. Babanejad, "Cryogels: Advancing biomaterials for transformative biomedical applications," *Pharmaceutics*, vol. 15, no. 7, 2023.
[59] Y. A. Skorik, "Biopolymers in drug and gene delivery systems," *Int. J. Mol. Sci.*, vol. 24, no. 16, p. 12763, 2023.
[60] J. Mehta, K. Gupta, S. Lavania, P. Kumar, V. Chaudhary, and P. Gupta, "Inherent roadmap in synthesis and applications of sustainable materials using oil based and microbial polymers," *Mater. Today Sustain.*, vol. 25, p. 100615, 2024.
[61] J. Baranwal, B. Barse, A. Fais, G. L. Delogu, and A. Kumar, "Biopolymer: A sustainable material for food and medical applications," *Polymers (Basel)*, vol. 14, no. 5, p. 983, 2022.
[62] U. Bulbake, S. Doppalapudi, N. Kommineni, and W. Khan, "Liposomal formulations in clinical use: An updated review," *Pharmaceutics*, vol. 9, no. 4, p. 12, 2017.
[63] M. K. Yeh, H. I. Chang, and M. Y. Cheng, "Clinical development of liposome based drugs: Formulation, characterization, and therapeutic efficacy," *Int. J. Nanomedicine*, p. 49, 2011.
[64] Y. K. Sung and S. W. Kim, "Recent advances in polymeric drug delivery systems," *Biomater. Res.*, vol. 24, no. 1, 2020.
[65] L. I. Atanase, "Micellar drug delivery systems based on natural biopolymers," *Polymers (Basel)*, vol. 13, no. 3, p. 477, 2021.

[66] T. Fazal et al., "Recent developments in natural biopolymer based drug delivery systems," *RSC Adv.*, vol. 13, no. 33, pp. 23087–23121, 2023.

[67] M. Mohammed, J. Syeda, K. Wasan, and E. Wasan, "An overview of chitosan nanoparticles and its application in non-parenteral drug delivery," *Pharmaceutics*, vol. 9, no. 4, p. 53, 2017.

[68] D. R. Sahoo and T. Biswal, "Alginate and its application to tissue engineering," *SN Appl. Sci.*, vol. 3, no. 1, p. 30, 2021.

[69] R. Naomi, H. Bahari, P. M. Ridzuan, and F. Othman, Natural-based biomaterial for skin wound healing (gelatin vs. collagen): Expert review," *Polymers (Basel)*, vol. 13, no. 14, p. 2319, 2021.

[70] M. Dovedytis, Z. J. Liu, and S. Bartlett, "Hyaluronic acid and its biomedical applications: A review," *Eng. Regen.*, vol. 1, pp. 102–113, 2020.

[71] M. J. Mitchell, M. M. Billingsley, R. M. Haley, M. E. Wechsler, N. A. Peppas, and R. Langer, "Engineering precision nanoparticles for drug delivery," *Nat. Rev. Drug Discov.*, vol. 20, no. 2, pp. 101–124, 2021.

[72] A. A. Yetisgin, S. Cetinel, M. Zuvin, A. Kosar, and O. Kutlu, "Therapeutic nanoparticles and their targeted delivery applications," *Molecules*, vol. 25, no. 9, p. 2193, 2020.

[73] A. Yusuf, A. R. Z. Almotairy, H. Henidi, O. Y. Alshehri, and M. S. Aldughaim, "Nanoparticles as drug delivery systems: A review of the implication of nanoparticles' physicochemical properties on responses in biological systems," *Polymers (Basel)*, vol. 15, no. 7, p. 1596, 2023.

[74] O. Afzal et al., "Nanoparticles in drug delivery: From history to therapeutic applications," *Nanomaterials (Basel)*, vol. 12, no. 24, p. 4494, 2022.

[75] S. Bhatia, "Nanoparticles types, classification, characterization, fabrication methods and drug delivery applications," in *Natural Polymer Drug Delivery Systems*, Cham: Springer International Publishing, 2016, pp. 33–93.

[76] N. Aminu, I. Bello, N. M. Umar, N. Tanko, A. Aminu, and M. M. Audu, "The influence of nanoparticulate drug delivery systems in drug therapy," *J. Drug Deliv. Sci. Technol.*, vol. 60, p. 101961, 2020.

[77] I. Chattopadhyay, "Application of nanoparticles in drug delivery," in *Model Organisms to Study Biological Activities and Toxicity of Nanoparticles*, Singapore: Springer Singapore, 2020, pp. 35–57.

[78] L. Palmerston Mendes, J. Pan, and V. Torchilin, "Dendrimers as nanocarriers for nucleic acid and drug delivery in cancer therapy," *Molecules*, vol. 22, no. 9, p. 1401, 2017.

[79] R. Gauro, M. Nandave, V. K. Jain, and K. Jain, "Advances in dendrimer-mediated targeted drug delivery to the brain," *J. Nanopart. Res.*, vol. 23, no. 3, p. 76, 2021.

[80] M. Nikzamir, Y. Hanifehpour, A. Akbarzadeh, and Y. Panahi, "Applications of dendrimers in nanomedicine and drug delivery: A review," *J. Inorg. Organomet. Polym. Mater.*, vol. 31, no. 6, pp. 2246–2261, 2021.

[81] D. Chenthamara et al., "Therapeutic efficacy of nanoparticles and routes of administration," *Biomater. Res.*, vol. 23, no. 1, p. 20, 2019.

[82] S. Khizar et al., "Nanocarriers based novel and effective drug delivery system," *Int. J. Pharm.*, vol. 632, p. 122570, 2023.

[83] F. Lai, M. Schlich, C. Sinico, and A. M. Fadda, "Liposomes as brain targeted delivery systems," in *Neuromethods*, New York, NY: Springer US, 2021, pp. 29–59.

[84] M. A. Farooq and N. L. Trevaskis, "TPGS decorated liposomes as multifunctional nano-delivery systems," *Pharm. Res.*, vol. 40, no. 1, pp. 245–263, 2023.

[85] A. Zielińska et al., "Polymeric nanoparticles: Production, characterization, toxicology and ecotoxicology," *Molecules*, vol. 25, no. 16, p. 3731, 2020.

[86] S. Perumal, "Polymer nanoparticles: Synthesis and applications," *Polymers (Basel)*, vol. 14, no. 24, p. 5449, 2022.

[87] E. Abbasi et al., "Dendrimers: Synthesis, applications, and properties," *Nanoscale Res. Lett.*, vol. 9, no. 1, pp. 1–10, 2014.

[88] M. Pérez-Ferreiro, A. M. Abelairas, A. Criado, I. J. Gómez, and J. Mosquera, "Dendrimers: Exploring their wide structural variety and applications," *Polymers (Basel)*, vol. 15, no. 22, p. 4369, 2023.

[89] A. Gagliardi et al., "Biodegradable polymeric nanoparticles for drug delivery to solid tumors," *Front. Pharmacol.*, vol. 12, p. 601626, 2021.

[90] N. Andrýsková, P. Sourivong, M. Babincová, and M. Šimaljaková, "Controlled release of tazarotene from magnetically responsive nanofiber patch: Towards more efficient topical therapy of psoriasis," *Appl. Sci. (Basel)*, vol. 11, no. 22, p. 11022, 2021.

[91] N. Sumrith, S. M. Rangappa, R. Dangtungee, S. Siengchin, M. Jawaid, and C. I. Pruncu, "Biopolymers-based nanocomposites: Properties and applications," in *Bio-based Polymers and Nanocomposites*, Cham: Springer International Publishing, 2019, pp. 255–272.

[92] S. Nitta and K. Numata, "Biopolymer-based nanoparticles for drug/gene delivery and tissue engineering," *Int. J. Mol. Sci.*, vol. 14, no. 1, pp. 1629–1654, 2013.

[93] S. Chandran, A. Pricillia, A. Natarajan, and G. Venkatesan, "Enhancing sustainability: Chitosan biopolymers with Ag nanoparticles for eco-friendly applications in food packaging," *Biomass Convers. Biorefin.*, 2024. https://doi.org/10.1007/s13399-024-05325-7

[94] P. Bala and S. N. Kale, "Smart biopolymeric nanocarriers for drug delivery applications," in *Advances in Bioengineering*, Singapore: Springer Singapore, 2020, pp. 183–197.

[95] D. C. Ferreira Soares, S. C. Domingues, D. B. Viana, and M. L. Tebaldi, "Polymer-hybrid nanoparticles: Current advances in biomedical applications," *Biomed. Pharmacother.*, vol. 131, p. 110695, 2020.

[96] N. Kučuk, M. Primožič, Ž. Knez, and M. Leitgeb, "Sustainable biodegradable biopolymer-based nanoparticles for healthcare applications," *Int. J. Mol. Sci.*, vol. 24, no. 4, p. 3188, 2023.

[97] K. Prabahar, Z. Alanazi, and M. Qushawy, "Targeted drug delivery system: Advantages, carriers and strategies," *Ind. J. Pharm. Educ.*, vol. 55, no. 2, pp. 346–353, 2021.

[98] P. Sirim, L. Zeitlmann, B. Kellersch, C. S. Falk, D. J. Schendel, and W. Kolanus, "Calcium signaling through the β2-cytoplasmic domain of LFA-1 requires intracellular elements of the T cell receptor complex," *J. Biol. Chem.*, vol. 276, no. 46, pp. 42945–42956, 2001.

[99] J. Wang et al., "Enhancement of scutellarin oral delivery efficacy by vitamin B12-modified amphiphilic chitosan derivatives to treat type II diabetes induced-retinopathy," *J. Nanobiotechnol.*, vol. 15, no. 1, 2017.

[100] M. Rakotoarisoa, B. Angelov, V. M. Garamus, and A. Angelova, "Curcumin- and fish oil-loaded spongosome and cubosome nanoparticles with neuroprotective potential against H_2O_2-induced oxidative stress in differentiated human SH-SY5Y cells," *ACS Omega*, vol. 4, no. 2, pp. 3061–3073, 2019.

[101] D. Nishimoto-Sauceda, L. E. Romero-Robles, and M. Antunes-Ricardo, "Biopolymer nanoparticles: A strategy to enhance stability, bioavailability, and biological effects of phenolic compounds as functional ingredients," *J. Sci. Food Agric.*, vol. 102, no. 1, pp. 41–52, 2022.

[102] N. K. Lotey, S. Pednekar, and R. Chaughule, "Hybrid nanoparticles in biomedical applications," in *Nanomaterials for Cancer Detection using Imaging Techniques and their Clinical Applications*, Cham: Springer International Publishing, 2022, pp. 365–400.

[103] D. Edgren, H. Leeper, K. Nichols, and J. Wright, "Controlled release technology, pharmaceutical," *Kirk-Othmer Encyclopedia of Chemical Technology*. Wiley, 2000.

[104] J. Y. Choi, R. K. Thapa, C. S. Yong, and J. O. Kim, "Nanoparticle-based combination drug delivery systems for synergistic cancer treatment," *J. Pharm. Investig.*, vol. 46, no. 4, pp. 325–339, 2016.

[105] B. Begines et al., "Polymeric nanoparticles for drug delivery: Recent developments and future prospects," *Nanomaterials (Basel)*, vol. 10, no. 7, p. 1403, 2020.

[106] S. Z. Alshawwa, A. A. Kassem, R. M. Farid, S. K. Mostafa, and G. S. Labib, "Nanocarrier drug delivery systems: Characterization, limitations, future perspectives and implementation of artificial intelligence," *Pharmaceutics*, vol. 14, no. 4, p. 883, 2022.

[107] L. Gutierrez, N. S. Cauchon, T. R. Christian, M. J. Giffin, and M. J. Abernathy, "The confluence of innovation in therapeutics and regulation: Recent CMC considerations," *J. Pharm. Sci.*, vol. 109, no. 12, pp. 3524–3534, 2020.

[108] V. M. Ragitha and L. K. Edison, "Safety issues, environmental impacts, and health effects of biopolymers," in *Handbook of Biopolymers*, Singapore: Springer Nature Singapore, 2022, pp. 1–27.

[109] Y. Choi, A. A. Vinks, and P. H. van der Graaf, "Novel therapeutic modalities: The future is now," *Clin. Pharmacol. Ther.*, vol. 114, no. 3, pp. 493–496, 2023.

[110] N. Singh, "Polypyrrole-based emerging and futuristic hybrid nanocomposites," *Polym. Bull. (Berl.)*, vol. 79, no. 9, pp. 6929–7007, 2022.

[111] Y. Jung and D. Kim, "Recent advances in a hybrid system of porous silicon nanoparticles and biocompatible polymers for biomedical applications," *Biomed. Eng. Lett.*, vol. 11, no. 3, pp. 171–181, 2021.

[112] R. A. Ilyas, S. M. Sapuan, and E. Bayraktar, "Current progress in biopolymer-based bionanocomposites and hybrid materials," *Polymers (Basel)*, vol. 14, no. 17, p. 3479, 2022.

Index

Pages in *italics* refer to figures and pages in **bold** refer to tables.

C

G

H

O

P

Q

R

S

T

U

V

W

X

Y

Z